# Controversies in Nephrology and Hypertension

# Controversies in Nephrology and Hypertension

Edited by

## Robert G. Narins, M.D.

Professor of Medicine
Chief
Renal Section
Temple University Health Sciences Center
Philadelphia, Pennsylvania

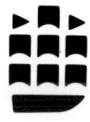

**CHURCHILL LIVINGSTONE**          1984
New York, Edinburgh, London, and Melbourne

Acquisitions editor: *Gene Kearn*
Copy editor: *Peggy Brigg*
Production editor: *Fred L. Kantrowitz*
Production supervisor: *Joe Sita*
Compositor: *Eastern Graphics*
Printer/Binder: *The Murray Printing Co.*

**© Churchill Livingstone Inc. 1984**

Distributed in the United Kingdom by Churchill Livingstone, Robert Stevenson House, 1-3 Baxter's Place, Leith Walk, Edinburgh EH1 3AF and by associated companies, branches and representatives throughout the world.

First published 1984

Printed in USA

ISBN 0-443-08238-3

9 8 7 6 5 4 3 2 1

**Library of Congress Cataloging in Publication Data**
Main entry under title:

Controversies in nephrology and hypertension.

   Includes bibliographies and index.
   1. Renal insufficiency. 2. Renal hypertension. 3. Renal insufficiency—Social aspects. 4. Renal insufficiency—Economic aspects. 5. Renal insufficiency—Moral and ethical aspects. 6. Medical policy—United States. I. Narins, Robert G. [DNLM: 1. Health Policy—economics—United States. 2. Hypertension—therapy. 3. Kidney Diseases—economics. 4. Kidney Diseases—therapy. WJ 300 C764]
RC918.R4C66   1984        616.6′1        84-7639
ISBN 0-443-08238-3
**Manufactured in the United States of America**

To Beatrice and Benjamin who made it all possible and to Barbara, Brigham, and David without whom the "possible" would be meaningless

# Contributors

**Zalman S. Agus, M.D.**
Associate Professor of Medicine, University of Pennsylvania School of Medicine; Chief, Renal-Electrolyte Section, Hospital of the University of Pennsylvania, Philadelphia, Pennsylvania

**Allen C. Alfrey, M.D.**
Professor of Medicine, University of Colorado Health Sciences Center; Chief, Renal Section, Veterans Administration Medical Center, Denver, Colorado

**Sharon Anderson, M.D.**
Research Fellow, Department of Medicine, Harvard Medical School; Renal Section, Brigham and Women's Hospital, Boston, Massachusetts

**Allen I. Arieff, M.D.**
Professor of Medicine, University of California, San Francisco, School of Medicine; Chief, Nephrology Service, San Francisco Veterans Administration Medical Center, San Francisco, California

**Stanley P. Ballou, M.D.**
Assistant Professor of Medicine, Case Western Reserve University School of Medicine; Rheumatologist, Cleveland Metropolitan General Hospital, Cleveland, Ohio

**Christine P. Bastl, M.D.**
Associate Professor of Medicine, Temple University Health Sciences Center, Philadelphia, Pennsylvania

**Ulrich Binswanger, M.D.**
Section of Nephrology, University Hospital, Zurich, Switzerland

**Christopher R. Blagg, M.D.**
Director, Northwest Kidney Center; Professor of Medicine, University of Washington School of Medicine, Seattle, Washington

**W. Kline Bolton, M.D.**
Associate Professor of Medicine, University of Virginia School of Medicine, Charlottesville, Virginia

**Barry M. Brenner, M.D.**
Samuel A. Levine Professor of Medicine, Harvard Medical School; Director, Renal Section, Brigham and Women's Hospital, Boston, Massachusetts

**Elizabeth M. Cameron, R.N.**
Assistant Director, Transplant Department, Hospital of the University of Pennsylvania, Philadelphia, Pennsylvania

**Jack W. Coburn, M.D.**
Professor of Medicine, UCLA School of Medicine; Medical Investigator, Veterans Administration Medical Center, Los Angeles, California

**Leslie P. Dornfeld, M.D.**
Clinical Professor of Medicine, UCLA School of Medicine, Los Angeles, California

**Gary D. Dubois, M.D.**
Clinical Instructor, Department of Medicine, University of Oklahoma; Staff Physician, Veterans Administration Medical Center, Oklahoma City, Oklahoma

**Renée C. Fox, Ph.D.**
Professor of Sociology, University of Pennsylvania, Philadelphia, Pennsylvania

**Stanley S. Franklin, M.D.**
Clinical Professor of Medicine, Associate Director of Hypertension, UCLA School of Medicine, Los Angeles, California

**Lawrence R. Freedman, M.D.**
Professor and Chairman, Department of Internal Medicine, UCLA School of Medicine; Veterans Administration Medical Center, Los Angeles, California

**Eli A. Friedman, M.D.**
Professor of Medicine, State University of New York; Chief, Renal Diseases Division, Downstate Medical Center-Kings County Hospital, New York, New York

**Edward D. Frohlich, M.D.**
Vice President, Education and Research, Alton Ochsner Medical Foundation, New Orleans, Louisiana

**Richard J. Glassock, M.D.**
Professor of Medicine, UCLA School of Medicine, Los Angeles, California; Chairman, Department of Medicine, Harbor-UCLA Medical Center, Torrance, California

**Clarence E. Grim, M.D.**
Professor of Medicine, Division of Endocrinology, Indiana University School of Medicine, Indianapolis, Indiana

**Constantine L. Hampers, M.D.**
Chairman of the Board, National Medical Care, Inc., Boston, Massachusetts

**O. Bryan Holland, M.D.**
Associate Professor of Medicine, Hypertensive Service, University of Texas Medical Branch, Galveston, Texas

**Howard I. Hurtig, M.D.**
Chief, Department of Neurology, University of Pennsylvania Graduate Hospital, Philadelphia, Pennsylvania

**Edward R. Jones, M.D.**
Assistant Professor of Medicine, Temple University Health Sciences Center, Philadelphia, Pennsylvania

**Norman M. Kaplan, M.D.**
Professor of Medicine, University of Texas Health Sciences Center,
Dallas, Texas

**Priscilla Kincaid-Smith, M.D., D.Sc.**
Professor of Medicine, University of Melbourne; Director of Nephrology, The Royal
Melbourne Hospital, Melbourne, Victoria, Australia

**Irving Kushner, M.D.**
Professor of Medicine, Case Western Reserve University School of Medicine; Chief, Division of Rheumatology, Cleveland Metropolitan General Hospital, Cleveland, Ohio

**David H. Lawson, M.D.**
Department of Clinical Pharmacology, Royal Infirmary, Glasgow, Scotland

**David T. Lowenthal, M.D.**
Professor of Medicine and Pharmacology, Likoff Cardiovascular Institute, Hahnemann
University, Philadelphia, Pennsylvania

**Edmund G. Lowrie, M.D.**
Senior Vice President, National Medical Care, Inc., Boston, Massachusetts

**Diana Marver, Ph.D.**
Assistant Professor of Medicine, University of Texas Health Sciences Center, Dallas,
Texas

**Morton H. Maxwell, M.D.**
Clinical Professor of Medicine, UCLA School of Medicine; Director, Hypertension
Services, Cedars-Sinai Medical Center, Los Angeles, California

**Timothy W. Meyer, M.D.**
Instructor in Medicine, Harvard Medical School; Associate Physician, Brigham and
Women's Hospital, Boston, Massachusetts

**Robert G. Narins, M.D.**
Professor of Medicine; Chief, Renal Section, Temple University Health Sciences Center, Philadelphia, Pennsylvania

**Michael D. Norenberg, M.D.**
Professor of Pathology and Neurology, University of Miami School of Medicine;
Neuropathologist, Jackson Memorial Hospital and Veterans Administration Hospital,
Miami, Florida

**Andrew C. Novick, M.D.**
Head, Section of Renal Transplantation, Department of Urology, Cleveland Clinic
Foundation, Cleveland, Ohio

**Charles Y. C. Pak, M.D.**
Professor of Medicine, University of Texas Health Sciences Center, Dallas, Texas

**Alan B. Retik, M.D.**
Associate Professor of Urology, Harvard Medical School; Chief, Division of Urology,
Children's Hospital Medical Center, Boston, Massachusetts

**Michael R. Rudnick, M.D.**
Clinical Associate Professor of Medicine, University of Pennsylvania School of Medicine; Chief, Section of Nephrology and Hypertension, University of Pennsylvania Graduate Hospital, Philadelphia, Pennsylvania

**Steven D. Saris, M.D.**
Assistant Professor of Medicine, Likoff Cardiovascular Institute, Hahnemann University, Philadelphia, Pennsylvania

**Donald E. Schwarten, M.D.**
Director, Cardiovascular Laboratories, Department of Radiology, St. Vincent Hospital and Health Care Center, Indianapolis, Indiana

**Judith P. Swazey, Ph.D.**
Executive Director, Medicine in the Public Interest, Boston, Massachusetts

**Robert C. Tomford, M.D.**
Assistant Professor of Medicine, Case Western Reserve University School of Medicine; Staff Nephrologist, Cleveland Metropolitan General Hospital, Cleveland, Ohio

**Rowan G. Walker, M.B., B.S.**
Nephrologist, The Royal Melbourne Hospital, Melbourne, Victoria, Australia

**Alan G. Wasserstein, M.D.**
Assistant Professor of Medicine, University of Pennsylvania School of Medicine, Philadelphia, Pennsylvania

**Myron H. Weinberger, M.D.**
Professor of Medicine, Director, Hypertension Research Center, Indiana University School of Medicine, Indianapolis, Indiana

**Robert S. Wright, M.D.**
Staff Physician, Santa Barbara Medical Foundation Clinic, Santa Barbara, California

# Foreword

The history of modern medicine is replete with controversy. That is just what one would have expected when medicine was young and facts were greatly outnumbered by theories. In the absence of facts established by clinical research, diverse opinions would have been expected to flourish and controversy to abound. But today's medical practice, although far more rigorously founded on facts, is no less controversial than that of a century ago. The questions have changed, but not the habit of disputation.

Contrary to common opinion, the advance of medical science does not eliminate controversy; it merely shifts the arguments. Progress in basic biology results in better understanding, which settles some disputes but also leads to new and more searching questions and hence to more controversy. Likewise, advances in clinical medicine may resolve differences about diagnostic or therapeutic interventions, but at the same time new techniques and new concepts evolve which generate fresh controversies.

Disputation is an integral part of medical research, an essential component of the process by which questions are propounded, examined, and ultimately resolved. It generates ideas, clarifies issues, and suggests possible solutions that can be tested by observation and experimentation. Since progress in medicine depends on the propounding and resolution of questions, controversy must be regarded as one of the main engines of clinical progress.

It follows from all of this that a survey of the controversies in a field should provide insight into many of the most important current ideas in that field as well as valuable clues to the direction of future developments. The present collection of *Controversies in Nephrology and Hypertension* is a convincing illustration of that point.

Dr. Robert G. Narins has assembled here a provocative yet highly informative collection of essays on some of the most important and contentious topics in nephrology and hypertension. The authors, all experts in their respective fields, defend their point of view on an issue of current interest. Sometimes there are direct confrontations; in other instances the authors discuss different aspects of a subject without ever locking horns. Whatever the style, the discussion is interesting and instructive, in a way that an ordinary review—however erudite—can rarely achieve.

Most of the topics Dr. Narins has chosen deal with technical, clinical questions of diagnosis, management, or pathophysiology. The three articles on Social, Economical, and Ethical Controversies in End-Stage Renal Disease (ESRD) are exceptions. They discuss broader policy issues of a kind that are increasingly impinging on the practice of medicine these days. Anyone interested in nephrology cannot fail to be concerned about the problems covered in these articles. As someone formerly involved in the treatment of patients with renal failure, and now, by virtue of new duties, struggling to understand national health policy issues, I found the contrasting essays in this section to be of particular interest.

Lowrie and Hampers develop and extend a theme they have introduced else-where: They argue for an expansion of for-profit entrepreneurship in the delivery of medical care to ESRD patients. As senior executives of a large investor-owned cor-poration that sells hemodialysis services and equipment, they contend that di-alysis treatment would be provided more efficiently and effectively if patients were paid a fixed sum per treatment by the federal government and then allowed to shop in a competitive commercial marketplace for the dialysis services they want at the price they are willing to pay. Profit incentives, they suggest, should be available to physicians as well as to the owners of the dialysis facilities.

Blagg, on the other hand, points out that there are no adequate data on the comparative medical performance of existing for-profit and not-for-profit dialysis facilities. Of special concern is the lack of good comparative data on patient mix, medi-cal management, treatment outcome, and patient satisfaction in the two kinds of facilities. Without such medical information, differences in economic performance cannot be interpreted, and equitable and effective national policies cannot be designed. It is astonishing that the federal government spends billions of dollars on the care of ESRD patients and yet has done so little to collect the information necessary to evaluate what is being done with this money and what results are being achieved.

In this respect, the debate over the ESRD program resembles the purely medical controversies that constitute the major part of this volume: It stems, at least in part, from incomplete information and from a lack of critical data. The imbalance between concept and fact, the inability to marshall decisive and reliable, factual answers to practical questions, accounts for most of the purely medical controversies, but for only part of the ESRD policy debate. The latter has an additional important element not to be found in the debates over the diagnosis and treatment of renovascular hyper-tension or the role of plasmapheresis in the management of nephritic sydromes. Ques-tions of ethics and social values loom large in the ESRD debate. Should health care be distributed by the market? Are the professional values of physicians compatible with their role as businessmen? Should everyone with ESRD, regardless of other considera-tions, be treated by dialysis or transplantation, simply because federal funds are avail-able? And, if not, should economic considerations be weighed in the balance? Who should make such decisions?

These and other related questions are widening the range of debate in *Controver-sies in Nephrology and Hypertension*. They suggest that tomorrow's nephrologists will have to be even more broadly educated than their predecessors, because they will deal with issues hardly imagined a decade or two ago.

*Arnold S. Relman, M.D.*

# Preface

Controversy energizes intellectual debate and investigation while providing the backdrop for an entertaining discussion. Accordingly, I have carefully selected topics for *Controversies in Nephrology and Hypertension*, and am most pleased to present an outstanding array of clinician-investigators to discuss them.

Nephrology, like few other specialties, cuts across the broad swath of Internal Medicine. Fluid-electrolyte and acid-base disorders, renal failure, and hypertension all affect many systems. The clinical nephrologist or the investigator who narrows his focus to only the kidney misses the intellectual and practical benefit of seeing the kidney and its related disorders in the broad perspective of their most important extrarenal effects.

With these points in mind, the topics were chosen to cover the broad range of currently "fiery subjects" in nephrology and hypertension. Socioeconomic issues and raging debates covering pathophysiology, diagnosis, and therapy, all have found a place. Our discussants have been culled from disciplines as disparate as the business world, sociology, and medicine. Hypertension is a "welcome guest in many houses" and our authorship reflects this diversity. Endocrinologists, cardiologists, surgeons, radiologists, and nephrologists have contributed to this section. Our contributors were chosen because of their well-known and strongly professed views on controversial issues. I have encouraged them to be as scorching in their debate as the bonds of civility allow. Some, as the reader will see, have taken the challenge while cooler heads recognized the durability of the written word and gravitated toward the middle. Nonetheless, each debate is well conceived and well written and provides the reader with entertaining insights into important topics.

Except for three of the seventeen chapters, a point-counterpoint format has been utilized. The case for or against a given issue is developed in each of these chapters.

Section one deals with economic, social, and ethical issues in end-stage renal disease (ESRD). Lowrie and Hampers review the evolution of how the Federal Government became financially responsible for ESRD and how the bureaucracy meting out this support is constructed. Additionally, these authors develop the case for competition and the profit motive as ensurers of cost-effective and adequate medical care. Blagg takes issue with this approach and makes his articulate argument for the importance of homecare and transplantation as being most cost-effective and medically superior.

Fox, Swazey and Cameron develop important and penetrating insights into several ethical and moral issues. The cycle of boisterous hope followed by quiet despair that each new immunosuppressive agent has initiated is outlined and applied to cyclosporin, transplantation's new champion against immunologic rejection. The concept and issues surrounding the donation of a kidney by family or friends are artfully and empathetically presented. The painful decisions involved in allocating ever-constricting federal resources and the changing role and problems faced by dialysis nurses round out their stimulating chapter.

Four controversies are trenchantly debated in the hypertension section. Kaplan and Frohlich argue the pros and cons, respectively, of nondrug therapy for hypertension. The former author outlines the shortcomings of pharmacologic therapy and the potential benefits of weight reduction, exercise, and relaxation therapies. Frohlich suggests that diastolic blood pressures ≥90 mm Hg ought to be treated in all-comers. Nonpharmacologic treatment is fine, but for only as long as it normalizes the pressure. Renal vein renin assays are the centerpiece for diagnosing renovascular hypertension according to Grim and Weinberger. Rudnick and Maxwell, however, use their thorough review of the literature to identify the striking limitations of this test. Interventional radiologist confronts surgeon as Schwarten and Novick take opposite positions regarding the relative merits of balloon angioplasty and arterial surgery in treating renovascular hypertension. Novick also draws upon his immense experience to present a lucid description of the various renal vascular lesions causing this disorder, their individual natural histories, and the various surgical options available for their correction. Finally, Hurtig and Franklin review the potential dangers of rapid lowering of severely elevated blood pressure. The former author, a neurologist, argues for a more cautious and slower decrease in pressure than Franklin, a nephrologist. The latter's chapter spells out, in practical terms, how and when to quickly lower pressure and to what level it should be lowered.

The next section treats two diagnostic issues. Lowenthal and Saris strongly advocate use of the renal biopsy as critical for proper diagnosis and therapy of many, if not most, renal diseases. Ballou and Kushner, using lupus nephritis as their prime example, authoritatively argue that renal biopsies yield information that adds little to what is already known from history, physical, and noninvasive tests. The "impalee" accrues disturbingly few benefits from the impaling! An extensive workup is required for those with nephrolithiasis and hypercalciuria, argues Pak, since a rational therapeutic approach can only be developed after defining the pathophysiology underlying the hypercalciuria. Wasserstein and Agus carefully review the literature and construct a compelling argument for a limited diagnostic approach.

The treatment of renal-electrolyte disorders is a hotbed of controversy and as such has spawned seven of our chapters. The potentially malignant cardiovascular effects of even mild hypokalemia are stressed by Holland as he convincingly argues for normalizing serum potassium concentrations in even asymptomatic hypertensives without apparent heart disease. The threat of iatrogenic hyperkalemia and the economic aspects of treating millions of hypertensives unnecessarily form much of Lawson's countervailing argument. Narins, Jones, and Dornfeld discuss the pros and cons of alkali therapy for keto- and lactic acidosis. They conclude that the weight of evidence clearly favors the judicious use of sodium bicarbonate, an argument strongly favored by the Editor! The rapid correction of hyponatremia predisposes patients to the threat of central pontine myelinolysis, writes Norenberg, who argues for a slower, more cautious return of serum sodium to normal. Not so, argue Dubois and Arieff who present an extensive review of the literature and some of their own animal research. They strongly profess rapidly correcting hyponatremia, which they conclude protects patients from permanent central nervous system disease. Bolton definitively reviews the world's literature regarding the aggressive use of high dose steroids in rapidly progressive glomerulonephritis (RPGN) and summarizes his own extensive experience. He clearly outlines his therapeutic regimen and builds a strong argument for the benefits of this approach. Glassock takes a somewhat more conservative view while expanding his review to cover other nephritic syndromes in addition to RPGN and reviews their response to steroids. Plasmapheresis is a widely used and highly touted therapy for many renal and extrarenal diseases which are refractory to other measures. Kincaid-Smith and Walker present their prodigious experience with this relatively new treatment and strongly advocate its use in a wide range of renal disorders. Friedman takes a step back and remembers that the glorious peal of bells and blare of trumpets that greet many new therapies in Medicine give way to a funereal dirge when the light of controlled studies is shed on these nostrums and operations. He is uncertain as to whether plasmapheresis will stand up to the test of time. Reflux nephropathy pits the internist against the urologist in developing the proper diagnostic and therapeutic approach to this disorder. Freedman articulately makes the case for a conservative approach whereas Retik develops the indications for a more aggressive surgical approach. The prophylactic use of 1,25-dihydroxycholecalciferol (1,25(OH)$_2$D$_3$) raises serum calcium, suppresses parathyroid hormone secretion, and protects bone from the ravages of ESRD, say Coburn and Wright. Binswanger argues that 1,25(OH)$_2$D$_3$ is an expensive way to create normocalcemia and indeed commonly causes hypercalcemia; he cautions against its use.

The last section discusses certain controversies in pathophysiology and physiology. Meyer, Anderson, and Brenner argue that glomerular hyperperfusion, a nonspecific adaptation to the loss of renal mass, progressively damages glomeruli and is a root-cause of the progression of renal disease. Alfrey and Tomford emphasize various metabolic, immune, and interstitial factors that follow the initial renal insult, and these factors, they suggest, cause inexorable progression to dialysis and transplantation. Finally, Bastl and Marver review their own work and that of others as they identify current and emerging controversies regarding the mechanism of action and effects of glucocorticoids and mineralocorticoids.

The Editor wishes to acknowlege the outstanding administrative and secretarial help provided by Ms. Kathleen Petruzzelli, Elsie M. Williams, Doris E. Snyder, and Melissa Stukes. Special thanks go to Gene Kearn and Churchill Livingstone for their help and continuing support.

*Robert G. Narins, M.D.*

# Contents

# Section I

## Social, Economic, and Ethical Controversies in End-Stage Renal Disease

# 1

# Dialysis for End-Stage Renal Disease

# Medicare's End-Stage Renal Disease Program: Historical and Policy Considerations

Edmund G. Lowrie, M.D.
Constantine L. Hampers, M.D.

The editor of this volume has asked us to write defending profit by physicians and institutions in the End-Stage Renal Disease (ESRD) program. We have done so previously,[32,33] and earning a profit needs no defense. Nonetheless, the purpose of this book is to stimulate thought, so we will try to be controversial as the title suggests.

The real issue in the ESRD program should involve caring for the greatest number of patients needing treatment (without regard to age, sex, race, or social status) using the best available therapy (considering the particular needs of the patient) at the lowest overall cost—not the earning of profits. This social goal can be accomplished either by using profit motives as incentives to efficiency or by direct "command and control" regulations—depending upon which system seems to work best. Unfortunately, the political and philosophical aspects of the "patient care and profit debate" have overshadowed the burning social, medical, and public health issues which form real and substantive roots of the ESRD program.

Just over 10 years ago Congress created a social experiment financing health care for a catastrophic illness. They authorized Medicare payments for patients—regardless of age—whose kidneys cannot sustain life. The legislation resulted in federal regulations and then more legislation, all of which affect the lives and activities of patients, physicians, and health care institutions. This entanglement of political and medical processes has evolved into what is known now as Medicare's ESRD program. But in spite of many problems, the program has been quite successful in many ways. While overall costs have increased, this has been due to treating more patients who need life-saving care. The cost per patient has increased very little and has actually decreased when adjusted for inflation.[32,33] This is not true for other areas of health care.[32,33] The cost of dialysis to government in freestanding units (i.e., nonhospital) has remained the same since 1974—an actual 50 percent decrease with inflation adjustment.

The organization of the ESRD program includes a *policy function* which resides in the Department of Health and Human Services (HHS). This receives advice from Congress and others and determines the goals and direction for the program. The organization also includes an *administrative infrastructure* located within and directed by the Health Care Financing Administration (HCFA) which implements policies through operating rules and procedures. Finally, the *medical care*

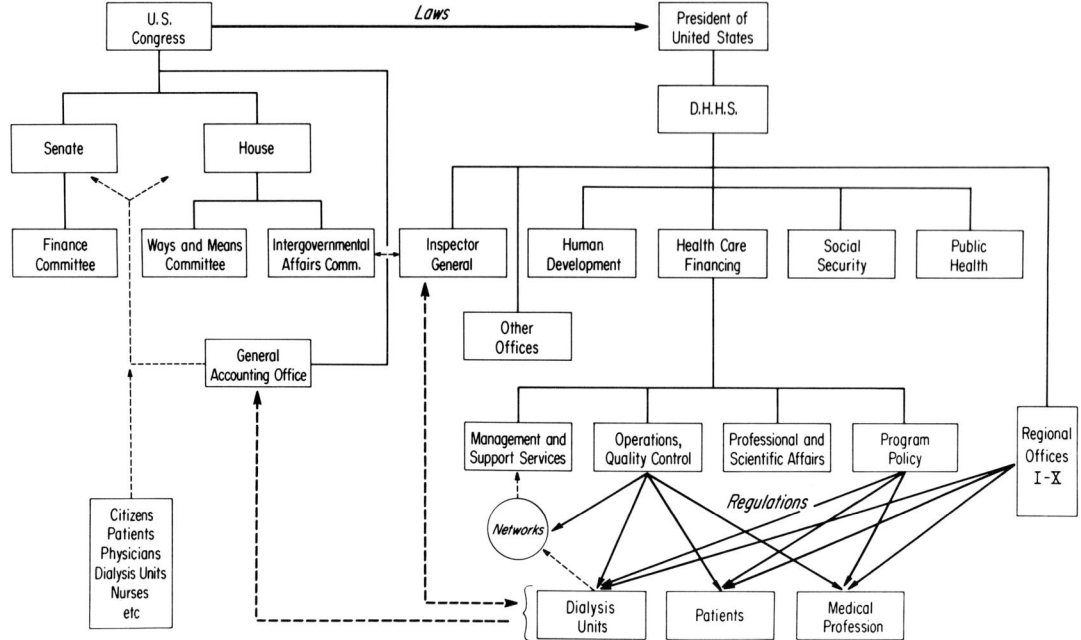

**Fig. 1-1.** Organization schematic of the ESRD system. Heavy solid arrows indicate a law or regulation. For example, Congress passes laws with which the Executive Branch of government, including the Department of Health and Human Services (DHHS) must comply. Administrations within DHHS and/or their subsidiary offices draft regulations which are promulgated by the Secretary of DHHS. These affect dialysis units, patients, and health-care personnel. Heavy dashed arrows show investigative functions which gather data from dialysis units, patients, and the medical profession and synthesize reports which are distributed to the Secretary and/or to Congress. The Inspector General of DHHS, though residing in DHHS, reports directly to Congress. Some program data flow to the Administrator for Management and Support Services, through "Networks" that are loose, provider organizations composed of patients, representatives from dialysis units, and other health care professionals. Patients, health care professionals and other citizens may make their views known to Congress through their elected representatives or through statements made to various Congressional committees.

*community* including consumers and health care providers rest at the base of the ESRD program's structure and must conform to the policy and administrative provisions. An organizational schematic is shown in Fig. 1-1. Not shown in this diagram are other organizations in HHS concerned with ESRD. These include the Food and Drug Administration, the Center for Disease Control, and the National Institutes for Health—all located within the Public Health Service. Fiscal intermediaries such as Blue Cross and Blue Shield, who contract with Medicare to pay the bills, also are not shown. Finally, insufficient space exists to show the third branch of government, the Judiciary, which interprets law and to which patients or health care professionals may appeal in their dealings with HHS. The policy functions mentioned in the text exist within the Office of the Secretary of DHHS and within certain elements of the Health Care Financing Administration (HCFA)—most notably the Associate Administrator for Policy. The administrative infrastructure also mentioned in the text exists within all of the major administrations of HCFA. Finally, the professionals forming the base of the ESRD program and patients are shown at the bottom of the chart. Program success, however, has been due to those who provide the care more than to sound Federal policy. Doctor Richard Rettig notes[42] that policy function within HHS has been fragmented, unstable, and has declined in capability over time:

> The result has been weak policy control over operations, confusion in the operational domain, and confusion among those who are delivering care.[42]

He then describes the success of the program:

> The organizational base of the ESRD program is the delivery system, which consists of treatment institutions and the health care professionals who run them. . . . Where clear policy exists, where Medicare administrative procedures are more traditional than new, those factors combined with competent professionals administering basically routine therapy on a daily basis essentially guarantee the delivery of high quality care.[42]

A brief review of the legislative and regulatory history of the program through New Year's Day, 1983 will be provided to paint a clearer picture of the interaction between government and the medical community as it has been.

# LEGISLATIVE AND REGULATORY HISTORY OF THE ESRD PROGRAM

A detailed chronology of the program through mid-1978 is available elsewhere.[41-43] We draw heavily on those reports focusing on major milestones while commenting on important events that affected policy.

The first involvement of government in dialysis occurred in the early 1960s when the Veterans Administration announced plans to establish dialysis centers. In 1964 Congress sponsored *research and development* in ESRD therapy by appropriating funds for the National Institutes of Allergy and Infectious Diseases to study transplantation immunology. One year later, it created the Artificial Kidney–Chronic Uremia Program within the National Institutes of Health to foster the development of better artificial kidneys. Congress then proceeded to fund clinical demonstration programs by appropriating funds to support 14 community dialysis centers. Dialysis therapy also grew spontaneously, without federal support, during the ensuing years and there was considerable legislative and executive resistance to government's expanding role in providing hemodialysis. In 1967, however, an ad hoc committee sponsored by the Bureau of the Budget released its report,[20] which recommended amending Title XVIII (Medicare) of the Social Security Act to finance the treatment of ESRD.

In 1970 the Congress added kidney disease to the legislative authority for Regional Medical Programs, thereby *stimulating new capacity to provide care.* Community dialysis centers could now receive federal support. Reluctance remained, however, to provide legislation that would finance patient care directly. That came later with the Social Security Amendments of 1972, much as an ad hoc committee[20] had recommended 5 years earlier. The "renal" portion of this bill (Sec. 299I of PL92-603) received less than one-half hour debate on the Senate floor. Speaking on its behalf, Senator Henry Jackson (Dem., Washington) said,

> I think it is a great tragedy in a nation as affluent as ours that we have to consciously make a decision all over America as to the

people who live and the people who will die. We had a committee in Seattle, when the first series of kidney machines were put in operation, who had to pass judgement on who would live and who would die. I believe we can do better than that. . . . (118 Cong. Rec. 33007 [1972]).

This humanitarian act provided lifesaving treatments that were beyond the financial means of most patients. A recent review[14] of patients before and after PL92-603 suggests that the dialysis population has changed from one that was largely young, white, male, and highly educated to one which more nearly approximates a cross section of American life. The law provided a model for the federal funding of catastrophic illness care which has received much more public attention than would usually be warranted by a program of its small size.

Political scientist Rettig comments[42] on this progression from research and development through demonstration and training to capacity building, but notes that the "technical logic" of policy development appears more rational in retrospect than it did at the time. The point is that we have passed now through simple capacity building into a period of direct reimbursement and that with payment has come a tangle of quasi-technical regulations which affect the way in which physicians and facilities provide care to patients. These regulations can be fashioned to restrict access to care, as we will see later. The medical profession and health care consumers, as well as health planners, should heed the lesson which emerges from ESRD program history.

*Interim regulations* implementing the provisions of Sec. 299I were published on June 23, 1973 to become effective only 3 days later. They addressed eligibility requirements for patients and facilities, but reimbursement was the primary focus. A distinction was made between hospital and nonhospital (also called independent or freestanding dialysis units). About three quarters of independents are operated for profit whereas virtually all of the hospitals are nonprofit. Hospitals were paid for *outpatient dialysis* on a cost basis, limited by a "screen" of $150 per treatment. Independents were reimbursed on a "reasonable charge" basis, not to exceed the screen. In certain cases the charge was calculated from the weighted average of all third party payments made to the independent unit during the previous 12 months. This method for calculating a charge was a special procedure introduced by Medicare for the ESRD program. It is not at all clear how the dollar value of the screen or the algorithm for selecting a lower value for certain independents was selected. Nonetheless, a novel approach was created within a system which theretofore had paid facilities for any and all costs. For the first time, Medicare had said, in effect, "this is what the service is worth and this is what we will pay" and, for the first time had created potential incentives for cost containment. Hedging a bit, they permitted exceptions to the screen if a facility could show hardship or that their *costs* exceed the screen—regardless of the rates paid to other nearby units. This poorly monitored loophole was the subject of ultimate abuse by hospitals and has permitted wide-ranging reimbursement rates exceeding $275 per dialysis treatment.

Payments for physician service were simply disallowed. Rettig, quoting a Medicare Intermediary Letter, summarizes the problem nicely:

The insult to physicians was stated this way: "Fee-for-service reimbursement for physicians' services in an out-of-hospital (as well as in-hospital) dialysis center shall be made only when an identifiable service to the patient is performed, e.g., the patient goes into shock, experiences severe chest pains, etc. Supervision by a physician of the dialysis "run" is part of the facility cost for the dialysis and is not reimbursable as a separate charge."* Alteration of the existing practice was bad enough; that the government should now attempt to specify how doctors should practice medicine was too much.[42]

The response was instantaneous. Two weeks after the screen was announced (with the regulations in June, 1973), a group of about 60 nephrologists met at an airport hotel. A number previously not interested in legislative and regulatory matters became interested and now well established professional association (Renal Physicians Association) grew out of that meeting. Protracted negotiations with HHS (then HEW) were frustrating and 8 months later (March, 1974) two groups of physicians filed suit against the Secretary.

The *final regulations* implementing Section 299I were long overdue by then. Six weeks after the suits were filed, their essential elements were announced at a press conference in New York. They were not published, however, until June 1, 1975—almost 3 years after the law was passed.

Those regulations described the organizational framework for the ESRD program and included a geographic network approach for administering care, minimum utilization rates for dialysis and transplant facilities, and an outline of mechanisms for reviewing the appropriateness of patient care. Important to physicians, however, was the inclusion of an *alternate method* for physician reimbursement. Instead of receiving payment from the dialysis unit and/or a traditional fee for service, the physician could receive a monthly capitation fee for providing care. Actually, the method was described first

in June 1974* following the physician suit. If the physicians in a unit selected the alternate method, the facility screen would be reduced by $12 per treatment (e.g., from $150 to $138). In principle, a monthly retainer (capitation fee) for medical service had been created. New ground had been broken again.

Congress passed another interesting piece of renal legislation two years later. Early in 1977 a bill was brought before the House of Representatives which would have required that 40 percent of all patients be treated with self-dialysis by October 1st, 1978 and that 50 percent be so treated by October 1st, 1980. The phrase "self-dialysis" was presumably a substitute for "home dialysis." At the time, about 13 percent of patients were being treated in the home, 1 percent were in home care training, and less than 1 percent were treated by self-dialysis in centers.[9] In slightly over 1½ years, then, the fraction of patients so treated was to triple according to legislative prescription. The fraction of home dialysis patients in 1979 was still only 13 percent.[10] By 1982 it had increased to 17 percent but much of this was due to continuous ambulatory peritoneal dialysis (CAPD) which was not available in 1977 and the fraction of home hemodialysis patients was still only 11 percent.

An analysis of HCFA data showed that the home dialysis population was much younger than center patients (home = 44 years; center = 53), was composed of far fewer black persons (12 versus 31 percent), and was generally characterized by less complicated medical illness (e.g., 7 percent diabetic versus 11 percent; 10 percent with hypertensive disease versus 21 percent).[33] While Senator Jackson's goals have been met and dialysis had been made available to all in need[13] passage of this legislation could well have

---

*Intermediary Letter 73-25(A)/73-22(B).

*Intermediary Letter 74-29(A)(3)

disadvantaged severely the aged, minorities, and the underprivileged.

Fortunately, some disliked quotas like 40 or 50 percent so Congress modified its directive to, "The maximum practical number of patients who are medically, socially and psychologically suitable candidates for home dialysis or transplantation should be so treated" (PL 95-292). Forgoing for this purpose a discussion of renal transplantation, home dialysis, or center dialysis, the important lesson is that certain members of Congress were willing to make judgments about what they considered suitable forms of medical treatment since they were paying the bill.

This legislation (Public Law 95-292) also added financial incentives for home dialysis by waiving the eligibility waiting period for home and transplant patients. Home dialysis, which was supposedly cheaper than center dialysis could be reimbursed at 70 percent of the center rate and payment made for a nurse or other unrelated aide to perform the treatment (it is interesting to speculate whether or not patients who receive such assistance are considered to be receiving "self-dialysis" in the sense of the original legislation) provided that the cost did not exceed the 70 percent limit. Finally, a policy statement which was both altruistic and pragmatic suggested incentive based reimbursement:

> Such regulations shall provide for the *implementation of appropriate incentives for encouraging more efficient and effective delivery of services* (consistent with quality care), and shall include, to the extent determined feasible by the Secretary, a system for classifying comparable providers and facilities, and prospectively set rates or target rates *with arrangements for sharing such reductions in costs as may be attributable to more efficient and effective delivery of service.* (PL 95-292) [Emphasis added].

HCFA regulators had difficulty responding to this challenge. Instead of breaking new ground—this time with legislative authority—they proposed[6] a reimbursement method that classified each facility by setting (urban or rural) and by ownership (hospital owned or not). Hospitals had reported labor costs which were 30 percent higher than independents and supply costs which were 13 percent higher. Of course, obtaining an exception to the $150 screen depended on reporting higher cost and exceptions were granted freely to hospitals. The justification for this segregation was unclear because HCFA said,[6] "We do not have sufficient information at this time to make reliable conclusions why hospitals show higher costs." HCFA readily admitted that there were no data to suggest that rural patients required more care than urban patients or that outpatients dialyzed in hospital owned units required more or less care than those dialyzed in facilities not owned by hospitals.[6] Instead of being innovative by creating an incentive-based system, HCFA had once again retreated to its comfortable and discredited Medicare Part A, cost-based reimbursement scheme.

Reaction to these September 1980 Proposed Rules was adverse, and presumably they were being revised when Congress passed the Omnibus Reconciliation Act of 1981 (PL 97-35) the following June. Much of the act was drafted in confusion by conference committees so that its provisions were not made public or debated openly. So it was with the Renal Section (Sec. 2145). Regulators were unable to conceive a system of "appropriate incentives for encouraging more efficient and effective delivery of service . . . with arrangements for sharing reductions in cost" as required by PL 95-292, so the language was simply stricken from the law.

It was difficult to defend on logical grounds the payment of a higher rate to hospitals because analysis of government data showed that there was, in fact, no difference in case mix or medical requirement between hospital treated and independent treated patients.[32,33] The solution was simple and the act now required that reimbursement screens differentiate between hospital and independent units. This posed the supposedly procompetitive Reagan administration with a dilemma. After all, the Office of Management and Budget was calling for a single, competitive reimbursement rate for home health agencies and skilled nursing facilities[35] while HCFA and Congress were talking about dual dialysis rates. The problem was symptomatic of the confusion surrounding the Act.

One last HCFA evaluation of possible case mix differences was undertaken.[8] Average age, sex, and race distributions were similar in hospitals and independent units. However, annual survival rates were superior in the independents (84 versus 79 percent on the average) for all age groups—particularly older patients. Independent treated patients were hospitalized less (19 percent fewer days of hospital care) than hospital treated patients but there was no significant difference in primary diagnoses. The author of the report noted that type and quality of treatment may affect patient morbidity and hospitalization. Certainly, a recent controlled clinical trial[34] supports that notion. He also noted that local medical custom, as well as case mix, may affect hospitalization rates. A hospital may well promote the use of its own resources. Reduced survival and increased frequency of hospitalization were nonetheless interpreted by HCFA bureaucrats to suggest that hospitals may, in fact, treat sicker outpatients in spite of similar age, sex, race, and primary diagnosis. Even so, using this argument to justify a higher rate for hospitals was effectively forestalled by

the finding that there was *no* correlation between the rate paid to a hospital and the frequency with which its patients were hospitalized. Reimbursement and case mix were not correlated in cost-reimbursed hospitals! The common claim that other outpatients seen in hospital clinics are sicker than those seen in private practice had also been disproved[31] and HCFA ultimately proposed a cosmetic "dual rate" with only a $4 spread.

The Act also increased the payment for home dialysis from 70 to 75 percent of the prevailing outpatient charge. It suggested, however, that a composite rate for dialysis be constructed in which the cost for home and center dialysis would be averaged. This sum would be paid to an institution on behalf of all of its patients, whether treated in center or in the home. Insomuch as the rate would be prospective, any surplus of revenue over expense (i.e., profit) could be retained by the institution whether or not it was "nonprofit."

A Notice of Proposed Rule Making implementing the renal provisions of PL 97-35 was published on February 12th, 1982,[7] and the following example shows how the rates would be calculated. If the fraction of patients on home dialysis were 15 percent and if Medicare determined (after excluding certain expenditures) that the costs were as follows:

> Facility labor cost (administrative and direct patient care)–$60
> Home dialysis labor cost (facility administrative—with no allowance for direct care)–$10
> Facility nonlabor cost–$80
> Home dialysis nonlabor–$90

Home and center costs would be averaged (weighted) and the labor and nonlabor components would be added.

| | | |
|---|---|---|
| Labor | $(85\% \times \$60) + (15\% \times \$10) =$ | $52.50 |
| Nonlabor | $(85\% \times \$80) + (15\% \times \$90) =$ | $81.50 |
| Composite Rate | = | $134.00 |

Facilities would be paid $134 for both center dialysis (which cost $60 + $80 = $140 in this example) and home dialysis (which cost $10 + $90 = $100). Losing $6.00 per center treatment for 85 percent of all treatments and profiting $34 per home treatment for only 15 percent of all treatments, facilities would be required simply to break even by exploiting the free labor of patients and their families. If the home dialysis percentage increased to 40 percent in this example, the screen would fall to $124 and units would lose $16 per center treatment while making $24 per home treatment. Again, they only break even! The greater the percentage on home dialysis the worse this problem becomes. HCFA's scheme was made quite clear by their statements,

> The resulting greater *profit margin for home dialysis* would create incentives for facilities to furnish home dialysis and to encourage patients to switch from in-facility to home dialysis. The composite rate would *pay marginally less than the full cost for in-facility dialysis* because of the home component formula.[7] [Emphasis added]

With respect to home patients and paid dialysis assistants,

> "Most of these (home patients) are assisted by family members who are *not paid* . . . a separate allowance for such costs (of a paid assistant) in the home component of the composite rate *would not be authorized*.[7] [Emphasis added]

So the home dialysis profit results from the fact that the person performing the treatment is unpaid. Ultimately, a patient would be unable to receive dialysis unless the family performed the treatment. Nonetheless, Dr. Christopher Blagg, a strong advocate of home dialysis, preferred this method, expressing his concern that 70 percent reimbursement would be "very tight"! That rendered

moot the argument that home hemodialysis is significantly less expensive than center dialysis in independent units if one considers labor.

The actual screens would reduce reimbursement for independents from $138 per treatment (net of a physician component) to $128 and would reduce the amount paid to hospital units from the then average rate of about $175 per treatment[33] to $132. The regulation stipulated that:

> The rates would result in reimbursing 46% of all hospital-based facilities and 28% of all independent facilities at a rate per treatment below their current cost.[7]

but they speculated that economies could be found in other ways.[7] The conjecture is not unlike the illogical notion that one can simply triple the fraction of home dialysis patients in 1½ years or that hospitals obviously treat sicker outpatients and are therefore due a higher rate. Even worse, the Government Accounting Office later found that the cost of home hemo- and peritoneal dialysis was substantially higher than HCFA had presumed and that 35 percent of home dialysis patients were experiencing costs which exceeded the proposed $128 screen.* Where, then, would be the home dialysis "profits" which were theoretically to compensate for paying "marginally less than the full cost" for in-facility dialysis?

Finally, the regulations virtually endorsed CAPD which had received only limited clinical trails. This was added after the original regulations were typed even though the Medicare estimated cost for CAPD was much higher than for home hemodialysis and dialysis in independent units.[7] The reason for the addition was unclear. However, testimony before the

---

*Letter to HSS Secretary Schweiker (HRD 83-28), January 21, 1983.

Health Subcommittee of the Senate Finance Committee* demonstrated that a major manufacturer† of CAPD solutions was marketing its product through a large number of lucrative consulting awards to prominent academic physicians. Lobbying efforts by the company supported by these physicians with undisclosed awards may have resulted in the HCFA endorsement.

The endorsement of CAPD was doubly embarrassing because it came at a time when large registry statistics showed that only 28 percent of patients remained on CAPD after 2 years and the patient mortality on CAPD was greater than in all other ESRD patients—even those 60 to 65 years old.[30] Even a preliminary NIH-sponsored study showed one-year treatment failure exceeding 40 percent. Finally, HCFA itself was sponsoring a study to evaluate dialysis and transplantation in terms of case mix, treatment type, and outcome. Data showed that CAPD patients, like home hemodialysis patients, were a highly selected group[12] and were younger, far more likely to be white, better educated, more likely to be married, and more likely to own their own home than center hemodialysis patients. Similarly, CAPD patients, like home hemodialysis patients, suffered from far fewer baseline co-morbid conditions than patients receiving treatment in centers. In spite of being highly selected, but unlike home hemodialysis patients, CAPD patients were less likely to be working than center treated patients. The study also used a variety of subjective self-reporting techniques to assess "quality of life."[13] Restricting the analysis to dialysis patients, only 5 of 17 measures showed any significant difference. Home hemodialysis

patients generally showed better scores. Unfortunately, many measures were intercorrelated and involved satisfaction with home, sex, and family life. Home ownership and marriage were not considered (statistically controlled for) in the analysis (about 50 percent of center patients owned their own home while 75 to 80 percent CAPD and home hemodialysis patients did so—the same percentages apply to marriage) so that these factors rather than treatment per se may have caused the result. In any event, the authors noted the lack of correlation of these subjective measures with objective outcomes. Finally, and perhaps most significant, CAPD patients required significantly more hospitalization even though they are a highly selected group, resembling home hemodialysis patients medically (in nights hospitalized per year, home hemodialysis = 8, center dialysis = 13, CAPD = 21). Thus, HCFA had officially endorsed for unknown reasons a new and unproven medical therapy that is, particularly with added hospitalization cost, more expensive than conventional treatment and is associated with more complications. But, as we have seen, government does not hesitate to indulge in medical decision making as a part of the political process.

Structuring the rate the way HCFA did while encouraging CAPD is doubly distressing considering the thesis of Prottas, Segal, and Sapolsky.[40] Briefly, they noted large differences in dialysis prevalence between Western countries. Norway, Finland, Ireland, and the United Kingdom, for example, were very low (31, 36, 47, and 53 per million, respectively) while Switzerland, France, Israel, and the United States were higher (127, 133, 144, and 209 per million, respectively). About one-half of the difference between the United States and the West European maximums was attributed to differences in the black/white composition of the pop-

*Hearings on the End Stage Renal Disease Program of Medicare; Subcommittee on Health of the Senate Finance Committee, March 15, 1982.
†Travenol Laboratories, Deerfield, Ill.

ulations and the high incidence of renal failure in black persons. Other differences between countries could be explained by policies which prohibit or severely limit access to dialysis for the elderly or other potentially disadvantaged patients in certain European nations. For example, the United Kingdom, which has one of the lowest dialysis prevalance rates, has been rationing treatment by constraining the resources allocated to patients with renal failure.[40] The British rely heavily on home dialysis without the assistance of a paid nurse, which results in more restrictive selection policies. This is indirect rationing of treatment, the specific detail of which is not governmentally directed for individual patients. In other words, the selection criteria in England are less a result of direct government regulations than of resource constraints, which makes selection necessary. To quote the authors,[40]

It is after all the selection policies of centers, *a combination of government resource allocation, and physician decisions,* that will ultimately affect treatment prevalence. [Emphasis added]

The consequence of resource constraint on physicians' decisions can be easily anticipated. After all, the Seattle Committee to which Senator Jackson referred in 1972 simply reflected an attempt to allocate a scarce resource.

Adding to this issue is the irrational, malignant, and pervasive bias against the private sector which we have encountered in many HCFA bureaucrats and auditors. They would seemingly sacrifice a health care system in pursuit of their own personal, political, and social goals. Nowhere was this better demonstrated than in the courtroom of Judge Harold Green last year where an HCFA bureaucrat may have perjured himself during National Medical Care instigated litigation. Said Justice Green to HHS lawyers about the Department's behavior,

Judging from what I heard in this court today and what I've seen about this case ever since it has been filed, I would have no confidence that anybody in your department (HHS) is going to do anything that is appropriate and that is fair. (Slifkin et al. vs. Schweiker; U.S. District Court for the District of Columbia; Case No. 82-383.)

These are the lessons which the medical profession and health care consumers should learn from the recent policy history of the ESRD program. Why would HCFA knowingly reimburse 46 percent of hospitals and 28 percent of indepdndent facilities below their costs and by direct legislation or economic coercion force rationing through home dialysis? If health rationing through resource constraint or elimination of the private sector is the choice of society, so be it. Surely there must be a better way. But if not, the decision should be made with full and open social debate, not by some backdoor set of regulations defended by ill-gotten data and weak or contrived arguments by people knowing little about the care of patients.

## AN ALTERNATIVE

Hopefully, ESRD care in the United States has not progressed through research and development, demonstration and training and finally capacity building as Rettig notes[42] only to enter now a phase of capacity contraction and resource rationing. But now the public pays for 43 percent of the health dollar compared to 25 percent only 20 years ago.[17] And how do we control the spiralling personal health care costs which have increased at 13 percent per year since 1965? The renal program itself may provide a key. The ESRD experiment was partially successful and per capita costs in the program have been much better contained than in other health care areas.[32,33] The "screen" provided a powerful incentive for cost containment to which limited care facilities responded by finding cost containing strategies. Hospitals, accustomed to the so-called cost-plus-reimbursement procedures embodied in Medicare law, responded by seeking exceptions through cost justification. HCFA acquiesced with a liberal exception policy.

HCFA now seeks to correct this historical error by choking the rest of the system while retreating to another form of cost reimbursement called prospective.[7] Congressman Richard Gebhart noted recently,[16]

> Prospective reimbursement, with which the Department (of Health and Human Services) is flirting, is merely a euphemism for rate setting and does not lead to price competition among providers.

Generally considered a liberal Congressman, he also notes that the current Medicare reimbursement system "removes the economic incentives for providers to compete in terms of price, protects the inefficient and underpays the efficient."

Medicare and certain other insurers have traditionally geared reimbursement to hospitals on a "cost" basis. Under this policy, an institution is paid for all of its costs while caring for beneficiaries if those costs are deemed "allowable." If hospital costs go up by a dollar, so do revenues, and there is no financial incentive to hold costs down.[11] A "disallowed" cost can be shifted easily in ways that lead to higher overall costs. For example, the hospital can encourage longer inpatient stays to spread overhead over more days when the patient is least ill, requiring less service at the same charge per day—which they have done.[47] It can encourage treatment in specialty units or performance of more ancillary tests such as admission electrocardiograms, chest x-rays, urinalyses, and blood counts. They also did

precisely that in response to Section 223 of the Social Security Amendments of 1972 which placed limits upon reimbursement for routine inpatient cost.[2]

Since there is no real incentive for anyone to contain costs under the current cost-based, Medicare system of payment,[11,37] what then has stopped them from spiralling upward? In fact, they have not been controlled and medical inflation has increased at a rate faster than the economy in general.[17] Instead of using incentives in the past, the Congress, HCFA, and state agencies have tried to contain costs by forced controls. Economist Enthoven[11] and others[24,37] reviewed the problems associated with these command and control regulations, which have been counterproductive and ineffective. The real problem may originate from the fact that authors of most regulations have not understood medical care or how it is delivered.[21,22] Enthoven says it nicely:

> In my view, the regulatory approach is like trying to make water run uphill, whereas in the competitive market approach the government is merely trying to channel the stream in its downhill course.[11]

In spite of administrative and policy problems, the original ESRD program architects sowed the seeds from which have emerged the elements of an incentive health delivery system. They set a dollar screen—only in part dependent on cost—which defined the dollar value of service. When evaluating lessons to be learned from the program, Rettig notes:

> Cost containment is controlled by the incentives created by the reimbursement system. When incentives can be established administratively without interference in the practice of medicine, *as they were for the screen on facility reimbursement*, cost control can be quite effective. A steady pattern of exceptions for higher cost treat-

ment, however, will obviously weaken these effects over time.[42] [Emphasis added]

How might these beginnings at an incentive-based, competitive cost containment system be developed further? Systems should be created so that patients, physicians, and providers are induced to weigh the relative risks, benefits, and costs of competing therapies and procedures to make appropriate "benefit/cost" decisions. Where therapies are otherwise equivalent, regulations should encourage by incentives, but not direct, that they be delivered by the least cost method.

There are three primary participants to whom incentives must be directed in the ESRD care system—physicians, facilities, and consumers. We have previously discussed physicians, facilities, and their complex interaction.[32] Hospital costs amount to about 40 percent of health expenditures[11,17] while physician services account for 18 to 19 percent. Physicians, who have no traditional incentive to control the cost of the services they prescribe, are the decision makers, however, and probably influence or control directly up to 70 percent of personal health care expenditures.[11] Any rational system must provide economic incentives for those who control most of the costs—in this case, the physician.

Harris[23] believes that health care institutions are essentially two separate but interacting firms—a demand division (medical staff) and a supply division (the administration). Physicians behave in economic ways but are not particularly interested in the cost of care because they have no responsibility for controlling it. Clearly, unless health care policy views the physician and the hospital in the same firm, so that their interests concerning cost control are similar, it will be doomed to failure. We have offered potential solutions to this problem previously[32] suggesting that physicians have a financial stake through profit sharing in the facilities they use to deliver care whether or not they are run for profit.

Incentives for consumers are complicated.[11,19,44] Current policy fosters first-dollar coverage by insurance plans. The premiums of these are not taxed to either an employer or employee, but when they are paid by a private citizen they are taxed. Most Americans (74 percent) receive either this employer-paid, tax-free, first-dollar medical insurance or government payment.[18] So there is no consumer incentive to control cost. Health insurance funded in this way resembles a prepaid, taxpayer-subsidized, installment purchase plan more than an insurance program. The cost of it is unimportant and relatively invisible to the consumer.

The consumers should stand to gain or lose economically in some way for the choices they make concerning their own health care consumption. Incentives to control cost are thereby created for consumers as well as physicians and institutions. Gebhardt noted, however, that any plan containing consumer incentives must not discriminate against the sick, the elderly, or the disadvantaged and incentives should not degenerate into "cream skimming" in the name of competition.[16] Such a policy would subvert the obligation to provide assistance to all who truly need care. The proposed renal regulations[7] would do just that because they compute the rate to be paid for service upon the cost of home dialysis (without a nurse) and the cost of center dialysis. Increasing the percentage of patients dialyzed at home without a nurse will increase the profits of an institution. However, the home dialysis population is young, white, male, and less medically complicated than other dialysis patients.[33] Therefore, institutions would be compelled to select young, white, male and less medically complicated individuals for care.

Structuring incentives for patients with a chronic, catastrophic illness may be somewhat more complicated than structuring incentives for routine medical care. A policy that created economic incentives for inadequate care would not be desirable. Inadequate dialysis may increase the probability of morbidity even though the cause and effect relationship may not be readily apparent.[34] Furthermore, the effect of underdialysis may not be easily reversible, exposing the patients to an increased risk of mortality even after they have returned to conventional therapy.[38] Policy should not encourage patients to accept long-term health risks in pursuit of a short-term economic gain.

Restricting the discussion to outpatient dialysis, consumers could receive an allocation of funds to their Medicare account which equals a fixed per-treatment fee—say, $150. Dialysis facilities would be free to charge what they wished, but could not allocate costs to other departments which received Medicare fees in order to subsidize dialysis activities. If a patient selected treatment in a more expensive unit he or she would be required to pay a portion of the difference which could not be covered by coinsurance. If, on the other hand, the patient elected treatment in a facility which charged less than $150 per treatment, he or she would receive a portion of the difference but a coinsurer could not deny payment because of this rebate. Home dialysis patients who did *not* employ a home dialysis nurse would receive a *larger* rebate than one who did. If home dialysis with a nurse were more expensive than limited care dialysis, the patient would pay more or receive a smaller rebate than the limited care patient. Figure 1-2 is a graphic display of such a plan. The screen

($150) could be adjusted periodically based upon actual expenditure experience which would reflect the choices of consumers in which they had both a financial and a medical stake. Both the public and patients would share in the cost-saving decisions patients make and future rate-setting activities would be market rather than cost oriented.

## PROFIT AND NONPROFIT

We have discussed this issue previously[32,33] but it may be of value to review the economic incentives of profit and nonprofit institutions. About 40 percent of dialysis units are independents and over three quarters of these are operated for profit. Few if any hospital units are for profit. Profit is defined simply as the amount by which income exceeds expenses. The tax code permits certain institutions to retain these "surplus revenues" without paying income, property, or (in most states) sales tax. These are nonprofit institutions. All other institutions must pay income tax (and other taxes) and are called profit making

The problem with both profit and nonprofit institutions is: How high should the profits be? Economists distinguish between normal and "excess profits" calling the latter "rents." The question here is the definition of "excess." What is average to one person may appear obscene to another. Economists define a "rent" as a return that exceeds opportunity cost, which is a complicated way of saying it is profit exceeding a return expected from the next best alternative use of resources. But rents are not necessarily bad or immoral. They may be earned by individuals because the value of their services exceeds that of competitors—superb athletes and entertainers earn superb salaries. They may

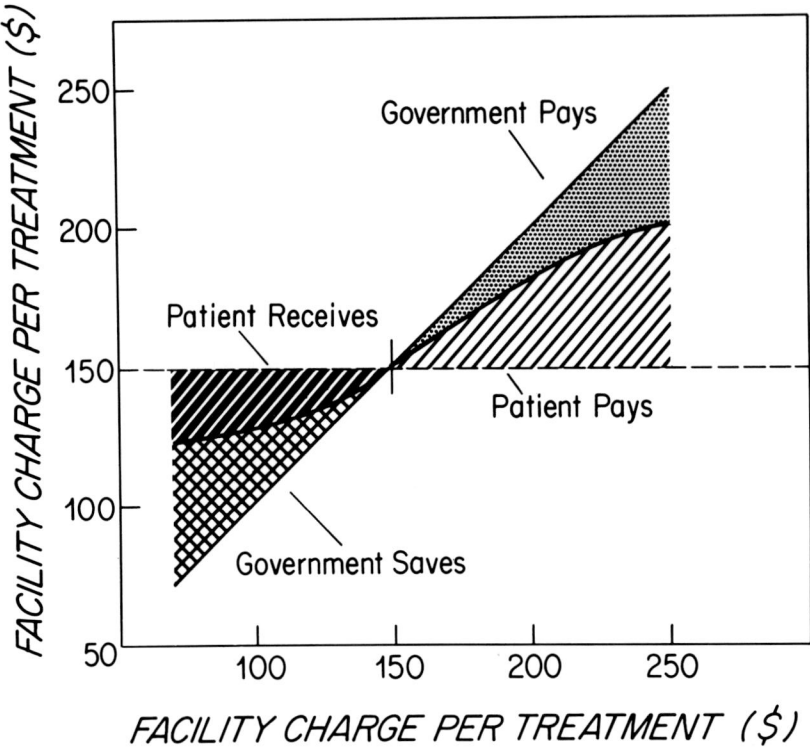

**Fig. 1-2.**   Graph showing a potential rebate–charge for consumers of dialysis. Both the ordinate and the abcissa show the facility charge per treatment and a diagonal line of identity is shown. Any profit or loss resulting from a difference between the screen and the actual charge would be shared by the patient and government. The horizontal, dashed line shows a possible HCFA authorized screen ($150 per treatment). The shaded areas describe the patient's and the government's liability or profit from the difference between the screen and the charge of the facility which the patient selects. For example: If the patients selects a facility with a $150 screen, neither the public nor the patient gains or loses relative to the screen. If (s)he chooses a facility with a $200 charge, the patient pays an additional $30 per treatment and Medicare pays an additional $20. If the patient selects a unit charging $100 per treatment, the patient receives a $20 credit and Medicare saves $30.

also be earned by companies even though their products or services are sold at market cost. Such companies may be highly efficient, enabling them to reduce production costs below that of their competitors. *If there is a desire to define a reasonable level of profit, we feel it should be that profit level which will be sufficient to attract enough capital (i.e., fixed resources) to finance the socially required level of care.* The level of profit is sufficient when there is enough capital in the system whether it is in profit or nonprofit institutions. In this regard, the rules used to calculate the most recent proposed dialysis rates eliminated return on invested capital as an allowable cost.[7] It is permitted in other areas and the elimination is but another indication of HCFA's intention to reduce treatment capacity.

What are the economic goals and

functional goals of profit and nonprofit centers? We assume that profit-making centers will seek to maximize profits. If operating in a noncompetitive environment (no other dialysis units in the area), they will seek to reduce costs if price is fixed. If operating in a competitive environment with other dialysis units in the area, they will expend much of their excess revenues on patient and physician amenities* in order to attract patients and physicians.[25] This describes a classical free market force.

The goals of nonprofit organizations are obscure and more difficult to predict.[35] Economists have therefore experienced trouble trying to model their behavior. Newhouse[34] and Feldstein[13] postulated that hospitals attempted to maximize the quantity and quality of service subject to certain budgetary constraints requiring them to "break even." Most models, however, ignore the central role of physicians in determining costs, as suggested by Enthoven.[11] Pauley and Redisch[39] view physicians as having effective control of hospital operations by controlling the demand for service. Services are then produced in such a way as to enhance physician income—but physicians generally have no stake in hospital costs.

Some suppose that nonprofit hospitals are nonprofit. This is simply not true. If it were, their profits should be zero on the average. Davis[5] found that nonprofit hospital revenues exceed expenses for every year from 1961 through 1969 except 1962. Reports from the American Hospital Association still show this profit.[32] Hospitals behave so as to maximize cash flow[5]—that is, revenue minus operating expenses other than depreciation. They acquire capital from philanthropies, contributions, government and charitable grants, and tax-exempt bond issues. Much of this contributed capital is risk free to the hospital and considering its amount, cash flows are likely to be large. These monies can be used to support research, pay for students, subsidize physicians who engage in other activities, and support other activities which are irrelevant to the service for which the payments were intended. The public is not aware of the disposition of these funds even though it pays for a large share of health care consumed through both tax subsidies and direct payments. Furthermore, the cost of these irrelevant activities is included in the cost of business so profits are even higher than commonly recognized. The point of all this is that tax-exempt, nonprofit institutions have been able to modify their behavior to realize profit consonant with their internal motives while not violating current provisions of the Internal Revenue Code. These motives are so complex as to defy the explicit understanding of health economists, let alone the general public.

It is interesting to note that many nonprofit hospitals now feel that they must be permitted to make a profit to ensure their economic viability.[4] This would permit them to maintain adequate working and reserve capital, meet debt requirement, and establish a credible credit position to receive borrowed or invested funds.[4] Financial simulation models showed,[4]

> The simulation demonstrated conclusively and dramatically the *need for profit* in Illinois hospitals if they are to maintain their service capacity (asset base) in an inflationary economy. . . . Thus hospitals must be able to generate *adequate profit* and cash flow to maintain and expand their service potential.[4] [Emphasis added]

---

*"Amenities" is a general term which may include such things as convenient scheduling, TV sets, transportation, physician conveniences, or other things which are perceived to be of value to patients or physicians. It could also include the concept of "quality" of care.

Regarding the desirable level of profit they say, "there was no clear answer to the right level of profitability for health care institutions." These concepts are remarkably similar to tax paying, private sector needs and goals. However, while wanting the privilege of profit, hospitals seek to retain their tax-exempt status. They are actively exploring complicated corporate reorganization schemes that would permit retention of profit without paying tax.[45,46]

The economic motives in for-profit centers seem clear as they relate to patient care. To reject patients or dialyze them at low and possibly inadequate levels may reduce future revenues. It is in the economic as well as the professional interests of these centers to accept patients for treatment and to provide a level of care that is sufficient to maintain life and health to avoid hospitalization. The ethical *similarities* of proprietary and nonprofit institutions have been stressed recently.[3] Quoting the author, "all institutions of healing have to attend to both the canons of ethics and the canons of economics" to survive in today's world.

Health economists Held and Pauley have reviewed recently the HCFA cost data for both profit-making and nonprofit hospitals and independents.[37] They note that trying to determine the "true cost" of dialysis is misdirected, if not futile. Actual costs will include optional physician and patient amenities which will be greater in a competitive than in a noncompetitive environment. Therefore, cost and profit are what the facility makes them in response to external demands and determining a cost required to perform dialysis may be impossible. Supporting this thesis, their analysis showed that competition eroded the profits of institutions. Furthermore, hospital dialysis centers were associated with higher profits, while for-profit ownership was associated with lower profits. While the finding is coun-

ter-intuitive on the surface, it is not surprising, because average hospital costs were about $175 per treatment in 1981 but reimbursement to independents remained at $138.[33]

Held and Pauly[27] also evaluated production functions for-profit and nonprofit dialysis units in high and low competitive environments. Production functions provide a mathematical description of the relationship between the physical inputs to and the outputs from a process such as dialysis. Their coefficients can be determined statistically and used to compare the production efficiencies of different units with respect to each and all of the inputs. Inputs for dialysis included labor, capital, and supplies. The analysis showed that the for-profit form of organization leads to greater production efficiency but that in competitive markets much of these efficiency gains are transferred to consumers in the form of greater amenities.

Held and Pauly had analyzed previously the resources used for dialysis in profit and nonprofit units.[26] They concluded that both commit the same level of real physical resources per patient. The finding was essentially similar to that of Kirsch and colleagues,[28,29] who evaluated patterns of patient selection and treatment methods in profit and nonprofit units in the California End-Stage Renal Disease Program. There was no difference in patient selection patterns but for-profit units tended to commit more resources, dialyzing equivalent patients more intensively than their nonprofit counterparts.

The foregoing shows that the production of service is more efficient in the for-profit environment and that quality has not suffered either in terms of technical competence or patient amenities. If nonprofit institutions are behaving more and more like their profit-making counterparts and vice versa,[3] perhaps it is time to revisit the tax-exempt status of hospitals.

The taxpayer is assuming a greater and greater responsibility for the direct funding of health care,[17] rendering unnecessary and duplicative the tax subsidies granted to hospitals. The tax code permits a convenient vehicle by which "arrangements for sharing (with government) such reduction in cost as may be attributable to the more efficient and effective delivery of service" as suggested by PL 95-292. As taxed institutions, the public—which provides most of the revenue to hospitals—would also share in any cost-saving strategies that they develop rather than simply transferring all of these profits for discretionary distribution by hospital physicians, administrators, and trustees.

Hospitals developed from the alms-houses of the past, which were a refuge for the sick who were unwanted by society. They provided little medical care and were supported only by donations and direct tax revenues. Thus, care of the sick has been a charitable activity since the Statute of Elizabeth in 1601. With the changing financial operation of hospitals and the changing needs of society, their privileged, tax-exempt status should be seriously reevaluated as an integral part of any health care reform proposal.

## THOUGHTS ABOUT POLICY

A cited reference[16] poses the question, "Do we need legislation. . . ?" Readers might presume that we would respond with a resounding "NO." But they would be wrong because it is needed if only to undo existing law and regulation concerning health in general and renal disease in particular. The law, however, while reflecting broad and consistent policy intent, should refrain from medical prescription. Similarly, implementing regulations, while creating the structure to make

the law work, should also refrain from medical prescription.

Law and regulation should address all parts of the health care system with which they are concerned in a global and not a piecemeal way to create incentives which will encourage the system to evolve in a socially desirable direction. Of the three participants in the ESRD system—institutions, physicians, and patients (consumers)—consumers have been totally ignored. The most recently proposed regulations[7] are a clear example and they even create an intense disincentive for physicians and institutions—both profit and nonprofit.

It seems to us that the now stricken language from PL 95-292 which is cited in this chapter is a laudable policy goal for reimbursement regulations in the ESRD program and other programs as well. The incentives must be direct to each ESRD program participant.

*Consumers.* Patients and their families must be induced to learn about the costs that they incur on their own behalf and to make appropriate cost/benefit (or amenity) decisions in their relationships with physicians and institutions considering their own personal circumstances. They will only do that if they are given a financial as well as a medical stake in the action. Laws and regulations must therefore address the interaction between patients and physicians and between patients and institutions.

*Physicians* must be induced to learn about and control the costs of the therapies they prescribe and must learn constraint in their prescriptive practice. Who else is better able to make the technical cost/benefit decisions that affect direct patient care? This can only occur if physicians stand to gain or lose economically as well as professionally from the medical-administrative decisions they make. This goal can be achieved through the interaction of physicians and institutions, by creating a "profit share" for physicians in the clinical departments they run whether or not the institution is run for profit. When modulated by other physicians and interested consumers, this arrangement cannot lead to abuse.

*Institutions* must be induced to maximum efficiency in their administrative functions such as billing, purchasing, and personnel management. In technical matters involving the interaction of the medical staff and administration, their mutual goals must be cost control with quality preservation. This can occur only if the Medicare Part A cost reimbursement procedures are abandoned and physicians have incentives. Patients and physicians who use the institution will modulate any unacceptable amenity reductions in pursuit of cost control by direct pressure and simply by going elsewhere.

Most of the health care dollar is spent in institutions—notably hospitals. The public is paying directly for an increasing fraction of health care and the fruits of the cost-saving efforts of hospitals should be shared with the public through taxing hospitals as other businesses are taxed.

For most of this chapter we have discussed government's role but have not said much about that in our concluding remarks. Government should create and monitor the system of incentives but it should refrain from medical decision making. If the incentives are properly balanced among the ESRD system participants an optimum price of service can be achieved reflecting the relative interests of all participants. Government can reevaluate price periodically in terms of the choices consumers make. Considering the proposed example, for instance, if consumers are choosing lower price treatment to achieve rebates, the price paid for dialysis (the screen) could be reduced. If, on the other hand, they are choosing higher priced treatment requiring undesirably high out-of-pocket expenditures,

the price can be increased. In this way, the rate-setting activities of government use market driven principles rather than the historic cost-based system. We hope that HCFA will provide new and innovative reimbursement guidelines for this small and easily analyzed ESRD program so that the "experiment" in funding care for catastrophic illness may be continued.

# CONCLUSION

Ignoring the vast majority of public comment, HCFA published on May 11, 1983 Final Rules for Dialysis Reimbursement in much the same form which they had proposed on February 12th—one year earlier. The average rate, however, was about $1 per treatment less. In forming their conclusions, HCFA placed great weight on their analysis showing that 114 new dialysis units had opened since the rates were first announced by HHS Secretary Schweiker in a press release on November 25, 1981. In her own release on March 25, 1983, the new HHS Secretary Heckler said, "I am convinced that these rates will be sufficient to maintain available service. Since the new rates were first proposed 114 new facilities have opened."

Analysis of HCFA's own data showed that HCFA counted as the opening date the month in which Washington received *notification* from its Regional Offices that the unit had opened and had been approved—not the actual opening date. Even so, they counted all notifications received in November—not just those received on or after November 25, 1981.

Of greater importance, however, is the fact that at least 51 of the units were really approved and operational *before* November 25, 1981. Of those approved after November 25th, 6 were government or inpatient only units (two stations in Pago

Pago, and so forth), 15 were transfers without service capacity change (hospitals reorganizing, etcetera) and 6 were satellites of existing units. This leaves 36 new units—42 if one includes the satellites—which were approved between the original HHS press release and March, 1983 (one and one-third years)—not 114 as announced by HCFA. In addition, the trend for new openings was clearly down because 30 units were approved in the 3-month period from November, 1981 through January, 1982, but only 8 units were approved in the three months from November, 1982 through January, 1983.

Perhaps this is another lesson we should learn from the history of ESRD regulation in this country. When it comes to policy decisions, one may not be able to take at face value government's analysis of its own data. Health care professionals and other citizens should demand and receive *full* technical disclosure to ensure the competency and objectivity of the summary information policy makers use to make their decisions. This short saga reminds us again of Justice Green's impressions about the fairness of government.

# REFERENCES

1. Anast D: Guest Interview, Doctor Christopher Blagg. Contemporary Dialysis, Oct. 1980, p. 17; Dec. 1980, p. 8.
2. Ashby JL: An analysis of hospital costs by center, 1971–1978. Health Care Financing Review 4 (No. 1):37, Sept. 1982.
3. Cunningham R: Changing philosophies in medical care and the rise of the investor owned hospital. New Engl J Med 307:817, 1982.
4. David IT: Why tax exempt hospitals need profit. Health Care Finan Man Sept. 1982, p. 46.
5. Davis K: Economic theories of behavior in non profit, private hospitals. Econ Bus Bull 24:1, 1972.
6. Department of Health & Human Services: Health Care Financing Administration, Medicare Program: Reimbursement for outpatient dialysis and self-care dialysis training. Fed Reg 45, No. 189, p. 64008, Sept. 26, 1980.
7. Department of Health & Human Services: Health Care Financing Administration, Medicare Program: End-Stage Renal Disease Program; Prospective Reimbursement for Dialysis Services. Fed Reg 37, No. 30, p. 6556, Feb. 12, 1982.
8. Eggers P: Analysis of indicators of case-mix differences between freestanding facilities and hospital based Medicare ESRD patients. Working Paper #OR38. Program Evaluation Group, Division of Beneficiary Studies/Office of Research/Office of Research & Demonstration/Health Care Financing Administration. May 14, 1982.
9. End Stage Renal Disease Medical Information System Facility Report No. 2, prepared for Health Care Financing Administration (Contract No. HSA-240-75-0123) by Value Engineering Co., 1976.
10. End Stage Renal Disease Second Annual Report to Congress, FY 1980, OESRD/OSP/HCFA/DHHS, U.S. Govt. Printing Office No. 1980-311-168/469.
11. Enthoven AC: Health Plan. Addison-Wesley. Reading, MA, 1980.
12. Evans R: Case mix, treatment modalities, and patient outcomes: Results of the National Kidney Dialysis and Kidney Transplantation Study. Submitted as Update Number 14 for the National Kidney Dialysis and Kidney Transplantation Study, Sponsored by ORD/HCFA/DHHS, Grant No. 95-P-97887/0-01, 1982.
13. Evans R: A comparison of the quality of life of patients undergoing treatment for chronic renal failure: Results from the National Kidney Dialysis and Kidney Transplantation Study. Submitted as Update No. 15 for the National Kidney Dialysis and Kidney Transplantation Study, Sponsored by ORD/HCFA/DHHS Grant No. 95-P-97887/0-01, 1982.
14. Evans R, Blagg C, Bryan F: Implications for health care policy: A social and demographic profile of hemodialysis patients in the United States. J Am Med Assoc 245:487, 1981.

15. Feldstein MS: Hospital cost inflation: A study of non profit price dynamics. Am Econ Rev 51:853, 1971.

16. Gephardt RA: Do we need legislation to achieve competition? Review of an advocate. Health Affairs 1:53, 1982.

17. Gibson R: National Health Expenditures, 1981. Health Care Financ Rev 4 (1):1, 1982.

18. Ginsberg P: Containing medical costs through market forces. Congress of the United States, Congressional Budget Office, May, 1982.

19. Ginzberg E: Competition and cost containment. N Engl J Med 303:1112, 1980.

20. Gottchalk C: Report of the Committee on Chronic Kidney Disease, United States Bureau of the Budget, Washington, D.C., Sept. 1967.

21. Halenor JF: Surprise! Bureaucrats don't trust doctors. Medical Econ Nov. 24, pp. 23–33, 1980.

22. Harris J: The internal organization of hospitals: Some economic considerations. Bell J Econ 8:467, 1977.

23. Harris JE: Regulation and internal control in hospitals. Bull NY Acad Med 55:88, 1979.

24. Havighurst CC: Prospects for competition under health planning-cum-regulation. In Pauly MV, Ed: National Health Insurance: What now, what later, what never? American Enterprise Institute for Policy Research, Washington, D.C., 1980.

25. Held P, Pauly M: Financial and policy goals of the End-Stage Renal Disease Program. Report prepared under Grant No. 18-97265/5-01 from HCFA/DHHS.

26. Held P, Pauly M: An economic analysis of the production and cost of renal dialysis treatments. Report to Health Care Financing Administration, Grant No. 18-97265/5-01, 1980.

27. Held PJ, Pauly MV: Competition and efficiency in the End Stage Renal Disease Program. Working Paper #3064-04. HCFA/HSS Grant No. 18-P-97516/3-01. The Urban Institute, Washington, D.C., Dec. 1982.

28. Kirsch L, Rowe J, Brown M, et al: Influence of dialysis center ownership characteristics and dialysis-to-population rates on patient selection and treatment. Kidney Int 10:519, 1976.

29. Kirsch L, Rowe J, Brown M, et al: Risk factors and patterns of patient selection, treatment and outcome in California's End Stage Renal Disease Program: Final Report to the California State Assembly. March, 1977.

30. Kramer P, Boyer M, Brunner FP, et al: Combined Report on Regular Dialysis and Transplantation in Europe, XII, 1981. Published by the European Dialysis and Transplant Association, Sept. 1982.

31. Lion J, Altman S: Case mix differences between hospital outpatient departments and private practice. Health Care Financ Rev 4:89, 1982.

32. Lowrie EG, Hampers CL: Success of Medicare's End-Stage Renal Disease Program. The case for profits and the private marketplace. N Engl J Med 305:434, 1981.

33. Lowrie EG, Hampers CL: Proprietary dialysis and the End Stage Renal Disease Program. Dial Transplant 11:191, 1982.

34. Lowrie EG, Laird NM, Parker TF, & et al: Effect of the Hemodialysis prescription on patient morbidity. Report from the National Cooperative Dialysis Study. N Engl J Med 305:1176, 1981.

35. Major Themes and Additional Budget Details, Fiscal Year 1983, Executive Office of the President, Office of Management and Budget, Feb. 8, 1982, p. 59.

36. Newhouse JP: Toward a theory of nonprofit institutions. An economic model of a hospital. Am Econ Rev 60:64, 1970.

37. Newhouse JP: The Economics of Medical Care, Addison-Wesley, Reading, Mass 1978.

38. Parker T, Laird N, Lowrie E: A comparison of study groups and a description of morbidity, mortality, and patient withdrawal. In Lowrie E, Laird N, et al: The National Cooperative Dialysis Study. Kidney Int.

39. Pauly M, Redisch M: The not-for-profit hospital as a physician's cooperative. Am Econ Rev 63:87, 1973.

40. Prottas J, Segal M, Sapolsky HM: Cross-National Differences in Dialysis Rates. Health Care Financ Rev 4:91, 1983.

41. Rettig RA: The policy debate on patient care financing for victims of End Stage Renal Disease. Law Contemp Prob 40:196, 1976.

42. Rettig RA: Implementing the End Stage Renal Disease Program of Medicare. Rand Publication No. 2505-HCFA/HEW, Rand Inc., Santa Monica, 1980.

43. Rettig RA: The politics of health cost containment: End Stage Renal Disease. Bull NY Acad Sci 56:115, 980.

44. Seidman LS: Income related consumer cost sharing: A strategy for the health sector. In Pauly MD, Ed: National Health Insurance: What Now, What Later, What Never? American Enterprise Institute for Policy Research, Washington, D.C., 1980.

45. Stonehill E, Ewell CM: Constraints and risks of corporate reorganization. Health Care Fin Manag Sept. 1982 26.

46. Tillet JW, Linkluter RB, Sucher RA: Survey reveals trends in corporate reorganization: 155 hospitals studied. Health Care Financ Manag Sept. 1982, 38.

47. Worthington M, Pero P: The effect of hospital rate-setting programs on volumes of hospital services: A preliminary analysis. Health Care Financ Rev 4:47, 1982.

# Cost-Effective Treatment of Chronic Renal Disease

## Christopher R. Blagg, M.D.

In 1982 the cost to Medicare of dialysis and transplantation for some 60,000 patients with end-stage renal disease (ESRD) in the United States was approximately $1.8 billion,[20] and the projected cost rises to more than $3 billion by 1984. This does not take into account contributions from private insurance, state funds, individuals, and other sources of coinsurance. The relatively large expenditure of Medicare funds, some four percent of the total Medicare budget, for a relatively small number of patients has become a matter of increasing concern in recent years. During 1982, for example, the Health Care Financing Administration (HCFA) published proposed rules for changes in reimbursement for dialysis, there were several congressional hearings on the ESRD program, and a number of lay publications criticized the program and its high costs.

The ESRD program, in microcosm, exemplifies many of the problems facing medicine in general in the United States and elsewhere. Cost has been an issue since maintenance dialysis became possible with development of the external arteriovenous shunt by Scribner and coworkers at the University of Washington in 1960. From the initiation of dialysis and renal transplant programs in the early 1960s until introduction of the Medicare ESRD program in 1973, lack of funds was the major cause of death for ESRD patients in the United States. Since 1973, with relatively ready availability of financial support, both the number of patients and total cost of the program have increased considerably. Over the same time period the number of ESRD patients treated in Europe and elsewhere also has increased, although usually not as dramatically as in the United States; and as one might expect, there is a statistical relationship between the gross national product of a country and provision of ESRD treatment for its citizens.[21]

Despite concern about the cost of the ESRD program, this clearly relates to the increase in the number of patients treated rather than to any increase in the cost of treatment per se, and early projections of program cost seriously underestimated the number of potential patients.[28] In fact, the cost to Medicare per patient in constant dollars has not changed significantly since 1973, despite a marked change in composition of the patient population, which now includes many more elderly patients and those with systemic diseases such as diabetes.[14] Such a change in patient population would be anticipated to increase the cost per patient because of more frequent hospitalization and other treatment than required for younger patients with uncomplicated renal diseases, but this has not been the case. Consequently, in terms of the cost per patient, the Medicare ESRD program has been relatively cost-effective.[23] Despite this, the administration and Congress continue to express interest in reducing health expenditures in the program and making it more cost-effective, although this issue is now being over-

**Table 1-1.** Cost of Dialysis—HCFA, 1982 Based on 1977–1979 Data

| | Median Costs per Treatment ($) | | |
| --- | --- | --- | --- |
| | Adjusted Labor Costs | Nonlabor Costs | Total |
| All facilities | 54.06 | 71.47 | 125.53 |
| Hospital-based | 61.17 | 73.94 | 135.11 |
| Freestanding | 40.79 | 66.87 | 107.66 |
| Home dialysis | 11.70 | 85.09 | 96.79 |

shadowed by the much greater problems with the cost of health care generally.

In order to examine the ESRD program in terms of cost-effectiveness, it is essential to look at both cost and outcome of treatment. If modification of reimbursement or other changes are to be made in the program, these must be based on information; yet one major shortcoming of the ESRD program has been the lack of reliable data on the results of treatment by dialysis and transplantation.[5] Limited survival data are beginning to become available from the Office of Research of HCFA, but this does not yet permit comparison of the various modalities of treatment. Similarly, there is presently little information on patient rehabilitation,[27] although a recent paper has suggested this is less than anticipated at the time the program was instituted.[17] There is also need for information about the effectiveness of different modalities of treatment in terms of rehabilitation and life satisfaction. The association between the various measures of outcome and treatment modality is complex; and in order to make policy judgments with regard to cost-effectiveness, all these forms of information need to be considered.

# COST OF TREATMENT

Discussion of cost-effectiveness must start with examination of the cost of providing the various modalities of treatment. Over the years, papers devoted to cost have been criticized because of lack of uniformity in accounting and patient selection; and there is difficulty in obtaining reliable cost data from hospitals so that the cost of transplantation and hospitalization is less well defined than that of dialysis.

Unfortunately, and at first sight surprisingly, cost data from HCFA are also remarkable for their lack of specificity and accuracy. The most recent published information on cost of dialysis comes from audits carried out on behalf of HCFA in 1980 involving 67 hospital-based facilities and 38 freestanding dialysis facilities (Federal Register, February 12, 1982). For home dialysis, 23 dialysis facilities and two state kidney programs were audited in 1981, representing 30 percent of all home dialysis patients in the United States. Summaries of the results of these audits are shown in Tables 1-1 and 1-2. These data have been roundly criticized following their publication in a Notice of

**Table 1-2.** Cost of Home Dialysis—HCFA 1982

| | Hemodialysis | IPD | CAPD |
| --- | --- | --- | --- |
| Number of home programs | 25 | 13 | 17 |
| Number of facilities providing full range of services | 10 | 3 | 8 |
| Median cost per treatment | $ 87 | $111 | $114 |
| Highest cost facility | $156 | $153 | $202 |
| Lowest cost facility | $ 63 | $ 74 | $ 54 |

**Table 1-3.** Cost to Medicare of Dialysis in 1979

| | |
|---|---|
| Outpatient dialysis | $22,700 |
| Home dialysis | $17,822 |

(Data from Eggers, P. Trends in incidence, prevalence, survival, and reimbursement in Medicare ESRD. Forum Meeting, April 13, 1982.)

Proposed Rule Making for prospective reimbursement because they are outdated and from selected facilities. More recently, the Office of Research of the HCFA has developed information on the average Medicare reimbursement for various modalities of treatment for the calendar year 1979. These data, shown in Tables 1-3 and 1-4, are based on Medicare billing data and so give a good general indication of cost to Medicare. It should be noted that Tables 1-1 and 1-2 relate to cost of the dialysis itself and not necessarily to charges made by a facility to Medicare for treatment, and do not take into account the cost of treatment for complications due to dialysis or other medical problems the patient may suffer. On the other hand, Tables 1-3 and 1-4 contain information on total Medicare reimbursement for patients based on charges, not costs, and are for all care received by patients treated by a given modality.

## Transplantation

Information provided to Congress by proponents of transplantation at the time of the original Medicare legislation in 1972 suggested that this would prove to be the most cost-effective form of treatment. With increasing availability of kidneys and ongoing developments in cadaver transplantation, it was anticipated that the number of patients treated by dialysis would be limited, rehabilitation following transplantation would be optimal, and the cost of transplantation would prove to be much less than that of dialysis. Unfortunately, to the present time, much of this has not proved to be the case.

Little information is available from individual programs on the cost of transplantation, but recently Belzer et al.[1] discussed costs at the University of Wisconsin. These data are summarized in Table 1-5, which shows costs for 20 selected patients in each of four subgroups: nondiabetic living-related recipient, diabetic living-related recipient, nondiabetic cadaver recipient, and diabetic cadaver recipient. A large university-based transplant program may be more efficient than smaller programs, but it should be pointed out that the cost of a cadaver kidney in the Wisconsin program is "artifi-

**Table 1-4.** Cost to Medicare of Transplantation in 1979

| | |
|---|---|
| All patients transplanted in 1979 | $36,411 |
| Patients transplanted in 1979 whose graft did not fail in 1979 | $32,067 |
| Patients transplanted in 1979 whose graft failed in 1979 | $44,639 |
| Patients transplanted in 1979 who died in 1979 | $36,662 (annualized) $\approx$ $60,000) |
| Patients transplanted prior to 1979 with functioning graft through 1979 | $ 4,079 |
| Patients transplanted prior to 1979 whose graft failed in 1979 | $30,189 |

(Data from Eggers, P. Trends in incidence, prevalence, survival, and reimbursement in Medicare ESRD. Forum Meeting, April 13, 1982.)

**Table 1-5.** Total Cost of Transplant (in Dollars)

|  | Living-Related Donor Nondiabetic | Living-Related Donor Diabetic | Cadaver Donor Nondiabetic | Cadaver Donor Diabetic |
|---|---|---|---|---|
| **First Admission** |  |  |  |  |
| Mean | 11125 | 12633 | 12717 | 15316 |
| S.D. | 1818 | 3087 | 4687 | 6838 |
| Maximum | 14855 | 23095 | 25277 | 37195 |
| Minimum | 7481 | 9619 | 8798 | 8596 |
| **Additional Admission Costs—First Year** |  |  |  |  |
| Mean | 1967 | 4104 | 4682 | 7561 |
| S.D. | 3212 | 7465 | 6843 | 9062 |
| Maximum | 10226 | 31733 | 19455 | 30986 |
| Minimum | 0 | 0 | 0 | 0 |

(Reprinted by permission from Belzer, F.O., Miller, D.T., Sollinger, H.W., & Glass, N.R. Renal transplantation—a view of the 1980s. Seminars in Nephrology, **2**, 99– 1982.)

cially low" and the true cost probably is about $2,500 greater. In addition, the costs for the year include hospital admission costs but do not include the cost of outpatient drugs or of outpatient dialysis for those patients whose transplants failed. Consequently, these costs are somewhat lower than actual costs.

The HCFA data from Table 1-4 are much more inclusive, and for patients transplanted in 1979, the cost of treatment to Medicare throughout calendar 1979, averaged $36,411. Unfortunately, separate information is not available on the cost of living-related and cadaver donor transplants, but approximately 70 percent of all transplants in the United States in 1979 were cadaver donor transplants. If the data from Belzer et al.[1] can be used as a guide, a cadaver transplant costs 21 percent more than a related donor transplant in nondiabetic recipients, and 37 percent more in diabetic recipients. Note that these HCFA costs include costs for any dialysis the patient may have undergone during the year. For those patients transplanted in 1979 whose kidney did not reject during the year, the cost was somewhat less—$32,067—whereas for those transplanted and whose graft failed, the cost averaged $44,639. For patients who were both transplanted and died during

1979, the cost averaged $36,662; but this differs from the preceding figure in that, because of death, it is not based on a full year of patient experience, and if annualized would be approximately $60,000. For patients who were transplanted prior to 1979 and who had a functioning graft throughout 1979, the cost to Medicare for the year averaged $4,079 per patient, and for those patients transplanted prior to 1979 and whose graft failed during that year, the cost to Medicare averaged $30,189 per patient. Note that these costs do not include the coinsurance for physician fees and outpatient services, including dialysis, and that Medicare does not pay for outpatient drugs.

Based on this information, some generalizations about the cost of transplantation can be made. With the relatively high success rate of related donor transplantation, the increased costs associated with transplantation as compared with dialysis likely will be compensated for within one to two years; and thereafter the cost of maintaining the successfully transplanted patient will be much less than that of any form of dialysis. For cadaver transplantation, the issue is less clear, but again, within two to three years the increased cost associated with transplantation is likely to be offset. For diabetic patients, the cost of transplantation is one-fifth to one-third higher, but the cost of maintaining diabetic patients on dialysis is also greater than that for nondiabetic patients. Thus it appears clear that transplantation generally is a more cost-effective treatment than dialysis for suitable patients. Nevertheless, because of the age of the majority of the dialysis population and the number of patients with multisystem diseases, at this time most dialysis patients are not candidates for transplantation. Perhaps this may change in the future with new advances in immunology.

## Outpatient Dialysis

In the United States outpatient dialysis is provided by facilities sited in hospitals and by freestanding out-of-hospital (limited care) units. Many of the latter are proprietary, owned either by corporations or by individuals. According to HCFA data, 55 percent of maintenance dialysis facilities are hospital-based, and 45 percent are freestanding or hospital satellite dialysis units. About 40 percent of all dialysis patients are treated in proprietary facilities.

The possibility of reducing the cost of routine dialysis in a low-overhead out-of-hospital facility with the minimum of staff was appreciated as far back as 1962 when the Seattle Artificial Kidney Center was established in a nurses' residence adjacent to a hospital. In 1968 in Boston a dialysis unit was established in a nursing home for similar reasons, and from this the first proprietary dialysis corporation was developed to provide dialysis facilities at a time when nonprofit institutions were reluctant to commit the necessary capital, space, and staff.[18] Because of capable administration and the limited range of services offered, proprietary dialysis units proved to be very efficient; and with the advent of Medicare support for dialysis patients, they have also proved to be a very sound financial investment. The reported cost of outpatient dialysis in a freestanding unit (Table 1-1) is such that the present screen rate for reimbursement of $138 per outpatient dialysis (exclusive of physician fee and including $5 for routine laboratory charges) still provides a significant margin of profit. This reimbursement rate was first established in 1973, and the very significant potential for profit from outpatient dialysis clearly has been a major factor in the proliferation of dialysis units throughout the United States.

The cost of outpatient dialysis in a hospital facility generally is higher than in a freestanding facility (Table 1-1). In part this may be due to inefficiency, as claimed by proponents of proprietary dialysis,[23] and it also relates to cost plus hospital reimbursement under Medicare. Nevertheless, two other explanations need consideration. First, because of the method of Medicare reimbursement to hospitals, indirect costs are distributed across all departments, and outpatient dialysis costs include costs from completely unrelated areas of the hospital. Second, and more difficult to document, at least some hospital outpatient dialysis units treat a higher-than-average proportion of sick patients. In some cities, one facility, usually hospital-based, takes a high proportion of the patients with serious medical and other problems who may require more nursing and other services during dialysis; and in such units the cost per dialysis would be expected to be greater. Recent HCFA data do show that hospital facilities treat patients who have a higher mortality and a higher hospitalization rate, and therefore presumably are sicker patients, but did not show a clear relationship between case mix and cost.[12] Medicare permits an exception to the screen rate for facilities if they can provide medical or other justification for higher costs; but until 1982 such exceptions were much too easily obtainable simply by a hospital reporting their costs to exceed the screen level. This has changed recently with adoption of better cost reporting by HCFA and a tougher exception policy.

As part of the same issue, the question has been raised whether freestanding dialysis units, and in particular proprietary units, may contribute to an uneven distribution of sick patients by "skimming," that is, retaining stable patients and referring sicker patients to a hospital unit. This is difficult to substantiate.

Clearly, it is essential to obtain more information on the cost of treatment in all facilities and on the medical characteristics of the patients treated. Unless a hospital facility does treat an abnormally large proportion of sick patients, there is no reason why its cost of outpatient dialysis should differ significantly from that in a freestanding facility. This issue of outpatient treatment costs and their justification will be a major issue facing hospital dialysis units in the future as cost-containment pressures increase and likely will result in conversion of some hospital units to separate nonprofit (i.e., freestanding) corporations within the hospital, or transfer of management or of the unit itself to a proprietary corporation.

### Home Dialysis

Home dialysis as a means of conserving health care funds was an issue before the start of the ESRD program,[4] and the controversy over the role of home dialysis has continued.[2,18,28] Home dialysis was developed in response to lack of funding for maintenance dialysis in the early 1960s; and while the cost saving with home dialysis is clear, at least to its proponents, for many patients home dialysis is preferable for other reasons, including encouragement of independence and better opportunity for rehabilitation. Tables 1-1 and 1-2 show the cost of home

dialysis based on HCFA data, including the cost of dialysis and of personnel and other costs for providing support to patient and family, but not including the cost of backup outpatient dialyses, hospitalization, or other treatment of complications, or provision of a home dialysis helper. In terms of equipment, home dialysis is more expensive than outpatient dialysis because one machine is used for one patient; the cost of supplies should be comparable; and with an increase in the practice of dialyzer reuse in both outpatient and home dialysis, supply costs can be reduced further. The difference in cost between home and outpatient dialysis represents primarily the saving associated with patient and spouse performing the treatment, together with saving on the use of expensive facility space. Lowrie and Hampers[24] have criticized this transfer of the labor component of dialysis to the patient's family as "subsidizing a portion of the ESRD program." However, with increasing health care costs generally, it seems clear that home treatment of the chronically ill and the aged will be more and more widely utilized in the future.

One issue often raised with regard to home dialysis is the cost of paid dialysis helpers or aides. These have been used by a number of home dialysis programs and generally are carefully selected, nonprofessional (i.e., non-R.N.) individuals trained to assist a specific patient to perform dialysis at home. The cost of a helper varies but usually is related to the services performed, and in our program averages $35 per dialysis for a helper who provides coverage throughout dialysis. Thus provision of a helper does increase the cost of home dialysis appreciably so that this may be only slightly less than the cost of outpatient dialysis in the most efficient facilities. Recently HCFA supported studies on the effect of making payment available for either helpers or family

**Table 1-6.** Cost of Home Dialysis with an Aide

| | Home Dialysis with Aide | Outpatient Dialysis— Same Facilities | Outpatient Dialysis— "Control" Facilities |
|---|---|---|---|
| Physician Costs | 3.82 (3%) | 13.75 (9%) | 13.37 (9%) |
| Other Salaries | 13.26 (11%) | 58.61 (38)% | 56.07 (39%) |
| Aides | 20.36 (17%) | — | — |
| Equipment | 10.95 (9%) | 4.93 (3%) | 4.15 (3%) |
| Supplies | 48.52 (41%) | 49.59 (32%) | 38.73 (27%) |
| Other | 22.09 (19%) | 27.57 (18%) | 32.26 (22%) |
| Total | 119.00 (100%) | 154.44 (100%) | 144.58 (100%) |

(Data from Orkand Corporation. Evaluation of the Home Dialysis Aide Demonstration. Contract HCFA 500-79-0054. Silver Springs, Md., 1982.)

members to perform home dialysis. These showed that the number of patients performing home dialysis could be increased significantly by availability of such funding, particularly in nonprofit facilities.[26] Cost data from these studies are summarized in Table 1-6. Although there was significant variation in the cost of home dialysis, helper costs averaged 17 percent of home dialysis costs. The cost of home dialysis with such an aide averaged $119, which was 77 percent of the cost of outpatient dialysis at the same facilities and 82 percent of the cost of outpatient dialysis at 23 "control" facilities. Thus it was possible for these to be funded to provide paid aides or family support without the cost of home dialysis exceeding that of outpatient dialysis in the facilities taking part in the study.

The other significant cost associated with home hemodialysis is that of training the patient, family member, and/or helper. No information about this is available from HCFA, but the cost is greater than that of outpatient dialysis because of increased personnel costs and the need for training materials. Information from 27 programs showed the cost of a training dialysis to be approximately 2½ times the cost of an outpatient dialysis.[26] The payback time to recover this extra cost of training from the savings resulting from use of home dialysis in 15 of the 22 facilities, even when paid helpers were provided, was one year or less. If helpers were excluded, the mean payback period was nine months.[26]

Initiation of the ESRD program in the United States had a significant impact on home dialysis in terms of the percentage of dialysis patients treated by this modality. This percentage dropped steadily from about 40 percent in 1972 to only 11 percent in 1977, and has since increased to 17 percent in 1982, mainly as a result of introduction of continuous ambulatory peritoneal dialysis (CAPD). While the fall in home dialysis percentage related in part to the change in patient population as a result of near universal access to care,[14] it also relates to the financial disincentives for home dialysis and relatively generous support for outpatient dialysis in the initial regulations. Use of the screen level for outpatient dialysis reimbursement resulted in cost-containment as the screen has not been changed in 10 years, but this also suggests that the level must have been relatively generous reim-

**Table 1-7.** Home Dialysis and For-Profit Facilities

|            | Total Patients | Home Hemodialysis (%) | Total on Home Dialysis (%) |
|------------|----------------|------------------------|-----------------------------|
| For Profit | 19,936         | 6.0                    | 7.6                         |
| Nonprofit  | 31,634         | 20.4                   | 26.7                        |

(Department of Health and Human Services, Health Care Financing Administration. Medicare program: end-stage renal disease program; prospective reimbursement for dialysis services. Federal Register **47**, 6556.)

bursement at the start of the program. Federal funding and the associated increased demand for services resulted in a rapid increase in the number of dialysis facilities at a time when there were financial disincentives for both patient and facility discouraging them from undertaking home dialysis. These disincentives were reduced by legislation in 1978 which resulted in the option of payment for each dialysis at home at a rate of 70 percent (recently 75 percent) of that for outpatient dialysis. This legislation was strongly opposed by proprietary dialysis corporations.[28] The most recently proposed regulations (Federal Register, February, 1982) would equalize reimbursement for a dialysis performed at home or as an outpatient with the intention of encouraging more home dialysis. These proposed regulations have been widely criticized by physicians, facilities, and patients; and it seems unlikely now that they will be published in final form. In any case, they are unlikely to have much direct impact on the use of home dialysis unless the reimbursement is so low as to make outpatient dialysis undesirable, an approach which would be politically unfeasible.

Since early in the ESRD program the question has been raised whether proprietary dialysis facilities discourage the use of home dialysis and transplantation. Data gathered by Gardner[16] showed a statistical relationship between the number of proprietary dialysis facilities in an ESRD network area and the percentage of patients transplanted or performing home

dialysis, and other HCFA data also illustrates this (Table 1-7). Certainly the most vocal critics of home dialysis have been representatives of proprietary dialysis corporations who have questioned its safety and its cost.[2,18,24,28] The involvement of proprietary organizations in all aspects of health care in the United States is rapidly increasing, and it would seem worthwhile to study the relationship of facility ownership to patient distribution and utilization of different modalities of treatment in the ESRD program in the hope that lessons can be learned from this for future policies.

The data available demonstrate that home dialysis usually is less costly than outpatient dialysis, even if performed with a paid helper. This belief is the general wisdom in many other countries. In Britain, where funds for treatment of end-stage renal disease are extremely limited, more than 50 percent of patients are treated by home dialysis and CAPD, and home dialysis is also used extensively in a number of other countries. In Canada, for example, 51 percent of all dialysis patients are treated by either home hemodialysis, self-care hemodialysis, or peritoneal dialysis. There is wide variation in the use of home dialysis in different regions of the United States, ranging from 6 to 44 percent, but controversy continues as to the percentage of patients who are suitable for home dialysis. In the VA system, 38 percent of patients are treated by home dialysis (range in different units of from 9.6 to 90 percent), which is double the rate in the Medicare program. This may be related to the absence of financial incentives for VA physicians and facilities to keep patients on outpatient dialysis.[32] Clearly, a significantly greater percentage of patients generally could be treated by home dialysis, with cost savings of about $5,000 a year per patient; and the problem for policymakers is how to encourage use of home dialysis to the greatest extent possible. This requires motivating both physicians and facilities to encourage home dialysis; and it has been shown that wide discrepancies in home dialysis and transplantation rates may occur in closely contiguous facilities, mainly reflecting physician attitude and patient experience when starting dialysis.[29]

### Continuous Ambulatory Peritoneal Dialysis

In the last several years the total percentage of patients treated by home dialysis in the United States has begun to increase again, but only as a result of the dramatic increase in the use of CAPD.[3] Unfortunately, little information on the cost of CAPD is available other than HCFA data (Table 1-2). When CAPD was introduced, its proponents emphasized the cost saving which would result from use of this modality of treatment, but without providing information to justify this claim.

There are two parts to the cost of CAPD. First is the cost of the fluid, the major cost of the treatment itself. Presumably, with several manufacturers now in this field and increasing pressures to reduce the cost of the ESRD program, the price of a bag of fluid will decrease. The second major cost associated with CAPD is that of treating its complications. The frequency of peritonitis is well recognized, and also the very significant dropout rate from CAPD;[22] but little information is available on hospitalization costs

and how these compare with those for patients treated by other modalities, although CAPD appears to be associated with more hospital-days per year than other treatments (see below). In addition, the cost of treating peritonitis as an outpatient is unknown, as Medicare does not pay for outpatient drugs. Unfortunately, led on by the claims of enthusiasts about the cost-effectiveness of CAPD, HCFA in effect endorsed CAPD in its most recent reimbursement regulations by stating that "CAPD is the preferred treatment for many patients . . ." (Federal Register, February, 1982). Further detailed cost data and experience must be acquired, and the emphasis should be on selection of patients for CAPD who will benefit the most without excessive complications. Meanwhile, CAPD is an effective but not necessarily cost-effective form of home dialysis for some patients.

### Inpatient Costs

In addition to the cost of providing dialysis treatment, another important contribution to the total cost of the ESRD program is hospitalization. The differences in cost between living-related and cadaver transplantation and between transplantation for diabetics and nondiabetics illustrated earlier relate in large part to duration of hospitalization and complications. Similarly, CAPD patients have frequent hospitalizations; and it would be anticipated that their inpatient costs will be higher, but no data are available from HCFA with regard to this. Conversely, home hemodialysis patients are hospitalized less frequently than patients dialyzing as outpatients. In our own program last year, reviewing more than 600 patients, those treated by outpatient hemodialysis averaged 19 days of hospitalization per year, as compared with 11 days per year for home hemodialysis patients and 20 days per year for CAPD patients.

These differences might relate to patient selection, but data from the National Kidney Dialysis and Kidney Transplantation Study[25] suggest that there are differences in hospitalization rates among various treatment modalities which persist even when findings are adjusted for case mix differences related to sex, race, age, education, diagnosis, associated medical complications, and duration of treatment (Table 1-8). Thus hospitalization rates are lowest in patients treated by home hemodialysis. In a cost-benefit analysis these differences in hospitalization rates should be taken into account.

# PATIENT SURVIVAL

In addition to cost, an important factor in making decisions on cost-effectiveness is the risk to the patient of the various modalities of treatment. For example, Stange and Sumner[30] showed that while transplantation was more cost-effective than hemodialysis, this was associated with a reduction in average life expectancy of between 7 and 20 percent. However, much of this reduction was due to the higher first-year mortality in transplanted patients; and with improvement in patient survival with cadaveric transplantation, this risk may well be much reduced.

Up-to-date information on patient survival in relation to modality of treatment for large patient populations is lacking in the United States. The Cox regression model[8] can be used to quantitate the effects of age, diagnosis, and associated complications on survival of patients with end-stage renal disease;[19] and this technique can also be applied to the various treatment modalities. Our own data show that patient survival when adjusted for age, diagnosis, associated diseases, and years of treatment, clearly is better for patients who receive a related donor transplant; but there is no significant difference in overall survival of patients treated by cadaver transplantation or hemodialysis.[31] Cynics have suggested that cadaver transplantation is the most cost-effective form of treatment because of a higher mortality; and this was a factor in the analysis by Stange and Sumner,[30] but this may have changed with improvements in technique.

Another issue raised in the past has been whether home dialysis has a lower survival rate than outpatient hemodialysis. Most published series have shown better survival with home dialysis, presumably representing patient selection, and the likelihood is that there is no significant difference. This issue was raised in the Senate hearings in 1977 related to legislation to provide incentives for home dialysis,[28] but no scientific support for an increased risk with home dialysis has been forthcoming. Nevertheless, the supposed risk with home hemodialysis was publicized to proprietary dialysis facilities and some of their patients, and may have been at least in part responsible for the patients' concern about the most recent regulations.

Another unresolved issue with regard to patient survival is whether CAPD carries a different prognosis from hemodialysis. Again, no information is available on this, although one unpublished study suggests there is no difference.[7]

# QUALITY OF LIFE AND REHABILITATION

Two years ago Gutman et al.[17] published a paper describing the poor rehabilitation in many patients treated by dialysis. This paper, together with the lack of knowledge about rehabilitation in the program in general, prompted a reexamination of rehabilitation and the quality of life in patients. As a result, HCFA supported

**Table 1-8.** Hospitalization Days by Modality of Treatment

| | Unadjusted Mean Scores | | | | | | Mean Scores Adjusted for Case Mix Difference | | | | |
|---|---|---|---|---|---|---|---|---|---|---|---|
| | | Home Hemo-dialysis | In-Center Hemo-dialysis | CAPD | Trans-plant | Failed Trans-plant | | In-Center Hemo-dialysis | CAPD | Trans-plant | Failed Trans-plant |
| Mean number of nights hospitalized in past 12 months | 12.2 | 8.2 | 13.4 | 20.6 | 11.4 | 12.7 | 8.9 | 12.1 | 17.7 | 13.7 | 13.7 |
| Percentage of patients hospitalized one or more times | 63.7 | 56.4 | 70.6 | 82.9 | 54.9 | 59.8 | 57.3 | 67.4 | 72.3 | 60.8 | 64.5 |

(From Mannien DL, Evans RW, Garrison LP, et al: Update number 18: Health services utilization and disability days: indicators of the quality of patient care among ESRD patients, National Kidney Dialysis and Kidney Transplantation Study, HCFA Grant 95-P-97887/0-01. Battelle Human Affairs Research Centers, Seattle, Washington, 1983.)

**Table 1-9.** Quality of Life Indicators and Dialysis Adjusted for Case Mix

| Quality of Life Index or Measure | Overall Ranking[a] | |
| --- | --- | --- |
| | Best | Worst |
| General well-being index | Home hemodialysis | In-center hemodialysis |
| Index of general affect | Home hemodialysis | In-center hemodialysis |
| Index of well-being | Home hemodialysis | In-center hemodialysis |
| Overall life satisfaction | Home hemodialysis | In-center hemodialysis |
| Positive affect scale | CAPD | In-center hemodialysis |
| Negative affect scale | Home hemodialysis | In-center hemodialysis |
| Affect balance scale | Home hemodialysis | In-center hemodialysis |
| General life satisfaction | Home hemodialysis CAPD | In-center hemodialysis |
| Satisfaction with marriage | CAPD | In-center hemodialysis |
| Satisfaction with sex life | Home hemodialysis | CAPD |
| Satisfaction with family life | CAPD | In-center hemodialysis |
| Satisfaction with savings | CAPD | Home hemodialysis |
| Satisfaction with standard of living | CAPD | In-center hemodialysis |
| Satisfaction with friendships | Home hemodialysis | In-center hemodialysis |
| Satisfaction with health | Home hemodialysis | In-center hemodialysis |
| Feeling about present life (hard, easy) | Home hemodialysis | In-center hemodialysis |
| Feeling about present life (tied down, free) | CAPD | In-center hemodialysis |

[a]Based on adjusted mean scores.

(From Evans, R. W., Manninen, D.L., Garrison, L.P., & Hart, G.L. Update number 15: a comparative assessment of the quality of life of patients undergoing treatment for chronic renal failure: results from the National Kidney Dialysis and Kidney Transplantation Study. National Kidney Disease and Kidney Transplantation Study, HCFA Grant No. 95-P-97887/0-01, Battelle Human Affairs Research Center, Seattle, Washington, 1982.)

a study of outcome with transplantation, home hemodialysis, outpatient hemodialysis, and CAPD in patients randomly selected from 11 major centers. One aim of the study was to quantitate quality of life in patients treated by the different modalities and to adjust for such factors as patient selection and any facility effect. While the results of the study are still being analyzed, it has been found that patients with a successful transplant generally score best in terms of quality of life and related areas, home hemodialysis patients are next, CAPD patients are third, and patients on outpatient hemodialysis have the least satisfactory results.[15] This distinction remains when the analysis is repeated taking into account the different patient mix associated with the several modalities of treatment (Table 1-9). Further validation of those findings is required, but the results of this and similar studies will be of great importance to physicians and policymakers. So far, the results appear to lend support to the impression held by physicians associated with home dialysis programs that encouraging patient independence, knowledge of their disease, and responsibility for their treatment may result in a better patient outcome. Perhaps this relates to compliance with the treatment regimen that a home dialysis patient has to assume, and which they continue to apply at home.

## COST-EFFECTIVENESS

At the time of passage of the original Medicare legislation, emphasis was placed on the utilization of home dialysis and transplantation as the most cost-effective forms of treatment and also as the treatments most likely to result in rehabilitation. The administration and Congress have continued to express support for these forms of treatment, although it took 5 years before legislation was passed to remove disincentives to home dialysis. Now, 1983, the intention is to make the ESRD program "more efficient" and to encourage greater use of home dialysis and transplantation. However, efforts to achieve this by financial means have failed so far, and there is need for a thorough analysis of all aspects of the program if appropriate changes in policy are to be made.

With regard to the cost of various treatments, the data show that transplantation and home hemodialysis are the least costly forms of treatment. Comparative survival data are not available, but it seems likely that, with the possible exception of related donor transplantation, modality of treatment may not have a significant impact on survival, the latter being more related to such factors as age and diagnosis. Information on the relationships among modality of treatment, quality of life, and rehabilitation is only beginning to become available but appears to suggest that transplantation and home dialysis, including CAPD, have advantages over outpatient dialysis.

The association between treatment modality and patient outcome in terms of mortality, morbidity, and rehabilitation is complex; and the need for better information is paramount because of the priority the federal government has placed on transplantation and home dialysis. This was stressed in Public Law 95-292 in 1978 which states that ". . . the maximum practical number of patients who are medically, socially, and psychologically suitable candidates for home dialysis or transplantation should be so treated," and is also inherent in the 1982 Notice of Proposed Rule Making for the proposed composite rate regulations and in testimony to Congress by the Health Care Financing Administration.[9] Thus the federal government believes that home dialysis, CAPD, and transplantation not only are less

costly treatments but may also be associated with benefits to patients in terms of rehabilitation. Whether implementation of the recent proposed regulations will have any effect on the distribution of patients remains uncertain. Certainly, the 1978 legislation had little effect in this regard, as while the proportion of patients on home dialysis has increased since then, this has been due to the increased use of CAPD, and use of home hemodialysis has not changed significantly.

From an economic viewpoint, the concept of efficiency assumes that the cost of providing a service is related to the efficiency with which it is delivered. Consequently, inefficiency will result in higher costs. However, determination of efficiency is complex because the efficiency with which a service is provided may also have an impact on the quality of care that a patient receives. As various services and amenities are eliminated in the name of efficiency, it becomes more and more important to ensure that the quality of care is maintained. If quality of care remains unchanged despite a reduction or elimination of services, then inefficiency existed previously; however, if quality of care is adversely affected, then the service provided, as shown by patient outcome, has changed for the worse. Thus, if patient outcome deteriorates, initiatives undertaken with the intent of increasing efficiency are simply a way of reducing the services provided and saving money, irrespective of the adverse effect. The dilemma faced by policymakers is how to create incentives for efficiency while encouraging home dialysis and transplantation, without harming patients who are not suited for these treatments, in a program with capital investment in more than 1200 facilities.

The dilemma is compounded by the overall problem with the cost of health care and the current emphasis is on moving some of this burden from the federal government to the private sector and the individual. A significant proportion of patients with end-stage renal disease do not have private insurance, and any reduction in Medicare reimbursement will create problems for facilities in terms of supporting such patients. In addition, proprietary dialysis facilities also face the dilemma of decreasing reimbursement and their duty to maintain profits on behalf of their stockholders, while at the same time maintaining quality of care for their patients. It is likely that the future will see more support for end-stage renal disease patients having to come from state governments and charitable organizations, perhaps some reduction in the number of medically marginal patients referred for treatment, and increasing discussion of the issues associated with rationing of expensive treatments. As funding becomes limited, we may also see again patients electing not to be treated because of the financial implications for their family.

Efficiency tends to be induced through competition, but it yet remains to be shown that competition in the dialysis marketplace does in fact improve cost-effectiveness without jeopardizing quality of care. There must be a limit to the efficiency with which providers can deliver services; and once this is attained, the only way to contain costs further will be to consider again the question of patient selection for treatment. Before reaching this point, it would seem essential for HCFA to provide incentives for home dialysis and transplantation and also to review the utilization of dialysis stations throughout the country. Many dialysis facilities are underutilized, and efficiency could be increased by greater utilization of existing stations. This would require more limitation on expansion of dialysis services, as the tendency at this time is to provide more stations rather than increase the number of patients utilizing existing stations by operating more patient shifts.

Not all patients are equally suitable for all treatment modalities. This may raise problems for patients who are not well suited to the less costly treatment modalities which are likely to be most emphasized in the future. No studies have been undertaken to show how patients fare if placed on a treatment for which they are unsuited, although it has been suggested that a patient inappropriately placed on home dialysis may be less adversely affected than a patient inappropriately placed on outpatient dialysis.[13] However, a patient who has problems as a result of an inappropriate treatment is perhaps more likely to require hospitalization, more frequent physician visits, and greater need for support from social and other services, and consequently will incur higher costs.

Scarcity of the resources necessary to make all desirable treatments available to the population as a whole is a basic premise underlying the need to compare the cost and the benefits to the community of alternative actions related to financing of medical care. In the past, decisions generally have been made either on the basis of one treatment clearly being more beneficial than another, irrespective of cost, or because one treatment clearly is cheaper than the other, irrespective of its benefit or otherwise to the patient. The first approach tends to be that of the physician, the latter that of the economist and politician. Because of increasing awareness of the scarcity of resources, government has to examine the impact of the cost of the various high-technology treatments on the availability of dialysis, transplantation, and other expensive health services. Unfortunately, to analyze the cost-effectiveness of treatment alternatives requires reliable data, not only on cost, but also on patient outcome in terms of survival, morbidity, and rehabilitation. Clearly, the medical aspects of such information are equally important as the economic information.

More difficult, perhaps, is the issue

of cost-benefit analysis and discussion of how limited resources should be used for the treatment of one condition versus another. This was first attempted for dialysis and transplantation by Buxton and West,[6] who compared the relative cost of home and hospital outpatient dialysis in terms of the cost to the community for extension of a patient's life by one year. They showed that the implied costs were significantly less for home dialysis than for outpatient dialysis and suggested that policymakers could compare such figures with the expense required to extend life for one year for patients with other diseases requiring expensive therapies. Stange and Sumner[30] performed a somewhat similar analysis and, based on data available at that time, predicted that a shift of 1000 patients from outpatient to home dialysis occurring for each of 10 years would not affect patient life expectancy but would reduce the cost of the program by $241 million. A similar number of patients changing from outpatient dialysis to cadaver transplantation would save between $279 million and $330 million, but associated with a reduction of 7 percent to 17 percent in life expectancy. A similar shift from home dialysis to transplantation would reduce total costs by $103 million to $142 million, and life expectancy by 10 to 20 percent. Such a study of the "trade-offs" between cost saving and life expectancy, extended to consider rehabilitation and using reliable current data, is necessary before further major policy decisions are made affecting the End-Stage Renal Disease Program.

# CONCLUSION

When one compares the cost of the various forms of dialysis in the treatment of end-stage renal disease, it is apparent that home hemodialysis is less expensive than outpatient hemodialysis. Similarly, outpatient dialysis at a freestanding facil-

ity is less expensive than outpatient dialysis in a hospital unit, although at least in some situations this relates to the different population treated in the hospital. The relative cost of CAPD is uncertain, but probably this is closer to the cost of outpatient rather than home hemodialysis. Successful transplantation is less expensive than dialysis, although this difference is less with cadaver transplantation. No good information is available to take into account the cost of complications and hospitalization associated with the various forms of therapy or the relationship of cost to patient mix. There is no indication that there are significant differences in survival with the various modalities of dialysis, and information on rehabilitation and quality of life with different modalities is only beginning to become available. However, this information would suggest that while successful transplantation is the best treatment, home hemodialysis has advantages over CAPD and outpatient hemodialysis.

At this time the ESRD program in the United States is in a state of flux. Composition of the patient population has changed significantly over the last 10 years, patient outcome in terms of survival and rehabilitation is significantly different than was anticipated at the time the legislation was passed, the cost of the program continues to increase, and no new dramatic changes in treatment have occurred. Budgetary pressures will be likely to continue to force the federal government to attempt to encourage specific forms of therapy by financial manipulation, but this is a clumsy and potentially harmful process. Future policymaking should be based on adequate and reliable information, and this must be available before there is any consideration of limiting resources for the treatment of end-stage renal disease in such a way that some patients may be denied treatment. Meanwhile, efforts to maximize the use of home dialysis and transplantation wherever appropriate would appear to be the most cost-effective treatment.

# REFERENCES

1. Belzer FO, Miller DT, Sollinger HW, Glass NR: Renal transplantation—a view of the 1980s. Semin Nephrol 2:99, 1982.
2. Blagg CR: Cui bono? A response to Drs. Hamper and Hager. Dial Transplant 8:501, 1979.
3. Blagg CR: Continuous ambulatory peritoneal dialysis. Am J Kidney Dis 2:378, 1982.
4. Blagg CR, Cole JJ, Irvine G, et al: How much should dialysis cost? Proceedings of the Workshop on Dialysis and Transplantation, American Society for Artificial Internal Organs, Seattle, April 16, 1972, p 54.
5. Blagg CR, Scribner BH: Medicare end-stage renal disease program: More than a billion dollar question. Ann Intern Med 93:501, 1980.
6. Buxton MJ, West RR: Cost-benefit analysis of long-term hemodialysis for chronic renal failure. Br J Med 2:376, 1975.
7. Capelli JP: Personal communication.
8. Cox DR: Regression models and life tables (with discussion). J Roy Statist Soc B 34: 187, 1972.
9. Davis CK: Statement in Hearings before the Subcommittee on Oversight of the Committee on Ways and Means, House of Representatives on proposed regulations governing reimbursement under the Medicare end-stage renal disease program. Serial 97-57. U.S. Government Printing Office, Washington, 1982, p. 171.
10. Department of Health and Human Services, Health Care Financing Administration: Medicare program: End-stage renal disease program; prospective reimbursement for dialysis services. Federal Register, February 12, 1982, 47: 6556, 1982.
11. Eggers P: Trends in incidence, prevalence, survival and reimbursement in Medicare ESRD. Forum Meeting, April 13, 1982a.
12. Eggers PW: Analyses of indicators of case-mix differences between freestanding facility and hospital based Medicare ESRD patients. Working Paper No. OR38, Program Evaluation Group, Division of Beneficiary

Studies, Office of Research, Office of Research and Development, Health Care Financing Administration, Baltimore, Maryland, 1982b.
13. Evans RW: Center or home dialysis? N Engl J Med 301: 1186, 1979.
14. Evans RW, Blagg CR, Bryan FA: Implications for health care policy: a social and demographic profile of hemodialysis patients in the United States. JAMA, 245: 487, 1981.
15. Evans RW, Manninen DL, Garrison LP et al: Update number 15: a comparative assessment of the quality of life of patients undergoing treatment for chronic renal failure: results from the National Kidney Dialysis and Kidney Transplantation Study. National Kidney Disease and Kidney Transplantation Study, HCFA Grant No. 95-P-97887/0-01, Battelle Human Affairs Research Center, Seattle, Washington.
16. Gardner KD, Jr.: Profit and the end-stage renal disease program. N Engl J Med 305: 461, 1981.
17. Gutman RA, Stead WW, Robinson RR: Physical activity and employment status of patients on maintenance dialysis. N Engl J Med 304: 309, 1981.
18. Hampers CL, Hager EB: The delivery of dialysis services on a nationwide basis—can we afford the nonprofit system? Dial Transplant 8: 417, 1979.
19. Hutchinson TA, Thomas DC, MacGibbon B: Predicting survival in adults with end-stage renal disease: an age equivalence index. Ann Intern Med 96: 417, 1982.
20. Iglehart JK: Health policy report: funding the end-stage renal disease program. N Engl J Med 306: 492, 1982.
21. Jacobs C, Broyer M, Brunner FP, et al: Combined report on regular dialysis and transplantation in Europe, XI, 1980. Proc Europ Dial Transp Assoc 18: 2, 1982.
22. Kramer P, Broyer M, Brunner FP, et al: Combined report on regular dialysis and transplantation in Europe, XII, 1981. Proc Europe Dial Transp Assoc, 19: 4, 1983.
23. Lowrie EG, Hampers CL: The success of the Medicare end-stage renal disease program: the case for profit and the private marketplace. N Engl J Med 305: 434, 1981.

24. Lowrie EG, Hampers CL: Proprietary dialysis and the end-stage renal disease program. Dial Transplant, 11: 191, 1982.

25. Manninen DL, Evans RW, Garrison LP, Hart LG: Update number 18: Health services utilization and disability days: indicators of the quality of patient care among ESRD patients. National Kidney Dialysis and Kidney Transplantation Study, HCFA Grant 95-P-97887/0-01. Battelle Human Affairs Research Centers, Seattle, Washington, 1983.

26. Orkand Corporation: Evaluation of the Home Dialysis Aide Demonstration. Contract # HCFA 500-79-0054. The Orkand Corporation, Silver Springs, Maryland, 1982.

27. Rennie D: Renal rehabilitation: where are the data? N Engl J Med 304: 351, 1981.

28. Rettig RA: Implementing the End-Stage Renal Disease Program of Medicare. Rand Publication No. 2505-HCFA/HEW. Santa Monica, California, Rand Corporation, 1980.

29. Smith MD, Hong BA, Michelman JE, Robson AM: Treatment bias in the management of end-stage renal disease. Am J Kidney Dis, 3: 21, 1983.

30. Stange PV, Sumner AT: Predicting treatment costs and life expectancy for end-stage renal disease. N Engl J Med 298: 372, 1978.

31. Vollmer WM, Wahl PW, Blagg CR: Survival with dialysis and transplantation in patients with end-stage renal disease. N Engl J Med, 308: 1553, 1983.

32. Wiegmann TB, Blumenkrantz M, Layard M, et al: Home dialysis and dialysis treatment modalities in the VA System. Am J Kid Disease, 3: 32, 1983.

# 2

# Social and Ethical Problems in the Treatment of End-Stage Renal Disease Patients

Renée C. Fox, Ph.D.
Judith P. Swazey, Ph.D.
Elizabeth M. Cameron, R.N.

This chapter, collaboratively written from a historical, sociologic, and nursing perspective, focuses on an array of social and ethical phenomena that are associated with end-stage renal disease, what it means, and how it is experienced and treated in the 1980s, particularly in American society.

Basic to the phenomena with which we are concerned is the current capacity of medicine to understand, prevent, and treat kidney disorders and kidney failure. However impressive the field of nephrology may be at present, the fact remains that knowledge of the underlying mechanisms of kidney disease, and ability to forestall, ameliorate, or cure chronic, progressive kidney disorders continue to be problematic. The evolution of hemodialy-

sis and renal transplantation has powerfully, even dramatically, contributed to the treatment of end-stage renal disease. But patients receiving these life-sustaining therapies are still permanently afflicted with a terminal illness. Furthermore, although immunology is one of the most dynamic areas in medicine today, and immunosuppressive therapy has made considerable progress, the rejection reaction continues to be the fundamental source of uncertainty and the major deterrent to transplantation. And despite the fact that increasingly effective agents to manage rejection have been developed over the past three decades, each has proven to have serious side effects as well as basic limitations. These aspects of the current stage of basic and clinical knowledge of kidney disease have significant social and ethical implications for patients, their families, medical professionals, and for the larger society as well.

Along with these medical "state of

Preparation of Dr. Fox's and Dr. Swazey's portions of this chapter was supported by a grant from the James Picker Foundation Program on the Human Qualities of Medicine.

the art" factors, there are certain structural and cultural features of the way that end-stage renal disease is viewed and dealt with in American society that have had profound and ramifying social and moral effects. Paramount among these are two societal responses:

1. Since the inception of clinical organ transplantation in the mid-1950s in our society, the process of giving and receiving organs has been defined as a "gift of life," biologically, psychosocially, and morally. With the passage of the Uniform Anatomical Gift Act in 1968, which strengthened and simplified the mechanisms through which cadaver organ donations can be made, the conception of organ transplantation as a gift of life-in-death became a legal one as well.

2. In 1972, after a long period of trial-and-error experimentation with how to justly allocate the scarce, expensive resources of chronic dialysis and renal transplantation, Public Law 92-603 was passed, which provided unprecedented federal coverage for these and other treatment costs of end-stage renal disease.

The major goal of this chapter is to describe and analyze some of the social and ethical concomitants of the ensemble of medical and nonmedical factors that have been called into play by the occurrence of end-stage renal disease in our society and its treatment through dialysis and transplantation. We shall do so by focusing consecutively on the emergence of cyclosporine, a new immunosuppressive drug, and some of the patterns accompanying it; on organ transplantation as gift exchange; on the problems of allocating scarce resources that dialysis has posed; and on how the changes in the silhouette of dialysis and dialysis care over the past 30 years are experienced by the nephrology nurse—the member of the renal team with the closest, most continuous rela-

tionship to what this treatment involves, technically and humanly.

## THE "ADVENT" OF CYCLOSPORINE AND THE THERAPEUTIC INNOVATION CYCLE

Ever since laboratory and clinical studies of the 1940s and 1950s progressively resulted in the definition of the phenomenon of rejection as an immune reaction to a foreign protein, one of the major strategies that medical researchers and clinicians have employed to deal with this reaction is to try to suppress it through a variety of means. In their pursuit of the "elusive goal" of developing "consistently effective and safe immunosuppression," and beyond that, "a truly predictable donor-specific immunosuppressive manipulation,"[7] transplanters have used a succession of agents. From early clinical trials with total body X-irradiation in the late 1950s, they moved on in 1959 to try the antileukemic drug 6-mercaptopurine. Subsequently, in the early 1960s, slightly better results were obtained with a related antimetabolite drug, azathioprine. At about the same time, it was noted that corticosteroids seemed to delay the rejection of both canine and human autografts. By 1962, it was realized that azathioprine and a steroid, prednisone, had an added or possibly synergistic effect. Their combined use, in the form of what became known as "double drug therapy," contributed to the emergence of clinical organ transplantation as a "serious therapeutic endeavor,"[8] and the opening up of what is considered to be its "modern era."[47] This drug combination became "the sheet anchor of clinical immunosuppression."[8] Between 1963 and 1979, a number of other immunosuppressive regimens were developed, virtually all of which were modifications of or additions to the original double drug therapy, without demonstrable improvement in immunosuppression. The one notable exception was the introduction of anti-lymphocyte and antithymocyte globulin preparations. Beginning in 1966, in some centers, antilymphocyte globulin was given as an adjunct to azathioprine and prednisone, to form a "triple drug therapy" that became the second most commonly used type of chemical immunosuppression.

Despite all the effort devoted to immunosuppression, and the progress made in this area, the incidence of transplantation rejection remained unchanged throughout the decade of the 1970s. Patient survival improved, but this was primarily due to the policy that transplanters adopted of sacrificing the grafted kidney when a severe rejection reaction occurred, and returning, the recipient to maintenance treatment on dialysis, rather than subjecting such patients to dangerously increasing doses of immunosuppression. The potential dangers of immunosuppression were associated with the major clinical drawback of all these agents: the fact that they do not suppress immunologic processes selectively, but interfere with synthetic processes and inhibit cell division throughout the body. Because of the nonspecific nature of the immunosuppression they achieve, these drugs cause a number of serious side effects: infections, growth retardation, and suceptibility to tumors, especially malignancy of the lymphoid system. In addition, bone marrow toxicity is a frequent complication of azathioprine; corticosteroids have a wide range of unpleasant side effects, including a cushingoid "moon face," crippling dissolution of bones, and the development of diabetes; and many patients develop hypersensitivity to antilymphocyte globulin.

The 1970s were characterized by "widespread discontent with all . . . available techniques of immunosuppression";[47] a persistent "search for better immunosuppression," with "hundreds of agents . . . investigated in the laboratory";[8] and failure to discover a drug more effective and safe than those already in use—until cyclosporin A, now known as cyclosporine, appeared on the scene.

In reviewing the development of immunosuppressive drugs in the "pre-cyclosporin era,"[47] one is struck by the phase-movements through which this clinical research process has repeatedly passed. A highly structured and recurring therapeutic innovation cycle is discernible within it.[19] This cycle appears to be more than an artifact of the intellectual and technical properties of the medical scientific research and clinical trials involved in the quest for immunosuppression. It also seems to have been shaped by the sentiments, values, and expectations of the research and transplant physicians who most actively participated in the quest, and by the way that their outlook was reported and conveyed to a larger medical and lay public through their scientific papers, professional publications, and the media.

Each time that what was deemed a "new," "interesting," and "highly promising" type of immunosuppressive agent was discovered it was greeted by clinical investigators and prominent transplanters with enthusiastic hope. Here finally, perhaps, was a singular, highly selective, powerful, and safe and predictable immunosuppressant, with minimal side effects and without the drawbacks and limitations of its predecessors, that would lead to dramatically improved results in the clinical transplantation of organs. Cautionary statements were made by investigators conducting the earliest clinical trials of such an agent about the fact that no matter how careful the assessment of a new drug in laboratory animals may be, when it is first used in the clinic on patients, uncertainties, dangers, and limitations may emerge that were not anticipated. But when certain unpredicted and undesirable characteristics of the drug were observed in patients at this stage in its development, the general tendency was to attribute them to inexperience in the clinical management of the drug (its mode of administration, dosages, combination or lack of combination with other drugs), rather than to the agent's inherent properties, or to the generic responses of the human organism. By and large these difficulties were dealt with and partially explained away through relevant changes that were made in the clinical protocol under which the drug was given. It was characteristically at this point in the new drug's evolution that excitement about its actual and potential capacities peaked. By this time, a larger number of physicians were participating in the clinical trials. With a certain baseline of investigative experience established, the drug in question was released for less experimental, more general clinical use. Professional publications on the agent as a new therapy for treating rejection, which already abounded, expanded greatly. Unanswered questions about the drug, its limitations, and its hazardous side effects were scrupulously discussed in the papers and articles that appeared, but often in a more sparse and muted fashion than the presentation of what were conceived to be its positive attributes. Claims were made that the drug was applicable to far more than the rejection reaction in the grafting of kidneys. Its use in the transplantation of other organs, particularly the heart and the liver, was affirmatively described, and many statements were made about the basic and clinical "spin-off" significance the agent might prove to have. Postoperative recovery and rehabilitation were reported to be accelerated and improved because of the drug, the frequency and severity of rejection episodes diminished, both organ and patient survival prolonged, and the quality of life of transplant recipients enhanced. The "good news" about the immunosuppressive drug was further broadcast by the media, which picked up and amplified the underlying optimism of most medical reports and the ardor of certain investigators and transplanters. It was not until the end of the 1960s that this upbeat mood and buoyant outlook gave way to what could be described as the more sober, somewhat disappointed, and growingly frustrated perspective on the established repertoire of immunosuppressive agents that characterized transplanters in the 1970s. And yet, in spite of widespread discontent with what was now regarded as the static "therapeutic *cul de sac*" state of immunosuppression, as one transplant surgeon put it, "it was necessary to hope for better immunosuppressive drugs. [But] this did not seem a realistic possibility until the advent of the drug cyclosporin A."[47]

The "advent" of cyclosporine, to which both the collective dissatisfaction and hope of physicians involved in the field of transplantation contributed, represents a renewal of the cycle of therapeutic innovation through which its predecessors passed. At this writing (January 1983), it has entered what is probably its zenith phase. Although it is still only available on an investigational basis from Sandoz, the pharmaceutical firm where it was discovered and developed, hundreds of medical articles have already been published about the properties and actions of this new immunosuppressive agent. "Clinical reports so far have ranged from lukewarm to lyrical."[42] But at this juncture, the "lyrical" accounts predominate. A sizable proportion of them suggest that cyclosporine is "the most exciting development in the field of immune suppression since the original antimetabolites were discovered in 1962," and that it may "herald a new era in organ grafting."[45]

The history of cyclosporine began in

1970, in the context of a screening program of fungal agents that was being conducted in the microbiology department of Sandoz in Basle.[5,6] Two new strains of *fungi imperfecti* producing antifungal metabolites were discovered. They were isolated and characterized as novel neutral polypeptides. In early 1972, one of these metabolites, cyclosporin A, which had been extracted from the fermentation broths of the fungi *Cylindrocarpon lucidum* and *Trichoderma polysporum* was discovered by J. F. Borel (in the Sandoz pharmacology department) to be immunosuppressive in rodents. After it was purified in 1973, Borel carried out further animal studies of the immunosuppressive activity of cyclosporine in mice, rats, and guinea pigs. In 1975, its structure was elucidated through x-ray studies. Biochemically, it was found to be a cyclic peptide of 11 amino acids (one of which had not previously been described) which were soluble in oil and alcohol, but insoluble in water. Toxicity studies conducted on rats and monkeys in 1976 showed that cyclosporine acted as an antilymphocytic agent: one that powerfully suppressed humoral as well as cell-mediated immunity in all animal species tested, with a selective and rapidly reversible action against T lymphocytes, and without the bone marrow depression associated with azathioprine. The first articles were published about cyclosporine in 1976, and in 1977, oral absorption was demonstrated in man. 1977 was also the year in which R. Y. Calne and his group in Cambridge published a series of articles on the unusual effectiveness of cyclosporine in prolonging the survival of heart, kidney, liver, and pancreas grafts in rats, rabbits, dogs, and pigs. Calne concluded from these studies that cyclosporine was "sufficiently nontoxic and powerful as an immunosuppressant to make it an attractive candidate for clinical investigation in patients receiving organ grafts."[10] In mid-1978, Calne and his co-workers carried out pilot clinical trials in seven patients who received kidney transplants from mismatched cadaver donors, and initially received cyclosporine as the sole immunosuppressive agent. During the same period, R. L. Powles and his colleagues conducted the first trials of cyclosporine to treat graft-versus-host disease in five patients with leukemia, at the Royal Marsden Hospital in Sutton, Surrey. Both Calne's and Powles' results were published at the end of 1978.[12,32] Their reports further intensified and expanded medical interest in cyclosporine. In the United States, "eager transplant teams" described themselves as "chafing to give it a try."[15] And when cyclosporine did become available for clinical trials in this country in late 1979, new teams undertook its use and evaluation with high expectations.

From the outset of its laboratory and clinical trials, cyclosporine has been described in the medical literature as an immunosuppressive agent that is "novel," "unique," "interesting," and "fascinating"; a drug that is "chemically different from any other previously investigated immunosuppressive agent"; an "extremely powerful" and "most effective" drug, that is both "superior" and "important." It has been portrayed as a "real advance"; "the most promising new pharmacological immune suppressant to emerge in recent years"; a drug that represents "the first step in a new generation of agents for clinically effective immunosuppressive therapy," and that has "opened a new chapter" in transplantation. Cyclosporine has been credited with "revitalizing" the field of transplantation, and with making a "more important impact on it than any other development in nearly two decades"—an impact that may eventually "change the face of transplantation" and alter its very "tenets."

This early exuberance about cyclosporine notwithstanding, the first year of its clinical trial was marked by what was described in the medical literature as certain "worrisome" and even "dangerous" episodes. These "troubling" and "disturbing" events, which were apparently not anticipated by the physician-investigators involved, were nonetheless classic for this stage of clinical research and therapeutic innovation. Calne himself explained that, "Despite careful assessment in animals, when a drug is first used clinically the patient embarks on an uncertain and possibly hazardous journey."[11] Nevertheless, he was not totally prepared for the side effects of cyclosporine, which proved to be "more serious than would have been expected from much experimental work in various species."[11] The most serious of these effects were nephrotoxicity and the development of lymphomas. The potential capacity of cyclosporine to cause *de novo* malignant tumors, especially lymphomas, received the most publicity. Other side effects that were encountered included infection, hepatoxicity, gum hyperplasia, tremor, regional flushing or vague abdominal discomfort right after taking the drug, and the development of breast fibroadenomas in women. The principal physicians who conducted the pilot clinical studies attributed these side effects to four facts: they were still searching for the optimal dose of cyclosporine; they had used it in combination with other immunosuppressive agents, particularly steroids and cytotoxic drugs; the "sobering" but "not surprising" consequences of immunosuppression; and some of the concomitants of the "lethal diseases" from which their patient-subjects suffered.

By the time a year had elapsed, physician-investigators had learned more about how to adjust and "cleverly manage" the dose of cyclosporine. The issue about whether it should be used as a single agent or in combination (which had had its counterparts in the "double dose" and "triple dose" therapy debates that

had occurred with regard to earlier immunosuppressive drug regimens) was further clarified, but not resolved. (Nor is it to this day.) But a certain degree of rapprochement was gradually effected between those physicians, like Calne, who had hoped that no immunosuppressive drug other than cyclosporine would be routinely needed, and was intent on being as "steroid sparing" as possible, and physicians such as Starzl, whose conceptual and methodological approach was that cyclosporine should be combined with steroid therapy from the outset.

The concern about the side effects of cyclosporine diminished as progress was made in using the drug. It was also conterbalanced by *ex post facto*, philosophical acceptance of "the developing risk of lymphoma [as] an inevitable consequence"[9] and "price"[48] of all immunosuppression, and by emphasis on the drug's powerful effectiveness and its superiority to "standard immunosuppressive treatment." The chief positive properties of cyclosporine that were underscored were its greater specificity than previous immunosuppressants; its "uniqueness" in exerting its effects without the profound suppression of the bone marrow that had been characteristic of the earlier drugs; the role it seemed to play in decreasing the frequency and clinical severity of rejection episodes; the ready reversibility of many of the rejection reactions that did occur; cyclosporine's reduction of infectious complications; the ease and pleasantness with which it could be administered to patients orally; and the shortening of hospitalization that it apparently effected. As experience with cyclosporine accumulated and spread, "the spectre of this drug being a spectacular tumor producer . . . receded."[48] Not only did the clinical trials with cyclosporine "escape" and overcome the "disillusionment of other promising developments in immunosuppression,"[48] but they reached a stage where the physicians using it experimentally affirmed that in every transplanted organ for which it had been tested—kidneys, hearts, livers, lungs, pancreases, bone marrow—it appeared to be better than all other existing immunosuppressive agents. Human heart-lung transplants were launched, and the transplantation team that carried them out attributed what they called their "early success" to the use of cyclosporine, as well as to the anatomical and physiologic advantages of combined heart-lung replacement.[35] Articles on the greatly improved survival of transplant recipients and of the organs they received appeared in the literature. Although the "pattern of predominantly early mortality" with liver transplants continued, Starzl's group reported that in comparison to their previous experience in what they described as "the pre-cyclosporin era," the survival of both adult and child recipients "has more than doubled."[47] Many transplant teams announced that they were able to attain an 80 percent or better one-year survival rate of cadaveric kidney transplants, as compared with the 50 to 55 percent rate of continued functioning that had formerly been the norm, and that the figures were as high as 90 percent for live kidney transplants. It became progressively apparent that the introduction of cyclosporine and the growingly positive attitudes toward it were major factors contributing to the discernibly revived interest in transplant surgery and the increased number of organ transplants of different types that were being performed. "In the first 6 months of [1982], for instance, 56 heart transplants were done in the United States, compared with an average yearly total of 22 throughout the 1970s."[2] Furthermore, experimental trials began to be made with cyclosporine in nontransplantation fields; for example, in connection with the visually impairing autoimmune eye condition, posterior uveitis.[31] By mid-1981, a medical journal of the stature of *The New En-*

*gland Journal of Medicine* had published an editorial-essay celebrating the "Cosmas and Damian"-like hope that cyclosporine offered:[24]

> To achieve this miraculous skill remains the elusive goal of workers in transplantation. Today, consistently successful cadaveric transplantation appears to be more within our grasp than at any time since chemotherapeutic immunosuppression with 6-mercaptopurine was introduced by Schwartz and Dameshek and clinical trials of its analog, azathioprine, were performed by Murray et al. nearly 20 years ago. The advent of cyclosporin A offers hope that the legendary success of the two third-century patron saints of the healing profession will become a fait accompli of modern medical practice.

By the end of 1982, under the byline of Lawrence K. Altman, *The New York Times* devoted two whole pages to stories on the fact that "Transplants Are Surging As Survival Rates Improve," and the role of cyclosporine in this "dramatic surge";[2] and as 1983 began, James H. Sammons, Executive Vice-President of the American Medical Association, cited cyclosporine as one of the major medical advancements that had occurred in 1982.[3] Even before it had ended its clinical trial period and been approved by the Food and Drug Administration for more general use, cyclosporine had reached what might be called its "wonder drug" phase in the therapeutic innovation cycle.

Social attitudes and values as well as biomedical factors have shaped the history of cyclosporine and the immunosuppressants that preceded it, structuring the stages through which these drugs have passed. There is no inherent biological reason, for example, why discovery of the beneficial properties of a new agent should take place before the identification of its limitations and negative characteristics, or why clinical investigators should be "surprised" and "disappointed" when they encounter untoward side effects. Research physicians knew well in advance of their experience with cyclosporine that "the developing risk of lymphoma"[9] is a biomedical consequence of all immunosuppression; and yet, when these side effects occurred during early clinical trials of cyclosporine, investigators reacted as if they had not expected such developments to take place with *this* drug. Belief that all-therapeutic, side-effect-free modes of treatment can be found, and questing after them, seems to be a common characteristic of clinical investigators, who participate in the therapeutic innovation process with a "hope springs eternal" outlook. An attitude of "institutionalized optimism" pervades their involvement, particularly at the outset of clinical trials, again during the period after side effects are discovered and overridden, and subsequently, when the nonexperimental use of the new therapy begins. Cultural factors seem to play a role in enhancing or tempering the optimism. In this connection, it is interesting to note that to a greater degree in British than in American medical journals, the optimism surrounding cyclosporine has been accompanied by appeals to caution. Furthermore, in contrast to the overall enthusiasm of American press accounts of cyclosporine, the British press and other media reacted so negatively to the initial medical reports of the occurrence of lymphomas in patients treated with cyclosporine, that Calne felt obliged to respond in a letter to the editor of *The British Medical Journal,* "so that an unbalanced reaction on the part of the media [would] not lead to pressure to discontinue this drug."[9]

As the foregoing suggests, the expectant, hopeful, accentuate-the-positive attitudes of research physicians are integral to the belief in medical progress that underlies their motivation to look for better ways of preventing, treating, and managing disease (and also the iatrogenic conse-

quences of their medical actions), and to their ability to persist in the face of the many uncertainties, problems, and setbacks that clinical investigation entails. The fact that their research subjects are also their patients—persons who are suffering from often lethal diseases for which these physicians ardently wish to provide efficacious treatment—contributes both to the biomedical difficulties that they encounter in evaluating a new therapy like cyclosporine, and to their attitudinal tendency to "herald" its "advent."

These important functions notwithstanding, the "ritualization of optimism" involved here, and the utopian belief in the existence of an ultimate "magic bullet" therapy, create a distinctive kind of moral dilemma. The stage in the therapeutic innovation cycle that cyclosporine has entered exemplifies this dilemma. The collective optimism of clinical investigators has helped to bring it to its current "wonder drug" status. But one does not need to be prophetic to predict that, like the immunosuppressants that came before it, after it has been in clinical use for some time, it will arrive at another phase in the cycle, where its side effects and limitations—its "non-wondrous" properties—will be felt more keenly and be more greatly emphasized. In turn, this dissatisfaction and restiveness may provide momentum for a continuing search for another new immunosuppressive drug, and for a different approach to the prevention and treatment of the rejection reaction in organ transplantation.

In effect, the built-in tendency to focus on the positive features of a new and promising agent during the pilot trials and early clinical stages of its experiment-to-therapy trajectory constitutes what will later come to be seen as an exaggerated set of therapeutic expectations and claims. It could be argued that the most ethical way for physicians to behave under the circumstances would be to recognize this pattern, and respond to it by trying harder to balance off their early optimism with active skepticism, and to moderate the affirmations that they make about a new therapy to their colleagues, patients, and the public at large. Yet, as with all things in medicine, the ethics of therapeutic innovation in general, and of immuno-suppression and cyclosporine in particular, are not that simple. For, the same optimism that may lead to inflated attitudes toward a new therapy also enables physicians to search and find and search some more, in an inherently ironic situation where their medical, scientific, and technological interventions create problems as well as solve them.

## ORGAN TRANSPLANTATION AS GIFT EXCHANGE

Since the beginning of clinical organ transplantation in the mid-1950s, physicians, nurses, donors, recipients, and their families have defined transplantation as a "gift of life." At first this was done metaphorically, with little awareness or analysis of what the implications of calling this surgical act a gift might be for the participants in it. Only gradually, through clinical experience, and with some interpretive input from psychiatrists and social scientists, did the psychological, social, and cultural meaning and implications of the gift-exchange aspects of transplantation become more apparent and better understood.[19]

Before examining what is involved in this process of giving and receiving human organs, the constituent elements of a gift need to be considered. Regardless of the nature of content of the gift, the occasion on which it is offered, the reasons for which it is proffered, or the particular social and cultural setting in which it occurs,

the exchange of gifts always has certain social characteristics:[28]

1. The giving of a gift is in part a symbolic act, and often a ceremonial one. Ideally, it is an offering of self that is supposed to express the sentiments that the giver feels about the person or persons to whom he or she is making the gift, and about the relationship that exists between them.

2. However expressive and sincere an act it may be, the giving of a gift is rarely completely spontaneous. One is socially expected to offer a gift to certain people on certain occasions, such as holidays, and rites of passage events like birthdays, graduations, and weddings. What sort of gift is appropriate for particular occasions, who should give what to whom, and what kinds of sentiments the gift is supposed to convey, are all highly influenced, structured, and regulated by norms and custom.

3. Another characteristic of gift exchange in all societies and social settings is that if a person or group is offered a gift, they are placed under a great deal of social pressure to accept it. Because a gift represents the *persona* and sentiments of the giver, and a statement about his (her) relationship to the recipient, the refusal to accept a gift can be delicate or even serious. For it is likely to signify and be interpreted as a rejection of the donor by the recipient, or at least a refusal to receive the sentiments and to agree to the definition of the relationship that the giver of the gift wishes to express.

4. Once a person receives and accepts a gift, he or she incurs a "debt" to the giver, which there is a social obligation to "repay" by offering an equal or equivalent gift in exchange. The return-gift may not have to be given immediately, but on some other appropriate occasion there will be an obligation for it to be repaid. Although the gift need not be

identical, usually there is an attempt to make it equal in meaning and worth to what has been previously received.

## Live Donor Gifts: Renal Transplantation

These norms of giving, receiving, and repaying are called into play by the fact that organ transplants are defined as gifts of life that are exchanged between a donor and recipient, and their families, and mediated by members of the medical profession.

In American medical contexts, the ideal live kidney donation is conceived to be one that is offered as voluntarily as possible, by a person who is neither overtly nor covertly subject to undue psychological, social, economic, or moral pressure to give in this way, and who is biologically related to the recipient with whom he or she is also well-matched genetically. Although in our family system one's spouse is defined as the closest relative in adult life, the medical profession generally considers husbands and wives ineligible to become live donors for one another because (due to the way that the incest taboo governs the choice of marriage partners), they are not biologically related. Intimate, kinlike friends, who may want to be screened as prospective live donors, are even less likely to be considered potential candidates by the transplant team.

The question of why live kidney donations have been confined to biological relatives is a complex one. When they are interviewed on this matter, transplant teams attribute their policy to the unlikelihood of very close genetic compatibility existing between a live, nonrelated donor and a recipient. They take this as a given fact, without investigating the possibility that by chance a good tissue match may exist in particular cases. Transplanters insist that the results from a nonbiologi-

cally-related live donor would probably be no better than those from a cadaver donor, and they imply that under these circumstances, the potential risk to the live donor that a transplant involves may not be sensible or justifiable to incur. Behind these biomedical explanations, there also appear to be sociological reasons that transplanters find it difficult to articulate. To begin with, it is not logically clear why a well-matched cadaveric donation is acceptable to transplanters, while a comparably good, nonrelated live donation is not. Below the surface of this position lies an unverbalized assumption that the gift of a live organ is not only extraordinary, and potentially hazardous for the donor, but that the medical-surgical act of taking it is a burdensome responsibility for the physicians involved. Another contributing factor is what physicians have self-critically referred to as their tendency to put "altruism in disrepute."[16] By this they mean that they have difficulty in accepting the idea that a person would genuinely and freely—out of motivation that is not psychopathological—want to give a gift of such magnitude to someone who is not a biological relative. In turn, this attitude is strongly connected to a biologically determined, reductionistic view of relatedness. Hidden underneath transplanters' insistence that an individual must be biologically related to a recipient to be an acceptable donor-candidate is their belief that no other human relationships are as meaningful and enduring. The most telling indicator of this implicit conviction that we have observed was a transplant team's definition of a prospective kidney recipient's adopted daughter as a *nonrelated* and therefore ineligible donor. In effect, whether or not they were aware of it, they were refusing to recognize donor and recipient as mother and daughter.

The idea of an unpressured, voluntary offer to donate a kidney is tempered by the reality of the fact that the situation in which such a gift is called for is one in which a parent, sibling, or child is dying of kidney disease. No matter what efforts the medical team may make to protect the members of a prospective recipient's family from feeling too coerced or self-coerced, the pressure to offer this gift of life is all but overpowering. For example, in the American kinship system, primary family obligations after marriage are to spouse and children (the family of procreation) and secondarily to parents and siblings (the family of origin). But irrespective of their kinship patterns, when contronted with a parent or sibling who is dying of end-stage kidney disease, not many persons can assert firmly and serenely that they have no doubts about their obligation to think ot their family-by-marriage first, or can insist unqualifiedly that they do not want to jeopardize their responsibility to it in any way by giving a kidney to their mother, father, sister, or brother.

The process of selecting a family donor involves two primary groups of decision-makers: the transplant team, usually "captained" by the surgeon, and the family members of the prospective recipient. Studies of live donor transplants have shown that once the possibility of a transplant is raised, a family member's decision about whether he or she personally wants to be a donor usually is almost instantaneous and relatively independent of the receipt of available medical information and other components of an informed consent transaction.[46]

If a family member does volunteer for histocompatibility testing, the ensuing donor eligibility screening process has psychological and social as well as biomedical components. Questions about the donor's motives, the voluntariness of his or her offer, and how well the organ exchange will be dealt with within the family if the recipient keeps the kidney, rejects it, or dies, often are difficult questions for the members of a transplant team to answer. They have learned, through experience, that these aspects of a live donor transplant need to be addressed, and that some donations may not be suitable for psychosocial reasons despite immunogenetic compatibility. They have also learned that telling a prospective donor that he or she has been judged psychosocially ineligible can have serious consequences for that person and for the family unit. It is for these reasons that transplant teams have adopted the normative policy of telling donors who are excluded on psychological or social grounds that they are not "compatible" with the recipient. Here, medical professionals have bent the language of immunology to apply to nonbiological factors, in an effort to protect the potential donor, recipient, and their family from anticipated psychological and social harm. Some moral philosophers have criticized this transplant practice, on the grounds that however clinically insightful and beneficiently intended it may be, it is nevertheless a form of lying.[4]

An example of a recurrent family dynamic that, if recognized during donor screening, may lead to a judgment of ineligibility, is what we have termed the "black sheep syndrome." It is perhaps the most literally sacrificial act in human organ transplantation. Here a family member who is considered to be particularly deviant offers himself or herself as a donor, or is in effect offered up by his (her) relatives. Collective punishment, expiation, and redemption enter into this at once vindictive, guilt-ridden, altruistic, and quasi-religious behavior. It underscores the complexity and fundamentally symbolic nature of what is being given and taken in organ exchange.

A second gift-exchange issue is whether or not the prospective recipient will be willing to accept the gift offered to him or her by a close relative. For, it should not be supposed that the recipient is necessarily eager to receive an organ from the particular person designated to be the donor. There are at least three major sets of reasons why someone may refuse such a potentially life-saving gift. First, the recipient may wish to spare or protect the donor from what is thought to be the degree of discomfort, risk, or sacrifice that a transplant entails. Second, the recipient may feel that such a gift is so extraordinary that he or she will never be able to repay it, and does not wish to be indebted to the donor in this way for the rest of his or her life. Third, the recipient may not want to accept such a gift because the characteristics and qualities of the donor candidate may not be ones the recipient likes or wishes to become a part of his or her body, person, or life. These are not superstitious ideas held only by persons of little education, who have traditional beliefs, cling to old customs, are peculiarly predisposed to magical thinking, and do not understand organ transplantation in a medical scientific way. What transplantation has revealed in this regard is that most people have quite deep, hidden, nonrational, even animistic feelings about various of their vital organs, and their body as a whole.

Another set of social phenomena associated with the gift-exchange aspects of live donor transplants flows from the often held belief of recipients that the donated organ is such an extraordinary gift, both literally and symbolically, that it is inherently unreciprocal. There is a fundamental sense in which the recipient can never repay the donor for offering a gift of life that is a vital part of his or her bodily self. As a consequence, donor and recipient may find themselves psychologically and sociologically locked in a creditor-debtor vise that binds them to one another in a mutually fettering way.

Because a part of him(her)self is inside the recipient, the donor may feel impelled to watch over the transplanted kidney and the life of the individual who now carries it. The recipient, in turn, may feel that his (her) debt to the donor is so enormous and unrepayable that the donor has the right to ask anything of him (her) and to participate illimitably in his (her) life. We have called these aspects of the gift-exchange dimensions of transplantation—which can occur as well with a cadaver donor's family and recipient—"the tyranny of the gift."

Two final examples of the intricate phenomena evoked by the giving and receiving of a live donor kidney relate to the death of the recipient or the rejection of the transplant. If the recipient dies without rejecting the kidney, the donor may not only mourn the recipient's death, but be both sad and angry that this gift has been "wasted" or given in vain. It has proven to be no more than a gift of ephemeral life. But, at the same time, the knowledge that something other than a rejection reaction was responsible for the recipient's death may provide the donor with a comforting sense of reassurance that his (her) gift was neither flawed nor a failure.

When the recipient lives but the transplanted kidney is rejected it has far more than a biomedical meaning for the recipient, donor, and their families. Socially and psychologically the rejection reaction can have a triple meaning. It involves, at least symbolically, the rejection of the donor as a person by the recipient—of his or her qualities, sacrifice, and intention to give a gift of life. The recipient, in turn, may believe that the rejection occurred because he or she did not have the "right attitude" about the donor and the kidney that was given. Finally, the donor may feel guilty and depressed because his (her) gift was "not good enough." It was quite literally rejected by the body of the person to whom it was given.

Live organ transplants are not always characterized by gift-exchange problems, however. There are innumerable cases where the acts of giving and receiving a kidney have not only had positive biomedical consequences, but human ones as well. These are the cases in which donor and recipient feel inspired and enriched by participating in a reciprocal act of generosity and sacrifice. Under these circumstances, the sense of esteem, worth, and meaning of both donor and recipient are enhanced. They may feel ennobled by the gift of life that has been offered, received, and accepted. And rather than binding donor and recipient to one another in a mutually tyrannical way, the gift of the transplanted organ may unify and free them in a transcending and transfiguring way.

## Cadaveric Donor Gifts

While we have focused upon gift-exchange aspects of live donor transplants, may of the same complex psychosocial phenomena are associated with cadaveric transplants—whether of kidneys, hearts, lungs, livers, or other organs. For these organs too are defined and experienced as gifts of life. The Uniform Anatomical Gift Act, the name of the law that has made it legally possible to will all or parts of one's body for organ transplants upon one's death, exemplifies this.[43]

Most cadaver organs are obtained from young, healthy persons, often fatally injured in a vehicular accident, or who have taken their own lives. These deaths are not only sudden and unexpected; they are also especially tragic and fraught with problems of meaning. The grief-stricken families may be powerfully pushed in the direction of offering organ donations by their intense need to make redeeming sense out of what they may otherwise experience as an existentially absurd event. The possibility of contributing the organs of their newly deceased relative may be seized upon by the family as a powerful, immediate way that they can endow the death that has occurred with some meaning.

Because of the deep significance that cadaver donation has for families, transplantation teams have repeatedly found that they may have a number of social and psychological problems to deal with posttransplant. The donor's family, for example, may be intensely interested in the recipient's personal history and his posttransplant course. If the identities of the donor family and recipient are known to each other, the donor's family may make personal contact with the recipient and become closely involved with his or her life. If a recipient dies or rejects the organ, donor families are prone to feel that the gift of life was futile, and the death of their family member meaningless. Grieving may occur again, both for the death of their donor-relative and for the death of the recipient.

Recipients, too, may be very interested in knowing about the cadaver donor and his or her family—for example, about the donor's sex, age, race, height and weight, marital status, education, occupation, religion, personal qualities, and life history. Even with kidneys, and particularly with hearts, which have special cultural symbolism, recipients have expressed the belief that some of the human and social as well as the biological qualities of the donor are transplanted into them with the organ. Recipients may also be very concerned about how they can repay this gift of life to the donor's family, with the result that they, too, become involved with the cadaver donor's family.

Because these gift-exchange relationships among the recipient, the cadaver donor, and the donor's family can be so complicated and emotional, transplant teams have gradually adopted a policy of anonymity about cadaver transplants. With some exceptions, the prevailing norm in transplant units is not to tell the recipient about the identity of the donor, and not to tell the donor's family who the recipient is. Another less consciously intended role that this patterned anonymity plays is that it insulates the members of the transplant team from the discomfort they may feel in having to deal with manifest expressions of the magical and religious symbolic significance of giving and receiving organs for donors, recipients, and their families.

### The Societal Significance of Transplantation

In our view, as long as transplantation is defined as a gift, it will be subject to the triple norms of giving, receiving, and repaying with their attendant psychological, social, and cultural functions and strains. These aspects of transplantation, in particular, raise complex questions about the relationship in a society between individual and group needs, desires, goals, rights, responsibilities, and duties. What obligations do we have to ourselves as individuals, to the various members of our family, to our close friends, colleagues, and acquaintances? And beyond these relationships, what are our obligations to the countless persons in our daily social life, and in our society, whom we do not know? Should we be able to give of ourselves to mere acquaintances or strangers in life and death, as we do to our families and intimate friends? Who is my brother, sister, mother, father, child? Who is my friend, and who my stranger? How are we related to one another? Where does our in-

dividuality end, and our interconnection and solidarity begin? These are difficult questions with which every society struggles, and for which each society seeks solutions in its own distinctive way. In the end, this is where we believe the largest, most important social meaning of organ transplantation as gift exchange lies.

## DIALYSIS AND THE ALLOCATION OF SCARCE RESOURCES

How a society, or its constituent parts, can most justly or fairly distribute its limited resources is an ancient question that has long been grappled with in philosophical and political arenas.[25] In medical care, the starkest form of widespread decisions that must be made about the allocation of scarce resources is framed by the question, "Who shall live when not all can live?" This question, as Childress observed over a decade ago, "is hardly new," but it "has been urgently forced upon us by the dramatic use of artificial internal organs and organ transplantation."[14]

The intertwined social, ethical, and political issues concerning the allocation of scarce, potentially life-saving medical resources that are paradigmatically embedded in the history of chronic dialysis have fallen into two phases.[19] In phase one, from the inception of chronic dialysis in 1960 to the passage of Public Law 92-603 in 1972, the central issues turned around the classic "lifeboat ethic" dilemma of deciding who lives and who dies when not all lives can be saved. Since the mid-1970s, with funding for the treatment of end-stage renal disease provided by Medicare and the concomitant expansion of dialysis capabilities, attention has gradually focused on two other clusters of allocation questions: the expenditure of large sums of public monies for a costly mode of long-term, palliative treatment like dialysis in relation to other health care needs; and even more difficult questions about who should decide whether and how to withhold or terminate such forms of treatment.

## Allocating Dialysis before Public Law 92-603

The development of the Scribner shunt in 1960, making possible chronic dialysis as an alternative or adjunct to the then nascent procedure of renal transplantation, rapidly created a classic problem of what philosophers term distributive justice.[49] Given a large population of patients with end-stage renal disease relative to a limited dialysis capability—including funds, machines, hospital beds, and medical personnel—and the great expense of chronic treatment, who should receive dialysis, who should make such decisions, and what criteria should be used?

Throughout the 1960s, individual physicians, patient selection committees, and hospitals thus were forced to deal with the medical–moral dilemma of selecting a limited number of medically eligible candidates to receive dialysis, knowing that those patients not chosen would soon die unless a transplant was possible. The type of decision that recurrently had to be made—what many involved ruefully called "playing God"—was as follows: This month our hospital's dialysis unit has space for one new dialysis patient, but there are four medically eligible candidates. How do we select the recipient? Those responsible for allocating dialysis used a variety of selection methods, which were based on one or more of six principles of social justice that can be used to provide a moral basis for distributing scarce resources.

1. A *meritarian* concept of social justice allocates limited goods or resources to individuals on the basis of their merits or deserts. Merits or deserts, in turn, can be defined by the distributors—for example, a dialysis selection committee—in many ways, such as a person's conduct, achievement, or contributions to society.

2. A *needs* principle seeks to justly allocate a limited resource such as dialysis according to the essential needs of individuals, leaving for further definition the question of what constitutes "essential needs."

3. An *ability* principle distributes a scarce resource on the basis of various criteria concerning an individual's ability. For example, in a fee-for-service system ability to pay can be the determinant of who receives care, and a selection committee thus could narrow a pool of dialysis candidates by eliminating those who cannot afford to pay for treatment.

4. A principle of *compensatory justice* would distribute resources to those who have previously suffered social wrongs that deprived them of those resources, such as a lack of access to medical care because of a low socioeconomic status. (This is the principle of social justice underlying Medicaid insurance.)

5. A *utilitarian "ethometrics"* principle seeks to provide the greatest benefit or good for the greatest number of persons. This is the principle behind quantitative cost–benefit analyses for the provision of various forms of health care, which often founder in efforts to define what variables should constitute the "greatest good"—for example, economic, personal, social—and to quantitatively calculate noneconomic "goods" such as health status.

6. An *egalitarian* principle of social justice, in American society, is often viewed as the most morally acceptable way to distribute scarce resources. There are, however, many ways to formulate egalitarian principles, and it is seldom easy to specify just what is meant by

them and consequently how one should act on them. In the arena of medical care, for example, many hold that we should "provide similar treatment for similar cases," which then leads to a panorama of questions about how one defines "similar treatment" and "similar cases." During the 1960s, a number of dialysis facilities selected patients by random lottery, believing that this form of egalitarian distribution was the fairest, most neutral way of determining who might live when not all could live.

As this brief discussion of the principles of social justice underlying the allocation of dialysis during the 1960s suggests, the need to make such decisions involves a host of complex, painful medical, moral, and social issues. None involved in selecting dialysis recipients welcomed their task, or were comfortable with the selection methods they adopted. All felt there was no really good way to make such decisions; rather, they sought to find what they felt was the "least worst" selection method.

## Public Law 92-603 and Its Implications

The magnitude of the problems posed both by chronic renal disease and the limited availability of treatment capabilities were recognized by the federal government in the mid-1960s with the formation of a Committee on Chronic Kidney Disease. Their report, issued in 1967, drew public attention to the fact that "until capability meets demand agonizing decisions concerning patient selection are inevitable at both the local and national level." "Approximately 5,000 patients with chronic uremia died in fiscal year 1967 because of lack of adequate treatment facilities," the Committee reported, "and by 1973 . . . a minimum of 24,000 additional medically suitable pa-

tients will have died without the opportunity for treatment by chronic dialysis or transplantation."[21]

To meet the "psychological, ethical, and political problems" created by the scarcity of treatment capabilities, particularly dialysis, the Committee recommended the establishment of a federally funded treatment program for end-stage renal disease. But its estimated cost—$800 million to $1 billion for the first 6 years—was viewed by Congress as prohibitively expensive.

Between 1967 and 1972 the number of patients receiving dialysis and transplantation increased and the costs of the procedures decreased, particularly with the advent of home dialysis programs in the late 1960s. Treatment capabilities, however, still fell far short of demand, and pressures mounted for a federal response to the economics of scarcity. As analyzed most fully by Rettig, the passage of PL 92-603, the 1972 Social Security Amendment Act, was a watershed in the provision of chronic dialysis.[38] Public law 92-603 included provisions extending Medicare insurance coverage to virtually all patients with end-stage renal disease, giving them what is perhaps their most distinguishing characteristic: They became the first, and thus far only, victims of catastrophic illness singled out for special coverage of their treatment costs by the federal government.

By largely removing the financial barriers to the provision and receipt of dialysis that created the majority of the allocation issues of the 1960s, the federal government in effect became the new "gatekeeper" of this treatment. The government's assumption of this complex role has had profound effects on the delivery of dialysis and raises a series of critical issues that extend far beyond the confines of this therapy alone.

One cluster of issues generated by the passage of PL 92-603 involves the why and how of macro-level policy decisions about the allocation of public funds within the health-care segment of the federal budget. Why renal disease should have been singled out for special coverage, and the implications of this action for the federal financing of other catastrophic illness and for the provision of a broader-based form of national health insurance are two interrelated sociopolitical and moral questions that have been debated for the past decade.

A related series of issues concern the effects of PL 92-603 upon the provision of dialysis services. Data on treatment patterns before and after 1972 have generated debate about the extent to which lowering or removing financial barriers does, in fact, resolve problems of equity of access to treatment. The data, as various analysts have emphasized, are still sparse and subject to varied interpretations. It is clear that the number of patients entering end-stage renal disease programs since 1972 is vastly greater than the estimates provided in 1967 by the Committee on Chronic Kidney Disease. Analyses of cross-national differences in the prevalence rate of dialysis treatment (home and facility) per million population show that the United States rate is more than 50 percent higher than in any Western European nation.[34] Data also indicate wide variability in the treatment prevalence rate within the United States.

As Prottas et al. point out, "variations in the prevalence of a treatment modality can be explained in three ways: (1) differences in treatment choices made by medical practitioners; (2) differences in public policy decisions affecting the availability of treatment options, and (3) differences in the incidence of the underlying illnesses, reflecting, among other things, demographic differences in the compared populations."[34] With respect to interstate differences in dialysis treat-

ment rates in the United States, for example, some analysts have found a socioeconomic explanation, attributing the differential rates primarily to the effects of higher treatment rates in areas where the "medical industrial complex" of proprietary dialysis centers are located.[36,37] An alternative analysis of the same data, however, points to basic epidemiological differences in the incidence of end-stage renal disease, and attributes geographic differences in rates of new referrals for dialysis primarily to age and racial characteristics of various populations that may also underlie the causes of this disease.[41] A similar interpretation has also been given to the marked differences in cross-national treatment prevalence rates: "About 50 percent of the difference . . . between [the] American experience and the European maximum can be attributed to differences in the black/white composition of the populations. Most of the remaining difference in rates appears to be due to European policies that prohibit or severely limit access to dialysis by elderly and those potential patients with significant medical complications."[34]

In 1982, some 60,000 United States citizens were receiving dialysis at an estimated cost of $1.8 billion. Many charges and countercharges have been levied about the percentage of this cost—which is far in excess of initial estimates —attributable to fiscal mismanagement, ranging from inadequate federal and local institutional controls to fraud.[33,39] But beyond these familiar, recurring problems of responsible management —which are hardly unique to the provision of dialysis—the end-stage renal disease provisions of PL 92-603 embody a rapidly escalating value conflict in our society.

There is a widely shared value in our society that all citizens have a "right" to health care, which should not be abridged by lack of financial resources.

Efforts to act on the belief that health care is a right which society, through its government, has a reciprocal responsibility to meet by providing services that are available, accessible, and affordable appear to be on a collision course with escalating concerns about the costs of such care. As "cost containment" becomes a dominant theme in health policy arenas, and the "ethics of cost containment" a leitmotif in biomedical ethics, as people reexamine the "costs and benefits" of chronic dialysis and consider the implications of new technologies such as the first permanent artificial heart implant in December 1982, we hear recurrent and increasingly impassioned references to the same kind of allocation of scarce resources' dilemmas that were generated by the development of chronic dialysis in 1960.

If questions and decisions about the allocation of scarce resources are to be dealt with in more than economic terms, as we would argue they inescapably must be, it is appropriate to end this section by raising questions about the noneconomic effects of PL 92-603 on the recipients and providers of chronic dialysis. As we think back to the intertwined medical, social, and moral issues that surrounded dialysis in the 1960s, such as patient selection, the stresses on physicians and nurses, and the quality of life issues posed for and by dialysis patients, it seems to us that those involved in dialysis in the 1980s are confronted by many of the same problems as their predecessors, albeit in sometimes more refined, subtle, and varied forms.

For end-stage renal disease patients, their families, and those who care for them, the option of dialysis continues to pose fundamental value questions that pivot around the "quality of life" issues that are not unique to this mode of treatment but which it frames with special clarity. In the early years of Seattle's dialysis program, one of its physicians reflected that

> Doctors now find themselves able from time to time to enter a gray, limbo-like area where they are able to prolong life without, however, being able to cure the disease or heal the injury . . . The first great anxiety, then, that one faces in approaching the question of hemodialysis is whether from the patient's point of view the whole procedure will turn out to be a blessing or merely a labored and painful hanging on to life.[30]

Though seldom made with equanimity, decisions not to initiate treatment are a facet of their work well known to medical professionals. Faced with the allocation pressures of the 1960s, the selection procedures for dialysis frequently used "medical eligibility" criteria as a first screen, to rule out candidates who, in the clinical judgment of their physician-gatekeepers, would fare so poorly on dialysis that it was not deemed in their best interests to initiate treatment. The financial relief afforded by PL 92-603 made it possible to abandon the use of other, more onerous selection criteria, such as those based on psychosocial judgments about merit or need. At the same time, in part as an understandable reaction against the "playing God" choices they had had to make, physicians also moved away from exercising more medically traditional biomedical criteria as well. For they felt that, as expressed by one nephrologist in 1977, "with payment guaranteed under Social Security, there is no way—morally—to turn anyone down anymore."[29]

For medical professionals and others concerned with end-stage renal disease and its treatment, medical–moral questions about whether all candidates *should* receive dialysis now that it is available and affordable are accompanied by concerns about the medical, psychological, and social course of many of their patients. Three major changes in the dialysis population that have occurred since 1972 are increased percentages of patients who are older, of a lower socioeconomic status, or sicker compared to the more selective population of recipients in the 1960s.[22] Not surprisingly, therefore, recent studies of clinical outcomes of chronic dialysis "suggest that a larger proportion of dialysis patients than previously suspected are severely debilitated . . . any discussion of benefits should consider concurrent morbidity and the degree of occupational and physical rehabilitation, as well as the duration of extended life currently being achieved."[22]

These concerns, in turn, have raised afresh, and on a larger scale, the same intense questions about the quality of life and about decisions to stop treatment that providers and patients and their families have grappled with since chronic dialysis became technologically possible. "Who shall live when not all can live?" "Should all those who can be kept alive live?" These are two faces of the moral and social dilemmas contained in the phrase, "the allocation of scarce resources," that will be increasingly troublesome in a world of finite resources and growing technological capacities in medicine.

# THE NEPHROLOGY NURSE AND DIALYSIS

Throughout the 30-year-long history of dialysis, the nephrology nurse has been directly and intimately affected by the technical, social, and economic changes that this life-sustaining treatment has undergone, and by its impact on patients with end-stage renal disease, their families, and on the complex medical team involved in their care. At pres-

ent, the nurse is the member of this team who has the most continuous, direct relationship to the patient, "over many years of illness, including dialysis . . . and subsequent life-long observation."[25] This relationship involves the continuous care of patients in chronic renal failure, associated with their progressive, potentially life-threatening kidney disease, who by virtue of dialysis exist in a "marginal," "in limbo" state between sickness and wellness, life and death.[26] These are patients who are maintained in life and in the capacity to function to varying degrees in their social roles through the intermediary of a machine, a dialysis partner if on home dialysis, and medical caretakers. In this framework, the nurse is usually the professional who sees, coordinates, supervises, and counsels patients most often and regularly in their treatment program.

## Dialysis and the Nurse in the 1950s

The role of the nurse has been greatly altered as the technology and sociology of dialysis has evolved. In the 1950s, the artificial kidney machine was still in the early, clinical trial stage of its development, and only efficacious in treating patients with acute renal failure. The few medical teams in the country that were conducting these pioneering trials "were confronted with an ever-swelling stream of . . . terminally ill patients with chronic, irreversible kidney failure, who were sent by their own physicians or who came on their own volition, urgently hoping to be treated and 'saved' by this 'wonder machine,' which had received a considerable amount of mass media as well as medical journal attention."[18] But there was as yet no way to offer such patients the continuous dialysis treatment that they needed to survive. Making a new "cut-down" for each run, the teams working with the still experimental artificial kidney machine dialyzed some of these patients with end-stage renal disease numerous times, until there was no usable vein left to provide vascular access. After a short-lived improvement, uremia took over again, and carried the patient to his or her death. The Kolff model of the artificial kidney that was then in use was run by physicians, assisted by nurses, in a hierarchically organized team, and a heroic atmosphere. The dialysis nurse continued in the traditional role of providing physical care to the patient, and measuring vital signs.

## Dialysis and the Nurse in the 1960s

In 1960, with the invention, trial, and adoption of the Scribner shunt, chronic intermittent dialysis became possible, and the era of long-term dialysis began.[44] In 1963, home dialysis was initiated in Boston, Seattle, and England. Subsequently, peritoneal dialysis was improved, and limited home treatment with this method was introduced. These technological developments progressively altered the role of the nurse in important ways. (At that time, a total of 50 dialysis nurses existed in the United States.) Following the procedure and regimen established by Scribner and the University of Washington, Seattle kidney center, physicians delegated to nurses the tasks of setting up the hemodialysis machine, monitoring patients during their treatment, weighing the dialysis chemicals, and changing the dialysis bath solutions.[44] The nurse also helped the physician to make the components of the Teflon access materials. As programs of home dialysis were developed, the nurse became the principal educator who taught patients and their families the essentials of this unprecedented form of self-care

—training them competently and responsibly to perform their own dialysis and to manage the medical aspects of their dialysis-maintained lives.[23]

Because of the pioneering status of chronic dialysis in the 1960s and what it asked of patients and their families, as well as the scarcity of resources problems it posed, the policy of renal teams in this era was to try to select patients who seemed to have the best prognosis for doing well on the artificial kidney machine, biomedically and psychologically. Among the criteria of selection most frequently used were: the absence of medical conditions other than primary renal disease; a relatively young age (the average age of dialysis patients in the 1960s was 30); the intelligence and emotional stability to understand the procedure, face it, and to bear the uncertainty and the possibility of crisis that it involved; the motivation to cooperate, collaborate, and persist in the treatment regimen; strong family support; a reasonable likelihood of resuming work; a good reputation as a citizen and a community member; and the capacity to assume the $20,000 a year costs of dialysis. Psychological disturbance, mental "deficiency," a troubled family environment, a poor employment history, a criminal record, and indigency were among the conditions most likely to lead to the exclusion of patients from dialysis.[40] As a consequence, the typical patient on dialysis was a youthful, well-educated, emotionally and financially secure person, energetic and highly motivated, with outstanding family relations.

D.P., a 30 year-old lawyer, commuted 100 miles, three times a week, to and from the nearest dialysis unit. He also worked 40 to 50 hours a week at his law office. When a home dialysis program was started in his area, he and his wife undertook this mode of treatment. They performed his dialysis at home for the next 10 years, at which time he received a successful transplant.

Dialysis nurses of the 1960s lived uneasily with the medical implications and moral dilemmas that the policy of not selecting less "ideal" patients for dialysis entailed. In addition, as continuous caretakers, supervisors, educators, and counselors of dialysis patients, nurses were particularly keenly aware of the physical, emotional, and social stresses that many patients experienced on dialysis despite its lifesaving and life-sustaining benefits. Progressive, end-stage renal disease, problems of access, serious side effects of the dialysis process itself, the fettering and dehumanizing sense of being dependent on a machine as well as on other persons, severe dietary and fluid intake restrictions, and the impact of all of this on their families as well as on themselves made life on dialysis hard for numerous patients.[1] Many of them sought "deliverance" from the illness and dependency of hemodialysis through a kidney transplant. These were the sentiments of K.F., for example, a young wife, mother, and nurse, with end-stage renal disease, who embarked on a renal transplant convinced that "the surgical trauma and anxiety of rejection could not compare with the physical discomfort and feeling of futility" that she experienced on dialysis. "Caught between the ambivalent feelings of fear and hopefulness, I still believed that the hazard of transplantation was worth the risk if I might be able to contribute to family life rather than be a dependent burden."

There was more than an occasional patient who came to feel that dying would be a lesser evil than continuing dialysis, and who did not regard transplantation as a "liberation" from the machine or an alternative to it. Some of these patients explicitly requested that their dialysis be stopped; others engaged in self-destructive or suicidal behaviors, among which ripping out shunts, missing dialysis sessions, going on food or drink binges, and taking overdoses of medication were the most prominent. All the members of the renal team, physicians as well as nurses, agonized over the "quality of life," "right to death," and "death with dignity" questions that such patients posed and personified. "Once a patient begins a life-sustaining treatment such as dialysis, is it ever permissible, acceptable, or even desirable to discontinue it? If so, who has the right to make this decision? And who decides who decides?"[17]

The continuous, first-hand relationship of nurses to the dialysis process, and to dialysis patients and their families exposed them more directly and constantly to the problems and questions that this life-sustaining treatment raised, than other members of the medical team. Not only were nurses in a position to notice the difficulties that patients were experiencing; they were also the medical professionals to whom patients and their families most frequently and consistently communicated their problems. Patients on in-center dialysis saw the dialysis nurse three times a week for treatment that lasted for 4 or more hours, and that could and usually did go on for many years. In most home dialysis programs, an active communication system developed between patients, families, and nurses. In both dialysis settings, it was usually the nurse whom the patient and family consulted first about the day-by-day medical, psychological, and/or social problems they were encountering. Under these circumstances, strong bonds tended to develop among nurses, patients, and families.

The scope, duration, and intensity of these relationships were not only important and satisfying to nurses, but also a source of considerable strain. This was particularly true because, despite the fact that during the 1960s, chronic dialysis became more technically "ordinary" and routinized (and dialysis technicians, a new group of paramedical professionals, joined nurses in conducting in-center dialysis), patients being treated on the artificial kidney machine were still ill with end-stage renal disease. Dialysis maintained them, but it did not cure their disease, and it generated its own side effects that added to the burdensomeness of the patient's medical condition.

These distinctive characteristics of the dialysis situation, and of the nurse's relation to it, were key factors in a phenomenon that began to develop in the 1960s, and that continues to be true to this day: the rapid "burnout" and turnover of nurses in this field. A staff survey of 200 nurses in one end-stage renal disease network, for example, revealed that the average time a nurse stayed in nephrology was 2 years.[13] Nurses not only recognized that the stresses to which they were collectively subject were associated with their high rates of turnover and burnout; they were also convinced that increased support from other members of the medical team would help to reduce, if not prevent them. In the staff survey cited, 80 percent of the nurses questioned recommended liaison psychiatry, social service rounds, and meetings with the physician team as ways of helping them to handle the emotional demands that the role of nephrology/dialysis nurse entailed.[13]

The establishment of the American Association of Nephrology Nurses and Technicians (AANNT) in 1969 was a direct outgrowth of the initiative taken by nurses to organize new forms of peer support, as well as to advance their professional education and expertise. Previous to this, nurses had attended the annual physicians' meeting of the American Society for Artificial Internal Organs (ASAIO). It was symbolically, as well as

organizationally significant that the first meeting of AANNT was partly funded by ASAIO. Some 450 persons attended this full-day meeting. From those relatively modest beginnings, the membership of AANNT has grown to 4,000.[20] Over the course of the past 14 years, the annual program of the AANNT has increasingly included presentations concerning the troubling psychological, social, and moral issues and dilemmas involved in the care of end-stage renal disease patients with which nurses have such strategic and unremitting contact. Psychiatrist Norman B. Levy has coordinated the International Conference of Psychonephrology which has provided nurses with an additional, highly valued forum where they can periodically discuss these facets of end-stage renal disease, and its treatment by dialysis and transplantation, and work together to try to deal with them in ways that will be more effective for patients, families, and for the professionals responsible for their care.[27]

## Dialysis and the Nurse in the 1970s

It is the passage of Public Law 92-603 with its accompanying "democratization of dialysis,"[19] more than new biomedical and technological developments in the process of dialysis that has intensified the preoccupation of nurses with psychological, social, and ethical questions during the past decade. It is true that over the course of the 1970s, arteriovenous fistulas introduced by Brescia and colleagues, and bovine and Gore-tex grafts largely have replaced the shunt, and helped with certain access problems. The artificial kidney became smaller, more elegant in appearance, and had more failsafe features incorporated into it. Work on a portable "suitcase kidney" and a wearable artificial kidney continued. An ambulatory form of peritoneal dialysis became a viable option. Progress also occurred in the management of medical problems associated with dialysis and with the underlying diseases and disorders from which patients on dialysis suffer, such as anemia, malnutrition, bone disease, and peripheral nerve disorders. In the course of the 1970s, the medical profession improved its capacity to dialyze patients with complicated, multiple disorders. The number (though not proportion) of patients on home dialysis increased in the 1970s. Dialysis also became "more of a helpmate and less of a rival of renal transplantation as transplant teams modulated their efforts to 'save the organ' from rejection by reducing the high doses of immunosuppressive drugs they previously had given patients."[17] But the basic principles of dialysis remained the same. Problems of access were still common. Serious side effects continued to occur. It remained exceedingly difficult to treat patients who were not only afflicted with end-stage renal disease, but with other chronic conditions as well. And no "breakthrough" advances in biomedical understanding of the mechanisms in kidney disease, its causes, prevention, and therapy were made.

Within this "state of the art" framework, as a consequence of Public Law 92-603, the patient population to which nurses now found themselves providing care was radically different—both medically and sociologically—from those they had dialyzed in the 1960s. The average age of patients undergoing dialysis treatment changed from 30 to 50 years. In addition to end-stage renal disease, many of the patients had other serious, chronic, and progressive illnesses.

L.C. is a 56-year-old man on hemodialysis at an outpatient facility. He has had diabetes mellitus since age ten, is blind, and has undergone bilateral amputations below the knee.

D.M. is a 60-year-old woman, with end-stage renal disease, on chronic dialysis at a hospital center. She has had eight access procedures in the last year due to graft clotting. She has also had two strokes which have left her aphasic. Between dialysis treatments, she is cared for in a local nursing home.

The social origins of dialysis patients now encompassed all economic, educational, and ethnic groups, with styles of life that ranged from stable, successful, and conventionally upright to downtrodden, disorganized, and deviant. Nurses were faced with the challenge of developing ways to ensure that this socially heterogeneous array of patients would receive equally good dialysis treatment, irrespective of their age, education, family situation, cultural background, or way of life:

H.F., a 21-year-old man with end-stage renal disease secondary to diabetes mellitus, was successfully taught to perform ambulatory peritoneal dialysis. After 3 months at home, he asked to be put on in-center hemodialysis. He had no family, lived alone, and had become clinically depressed by the isolation of home care without the continuous support of the nursing staff.

F.S. is a 35-year-old woman with end-stage renal disease due to malignant hypertension. In the course of her evaluation for a kidney transplant, she explained that she had not been taking her antihypertension medications because it was "too complicated." Her difficulties stemmed from the fact that she did not have basic arithmetic and reading skills. Once this was discerned, the nurses taught her elementary addition and subtraction, and designed medication cards that would assist her in taking her daily medications regularly.

Two kinds of sociological difficulties that PL 92-603 brought in its wake proved to be the most disturbing to nurses. When they observed that many patients from deprived socioeconomic backgrounds, certain minority groups, or troubled families did not respond as well to dialysis as patients from more privileged environments, nurses felt concerned about these inequitable results. They were inclined to attribute the relatively poor response of such patients to their failure as nurses to relate to them in a prejudice-free, egalitarian, and effective way.

Harder still for nurses was the fact that some of the patients they were dialyzing and to whom they were obligated to give excellent care were leading deviant, exploitive, even criminal lives. For example, in one dialysis program we studied, nurses had a hard time justifying to themselves the care they gave to a patient who sold illicit drugs, to another who belonged to the "numbers racket," and to a third who was a procurer. Nurses have also had to treat menacing prisoners, brought to the dialysis unit three times a week by special transportation, and watched over by assigned guards.[17]

Nurses and physicians have always been called upon to care for all those who need their medical help, regardless of the origins, character, personality, values, beliefs, and behavior of the persons who are their patients. But, in contrast to most other forms of medical care, dialysis requires practitioners, especially nurses who are on the "front lines" of dialysis therapy, to treat patients, including those who are reprehensible or threatening to them, several times a week, for sessions that last from 4 to 6 hours, over a period of years, until the patient receives a kidney transplant, or succumbs to his or her disease. Under the circumstances, fulfilling one's professional obligations to patients in a universalistic way can be particularly stressful.

In the early 1980s, nurses still grapple daily with these sociomedical phenomena, and with questions about who rightfully should and should not be treated, about the quality of life of the patients receiving care, and about their own attitudinal as well as technical adequacy as nurses to treat these patients. Neither federal legislation, bioethical consultation, nor biomedical and bioengineering advances have dispelled these problems and questions associated with end-stage renal disease and its treatment.

# CONCLUSION

Through four interconnected case studies—of the advent of cyclosporine, organ transplantation as gift exchange, the democratization of dialysis, and the evolution of nephrology nursing—we have tried to show how psychological, social, and ethical factors, along with biomedical and technological ones have shaped and altered some of the problems with which patients, families, medical professionals, and American society more broadly have been faced over the past three decades, in their continuing attempt to deal competently, humanely, and morally with end-stage renal disease, and its treatment by dialysis and transplantation.

# REFERENCES

1. AANNT Testimony to the Health Subcommittee of the U.S. Senate Finance Committee, 28 September 1981.
2. Altman LK: Transplants are surging as survival rates improve. The New York Times (Science Times section), October 5, 1982, C1-C2.
3. Artificial heart among many '82 health gains. The New York Times, January 2, 1983, 25.
4. Bok S: Lying: Moral Choices in Public and Private Life. Pantheon Press, New York, 1978.
5. Borel JF: From our laboratories: Cyclosporin A. Triangle, 20:97, 1981.

6. Borel JF: Immunosuppressive properties of Cyclosporin A. Transpl. Proc., 12:233, 1980.
7. Calne RY: Cyclosporin (Editorial), Nephron, 26:57, 1980.
8. Calne RY: Transplant surgery: current status. Brit J Surg, 67:765, 1980.
9. Calne RY, McMaster P, Evans DB: Cyclosporin A and the media. Br Med J 280:43, 1980.
10. Calne RY, Rolles K, White DJG, et al: Prolonged survival of pig orthotopic heart grafts treated with cyclosporin A. Lancet 1:1183, 1978.
11. Calne RY, Rolles K, Thiru S, et al: Cyclosporin A initially as the only immunosuppressive in 36 recipients of cadaveric organs: 32 kidneys, 2 pancreases, and 2 livers. Lancet 2:1033, 1970.
12. Calne RY, Thiru S, McMaster P, et al: Cyclosporin A in patients receiving renal allografts from cadaver donors. Lancet, 2:1323, 1978.
13. Cameron EM, Neff ML, Eyer J, et al: Staff survey of ESRD Network #24. Presented at AANNT Annual Meeting, Chicago, 1982.
14. Childress JF: Who shall live when not all can live? Soundings, 43:339, 1970.
15. Eiseman B, Hanbrough J, Weil R: New approaches for immune suppression. Amer. Surgeon, 1:24, 1980.
16. Fellner CH, Marshall JR: Altruism in disrepute: Medical vs. public attitudes toward the living organ donor. N Engl J Med 284, 582, 1971.
17. Fox RC: Exclusion from dialysis: A sociologic and legal perspective. Kidney Int. 19:739, 1981.
18. Fox RC: The medical profession's changing outlook on hemodialysis (1950–1976). p.122. In Fox RC: Essays in Medical Sociology. John Wiley, New York, 1979.
19. Fox RC, Swazey JP: The Courage to Fail: A Social View of Organ Transplantation and Dialysis. 2nd Ed. Rev. University of Chicago Press, Chicago, 1978.
20. Fulton BJ, Cameron EM: History of AANNT. Presented at the AANNT Tenth Annual Meeting, April, 1979.
21. Gottschalk CW: Report of the Committee on Chronic Kidney Disease. U.S. Government Printing Office, Washington D. C., 1967.
22. Gutman RA, Stead WW, Robinson RR: Physical activity and employment status of patients on maintenance dialysis. N Eng J Med 304:309, 1981.
23. Hampers CL, Merrill JP, Cameron EM: Hemodialysis at the home. Trans Am Soc Artif Intern Organs 11:3, 1965.
24. Kahan BD: Cosmos and Damian in the 20th century? N Engl J Med 305:280, 1981.
25. Kintzel J, Silberman H, Cameron EM: Care of the patient with renal failure. In Kintzel KD: Advanced Concepts in Clinical Nursing. 2nd Ed. J. P. Lippincott, Philadelphia, 1977, p 582.
26. Landsman M: The patient with chronic renal failure: A marginal man. Ann Intern Med 82:268, 1975.
27. Levy NB, Ed: Psychological Factors in Hemodialysis and Transplantation. Plenum, New York, 1981.
28. Mauss M: The Gift: Forms and Functions of Exchange in Archaic Societies. I. Cunnison, Trans Free Press, Glencoe, 1954.
29. McLaughlin L: Self-care dialysis center planned in Boston. Boston Globe, May 18, 1977, p. 50.
30. Norton CE: Chronic hemodialysis as a medical and social experiment. Ann Intern Med 66:1267, 1967.
31. Nussemblatt RB, Rodrigues MD, Gery I, et al: Cyclosporin A inhibition of experimental autoimmune uveitis in Lewis rats. J Clin Invest 67:1228, 1981.
32. Powles RL, Clink H, Sloane J, et al: Cyclosporin A for the treatment of graft-versus-host disease in man. Lancet, 2:1327, 1978.
33. Prottas JM, Sapolsky HM: Administrative problems in the end-stage renal disease program. University Health Policy Consortium PA-5, November 1981.
34. Prottas JM, Segal M, Sapolsky HM: Cross-national differences in dialysis rates. University Health Policy Consortium DP-39, November 1981.
35. Reitz BA, Wallwork JJ, Hunt SA, et al: Heart-lung transplantation: successful therapy for patients with pulmonary vascular disease. N Engl J Med 306:557, 1982.

36. Relman AS: Race and end-stage renal disease. N Engl J Med 306:1290, 1982.
37. Relman AS, Rennie D: Treatment of end-stage renal disease: free but not equal. N Engl J Med 303:996, 1980.
38. Rettig RA: Valuing lives: the policy debate on patient care financing for victims of end-stage renal disease. Rand Corporation, Washington, D.C., 1976.
39. Robinson D: Kidney dialysis: A taxpayers' nightmare. Readers Digest, October 1982, p. 149.
40. Rosenbaum I, Atcherson E, Corry R: Rehabilitation and the transplant patient. Dialysis Transpl 10:136, 1981.
41. Rostand SF, Kirk KA, Rutsky EA, et al: Racial differences in the treatment for end-stage renal disease. N Engl J Med 306:1276, 1982.
42. Russell PA: Transplantation today. Presentation to the American Association of Immunologists, April 1982.
43. Sadler AM, Jr, Sadler BL, Stason EC: The uniform anatomical gift act: A model for reform. JAMA 206:2501, 1968.
44. Scribner BH, Buri R, Canner JEZ, et al: The treatment of chronic uremia by means of intermittent hemodialysis: A preliminary report. Trans Am Soc Artif Intern Organs 6:114, 1960.
45. Sheil AG: Cyclosporin A: A new immune suppressive agent. Med J Austral 1:37, 1982.
46. Simmons RC, Klein SD, Simmons RL: Gift of Life: The Social and Psychological Impact of Organ Transplantation. John Wiley & Sons, New York, 1977.
47. Starzl TE, Shunzaburo I, Van Theil DH, et al: Evolution of liver transplantation. Hepatology, 2:614, 1982.
48. Starzl TE, Shunzaburo I, Klintmalm GBG, et al: Human organ transplantation under Cyclosporin A and steroids. In Touraine, J, Traeger H, Betuel H, et al, Eds: Transplantation and Clinical Immunology. Vol. 13. Excerpta Medica, Amsterdam, 1981.
49. Swazey JP: The Scribner dialysis shunt: ramifications of a clinical-technological innovation. In Abernathy WJ, Sheldon A, Prahalad CK, Eds: The Management of Health Care. Ballinger Publishing Co., Cambridge, MA, 1974, p. 229.
50. Veatch RM, Branson R, Eds: Ethics and Health Policy. Ballinger Publishing Co., Cambridge, MA, 1976.

# Section II

## Controversies in Hypertension

# 3

# Treatment of Hypertension

# The Case for Nondrug Treatment

## Norman M. Kaplan, M.D.

In treating hypertension, physicians prefer to use pills rather than nondrug therapies. The reasons for this preference are multiple and fairly obvious and they can be grouped into four main categories:

1. The dangers of untreated hypertension: We and the public have become increasingly aware of the dangers of the "silent killer" so that more and more expect—even demand—that something be done to lower any elevated pressure.

2. The benefits of treatment: Most practitioners believe that reduction of even minimally elevated pressures will save lives and prevent disease.

3. The efficacy and safety of drugs: We are virtually certain that one or more of the steadily growing number of antihypertensive agents will lower the blood pressure of every hypertensive, and we believe that most hypertensives can and do take medications with little if any difficulty.

4. The questionable efficacy of and poor adherence to nondrug therapies: We are much less certain of the efficacy of nondrug therapies and believe that most people will not make the necessary changes in lifelong habits that are needed to make them work.

I will examine these four issues with the intention of convincing the reader

that there is a strong case for the routine use of nondrug therapies, while, of necessity, showing that drugs are not always indicated and may be harmful.

This discussion will relate primarily to the large majority, approximately two-thirds of hypertensives, with diastolic blood pressures (DBP) between 90 and 100, commonly referred to as "mild" hypertension. As we shall see, the evidence that drug therapy is usually indicated for those with DBP persistently above 100 is so strong that it needs no further debate.[15] Those with DBP over 100 also deserve and need nondrug therapies but antihypertensive drugs will almost always be the primary mode of their treatment.

## THE DANGERS OF UNTREATED HYPERTENSION

Hypertension has deservedly received a great deal of attention as one of the major risk factors for premature cardiovascular disease. Data from Framingham[13] and life insurance actuarial statistics[37] have demonstrated that even minimally elevated pressures are associated with significant increases of coronary, cerebral, and other vascular diseases. Even though the absolute degree of risk for each patient with mild hypertension is relatively small, since they comprise the majority of the hyperten-

Supported in part by an Academic Award in Preventive Cardiology from the NIH (5K07-HL00596).

sive population they contribute the largest share of the overall societal burden (Fig. 3-1).

## The Distribution of Risk

Even though mild hypertensives will suffer most of the premature cardiovascular diseases associated with hypertension, the risk is not equally distributed among them. The Framingham data have been tabulated to demonstrate the likelihood of a coronary event in the next eight years for both men and women at various ages from 35 to 65 with varying degrees of hypertension (using systolic levels) in association with the other known risk factors: cigarette smoking, hypercholesterolemia, glucose intolerance, and left ventricular hypertrophy (LVH) by electrocardiography (ECG). With each increment of blood pressure at every configuration of concomitant risk factors, the risk for a coronary event increases (Fig. 3-2). But note, as shown here

for a 40-year-old man, how the risk grows with the addition of more and more other risk factors. On the far left, the risk is shown to increase from about 1 percent to 4.6 percent as the systolic blood pressure increases from 105 mm Hg to 195 mm Hg in a 40-year-old man otherwise at "low risk." On the far right, the risk for a coronary event in eight years is shown to go from about 35 percent to as high as 70.8 percent for the same 40-year-old man with the same range of blood pressure but with the addition of the other factors placing him at "high risk." So, for the same systolic blood pressure of 195 mm Hg, the 8-year risk goes from 4.6 to 70.8 percent.

Most patients are somewhere in the middle, having moderate degrees of overall risk. But the point of Figure 3-2 should be obvious: The level of the blood pressure is only one determinant of risk; as important as it is, the other determinants need to be taken into account. In addition to those used in the Framing-

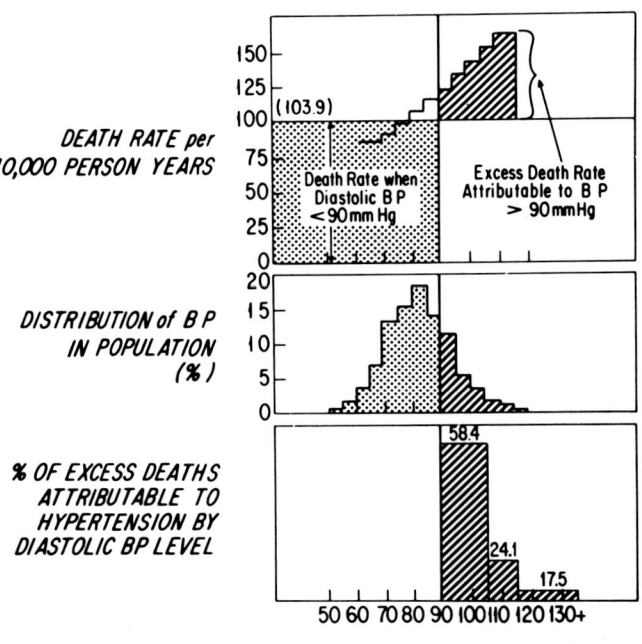

**Fig. 3-1.** The percentage of excess deaths attributable to hypertension by diastolic blood pressure level (bottom), based upon the death rate observed in Framingham (top) and the distribution of the blood pressure found in the HDFP population (middle) (from The Hypertension Detection and Follow-up Program. Circ. Res. 40 (5): May 1977 by permission of the American Heart Association, Inc.).

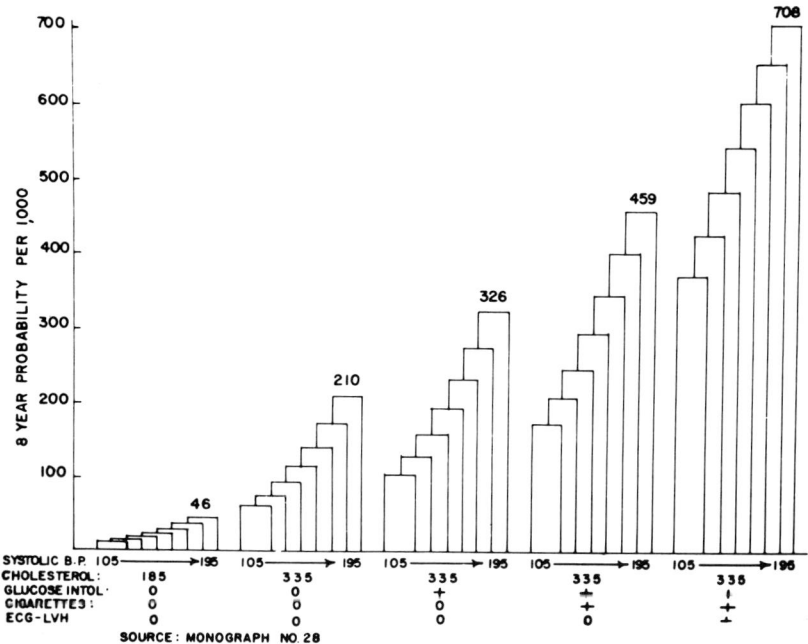

**Fig. 3-2.** The eight year risk of cardiovascular disease for 40-year-old men in Framingham according to progressively higher systolic blood pressure at specified levels of other risk factors. (From Kannel WB. In Genest J, Koiw E, Kuchel O (Eds): Hypertension: Physiopathology and Treatment. McGraw-Hill, New York, 1977. © 1977. Used with the permission of the McGraw-Hill Book Company.)

ham analysis, the patient's race, family history of premature cardiovascular disease, and the presence and degree of target organ damage, such as retinopathy and renal impairment, should also be considered. Dr. Edward D. Freis has composed a simple "Risk Factor Scoring System" for deciding upon the need for treatment of patients with diastolic pressures averaging 90 to 99 mm Hg (Table 3-1). This scoring system need not be used as a rigid rule but should be a helpful guide. Even better, each patient's likelihood for having a coronary event in the next 6 years can be found in the American Heart Association's Coronary Risk Handbook or by use of one of the slide rules provided by the Merrell-Dow and Pfizer pharmaceutical companies.

## The Variable Fall in Pressure

One reason why the risks for hypertension will vary is the variable nature of the blood pressure, rising to even more hazardous levels in some, changing little in others but spontaneously falling to safer levels in many. This tendency for the blood pressure to fall can be nicely seen from the experience of the largest population of untreated mild hypertensives yet observed, the placebo-treated half of the patients enrolled in the Australian therapeutic trial.[22] Over four years, the diastolic blood pressure, which averaged between 95 and 109 mm Hg on the second pair of two initial sets of readings, rose above 110 mm Hg in 12.2 percent, remained between 95 and 109 mm

**Table 3-1.** Risk Factor Scoring System (for patients with diastolic pressure averaging 90 to 99 mm Hg on repeated measurements)

| Risk Index | Score |
| --- | --- |
| Smoking | 1 |
| Diabetes | 1 |
| High Cholesterol-Low HDL | 1 |
| Average Systolic Pressure > 165 | 1 |
| Average Diastolic Pressure > 95 | 1 |
| Target Organ Disease (LVH, etc.) | 2 |
| Age < 45 | 1 |
| Black | 1 |
| Severe Hypertension in Family | 1 |
| TREAT IF AVERAGE DIASTOLIC PRESSURE IS | IF RISK SCORE IS |
| 90–94 mm Hg | 3 or more |
| 95–99 mm Hg | 2 or more |

(From E.D. Freis, personal communication.)

Hg in 32.5 percent and fell below 95 mm Hg in 47.7 percent. In fact, a significant number of those on placebo had average DBP below 90 over the next four years, including 11 percent of those who started with DBP between 105 and 109 mm Hg (Fig. 3-3). Obviously those whose pressures fall to below 90 mm Hg need not be given any antihypertensive therapy. There is then clearly a need to watch those with mildly elevated pressures for at least a time during which nondrug therapies may be reasonably used to hopefully bring even more to a safe level.

This frequent tendency for an initially elevated pressure to fall does not counter the considerable evidence from Framingham and elsewhere[13] that even one high pressure presages trouble, in the population at large. But what is true for the masses need not apply to each individual. Therefore there is a need to monitor each person's pressure over a prolonged time if the initial level is not above 100 mm Hg.

### Absolute versus Relative Risk

One further important point should be made about the risks for any level of elevated blood pressure: though the relative risk may be markedly increased, the ab-

solute risk may be only slightly increased. As shown on the top of Figure 3-1 increasing levels of diastolic blood pressure are associated with increasing death rates. But notice that this death rate rises from about 100 per 10,000 person years (or 1.0 percent per year) at a DBP of 80 mm Hg to about 140 per 10,000 person years (or 1.4 percent per year) at a DBP of 95 to 100. This is a 40 percent increase in *relative* risk, and this figure is often used to indicate the dangers of even mild hypertension. But in terms of *absolute* risk, the presence of the higher blood pressure means that another 40 out of 10,000 persons (or 0.4 percent) would die in the next year.

These 40 excess deaths per 10,000 people should not be disregarded. If there are 30 million people with mild hypertension in the United States, that would translate into 120,000 excess deaths in a year. But as bad as 120,000 may be, it means that less than one-half of one percent of the hypertensive population would die in the next year as a result of their elevated blood pressure, hardly the 40 percent increase that some may assume from the relative risk figures.

## THE BENEFITS OF TREATMENT

Most presume that these excess deaths associated with elevated blood pressure can be largely, if not totally, prevented by lowering of the pressure. That seems logical but the evidence now available shows only a partial degree of protection, particularly from coronary artery disease.

### The Australian Trial

Once again, the best evidence comes from the Australian trial, since it was de-

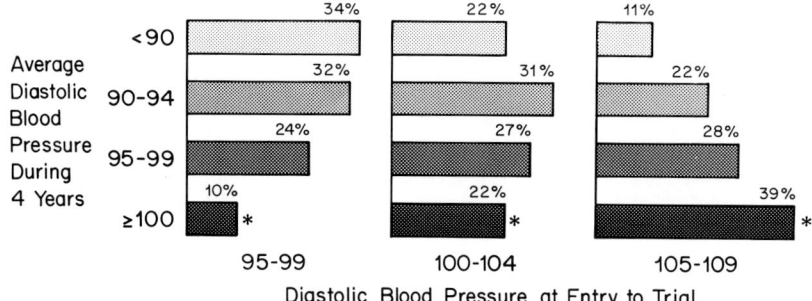

**Fig. 3-3.** The average diastolic blood pressure (DBP) during the four years of the Australian Therapeutic Trial in the 1,617 patients treated without drugs divided into three ranges of DBP entry. Note that the majority of those with initial DBP from 95 all the way up to 109 ended with DBP below 100 and that excess complications were noted only in those whose end DBP was above 100. (From Management Committee, 1980) (Reprinted from Kaplan, N.M.: Clinical Hypertension, 3rd edition. © 1982, The Williams & Wilkins Co., Baltimore.)

signed specifically as a trial of the efficacy of antihypertensive drug therapy for the prevention of cardiovascular mortality and morbidity.[21] The results were clear: the half given drug therapy had significantly lower rates of mortality and morbidity, that is, fewer total endpoints, from cardiovascular causes than did the half receiving placebo. However, at any level of blood pressure the rate of cardiovascular complications remained greater among those who achieved that level of blood pressure with drugs than among those whose pressures fell to that level with placebo (Fig. 3-4). In other words, reduction of the blood pressure by drugs did not lower the rate of complications to that observed among those on placebo with the same levels of blood pressure.

There are a number of possible explanations for this discrepancy.[14] One is that more of those whose pressures were brought down to a certain level with drugs started with higher levels of blood pressure than did those who reached that level on placebo, a fact that is documented by the smaller number of placebo-treated patients who ended the trial with pressures below 100 mm Hg (Fig. 3-4). Those who started with higher pressures would be expected to have a worse prognosis, which might not be completely reversible by a reduction of their blood pressure. However, all of these patients were free of demonstrable target organ damage at entry into the study, so they should be about as homogeneous a population as could be found, despite varying levels of blood pressure. Furthermore, it is statistically hazardous to compare two groups of different sizes who may not have been comparable to start with.

Another explanation for the higher rate of complications among the drug-treated half, however, cannot be discounted, namely, that the drugs themselves may engender a certain risk which partially removes the benefits of a lower blood pressure. As I have detailed elsewhere,[15] there are side effects, both immediate and long-term, with every antihypertensive drug and there may be particularly bothersome long-term problems with diuretics which were the first and often sole drugs used in the Austra-

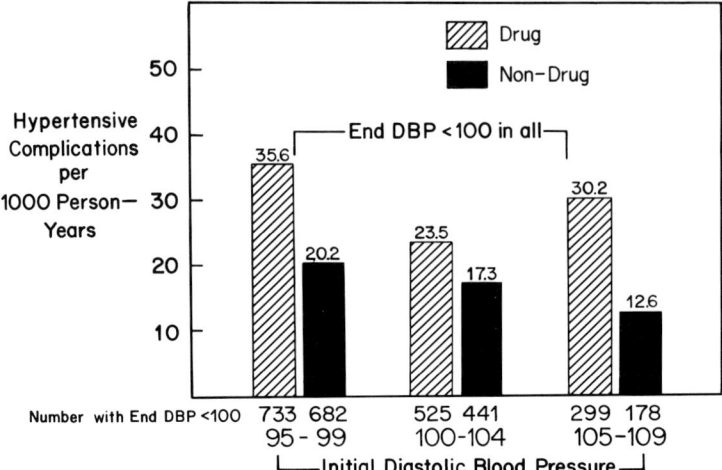

**Fig. 3-4.**   The cardiovascular complications per 1,000 person years among those receiving drugs and those receiving placebo during the Australian Therapeutic Trial. Note that for those whose average diastolic blood pressure (DBP) was below 100, regardless of the initial DBP range, the complication rates were lower in those not on drugs. More of those from each initial DBP group who were on drugs achieved an end DBP below 100 (composed from Report of the Management Committee, Lancet 1:1261, 1980) (Reprinted from Kaplan, N.M.: Clinical Hypertension, 3rd edition. © 1982, The Williams & Wilkins Co., Baltimore.)

lian trial and all the other therapeutic trials which have been completed as of early 1983.

## The MRFIT Study

The potential hazards of diuretics, particularly in the high doses used in most of the trials started in the early 1970s, have been invoked to explain the higher mortality rates among the more heavily treated half of the Multiple Risk Factor Intervention Trial (MRFIT).[28] As shown in Table 3-2, the mortality from coronary heart disease (CHD) as well as total mortality was lower in those who started with diastolic pressures of 100 or higher among those given more intensive therapy, the Special Intervention (SI) half. Among those who started with DBP of 95 to 99 mm Hg, the rates were equal. But among those who started with DBP

of 90 to 94 mm Hg, more deaths were seen among those more heavily treated. Notice the even more strikingly higher mortality among the SI half if their initial ECG was abnormal, suggesting that diuretic-induced hypokalemia may have been involved in their high rate of sudden death (see Chapter 9). We await detailed analyses of these mortality data to explain the differences.

## Benefit Minus Risk

At this time, however, the results of the Australian trial and the MRFIT study can be used to formulate a general statement about the benefits to be expected from drug therapy of hypertension. This statement fixes a certain hazard to drug therapy; for the sake of our discussion, let us accept a 10 percent increase in the risk of coronary death from drug ther-

**Table 3-2.** MRFIT: Mortality in Hypertensives Given Therapy

| Initial BP | Number | | CHD[a] Deaths Per 1,000 | | Total Deaths Per 1,000 | |
|---|---|---|---|---|---|---|
| | SI[b] | UC[c] | SI | UC | SI | UC |
| Receiving treatment at entry | 1261 | 1227 | 28 | 26 | 59 | 54 |
| Not receiving treatment at entry | | | | | | |
| 90–94 | 1157 | 1181 | 14.7 | 10.2 | 40.6 | 26.2 |
| 95–99 | 830 | 846 | 22.9 | 22.5 | 51.8 | 46.1 |
| ≥ 100 | 771 | 739 | 20.8 | 29.8 | 32.4 | 60.9 |
| Normal ECG | 2785 | 2808 | 15.8 | 20.7 | 35.9 | 43.4 |
| Abnormal ECG | 1233 | 1185 | 29.2 | 17.7 | 60.0 | 39.7 |

[a]CHD: Coronary heart disease.
[b]SI: Special intervention.
[c]UC: Usual care.
    (Adapted, excluding nonhypertensives, from MRFIT: Multiple risk factor intervention trial. JAMA 248: 1465, 1982. Copyright 1982 American Medical Association.)

apy. If the population being treated begins with diastolic blood pressures greater than 100 mm Hg and therefore has a 50 percent higher risk of coronary death, the application of drug therapy would prove beneficial. By the removal of the 50 percent excess by reduction of the pressure, patients would be benefited despite the 10 percent risk added by the therapy. On the other hand, if the population being treated starts with a 90 to 94 mm Hg diastolic pressure which has, for the sake of our discussion, only a 10 percent inherent risk, it is obvious that even if all of that risk could be removed, the 10 percent risk added by the treatment would wipe out all of the gain.

## HDFP Results

Data from the Hypertension Detection and Follow-up Program (HDFP)[12] might be taken to refute this argument, since there were significant reductions in mortality among the more intensively treated Stepped-Care (SC) half of those who entered the study with diastolic pressures in the "mild" range, that is, 90 to 104 mm Hg (Table 3-3). This table provides the data about those in the 90 to 104 range who were not on therapy and who had no evidence of target organ damage at entry into the trial, a popula-

tion comparable to those in the Australian trial.

Note that mortality was reduced 28.6 percent in the more intensively treated SC half, with the highest percentage of fall in those with the lowest DBP on entry, the 90 to 94 group who had a 34 percent reduction.

There are two points about these data that need to be remembered, one that puts them into question as evidence for the benefit of drug therapy per se, the other that puts them into a different perspective as to the degree of benefit they demonstrate. The first, developed elsewhere,[9,15] simply is that the HDFP was designed as a test of the ability to control the masses of hypertensive patients, not as a trial of drug therapy per se. Thus, the reduction in cardiovascular mortality, which could be attributable to the greater lowering of blood pressure achieved by more intensive drug therapy, was accompanied by a significant reduction in mortality from noncardiovascular causes which cannot logically be attributed to drug therapy per se. The SC half received much more intensive medical attention and care, so that their lesser cardiovascular mortality could reflect, at least in part, the benefits of more health care as well as the benefits of more drug therapy.

The second point about the HDFP goes back to the earlier discussion about relative versus absolute rates. Notice from Table 3-3 that in absolute numbers the reduction in mortality between the two groups was 3.2 per 1,000 person years or 0.32 percent per year. That looks a lot less impressive than the 28.6 percent relative difference between the two groups. Once again, we should not disregard the 0.32 percent difference, since for 30 million hypertensives that translates into 96,000 fewer deaths per year.

But it also means that to save one life per year, 300 hypertensives would have to be treated with drugs, 299 to receive no obvious immediate benefit, and likely to suffer from some side effects. Thus, we are left with a dilemma: Only a few patients will benefit while many more are bothered. One obvious way out of the dilemma is to restrict drug therapy to those who are at relatively higher overall risk, as defined earlier in this presentation. If only the higher-risk patients were included, more would likely benefit and fewer would be unnecessarily bothered (and put at some risk), so that the benefit-risk balance would be much more favorable.

## THE EFFICACY AND SAFETY OF DRUGS

Much of the preceding relates to this issue, so that little additional evidence need be given. There is no reason to question the efficacy of currently available drugs to lower the blood pressure, if patients take them. The question of the benefits to be derived from the effective reduction of the blood pressure has been addressed. But a bit more should be said about the patient acceptance of drug therapy.

Perhaps 5 to 10 percent of patients will have rather immediate side effects which preclude their taking the medications, the number likely greater with nondiuretic drugs than with diuretics. Over a five-year period, from 15 percent to 40 percent of patients will have adverse reactions which cause them to stop therapy. In the Australian trial, one-third prematurely stopped their regimen, including a significant number of those on placebo.[21] In the HDFP, 36.8 percent of those on the stepped-care regimen had adverse drug reactions severe enough to cause them to discontinue their drug over the five years of the study.[7] The incidence of adverse reactions was 17 percent in year 1 and fell to 6.5 percent in year 5. Most reactions required no therapy save discontinuation of the drug and there were no deaths due to adverse reactions.

The type of side effects seen with either a diuretic or a beta-blocker has been reported from another large-scale therapeutic trial that is still in progress, the English Medical Research Council (MRC) trial.[23] Over the first 5 years, about 18 percent of those treated with either drug withdrew, compared to five percent of those on placebo tablets. The principal reasons for withdrawal were pretty much in keeping with what is known about the side effects of these two types of drugs, other than for a surprisingly high incidence of impotence among the diuretic-treated men.

### Trials versus Ordinary Practice

Remember that these dropouts occurred in populations who were being encouraged to remain under therapy, often utilizing techniques to encourage adherence including provision of medication at no cost, home visits, and involvement with nonphysician health professionals.

Individual practitioners may do as well but it's likely that they are doing

**Table 3-3.** HDFP: Reduction in Mortality in Patients with Diastolic Pressure 90 to 104 mm Hg Not on Drug Therapy and Free of End-Organ Damage on Entry

| Entry Diastolic BP (mm Hg) | Stepped Care (Rate per 1,000 Patient-Years) | Referred Care (Rate per 1,000 Patient-Years) | Reduction in Mortality | |
|---|---|---|---|---|
| | | | Percentage | Absolute Number per 1,000 Patient-Years |
| 90–94 | 7.0 | 10.6 | 34.0 | 3.6 |
| 95–99 | 8.4 | 11.6 | 27.6 | 3.2 |
| 100–104 | 9.3 | 11.6 | 19.8 | 2.3 |
| 90–104 | 8.0 | 11.2 | 28.6 | 3.2 |

(Reprinted, by permission of the New England Journal of Medicine, from: Hypertension Detection and Follow-up Program Cooperative Group: The effect of treatment on mortality in "mild" hypertension. N. Engl J Med 307: 976, 1982.)

worse. Data from the National Health and Nutrition Survey of 1976–1980 show that in the United States, of all people previously diagnosed as being hypertensive, 23.4 percent were on no treatment, and 30.1 percent were on treatment but were not under adequate control, that is, they had a blood pressure above 160/95.[35]

Thus, despite all of our attempts to improve adherence to therapy, fewer than half of those who are aware of their diagnosis are being effectively treated. That number, 46.5 percent, is much better than measured in earlier surveys, but it points to the persisting problems of keeping patients on adequate antihypertensive drug therapy for prolonged periods.

## THE QUESTIONABLE EFFICACY OF AND POOR ADHERENCE TO NONDRUG THERAPIES

We finally come to the major issue: Regardless of how well drugs work, what about the value of nondrug therapies? A critical analysis of the efficacy of the various nondrug therapies in mild hypertension has been performed, examining 37 published reports in which means and standard deviations could be calculated.[2] The effects of treatment were expressed as an "effect size" calculated from the difference between mean blood pressures in treated and control groups, standardized by the variability of blood pressure in the control group (Table 3-4). According to the authors, the effect size is "a measure of the extent of improvement in standard deviation units"; an "effect size of one indicates that after treatment the distribution of blood pressures for the treated group would be reduced by one standard deviation; the average treated patient would then be better off than 84 percent of untreated patients."

Note that weight loss, yoga, and muscle relaxation have an effect size roughly half as great as drug therapy, whereas the overall impact of meditation, biofeedback, exercise, and salt restriction was no greater than that found for placebo. Without attempting to critique this analysis, it should be noted that some of the better studies on weight loss, exercise and salt restriction had not been published in time for inclusion in this survey. They will be discussed below.

### Modification of Diet

**Caloric Restriction.** Significant effects have been reported with weight loss, both in moderately and massively overweight hypertensives. Among 212 hypertensives who started at least 10 per-

**Table 3-4.** Effects of Treatment on Hypertension (Effect size of 1.0 = Decrease of BP by 1.0 SD)

|  | No. of Studies | Mean Effect Size |
|---|---|---|
| Drugs | 14 | 2.9 |
| Weight loss | 8 | 1.6 |
| Yoga | 23 | 1.4 |
| Muscle relaxation | 9 | 1.4 |
| Meditation | 21 | 0.7 |
| Exercise | 6 | 0.7 |
| Biofeedback | 13 | 0.7 |
| Salt restriction | 10 | 0.6 |
| Placebo | 5 | 0.6 |

(From Andrews G, MacMahon SW, Austin A, et al: Hypertension: Comparison of drug and non-drug treatments. Br Med J 284: 1523. Reproduced by permission of the Authors and Editors of the British Medical Journal.)

cent above ideal weight, 128 (58 percent) remained on a 1080 calorie diet long enough to reduce their percent of excess weight by five percent.[8] With each 1 percent fall in percentage overweight, they had about a 2.2 mm Hg fall in systolic BP and a 1.4 mm Hg fall in diastolic BP. The patients were advised not to reduce their sodium intake and their daily sodium excretion at the end of the study was not below that of a control group. Thus, the fall in blood pressure was likely attributable solely to the weight loss.

Similar falls in blood pressure were seen among more massively obese patients who lost an average of 20 kg during 12 weeks on a 320 calorie per day diet.[41] Those given 120 mmol/day of sodium had just as much of a fall in blood pressure as did those on a 40 mmol/day total intake.

In the Multiple Risk Factor Intervention Trial (MRFIT), 879 hypertensive men (DBP 90 to 104) who were 15 percent or more above their desirable weight followed a fat-modified eating plan for up to 16 weeks.[6] Of the 879, 370 had a fall of their DBP to below 90 mm Hg and 35 percent of the entire group had not required the institution of drug therapy when seen at the fourth annual visit.

In the MRFIT trial, the use of both diuretics and beta-blockers to treat hypertension caused a rise in plasma triglycer-

ide and a fall in high-density lipoprotein cholesterol (HDL-C) levels.[39] Moderate long-term weight loss prevented these unfavorable lipid changes.

With weight loss achieved by caloric restriction, various hormonal systems are quieted, which may help explain the lowering of blood pressure. In 20 obese patients, weight loss was accompanied by falls in plasma norepinephrine, epinephrine, renin activity and aldosterone.[38]

**Moderate Sodium Restriction.** A large body of evidence incriminates the greatly excessive intake of sodium in most modern diets as being necessary though not sufficient cause for primary hypertension.[15] Most acculturated people ingest amounts of sodium far in excess of any possible physiological need. Such high sodium intake is likely part of the pathogenesis of hypertension and it complicates the treatment of the disease.

Rigid salt restriction was shown to lower the blood pressure at a time (the 1940s) when little else was available for therapy. Kempner's rice diet was effective because it was so low in sodium.[42] But Watkin et al. concluded that "protracted effective maintenance of the Kempner regimen . . . imposes such hardship upon the patient and so much difficulty in control as to make it virtually impractical for general use."[42]

After thiazides were introduced dur-

**Table 3-5.** Modest Sodium Restriction in Hypertension

| Reference | No. | Sodium Excretion (mmol/day) | | Duration | Blood Pressure (mm Hg) | |
| --- | --- | --- | --- | --- | --- | --- |
| | | Pre | Post | | Pre | Post |
| Parijs (1973) | 17 | 191 | 93 | 4 wks | 147/98 | −9/6 |
| Carney (1975) | 19 | 205 | >120 (3) <120 (12) | 8 wks | 163/106 | −15/7 |
| Magnani (1976) | 37 | | | 15–21 mo | 166/105 | −14/14 |
| Morgan (1978) | 28 | 191 | 157 | 24 mo | 160/97 | DBP<95 in 55% |
| | | | | | DBP | DBP |
| Morgan and Myers (1981) | 12M < 105 | 197 | 78 | 8 wks | 97 | 87 |
| | 12F < 105 | 146 | 58 | | 95 | 89 |
| | 12M > 105 | 171 | 85 | | 115 | 103 |
| | 12M > 105 | 125 | 64 | | 111 | 101 |
| MacGregor (1982) | 19 | 191 | 86 | 4 wks | 156/98 | −12/6 |

ing the late 1950s and their mode of action shown to involve a mild state of sodium depletion, both physicians and patients eagerly adopted this form of therapy in place of dietary sodium restriction. But the changeover was too sweeping and in many instances proved detrimental. In discarding rigid salt restriction, physicians disregarded the benefits of modest restriction both for its inherent antihypertensive effect and for its potential of reducing diuretic-induced hypokalemia. Moreover, many fail to realize that the amount of salt ingested by many patients, 15 to 20 g per day, may completely overcome the antihypertensive effectiveness of diuretics.

There are two main benefits of moderate sodium restriction to a level of 2,000 mg of sodium or 5 g of sodium chloride per day, approximately half of our usual intake.

**Antihypertensive Effect.** Such modest restriction of dietary sodium intake may cause the blood pressure to fall 5 to 10 mm Hg (Table 3-5). In those subsequently given a diuretic, the lower sodium intake also potentiates the effect of the diuretic. Notice that even less sodium restriction may be effective: In the Morgan et al 1978 study, 28 patients who reduced their average sodium excretion from 195 to 157 mmol/day over a 2-year interval

had a 7.3 mm Hg fall in DBP whereas a control group had a 1.8 mm Hg rise.[26]

Perhaps the best published study of moderate sodium restriction is that of MacGregor et al.[19] (Fig. 3-5). In this study, 19 mild hypertensives (average initial BP = 156/98) all ingested a diet moderately restricted in sodium, lowering their daily urinary sodium excretion from 191 to 86 mmol. Thereafter they were randomly given, in a double-blind manner, either placebo tablets or enough sodium chloride tablets to bring their daily sodium intake up to 162 mmol. After 4 weeks on one regimen, they were crossed over to the other. Notice the lowering of the blood pressure by an average of 12/6 mm Hg on the moderate sodium restriction, and the prompt return of the pressure to initial levels with reinstitution of the higher sodium intake. It should be noted that 7 of the 19 patients did not have a fall in BP on the lower sodium intake.

The manner by which such moderate sodium restriction usually lowers the blood pressure may involve a number of mechanisms. When the dietary sodium intake was reduced from 200 to 50 mmol/day for two weeks in a group of normotensive subjects, the following were observed: (1) a lesser pressor response to exogenous norepinephrine; (2) a lesser pressor response to mental stress; and,

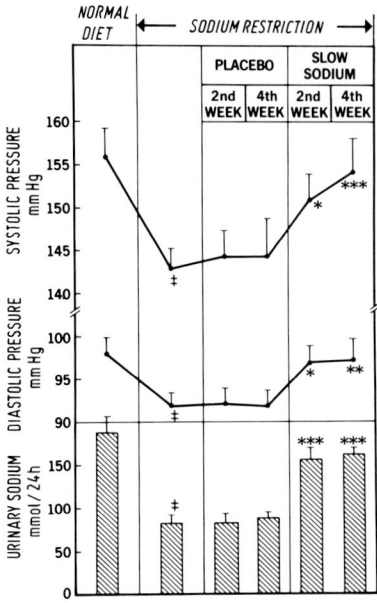

**Fig. 3-5.** The average systolic and diastolic blood pressure and urinary sodium excretion on a normal diet, two weeks after dietary sodium restriction, and at two-weekly intervals during the randomized crossover trial of placebo or sodium chloride tablets (Slow Sodium) (*p < 0.05, **p < 0.01, ***p < 0.001 comparing equivalent measurements of slow sodium to placebo; ≠p < 0.001 comparing measurement on normal diet to two weeks of dietary sodium restriction). (From MacGregor GA, Markandu ND, Best FE, et al: Double-blind randomised crossover trial of moderate sodium restriction in essential hypertension. Lancet 1: 351, 1982.)

(3) a rise in plasma norepinephrine levels.[36] When 25 young borderline hypertensives were randomly given either a 6- to 10-g or a 3- to 5-g sodium diet for 6-week intervals, they experienced little fall in blood pressure at rest while on the lower sodium intake but had significantly lesser rises in both systolic and diastolic

pressures during both mental and physical stress.[1] Moreover, the sodium content of lymphocytes, high in the untreated hypertensives, fell on the lower sodium intake and the diastolic blood pressure changes during stress were tightly correlated with the sodium content of the lymphocytes. Higher intracellular sodium, either from genetically determined changes in sodium transport[24] or from acquired increases in a circulating inhibitor of sodium transport[15] may be a primary mechanism in the pathogenesis of hypertension. Perhaps dietary sodium restriction will reverse or at least reduce the abnormality.

**Protection from Diuretic-Induced Potassium Loss.** The second benefit of sodium restriction is a reduction in diuretic induced potassium wastage. Unlimited access to dietary sodium and the daily intake of a thiazide diuretic makes every patient vulnerable to the major side effect of diuretic therapy—hypokalemia. The diuretic inhibits sodium reabsorption at the cortical diluting segment, a more proximal part of the distal convoluted tubule, thereby causing more sodium to reach the lower portions of the distal tubule where exchange of potassium for sodium occurs. When thiazides are given daily while the patient ingests large amounts of sodium, the initial diuretic-induced sodium depletion shrinks plasma volume, activating renin release and secondarily increasing aldosterone secretion. The increased amounts of aldosterone increase sodium reabsorption at the distal exchange site, thereby increasing potassium secretion into the urine. On daily diuretic therapy, the plasma potassium falls an average of 0.6 mmol/L.[25] With such diuretic-induced hypokalemia, increased ventricular ectopic activity has been recorded (see Chapter 9).[11]

With modest sodium restriction, less sodium would be delivered to the distal exchange site and therefore less potassium swept into the urine. This modest restriction should not further activate the renin-angiotensin-aldosterone mechanism to cause more distal tubular sodium-for-potassium exchange since such activation usually occurs only with more rigid sodium restriction. More rigid sodium restriction, impractical as it is, could be counterproductive: by inducing further secondary aldosteronism, more potassium would be wasted as the diuretic continues to deliver sodium to the distal exchange site.[18]

When this postulate was tested in 12 hypertensive patients, the results were confirmatory.[31] The patients were given one of three diuretics for 4-week intervals while ingesting a diet with either 72 mmol/day or 195 mmol/day of sodium. While on the modestly restricted diet, total body potassium levels fell only half as much.

To improve patient's adherence to dietary sodium restriction, two techniques for easier monitoring of urinary sodium content have been helpful: (1) the use of overnight rather than 24 hour urine collections; and, (2) the performance of an immediate assay or urine sodium using the Ames Quantab Chloride Titrator sticks.[16] With these, patients can be advised immediately of their degree of adherence and given additional counseling if needed.

With less sodium in the diet, more potassium will usually be present, since foods with little sodium usually have high potassium. Salt substitutes may be either half (i.e., Lite-Salt) or pure (i.e., No-Salt) potassium. Other than for patients with renal insufficiency who may be unable to handle potassium loads, the extra potassium may be helpful.

Beyond the prevention of diuretic-induced hypokalemia, there may be an extra benefit from increasing dietary potassium and that is a lowering of the blood pressure. In a study of 20 normo-tensives, the intake of 200 mmol per day of potassium reduced the blood pressure by at least five mm Hg in half and, when combined with a 50 mmol per day sodium intake, prevented the rise in plasma catecholamines seen with the lower sodium diet when used without the extra potassium.[36] These beneficial effects of extra potassium were related to a natriuresis and an increased sensitivity of the baroreceptor reflex. For many years, some have advocated a higher potassium intake along with a lower sodium intake in hopes of preventing hypertension.

**Other Dietary Changes.** There may be beneficial effects of changes in diet beyond caloric and sodium restriction: a high fiber intake for four weeks was accompanied by a 3 to 5 percent reduction in blood pressure[43] and an increase in dietary polyunsaturated fatty acids for 6 weeks lowered the blood pressures of another group of hypertensives.[32] The effect of the high fiber intake may be related to a decrease in sodium intake, whereas the effect of the higher polyunsaturated fat intake was attributed to a possible increase in vasodilatory prostaglandin synthesis. Vegetarians had 5 to 10 mm Hg lower blood pressures than age-, sex-, and weight-matched omnivores.[34]

## Relaxation Therapies

Various relaxation techniques—including transcendental meditation (TM), yoga, biofeedback and muscle relaxation—have all been shown to reduce the blood pressure of hypertensive patients at least transiently. Recall the survey of Andrews et al. (Table 3-4) showing that yoga and muscle relaxation have been found to have significant blood pressure lowering effect but meditation and biofeedback have not.

Recent studies have examined the duration of effect and the applicability of

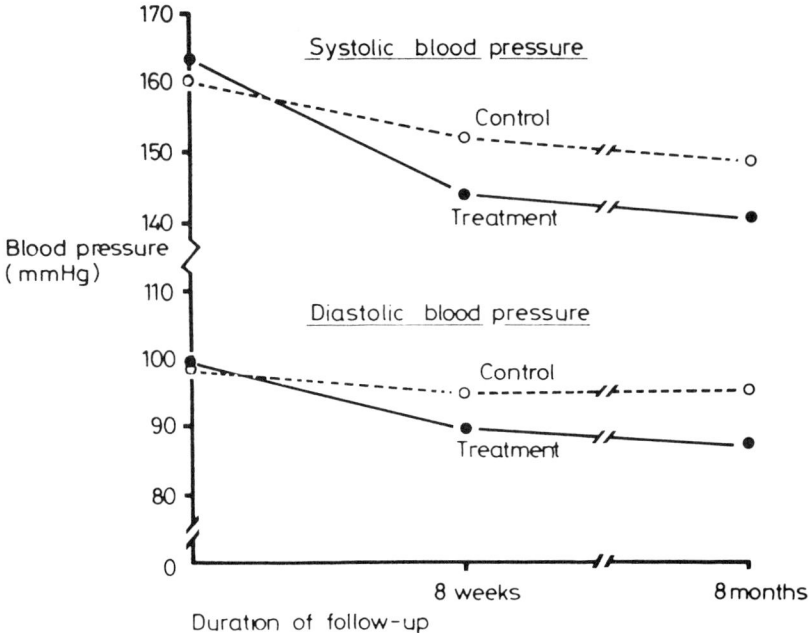

**Fig. 3-6.** The changes in systolic and diastolic blood pressures at eight weeks and eight months in a group of 50 hypertensives who received biofeedback-aided relaxation therapy for the initial eight weeks compared to a control group of 43 hypertensives (from Patel C, Marmot MG, Terry DJ: Controlled trial of biofeedback-aided behavioural methods in reducing mild hypertension. Br Med J 282:2005, 1981. Reproduced by permission of the Authors and Editors of the British Medical Journal)

such procedures to the general hypertensive population. Perhaps the most impressive study is that of Patel et al.[30] who identified hypertensives in a screening program at an English industrial firm and randomly assigned half to a biofeedback-aided relaxation program for eight weeks, while the other half served as controls. Both at the end of the active relaxation program and 6 months later (during which time the subjects had been asked to continue to practice relaxation but had not been seen), the blood pressures of the treated group were significantly lower (Fig. 3-6). Moreover, both plasma renin and aldosterone levels were lower at eight weeks in those undergoing relaxation, suggesting the changes were occurring in at least one of the mechanisms controlling the blood pressure. Pa-

tients who elicit the relaxation response have higher plasma norepinephrine levels after stress but no greater rises in pulse or blood pressure, suggesting a lesser end-organ responsivity to adrenergic stimulation.[10] My conclusion about all of this is that if it is available and acceptable to the patient, one or another form of relaxation therapy should be tried. There seems little to lose and perhaps a great deal to gain, although patients should be forewarned that short-term effects may not be maintained, so that continued surveillance is needed.

## Exercise

Many people are walking, jogging, and performing various other exercises in hopes of achieving various goals related to cardiovascular fitness. A reduction in elevated blood pressure may be one of these goals.[3] Though the evidence doesn't prove that this will happen (see Table 3-4), there seems no reason to curtail reasonable isotonic exercise in patients with mild to moderate hypertension. On the other hand, isometric exercise may be harmful. During isometric or static exercise—pushing, pulling, lifting—both the diastolic and systolic pressures and heart rate increase, in response to reflexes which abruptly withdraw vagal tone and increase peripheral resistance.[33] Since there are no good effects of isometric exercise and the high pressures attained during sustained muscular contraction may precipitate angina, congestive failure, and cerebral hemorrhage, hypertensives should be warned not to perform isometrics. This is particularly necessary since advertisements for isometric devices which falsely offer improved cardiovascular fitness may entice hypertensive patients who are concerned about their health.

### Moderate Alcohol Consumption

Heavy alcohol consumption, that is, more than 3 oz of ethanol per day, either causes or aggravates hypertension, in addition to increasing overall and cardiovascular mortality.[17] Some studies purport to show a deleterious effect of any degree of alcohol consumption on the blood pressure but a critical review reveals that this appears to be true only for heavy drinking and mainly among men.[5] The regular consumption of light to moderate amounts of alcohol, equivalent to one to two ounces of ethanol per day, has been shown to be associated with lower rates of coronary heart disease.[17] This may reflect a rise in HDL-cholesterol. Therefore, light to moderate consumption of alcohol may help hypertensives improve their overall cardiovascular

risk status, while likely not altering their blood pressure.

## THE PROBLEM OF COMPLIANCE

These various nondrug therapies will reduce the blood pressure of many hypertensives, in some to a level that is safe enough to eliminate the need for drug therapy. One or more of these nondrug therapies should be tried in all patients. Those with mild hypertension may thereby be able to stay off drugs, those with more severe hypertension may need less medication.

Part of what appears to be an antihypertensive effect of these nondrug therapies may be attributable to the "natural" fall in blood pressure seen when repeated readings are taken. Such falls may reflect a statistical regression toward the mean, a placebo effect, or a relief of anxiety and stress with time. The same phenomenon is likely responsible for much of the initial response to drug therapy as well, so both drugs and nondrugs may be given credit not deserved by either.

Many practitioners, though they recognize the potential benefits of these nondrug treatments, do not use them because they are too much trouble. The time and effort needed to instruct and motivate patients to use these therapies is undoubtedly greater than that needed to write a prescription. But various nonphysician practitioners—nurses, dieticians, psychologists—are available in most places to help in the effort. Numerous pamphlets, books, and audiovisual materials are also available to help instruct and motivate patients. Among these is "Prevent Your Heart Attack" (Scribner's and Sons, New York, 1982), which provides practical advice on following all of the nondrug therapies described earlier.

Despite all of these aides, it's true that many patients won't adhere to non-drug therapies. But remember that poor compliance is also a major problem with drug treatment as well. The same techniques known to improve compliance to drug therapy should be used with non-drug therapies: a gentle seduction, not a massive onslaught, should be used. Too many and too drastic changes in life-style may be counterproductive: though perhaps good for the patient, they may be more than many are willing to accept and they may reject all therapy. Therefore, nondrug therapies should be introduced gradually and gently.

## SUMMARY

This seems to be a reasonable approach to the use of nondrug therapies in the treatment of hypertensive patients:

1. Obese patients should be encouraged to follow a low calorie diet, and all should be asked to decrease their intake of saturated fats and cholesterol.

2. A moderately restricted sodium intake of 4 to 6 g of sodium chloride (2 g or 70 to 100 mmol of sodium) daily should be tried in all patients—more rigid restriction may be needed in those with renal insufficiency or heart failure.

3. Relaxation and relief of stress, by one or another technique, may be helpful. Tranquilizers and sedatives, though they do not lower the pressure permanently, may be helpful in getting extremely tense patients over the initial stress of the discovery of their hypertension.

4. Isotonic exercise may lower the blood pressure. Isometric exercise is potentially harmful and should be discouraged.

5. Alcohol intake should be moderated. Those who drink one to two ounces a day need not be asked to stop.

6. Attention should be given to other risk factors for cardiovascular disease; smoking, in particular, should be discouraged.

If introduced with enthusiasm and carefully monitored, such nondrug therapies will work.[40] In a 5-year study of a group of 67 obese hypertensive men given nutritional advice about calories, fat and sodium, encouraged to exercise and to stop smoking, success was accomplished—without drugs. The men lost an average of 10 pounds, had a fall of 12/9 mm Hg in blood pressure and 25 mg/dl in cholesterol. Thus, nondrug therapies should be enthusiastically tried in all hypertensives since they have a potential for great benefits with no risks.

## REFERENCES

1. Ambrosioni E, Costa FV, Borghi C, et al: Effects of moderate salt restriction on intralymphocytic sodium and pressor response to stress in borderline hypertension. Hypertension 4:789, 1982.
2. Andrews G, MacMahon SW, Austin A, et al: Hypertension: Comparison of drug and non-drug treatments. Br Med J 284:1523, 1982.
3. Bjorntorp P: Hypertension and exercise. Hypertension 4 (suppl III): 1982.
4. Carney S, Morgan T, Wilson M, et al: Sodium restriction and thiazide diuretics in the treatment of hypertension. Med J Aust 1:803, 1975.
5. Celentano DD, Martinez RM, McQueen DV: The association of alcohol consumption and hypertension. Prev Med 10:590, 1981.
6. Cohen JD, Rossa R, Smith K: Weight reduction for the initial management of mild hypertension—The Multiple Risk Factor Intervention Trial (MRFIT) Results. Circulation 64 (suppl IV) (abstr): 214, 1981.
7. Curb JD, Borhani NO, Blaszkowski T, et al: Adverse reactions to antihypertensive drugs in the Hypertension Detection and

Follow-up Program (HDFP). Circulation 66 (suppl II) (abstr): 328, 1982.

8. Eliahou HE, Iaina A, Gaon T, et al: Body weight reduction necessary to attain normotension in the overweight hypertensive patient. Int J Obes 5 (suppl 1):157, 1981.

9. Freis ED: Should mild hypertension be treated? N Engl J Med 307:306, 1982.

10. Hoffman JW, Benson H, Arns PA, et al: Reduced sympathetic nervous system responsivity associated with the relaxation response. Science 215:190, 1982.

11. Holland OB, Nixon JV, Kuhnert L: Diuretic-induced ventricular ectopic activity. Am J Med 70:762, 1981.

12. Hypertension Detection and Follow-up Program Cooperative Group: The effect of treatment on mortality in "mild" hypertension. N Engl J Med 307:976, 1982.

13. Kannel WB: Importance of hypertension as a major risk factor in cardiovascular disease. In Genest J, Koiw E, Kuchel O, Eds: Hypertension Physiopathology and Treatment. McGraw-Hill, New York, 1977, pp. 888–909.

14. Kaplan NM: Whom to treat: The dilemma of mild hypertension. Am Heart J 101:867, 1981.

15. Kaplan NM: Clinical Hypertension. 3rd Ed. Williams and Wilkins, Baltimore, 1982.

16. Kaplan NM, Simmons M, McPhee C, et al: Two techniques to improve adherence to dietary sodium restriction in the treatment of hypertension. Arch Intern Med 142:1638, 1982.

17. Klatsky AL, Friedman GD, Siegelaub AB: Alcohol and Mortality. Ann Intern Med 95:139, 1981.

18. Landmann-Suter R, Struyvenberg A: Initial potassium loss and hypokalaemia during chlorthalidone administration in patients with essential hypertension: the influence of dietary sodium restriction. Eur J Clin Invest 8:155, 1978.

19. MacGregor GA, Markandu ND, Best FE, et al: Double-blind randomised crossover trial of moderate sodium restriction in essential hypertension. Lancet 1:351, 1982.

20. Magnani B, Ambrosioni E, Agosta R, et al: Comparison of the effects of pharma-cological therapy and a low-sodium diet on mild hypertension. Clin Sci Mol Med 51:625s, 1976.

21. Management Committee: The Australian Therapeutic Trial in Mild Hypertension. Lancet 1:1261, 1980.

22. Management Committee: Untreated mild hypertension. Lancet 1:185, 1982.

23. Medical Research Council Working Party: Adverse reactions to bendrofluazide and propranolol for the treatment of mild hypertension. Lancet 2:539, 1981.

24. Meyer P, Garay RP, Nazaret C, et al: Inheritance of abnormal erythrocyte cation transport in essential hypertension. Br Med J 282:1114, 1981.

25. Morgan DB, Davidson C: Hypokalaemia and diuretics: An analysis of publications. Br Med J 280:905, 1980.

26. Morgan T, Adam W, Gillies A, et al: Hypertension treated by salt restriction. Lancet 1:227, 1978.

27. Morgan TO, Myers JB: Hypertension treated by sodium restriction. Med J Aust 2:396, 1981.

28. Multiple Risk Factor Intervention Trial Research Group: Multiple risk factor intervention trial. JAMA 248:1465, 1982.

29. Parijs J, Joossens JV, der Linden LV, et al: Moderate sodium restriction and diuretics in the treatment of hypertension. Am Heart J 85:22, 1973.

30. Patel C, Marmot MG, Terry DJ: Controlled trial of biofeedback-aided behavioural methods in reducing mild hypertension. Br Med J 282:2005, 1981.

31. Ram CVS, Garrett BN, Kaplan NM: Moderate sodium restriction and various diuretics in the treatment of hypertension: Effects on potassium wastage and blood pressure control. Arch Intern Med 141:1015, 1981.

32. Rao RH, Rao UB, Srikantia SG: Effect of polyunsaturate-rich vegetable oils on blood pressure in essential hypertension. Clin Exp Hypertension 3:27, 1981.

33. Riendl AM, Gotshall RW, Reinke JA, et al: Cardiovascular response of human subjects to isometric contraction of large and small muscle groups (39630). Proc Soc Exp Biol Med 154:171, 1977.

34. Rouse IL, Armstrong BK, Beilin LJ: Vege-

tarian diet, lifestyle and blood pressure in two religious populations. Clin Exp Pharmacol Physiol 9:327, 1982.

35. Rowland M, Roberts J: Blood pressure levels and hypertension in persons ages 6–74 years: United States, 1976–80. Advance Data 84:1, 1982.

36. Skrabal F, Aubock J, Hortnagl H: Low sodium/high potassium diet for prevention of hypertension: Probable mechanisms of action. Lancet 2:895, 1981.

37. Society of Actuaries and Association of Life Insurance Medical Directors of America: Blood Pressure Study 1979, Recording and Statistical Corp., 1980.

38. Sowers JR, Nyby M, Stern N, et al: Blood pressure and hormone changes associated with weight reduction in the obese. Hypertension 4:686, 1982.

39. Stamler J, Caggiula A, Christakis G, et al: Smoking, antihypertensive medication and diet-induced falls in plasma lipids-lipoproteins: 4-Year experience in the multiple risk factor intervention trial (MRFIT) (abstr). Circulation 64:IV-42, 1981.

40. Stamler J, Farinaro E, Mojonnier LM, et al: Prevention and control of hypertension by nutritional-hygienic means: Long-term experience of the Chicago coronary prevention evaluation program. JAMA 243: 1819, 1980.

41. Tuck ML, Sowers J, Dornfeld L, et al: The effect of weight reduction on blood pressure, plasma renin activity, and plasma aldosterone levels in obese patients. N Engl J Med 304: 930, 1981.

42. Watkin DM, Froeb HF, Hatch FT, et al: Effects of diet in essential hypertension: I. Baseline study: Effects in eighty-six cases of prolonged hospitalization on regular hospital diet. Am J Med 9:428, 1950.

43. Wright A, Burstyn PG, Gibney MJ: Dietary fibre and blood pressure: Br Med J 2:1541, 1979.

# The Case for Pharmacological Treatment

## Edward D. Frohlich, M.D.

Scarcely 30 years ago, discussions concerning treatment of high blood pressure were concerned primarily about whether its therapy would be of value in patients with malignant hypertension. Over the ensuing years, we have come to accept the efficacy of pharmacological therapy not only for the patients with the most severe forms of high blood pressure (i.e., diastolic pressures more than 129 mm Hg[56]) but also for patients with diastolic pressures over 114 mm Hg,[57] and from 90 through 114 mm Hg.[58] Moreover, we now generally hold that antihypertensive therapy is both safe and efficacious in all patients who demonstrate persistently elevated diastolic arterial pressures in excess of 104 mm Hg.[23,58] Therefore, few authorities now doubt that pharmacological therapy for these patients is acceptable and valid. [10,23,26,41,49,56,57–58]

What remains for debate at this time is whether the patient with the milder expression of hypertension merits antihypertensive therapy at all. But, to engage in this dialogue would be pointless unless we define the terms used: treatment, antihypertensive and pharmacological therapy, and mild hypertension. Even with such a precise measurement and physiologically identifiable point as a diastolic pressure of 104 mm Hg, more specific definition is necessary. Even if authorities agree with these definitions, we must inject the usual caveats that all of the data required for support of both points of view of this discussion are not yet available. Several important ongoing, prospective clinical and epidemiological studies remain to be reported.

Nevertheless, I believe that sufficient evidence is already available to permit these definitions; and if the terms are mutually acceptable, I believe they provide support for the proposition that patients with mild hypertension are at sufficient risk of increased morbidity and mortality to warrant effective therapy to reduce diastolic pressure to levels less than 90 mm Hg. To be more specific, I cannot visualize any worker in the hypertension "vineyards" over these years who would deny the inescapable conclusion: All patients with mild hypertension should come under vigorous medical management of their elevated arterial pressures. To my way of thinking, the only remaining question to this major medical concern is, *"How?"* It is the purpose of this thesis to justify the safety and merit of pharmacological therapy under certain circumstances.

## DEFINITIONS

One need not be a longstanding member of a first-rate debating society to know that before embarking on a debate of any controversial subject he must carefully and precisely define the terms he will use.

### Any Specific Level of Arterial Pressure (in mm Hg)

At first thought, it might be concluded that whenever a level of arterial

93

pressure is specifically defined to the millimeter of mercury, it is a very precise point. However, it is not sufficiently precise unless the conditions of pressure measurement are defined. If we are to say that diastolic pressures of 90 mm Hg and higher in any patient should be treated, a variety of assumptions must be made that take into consideration certain presuppositions. For this discussion, I have chosen to define the level of 90 mm Hg and higher according to the following conditions: (1) the patient must have been at rest for at least 5 minutes; (2) the pressure should be taken in the supine or sitting position; (3) the sphygmomanometer (preferably a mercury column instrument) must have been calibrated and fixed at a level appropriate for the patient; (4) the pressure cuff must be appropriate for the size of that patient's arm; (5) the patient must not be receiving any form of medication (including oral contraceptives, nosedrops, etc.) that might affect the arterial pressure reading; (6) the pressure must be the same in both arms (or the higher of the two arms); (7) the patient must not have any occluding clothing around the arm that would preclude valid pressure measurement; (8) the patient should not have smoked a cigarette or ingested any drug, including caffeine-containing beverage, within 30 minutes of the measurement; (9) under the foregoing conditions, this level of pressure elevation must have been confirmed on three separate occasions on an outpatient basis; and (10) confirmed under the same conditions each time. Thus having demonstrated diastolic pressure levels of 90 mm Hg or more, I would then agree that this indeed is a patient with sustained diastolic pressure elevation above 89 mm Hg. This individual is already at an increased risk of morbidity and mortality.[25,39,60]

## Mild Hypertension

The foregoing having been stated, I strongly believe that no specific level of arterial pressure confers upon any *individual* patient a prognostic state of severity that relates to his hypertensive vascular disease. We have all seen patients under usual office conditions (even if in the hospital) whose diastolic pressure was 120 mm Hg, or more, and who had no evidence of target organ involvement. We have similarly followed patients with diastolic pressures far lower who had definite and unequivocal evidence of target organ involvement from hypertension. Nevertheless, for the sake of this controversial dialogue, I accept the definition that patients whose diastolic pressures on three different occasions exceeded 90 mm Hg but were less than 105 mm Hg have *mild hypertension*. Patients with this degree of arterial pressure elevation are

**Table 3-6.** Summary of the Major Prospective Multicenter Antihypertensive Therapeutic Trials Involving Patients with Mild Essential Hypertension

| Study | Patients (number) | Diastolic Pressure (mm Hg) | Control for Step-Care | Reduced Complications (%) |
|---|---|---|---|---|
| VA Cooperative Study (1970) | 170 | 90–104 | Placebo | 35 |
| USPHS (1977) | 389 | 90–104 | Placebo | 44 |
| HDFP (1979) | 7825 | 90–104 | "Referred care" | 20 |
| Australian (1980) | 3427 | 95–109 | Placebo | 30 |
| Oslo (1980) | 785 | 90–109 | No treatment | 25 |
| MRFIT (1982) | 8012 | 90–120 | "Usual care" | 2 (increase) |

(Adapted from Kaplan NM: Therapy for hypertension: Toward a more balanced view. JAMA 249:365, 1983. Copyright 1983, American Medical Association.)

still included in prospective clinical trials designed to determine the efficacy of antihypertensive therapy. Moreover, this is the same definition accepted by other cooperative multicenter trials that I believe permits the justification of treatment.[60]

### Treatment

Certain, possibly obvious, premises need to be stated: all "treatment" is not drug therapy; all therapy need not be pharmacological or even dietary; and, furthermore, any professional interaction between a patient and his physician involves patient management and, as such, is treatment. Every effort will be made in this discussion to define precisely my concept of the role of pharmacological therapy in hypertension.

# HISTORICAL PERSPECTIVE

As indicated, the first prospective data to demonstrate the efficacy of treating hypertension with drugs were provided by treatment programs involving potent antihypertensive agents that, admittedly, produced a plethora of side effects.[51] With time, fortunately, treatment programs were devised that included agents with less disturbing side effects; and the introduction of newer, more specific agents with less bothersome side effects continues to this date.

Efficacy and improvement of antihypertensive agents have been demonstrated by several multicenter studies (Table 3-6). Certain of the studies were designed to specifically evaluate the safety and efficacy of the drugs while others were aimed at studying the therapeutic value of lowered blood pressure.

### V.A. Cooperative Studies

Over these years, under the meticulous supervision of Dr. Edward D. Freis,

a series of landmark multicenter studies were reported that demonstrated the efficacy of antihypertensive drug therapy.[56,57,58] Each of these studies involved randomized allocation of male patients with essential hypertension into pharmacological treatment and placebo groups. The first study reported that drug therapy significantly reduced arterial pressure in patients with severely elevated pressures.[56] Later morbidity and mortality were shown to be reduced in patients whose entry diastolic pressures ranged from 114 through 129 mm Hg.[57] Subsequent studies showed similar efficacy in patients whose diastolic pressures ranged from 90 through 114 mm Hg.[58] However, the conclusions were cautiously interpreted since: (1) only male patients were studied, and (2) there were relatively few patients whose entry diastolic pressures ranged from 90 through 104 mm Hg. Further, and this must be emphasized clearly, the average entry age of the matched groups of patients was 47 years.

Nevertheless, the conclusions were inescapable and the National High Blood Pressure Education Program (HBPEP) recommended that all patients whose repeatedly confirmed diastolic pressures were in excess of 104 mm Hg should be treated pharmacologically.[44] Moreover, a systematized treatment program employing a sequential stepped-care introduction of pharmacological agents was recommended[44] which now includes all patients whose diastolic pressures *repeatedly* (at least on three successive and independent outpatient visits) exceed 89 mm Hg.[23]

The treatment program includes initiating therapy (after an appropriate series of outpatient visits to confirm diastolic pressures of 90 mm Hg and higher) with a thiazide diuretic. To be added in successive stepwise therapeutic increments are any of a variety of adrenergic inhibiting compounds and vasodilators, with the more potent agents being reserved for a final, fourth step.[58]

## U.S. Public Health Service Study

Fortunately, this multicenter clinical trial was begun contemporaneously with the V. A. Cooperative Study for had it been initiated after the above results were reported, the study would not be possible to conduct; placebo "therapy" for study patients would have been deemed unethical. Nevertheless, this randomized clinical trial with patients receiving active and placebo therapy was conducted and yielded very similar results, further supporting the efficacy of antihypertensive therapy in not only reducing mortality but also of morbid events including the development of evidence of hypertensive heart disease.[52] Moreover, this study, like the VA Cooperative Study, failed to show a reduction in events from coronary artery disease.

## V.A.–NIH Cooperative Study

Because of the equivocal nature of the V. A. Cooperative Study results concerning patients whose diastolic pressures ranged from 90 through 104 mm Hg, a new study was initiated to determine the feasibility of a long-term randomized study of these patients with step-one and step-two agents and placebo. This study emphasized the difficulty of recruiting these patients with mild hypertension; repeated outpatient pressures demonstrated a high rate of reduction of diastolic pressure to levels lower than 90 mm Hg (i.e., the phenomenon of regression to the mean).[45] Moreover, this study demonstrated that these patients, often treated with just a single diuretic agent, had more side effects and notable "treatment end-points" than the placebo-treated individuals.[59]

## Hypertension Detection and Follow-Up Program (HDFP)

Nevertheless, still another large-scale multicenter study was initiated. This study randomly allocated approximately 11,000 patients (from over 158,000 screened) into two treatment groups: the stepped-care (SC) group received the specific, antihypertensive stepped-care program (outlined above) including general medical follow-up and vigorous encouragement to remain in therapy and return for clinic visits; the referred-care (RC) group was sent to their personal physicians for routine medical treatment.[19,20] The results of this study were striking. Despite reduction in pressure of both groups of patients to average diastolic pressure levels of less than 90 mm Hg, the SC group demonstrated significantly lower cardiovascular *and* total mortality rates.[19,20] Moreover, in a subsequent report from this study concerning only patients treated for "mild" hypertension (i.e., diastolic pressures ranging from 90 to 104 mm Hg) there was a 28.6 percent reduction in mortality in those patients treated in the SC group.[19–21] Most striking were the differences between the SC and RC groups of patients of stratum I (diastolic pressures of 90 through 104 mm Hg). Specifically, the data point out that 30 myocardial infarctions occurred in the SC group, whereas 56 occurred in the RC group. These data, although not emphasized specifically, point to development of half the number of heart attacks in vigorously treated patients.[19] Also striking was the occurrence of 17 strokes in the SC group and 31 in the RC group. It is important to note that the reduction in mortality was greater in patients whose diastolic pressures ranged from 90 to 104 mm Hg than in the 100 to 104 mm Hg group and not much different in the 90 to 94 mm Hg as compared with the 95 to 99 mm Hg group[6,21] (Ta-

**Table 3-7.** Five-Year Mortality Rates (per 100) Participants in Patients with Mild Hypertension

| Entry Diastolic Pressure (mm Hg) | Stepped-Care (SC) Patients (no.) | | | Referred Care (RC) Patients | | | Decreased SC Deaths (%) |
|---|---|---|---|---|---|---|---|
| | Sample | Deaths | Death Rate | Sample | Deaths | Death Rate | |
| 90–104 | 3903 | 231 | 5.9 | 3922 | 291 | 7.4 | 20.3 |
| 90–94 | 1474 | 84 | 5.7 | 1467 | 107 | 7.3 | 21.9 |
| 95–99 | 1390 | 69 | 5.0 | 1341 | 87 | 6.5 | 23.1 |
| 100–104 | 1039 | 78 | 7.5 | 1114 | 97 | 8.7 | 13.8 |

(From Hypertension Detection and Follow-up Program Cooperative Group: Five-year findings of the Hypertension Detection and Follow-up Program. II. Mortality by race, sex, and age. JAMA 242:2572, 1979. Copyright 1979, The American Medical Association.)

ble 3-7). It was this study and these impressive data that prompted the change in recommendations of the HBPEP to include patients whose confirmed diastolic pressures ranged from 90 through 104 mm Hg.[58] This increased the projected number of potential hypertensive patients in the United States that merited therapy from 23 to 60 million.

## Australian Trial

Soon after publication of the HDFP study, a well-designed multicenter trial was reported from Australia that involved active and placebo-treated patients with mild hypertension whose pressures ranged from 95 through 109 mm Hg.[31,32] Active therapy was similar to VA Cooperative and HDFP studies. Rates of morbidity and mortality were 30 percent lower in the actively treated group. The results also indicated higher rates of cardiovascular complications in those patients having certain pressure levels achieved by drugs as compared to placebo-"treated" patients having the same pressures. These are very subtle, but important, revelations and their implications are obviously controversial. However, one must take into consideration from which pressure levels the "treated" pressures come—not only the comparison of endpoints at the same levels of pressure. Thus, the actively treated patients at a specific pressure level presumably had higher pressures (and over

a longer period of time) than the placebo-treated individuals. Those individuals reporting on the implications of these data have suggested that this study supports the thesis that drug treatment of mild hypertension was shown to be of benefit only in those patients whose diastolic pressures averaged above 95 mm Hg. This argument is not entirely valid since only patients whose diastolic pressures were greater than 95 mm Hg were entered into the study—albeit in some patients pressure fell below 95 mm Hg during follow-up. This phenomenon of regression to the mean* has been observed in all large multicenter studies involving placebo.

## Oslo Study

Another multicenter study involving two groups actively treated or placebo-treated patients with mild and moderately severe hypertension has been reported from Norway.[15] This study, like each of the above placebo-controlled trials (V.A., USPHS, and Australia), showed a reduction in cardiovascular mortality in the treated patients although deaths from myocardial infarction were not reduced. However, there are no data available for analysis concerning patients

---

*Regression to the Mean: A specific statistical term referring the lowering of blood pressure with repeated measurements in untreated patients so that the successive pressures approach the mean for the untreated group.

whose diastolic pressures ranged from 90 through 99 mm Hg at the time of entry into the study.

## MRFIT Study

This multicenter study, the Multiple Risk Factor Intervention Trial (MRFIT), was initiated almost contemporaneously with the HDFP trial in order to determine whether a "special intervention" (SI) program would reduce morbidity and mortality through reducing known predisposing risk factors. The results of this SI group were compared with a randomly assigned second group of patients who were referred to their personal physicians for "usual care" (UC). The results of this long-term study showed a significant reduction in deaths from coronary heart disease (CHD) (and all causes of death) in the SI group.[42] However, this reduction in deaths did not hold for patients with hypertension whose diastolic pressures at the outset of the study were less than 100 mm Hg; and, in fact, those patients whose pretreatment diastolic pressures were between 90 and 94 mm Hg seemed to have more deaths than the patients receiving UC (Table 3-8). It is important to underscore two points related to this study. First, the patients in the SI group, like most of the other stud-

ies, were treated with diuretics as a first step of antihypertensive therapy (usually hydrochlorothiazide or chlorthalidone); and this was probably the only medication received by those patients with 90 to 94 mm Hg at the outset of the study. Second, the private physicians following the UC patients were also treating their patients—albeit, perhaps, less vigorously.

## Other Studies

In addition to the above studies that were concerned with mild hypertension, other multicenter studies have been (and remain) in progress. In Great Britain, a Medical Research Council Study is being conducted.[34] In western Europe, a European Workers Party group study of hypertension in the elderly is ongoing,[2] but it is too early to comment on their results. However, one study reported from Sweden did, in fact, show that treatment of patients with mild hypertension did result in a reduced incidence of CHD.[3] Although questions have been raised concerning several methodological points in this latter study, it is of importance to note that this is the only study (of all discussed) that involved treatment for mild essential hypertension with beta-adrenergic receptor blocking drugs.

**Table 3-8.** Number of CHD and Total Deaths (and mortality rates per 1,000) in Normotensive and Hypertensive Patients of the MRFIT Study

| BP Status at Baseline | Participants (no.) | | CHD Deaths | | Total Deaths | |
|---|---|---|---|---|---|---|
| | SI | UC | SI | UC | SI | UC |
| Normotensive | 2409 | 2445 | 35(14.5) | 45(18.4) | 91(37.8) | 91(37.2) |
| Hypertensive[a] | 4019 | 3993 | 80(19.9) | 79(19.8) | 174(43.3) | 169(42.3) |
| 90–94 mm Hg | 1157 | 1181 | 17(14.7) | 12(10.2) | 47(40.6) | 31(26.2) |
| 95–99 mm Hg | 830 | 846 | 19(22.9) | 19(22.5) | 43(51.8) | 39(46.1) |
| ≥100 mm Hg | 771 | 739 | 16(20.8) | 22(29.8) | 25(32.4) | 45(60.9) |
| Total Group[a] | 6428 | 6438 | 115(17.9) | 124(19.3) | 265(41.2) | 260(40.4) |

[a]Includes patients with hypertension receiving treatment at their second screening visit.

(From Multiple Risk Factor Intervention Trial Research Group: Multiple Risk Factor Interventional Trial. Risk factor changes and mortality results. JAMA 248:1465, 1982. Copyright 1982, The American Medical Association.)

# CRITICISMS AND COMMENTS

In the aftermath of the publication of these multicenter studies, a number of questions have been raised by various authorities. It is important to point out that these leaders in the hypertension area impugn the use of antihypertensive drugs for patients whose diastolic pressures *are less than* 104 mm Hg, *although* some define their "dividing lines" at 95, 100, and 104 mm Hg.[1,10,27,28] The important points upon which all agree are that: (1) therapy is still safe, effective and indicated for all patients whose pretreatment diastolic pressures exceed their respective dividing lines; (2) those patients whose diastolic pressures fall between 90 mm Hg and their respective dividing lines are at increased risk; and (3) patients with mild hypertension are not to be referred to as being "normotensive." However, the major and important concerns that they raise are as follows:

1. Do risks from antihypertensive pharmacological treatment exceed the benefits to be derived from treatment in patients whose diastolic pressures fall below their dividing lines (usually 100 mm Hg)?

2. The "awesome number" of people involved—i.e., in the upwards of 40 million individuals—would severely stress the economy of the involved patients (and their countries) were they to receive drug treatment.

3. They question whether certain methodological flaws are present in the multicenter studies. For example, (a) the VA studies only included men; (b) the HDFP study was not designed to test the effects of pharmacological therapy on mortality; (c) why were total deaths ("all deaths") significantly reduced in the SC and SI groups in the HDFP and MRFIT groups—did certain nonidentified cause(s) for this additional reduction in total mortality also affect the cardiovascular mortality results?

4. All suggest that antihypertensive therapy failed to reduce the prevalence of CHD deaths in the treated patients with mild essential hypertension. These and other well-conceived questions and issues have been raised.

Clearly, answers to these questions are necessary. Unfortunately, these answers will require: time; publication of results from ongoing studies; large amounts of public funds; and modification of existing concepts concerning the ethical issues that they raise.

## Risk/Benefit Ratio of Pharmacological Therapy

We must acknowledge that the greater mortality of the treated patients with mild hypertension was not related to *pharmacological* therapy, per se. For those patients with mild hypertension, therapy was the first step agent, a diuretic, chlorthalidone. The protocols of the V.A., USPHS, HDFP, and MRFIT clearly spelled out the selection of either hydrochlorothiazide or chlorthalidone. Moreover, while serum potassium levels were monitored by the study centers, there was no specified dictum followed in a uniform fashion for repair of potassium deficiency.

In contrast, the physician in the community (the RC, referred care, or UC, usual care, provider) was responding to the ongoing high blood pressure education program in a remarkable fashion. He was screening and detecting increasing numbers of patients with hypertension; and, as a result, greater numbers of patients with hypertension were coming under this management and followup.[30] A cursory review of pharmaceutical sales listings for the "best sellers" reveals their greater attention to the need for repair of hypokalemia. Moreover, the practicing physician had been using the beta-adrenergic receptor blocking drugs for the first-step treatment of hypertension. Thus, one must not focus solely upon data of the SC and SI groups for the higher rates of CHD and total mortality for the mild hypertension. It is indeed possible that intensive diuretic therapy might account for those higher rates; but we must also consider the possibilities of better attention to serum potassium levels by the RC and UC physicians in the community and to their increasing use of the beta blocking drugs.

Moreover, the precise nature of the cardiovascular (or CHD) deaths was not detailed. Presumably, these data can be retrieved by the investigators if funds permit. We must know whether these deaths were related to hypokalemia. What were the serum potassium levels of these patients? Did they have cardiac involvement at entrance to the study (see below)? What were the types of CHD deaths—sudden death, myocardial infarction, aneurysmal rupture, stroke?

## Hypokalemia (See Chapter 9)

A number of prospective clinical studies have demonstrated a greater number of premature cardiac beats in hypokalemic patients treated with diuretics.[17,22,40] Other studies have shown that even untreated patients with hypertension—even with early evidence of cardiac involvement—have a greater incidence of ectopic cardiac beats.[35] It is not, therefore, unreasonable to raise alternative questions: (a) were the greater number of CHD deaths due to hypokalemia induced by diuretics; (b) if so, were these deaths more prevalent in patients with early hypertensive heart disease (and the study designs do not permit retrieval of these data); and (c) would these deaths

have occurred if the patients had been treated with beta-adrenergic blocking drugs or slow-channel calcium blocking drugs or any other antihypertensive agent? Clearly, the last question is of a more rhetorical nature but it should be raised and considered broadly. Answers for these questions may be forthcoming from more penetrating analysis of data derived from the patients involved. Thus, it seems unwise to condemn pharmacological therapy because of possible complications from one class of agents used while excluding other means of effective pharmacological therapy.

## Preexisting Cardiac Disease

Patients with hypertension are predisposed to what I term "dimorphic" heart disease: ischemic, atherosclerotic, or coronary heart disease and hypertensive heart disease. A third cardiac problem is also possible, since hypertensive heart disease is frequently complicated by exogenous obesity.[36,37] Nevertheless, the studies referred to above made no attempt to identify the role of each. The electrocardiographic (ECG) analyses identified either gross evidence of left ventricular hypertrophy or were more concerned with criteria for ischemic heart disease. None of the tabulated data demonstrated incidence of: atrial arrhythmias, left atrial abnormality, differences in these as well as other possible abnormal ECG findings at entrance to the study and during the study—particularly in those patients who died. These are of critical importance if one is to impugn the wisdom of contraindicating *all* pharmacological therapy of patients with mild hypertension. It is imperative for these study groups to retrieve these data and subject them to critical analysis.

It is true that in none of the above-cited studies (except for the one in Sweden) was there a significant reduction in CHD deaths in the treated patients. But, it is appropriate to ask whether, in fact, it is realistic to expect that patients with preexisting CHD at entrance to the study should demonstrate improvement in mortality with all depressor agents. Already discussed is the potential of hypokalemia-inducing agents to aggravate cardiac arrhythmias and thus, perhaps, lead to sudden death. In addition, the age of the patients at the entrance to each of these multicenter studies was greater than 45 years—an age at which significant CHD occurs, even in those individuals who are normotensive. Even in 18- to 21-year-old men who were killed in the Korean and Vietnam wars, there was already significant evidence of atherosclerotic coronary arterial involvement.[9,33] With an agent such as a diuretic that reduces arterial pressure but has no known other "myocardial preserving" potential, why should the natural history of CHD be altered? In contrast, the Swedish study involving the use of beta-adrenergic blocking drugs may have shown a reduction in deaths from CHD.[3] These observations have been reinforced by data from several reports that demonstrated significant reduction in deaths from CHD and reinfarction in those patients with one documented myocardial infarction.[4,16,43]

## Costs of Therapy

It is true that the numbers of patients with treatable hypertension were increased dramatically from 23 to 60 million Americans when the treatable diastolic pressure level was reduced from 105 to 90 mm Hg. Because of this admittedly "awesome" number of patients, the "compliance" problems in asymptomatic patients, and the costs involved, Freis emphasized that we must be absolutely convinced that the potential benefits of therapy outweigh the disadvantages and risks.[10]

Admittedly, the numbers of mildly hypertensive patients are impressive: 40 million people is indeed an "awesome" number. While we know that the incidence of strokes was significantly reduced by therapy in the V. A. studies[56–58] and in the HDFP study,[19] we do not have precise data concerning this complication in the patients with mild hypertension in these reports, nor in the HDFP, MRFIT, and Australian trials. However, we do know that since the widespread emphasis in this country on the treatment of hypertension, there has been a 38 percent reduction in strokes.[30] Such an impressive reduction cannot be accounted for solely on the basis of lowering the blood pressure of only 10 to 25 percent of patients with only moderate and severe hypertension.

Further, the HDFP demonstrated 3.2 deaths per 1,000 person years of treatment. Whether one assumes there are 23 million or 60 million persons who would be the beneficiaries of such treatment, this would account for *an annual* mortality salvage of from 73,600 to 192,000 people. Would not their work productivity, the direct and indirect taxes derived from their work, the prevented hospitalizations, etc., outweigh their costs of medical management and medications—even excluding from our present consideration other humane concerns. Moreover, were therapy to be applied more specifically (and only once daily), problems of side effects (e.g., hypokalemia, hyperuricemia, hyperglycemia) and added medication for their correction would be reduced. Thus, even if we consider the lower 23 million figure, the mortality salvage over the next 20 years would approach 1.5 million Americans!

## Criticisms of Study Design

It is true that the VA studies did not include female patients, but several of the other studies have included women and the same conclusions were reached, at least for patients whose diastolic pressures exceeded 104 mm Hg. It is also true that the HDFP was designed to determine whether vigorous stepped-care treatment was more effective than the regular treatment group. Nevertheless, the SC group did have a lower treatment pressure than the RC group and this was associated with lower cardiovascular and total mortality.

The foregoing is not to disparage the usual treatment provided in the 14 communities, for pressures achieved by the referral physicians in their patients reduced pressure to less than 90 mm Hg. And, this is not to say that these physicians did not treat patients. The reduction in pressure reflected, among other things, the widespread hypertension education programs in the community already discussed above.

A similar argument may be advanced for the results of the UC group of the MRFIT study. Indeed, it is highly likely that if those physicians had not treated their patients with mild hypertension, the treatment pressures of the mildly hypertensive patients would have been significantly higher. And, perhaps, as also suggested above, if they used more beta-adrenergic receptor blocking drugs than the therapists of the SI study group, this also could explain the lower CHD of their group. Clearly, these data are available and should be evaluated carefully by the investigators. The relatively small additional expenditure of funds necessary to do this would be well justified.

### Other Therapy

These personal responses to questions that have been raised do not provide the answers to the criticisms raised. Public funding, being what it is these days, will hardly provide the support required of the studies aimed at obtaining these answers. Studies involving younger patients (under 30 years of age) with hypertension require tremendous numbers to be enrolled; many more people to be screened before patients can be entered; and, in the final analysis, will be fraught with ethical questions that will inevitably be asked by those of the other "school of thought" (i.e., is it ethically justified to withhold therapy that might prove efficacious?). During many of the years involved while the above studies were being conducted, we even delayed acceptance of beta-adrenergic receptor blocking therapy for clinical use for hypertension in the United States. Even now (unlike the rest of the world), we remain reluctant (or, at best, "conditionally tentative") to recommend its use as a first-step approach to therapy—even in some patients.[23]

Now that we have data suggesting that beta-adrenergic receptor blocking drugs are effective in some individuals and that the slow-channel calcium blocking drugs may be effective in patients at the other end of the therapeutic spectrum (e.g., white versus black, young versus old, men versus women, high renin versus low renin etc.), it may be that some answers are at hand. While both forms of therapy lower arterial pressure and are indicated for patients with CHD, they also have been shown to reduce cardiac mass (unlike the diuretics) at least experimentally.[13,14,29] Only time will tell whether this is another unwanted feature of therapy for the patient with mild hypertension.

## RECOMMENDATIONS

At this point in the discussion, I am prepared to suggest my approach to the patient with mild hypertension. This was done with the proviso that we are all entitled to alter our thinking as more knowledge and experience become available.

(1) Patients should not be treated for hypertension with pharmacotherapy until there is repeated documentation of a sustained elevation of diastolic pressure (i.e., greater than 89 mm Hg). Most authorities agree—even those who do not advocate pharmacotherapy of mild hypertension—that this diastolic pressure elevation should be documented on at least three temporally distinct and separated occasions.

(2) Having demonstrated a sustained elevation of diastolic pressure (90 mm Hg and over) the patient should be advised of *all* therapeutic alternatives. These would include nonpharmacological as well as pharmacological therapy. At this time, the advantages and disadvantages of both modalities should be outlined.

We have already outlined the benefits and disadvantages of drug therapy. It is clear that nonpharmacological therapy is advantageous for a variety of obvious reasons. The disadvantages of nonpharmacological therapy are also many: in patients who eat most of their meals out; in inconvenience of label-studying and finding appropriate foods and stores; in possibly higher costs, etc.

(3) Nevertheless, in some individuals nonpharmacological therapy is of value and should be recommended as enthusiastically as drug treatment. In this regard, we must discuss the options.

*Relaxation Therapy.* Whether this be scientific biofeedback techniques or yoga, the reduction in pressure is slight[50] and requires continuous reinforcement and participation—just as with pharmacotherapy. However, at this time, data are not available to warrant this as an acceptable alternative. At best, it is still an experimental approach to the therapy of patients with mild hypertension and is certainly unacceptable for patients with sustained diastolic pressure elevation in excess of 104 mm Hg.

*Exercise Therapy.* Isotonic exercise (e.g., jogging, swimming) has been shown to reduce arterial pressure only slightly in patients with mild hypertension.[5] If this works in the individual patient, fine; but if after a reasonable period of time pressure is not reduced, I would not temporize. My concern is that isotonic exercise increases myocardial mass by volume-loading (i.e., eccentric hypertrophy), whereas the cardiac mass of the patient with hypertension is increased by pressure-loading (i.e., concentric hypertrophy). Already, the cardiovascular risk of other volume- and pressure-loaded individuals (patients with obesity hypertension) is significantly increased.[36,37] We do not know the long-term effects of such exercise therapy on cardiovascular risk and, at least, this point should be raised. In contrast to isotonic exercise, isometric exercise is not well-suited for patients with hypertension. This is a form of cardiovascular stress that not only increases the cardiac output through increasing venous return but also increases arterial pressure through an increased total peripheral resistance.[8,53] To my way of thinking, this is totally unacceptable, clinically or physiologically, in a patient with hypertension.

*Dietotherapy.* Several approaches to dietotherapy remain for discussion. Excess body weight is a physical characteristic of any population of patients with hypertension.[24] In these individuals whose body weight is distinctly abnormal (> 15 percent of ideal body weight), a fair trial of *weight reduction,* even if associated with sodium restriction, is indicated.[47] Arterial pressure in these individuals is reduced by lowering cardiac output[48] and may be independent of reduced sodium intake.[47] In addition, *dietary sodium restriction,* approximately 5 g

(85 millimoles) NaCl daily, is appropriate and not unreasonable. Sodium restriction of this degree may be sufficient by itself to reduce arterial pressure in a large number of patients with mild essential hypertension.[18] Moreover, problems of hypokalemia may be significantly reduced by sodium restriction in those receiving diuretics.[46]

(4) If diastolic pressure is not reduced to levels of less than 90 mm Hg on the above treatment programs, I believe it is not unreasonable to pursue a pharmacological approach for the control of arterial pressure. These patients with persistently but mildly elevated diastolic pressures (90 through 104 mm Hg) are at a distinctly higher cardiovascular risk and their pressures may be controlled easily with one medication administered once daily. This is of particular importance in the patient with a family history of hypertension or premature death, myocardial infarction, or stroke and, certainly, if the patient himself has had a history of myocardial infarctions or stroke or if the patient is black or has diabetes mellitus. Moreover, as reported by Hunt, most patients with mild hypertension would respond to sodium restriction; however, he estimated that 97 percent of the total group would demonstrate control of pressure with the addition of a diuretic agent.[18] More recent information indicates that it is not necessary to restrict monotherapy to this class of antihypertensive agents[18]

*Diuretics.* It is unnecessary to prescribe a thiazide diuretic more than once daily to a patient with uncomplicated hypertension. Over the years, as indicated, we in the United States have come to prescribe the thiazide as a first step in antihypertensive therapy twice daily (e.g., hydrochlorothiazide, 50 mg twice daily). It is more reasonable to initiate therapy with 25 mg in the morning and then, if indicated, to increase this morning dosage by 25 mg. Those patients who are most likely to respond to this modality of therapy are patients whose hypertension has been shown to be more volume-dependent (and, therefore, thiazide or diuretic responsive). These include patients with history of repeated pyelonephritis even if renal function remains normal;[12] who are older (38) or obese[36,37] or black;[7] and who have low plasma renin activity[11] With the preliminary experience reported from the HDFP and MRFIT studies, it is not inappropriate to add a potassium-sparing agent (i.e., amiloride or triamterene) to control serum potassium levels. Since most mildly hypertensive patients will respond to dietary management (sodium restriction and/or weight reduction) and the remainder of these patients will respond to the addition of a diuretic, the number requiring the second, potassium-sparing agent should be less than 10 percent (a likely overestimation).[18] But, even even the number of these patients may be reduced by prescribing first a beta-adrenergic receptor blocking agent.

*Beta Blockers.* Which patients, then, would one select for monotherapy (once daily) of a beta-adrenergic receptor blocking drug? In general, we would start therapy in patients representing the opposite end of the spectrum described above for patients chosen for diuretic therapy: those who are younger,[11] with lean body mass,[36,37] white,[7] without a history of renal infections,[12] and with a medium or high plasma renin activity.[54] In addition, patients with symptoms of a rapid heart action, palpitations, ectopic cardiac beats, and chest discomfort would also be logical responders to this treatment program.[11] Ideally, it would be wise to prescribe a once-daily administered agent and this would include compounds such as atenolol or nadolol (starting with 50 or 40 mg, respectively). Other available beta-adrenergic receptor inhibitors (metoprolol, propranolol) have recently been approved by FDA for once daily administration.

*Calcium Entry Blockers.* Recent reports have indicated that certain patients who might be expected to respond to diuretic therapy may also respond to the administration of a slow-channel calcium influx inhibitor.[55] While many of these agents are presently available for the treatment of hypertension, none of the three available in the United States has FDA approval, at this time, for the treatment of hypertension. Moreover, none of these agents is presently available as once-daily administered agents.

# CONCLUSIONS

Attitudes of physicians toward the treatment of hypertension have become increasingly more sophisticated over these past three decades. Pharmacotherapy is now accepted broadly for all patients whose diastolic pressures exceed 100 or 104 mm Hg. Remaining for resolution is the question of treating those individuals whose diastolic pressures fall between 90 and 100 or 104 mm Hg. These patients are at greater risk for cardiovascular complications and premature death. However, some authorities argue that this risk is exceeded by the inherent risks of pharmacotherapy.

In this discussion, I took the position that any patient whose diastolic pressure persistently exceeds 90 mm Hg should come under continuous medical management. However, before *any* therapeutic decision is made, the advantages and disadvantages or the risks and benefits of *all* therapeutic options should be presented to the patient. Essential to this presentation is a frank and complete disclosure of nonpharmacological as well as pharmacological therapy.

If nonpharmacological means are pursued, this should only be for a finite time—limited by demonstrated control of arterial pressure levels below 90 mm Hg diastolic pressure. This is particularly applicable for patients who have a personal history of myocardial infarction, stroke, diabetes mellitus, or cardiac dysrhythmias; who are black; or who have a family history of hypertension, premature death, myocardial infarction, or stroke.

Pharmacotherapy *in no way* means that only the diuretic is an option for the first step of therapy. The beta-adrenergic receptor blocking drugs and (hopefully, soon in this country) the slow-channel calcium influx inhibitors are available for antihypertensive therapy. These compounds present distinct advantages in certain patients over the diuretics. Let us not condemn an entire means of effective and safe control of arterial pressure (i.e., pharmacotherapy) by equating this alternative with only one class of drugs that may have been best in the 1950's and 1960's. This is 1983 and the next millennium is soon upon us! Furthermore, let us not be turned away from effective mass control of a threatening disease and host of disastrous complications therefrom by the consideration of costs inherent in its treatment. Over these next 20 years, effective antihypertensive therapy of these patients with mild hypertension should permit the continued personal, national, and economic productivity of 1.5 million Americans who would otherwise be doomed to death associated with mild hypertension.

# REFERENCES

1. Alderman M: Mild hypertension: New light on an old clinical controversy. Am J Med 69:653, 1980.
2. Amery A, DeSchaepdryver A: European

Working Party on high blood pressure in elderly (EWPHE): Organization of a double-blind multicenter trial on antihypertensive therapy in elderly patients. Clin Sci Mol Med, 45:suppl. I, 71s 1973.

3. Berglund G, Sannerstedt R, Anderson O: Coronary heart disease after treatment of hypertension. Lancet, 1:1, 1978.

4. Beta-Blocker Heart Attack Study Group: The beta-blocker heart attack trial. JAMA, 246:2073, 1981.

5. Bjorntorp P: Hypertension and exercise. Hypertension, 4:[suppl. III]: 56, 1982.

6. Borhani NO: Should mild hypertension be treated? In Berlyne GM, Ed: Contributions to Nephrology. Vol. 33. Karger, Basel, 1982, p.239.

7. Chrysant SG, Danisa K, Kem DC, et al: Racial differences in pressure, volume and renin inter-relationships in essential hypertension. Hypertension 1:136, 1979.

8. Dunn FG, de Carvalho JGR, Frohlich ED: Hemodynamic, reflexive, and metabolic alterations induced by acute and chronic timolol therapy in hypertensive man. Circulation, 57:140, 1978.

9. Enos WF, Holmes RH, Beyer J: Coronary disease among United States soldiers killed in action in Korea. Preliminary report. JAMA, 152:1090, 1953.

10. Freis ED: Should mild hypertension be treated? N Engl J Med, 307:309, 1982.

11. Frohlich ED: Beta-adrenergic blockade in the circulatory regulation of hyperkinetic states. Am J Cardiol, 27:195, 1971.

12. Frohlich ED, Tarazi RC, Dustan HP: Hemodynamic and functional mechanisms in the two renal hypertensions: Arterial and pyelonephritis. Am J Med Sci, 261:189, 1971.

13. Frohlich ED: Hemodynamics and other determinants in development of left ventricular hypertrophy: Conflicting factors in its regression. Fed Proc 42:2709, 1983.

14. Frohlich ED: The heart in hypertension. In Genest, J, Kuchel O, Hamet P, et al Eds: Hypertension: Physiopathology and Treatment. 2nd Ed. McGraw-Hill Book Company, New York, 1983, p.791.

15. Hegleland A: Treatment of mild hypertension: A five-year controlled drug trial. The Oslo study. Am J Med, 69:725, 1980.

16. Hjalmarson A, Herlitz J, Malek I, et al: Effect on mortality of metoprolol in acute myocardial infarction: A double-blind randomized trial. Lancet, 2:823, 1981.

17. Holland OB, Nixon JF, Kuhnert L: Diuretic-induced ventricular ectopic activity. Am J Med, 70:762, 1981.

18. Hunt JC, Margie JD: The influence of diet on hypertension management. In Hunt JC, Cooper T, Frohlich ED, et al: Eds: Hypertension Update: Mechanisms, Epidemiology, Evaluation, Management. Health Learning Systems, Inc., Bloomfield, Ill. 1980, p 197.

19. Hypertension Detection and Follow-up Program Cooperative Group: Five-year findings of the Hypertension Detection and Follow-up Program. I. Reduction in mortality of persons with high blood pressure, including mild hypertension. JAMA, 242:2562, 1979.

20. Hypertension Detection and Follow-up Program Cooperative Group: Five-year findings of the Hypertension Detection and Follow-up Program. II. Mortality by race, sex and age. JAMA, 242:2572, 1979.

21. Hypertension Detection and Follow-up Program Cooperative Group: The effect of treatment on mortality in "mild" hypertension. N Engl J Med, 307:976, 1982.

22. Johansson BW, Ed: Electrolytes and cardiac arrhythmias. Acta Med Scand Suppl 647:1, 1980.

23. Joint National Committee on Detection, Evaluation, and Treatment of High Blood Pressure: The 1980 report of the Joint National Committee on Detection, Evaluation, and Treatment of High Blood Pressure. Arch Intern Med 140:1280, 1980.

24. Kannel WB, Brand N, Skinner JJ, Jr, et al: The relation of adiposity to blood pressure and development of hypertension: The Framingham Study. Ann Intern Med, 67:48, 1967.

25. Kannel WB, Gordon T, Schwartz MH: Systolic vs diastolic blood pressure and risk of coronary heart disease: The Framingham Study. Am J Cardiol 27:335, 1971.

26. Kaplan NM: Whom to treat: The dilemma of mild hypertension. Am Heart J, 101:867, 1982.

27. Kaplan NM: Mild hypertension: When

and how to treat. Arch Intern Med, 143:255, 1983.

28. Kaplan NM: Therapy for mild hypertension: Toward a more balanced view. JAMA, 249:365, 1983.

29. Kobrin I, Sesoko S, Pegram BL, Frohlich ED: Reduced cardiac mass by nitrendipine is dissociated from systemic or regional hemodynamic changes in rats. Cardiovasc. Res. (In Press).

30. Levy RI, Moskowitz J: Cardiovascular research: decades of progress, a decade of promise. Science 217:121, 1982.

31. Management Committee: The Australian therapeutic trial in mild hypertension. Lancet, 1:1261, 1980.

32. Management Committee of the Australian Therapeutic Trial in Mild Hypertension: Untreated mild hypertension. Lancet, 1:185, 1982.

33. McNamara JJ, Molot MA, Stremble JF, et al: Coronary artery disease in combat casualties in Vietnam. JAMA 216:1185, 1971.

34. Medical Research Council Working Party: Adverse reactions to bendrofluazide and propranolol for the treatment of mild hypertension. Lancet, 2:539, 1981.

35. Messerli FH, Glade LB, Elizardi DG, et al: Cardiac rhythm, arterial pressure, and urinary catecholamines in hypertension with and without left ventricular hypertrophy (abstr) Am J Cardiol, 47:480, 1981.

36. Messerli FH, Christie B, de Carvalho JGR, et al: Obesity and essential hypertension: Hemodynamics, intravascular volumes, sodium excretion, and plasma renin activity. Arch Intern Med, 141:81, 1981.

37. Messerli FH, Ventura HO, Reisin E, et al: Borderline hypertension and obesity: Two different prehypertensive states with high cardiac output. Circulation, 66:55, 1982.

38. Messerli FH, Sundgaard-Riise K, Ventura HO, et al: Essential hypertension in the elderly: Hemodynamics, intravascular volume, plasma renin activity and circulating catecholamine levels. Lancet 2:983, 1983.

39. Metropolitan Life Insurance Company: Blood Pressure: Insurance experience and its implication. New York, 1961.

40. Morgan DB, Davidson C: Hypokalemia and diuretics: An analysis of publications. Br Med J 280:905, 1980.

41. Moser M: "Less severe" hypertension: Should it be treated? Am Heart J, 101:465, 1982.

42. Multiple Risk Factor Intervention Trial Research Group: Multiple Risk Factor Intervention Trial. Risk factor changes and mortality results. JAMA, 248:1465, 1982.

43. The Norwegian Multicenter Study Group: Timolol-induced reduction in mortality and reinfarction in patients surviving acute myocardial infarction. N Engl J Med 304:801, 1981.

44. Perry HM, Chairman: Recommendations for a National High Blood Pressure Program Data Base for Effective Antihypertensive Therapy. Report of Task Force I, DHEW Publication No. (NIH) 75-593, U.S. Dept. of Health, Education and Welfare, Bethesda, 1973.

45. Perry, H.M., Jr., Goldman, A.I., Lavin, M.A., Schnaper, H.W., Fitz, A.E., Frohlich, E.D., Steele, B. and Richman, H.G.: Evaluation of drug treatment in mild hypertension: VA-NHLBI feasibility trial. p. 267. In Perry, H.M., Jr., Smith, W.M., Eds,: Mild Hypertension: To Treat or Not to Treat. Ann NY Acad Sci 304:1978.

46. Ram CVS, Garrett BN, Kaplan NM: Moderate hypertension: Effects on potassium wastage and blood pressure control. Arch Intern Med 141:1015, 1981.

47. Reisin E, Abel R, Modan M, et al: Effect of weight loss without salt restriction on the reduction of blood pressure in overweight hypertensive patients. N Engl J Med 298:1, 1978.

48. Reisin E, Frohlich ED, Messerli FH, et al: Cardiovascular changes following weight reduction in obesity hypertension. Ann Intern Med 98:315, 1983.

49. Report of WHO Expert Committee: Arterial hypertension. World Health Organization Technical Report Series, No. 628. Geneva, Switzerland, 1978.

50. Shapiro AP, Schwartz GE, Ferguson DCE, et al: Behavioral methods in the treatment of hypertension. Ann Intern Med, 86:626, 1977.

51. Smirk FH: High Arterial Pressure. Charles C. Thomas, Springfield, IL, 1957.

52. Smith McFW, US Public Health Service

Hospitals Cooperative Study Group: Treatment of mild hypertension. Results of a 10 year intervention trial. Circ Res (suppl I) 40:98, 1977.

53. Suarez DH, Messerli FH, Ventura HO, et al: Baroreceptor stimulation and isometric exercise in normotensive and borderline subjects. Clin Sci Mol Med, 62:307, 1982.

54. Vaughan ED, Jr, Laragh JH, Gavras I, et al: Volume factor in low and normal renin essential hypertension. Treatment with either spironolactone or chlorthalidone. Am J Cardiol, 32:523, 1973.

55. Ventura HO, Messerli FH, Oigman W, et al: Immediate hemodynamic effects of a new calcium channel blocker (nitrendipine) in essential hypertension. J Cardiol 51:783, 1983.

56. Veterans Administration Cooperative Study Group on Antihypertensive Agents: A double-blind control study of antihypertensive agents. I. Comparative effectiveness of reserpine and hydralazine and three ganglionic blocking agents. Arch Intern Med, 106:81, 1960.

57. Veterans Administration Cooperative Study Group on Antihypertensive Agents: Effects of treatment on morbidity in hypertension. Results in patients with diastolic blood pressure averaging 115 through 129 mm Hg. JAMA, 202:1028, 1967.

58. Veterans Administration Cooperative Study Group on Antihypertensive Agents: Effects of treatments on morbidity in hypertension. II. Results in patients with diastolic blood pressure averaging 90 through 114 mm Hg. JAMA, 213:1143, 1970.

59. Veterans Administration-National Heart, Lung, and Blood Institute Study Group for Cooperative Studies on Antihypertensive Therapy: Mild Hypertension: Treatment of mild hypertension. Preliminary results of a two-year feasibility trial. Circ Res 40 (suppl I): 180, 1977.

60. WHO/ISH: Mild Hypertension Liaison Committee: Trials of the treatment of mild hypertension: an interim analysis. Lancet, 1:149, 1982.

# 4

# Diagnosis of Renovascular Hypertension

# The Case for Renin Assays

Clarence E. Grim, M.D.
Myron H. Weinberger, M.D.

The accurate determination of plasma renin activity (PRA), if performed properly, can play an important role in the diagnostic evaluation of patients with hypertension. When renal artery stenosis is present, the careful measurement of renal vein renin activity allows the physician to identify those patients likely to benefit from treatment of renal artery stenosis and thus spare the patient who will not benefit from treatment unnecessary, expensive, and risky procedures on the renal artery.

## INTRODUCTION

Proof that renal artery stenosis is the cause of hypertension suggests certain specific methods of treatment[2,8] and alerts the physician to follow the patient carefully for changes in renal function. The goals of treatment are both to control blood pressure and to maximize renal function. Current evidence suggests that patients with hypertension secondary to renal artery stenosis (i.e., renal vascular hypertension, RVH) have improved survival if the renal artery stenosis is corrected by surgical repair than if the hypertension is treated medically.[24] Furthermore partial or total correction of renal artery stenosis by surgery or percutaneous transluminal angioplasty (PTA) results in the elimination of a need for medical therapy in approximately 50 percent of the patients and an additional 30 percent of patients have a decrease in the amount of medication needed for adequate control. Unfortunately about 20 percent of reported cases do not respond to PTA or surgery at all, but are exposed to the morbidity and mortality associated with the procedures.[18] Identification of those likely to benefit from intervention is therefore important. Untreated renal artery stenosis is usually a progressive disease (see chapter 5) since recent evidence from Vanderbilt University[12] has demonstrated that nearly one-third of patients with atherosclerotic renal artery stenosis showed a progressive decrease in kidney size over a 3-year period even though blood pressure was well controlled with antihypertensive medication. In our own experience, approximately 50 percent of patients over age 60 with this disease are found to have one renal artery totally occluded by the time the disease is diagnosed. Earlier diagnosis and treatment could prevent this loss of renal mass. Finally, the availability of specific medical therapy, such as angiotensin-converting enzyme inhibitors (captopril) directed at the disturbance of the renin-angiotensin-aldosterone system (RAAS) engendered by a significant stenosis of the renal artery allows specific pharmacologic therapy in these patients which may avoid the side effects of higher doses of standard antihypertensive regimens that many of these patients require.[2]

## SCREENING FOR RENOVASCULAR HYPERTENSION

The value of routine use of peripheral renin measurements in screening hypertensive patients for secondary causes lies not only in the fact that an elevated renin level suggests RVH[3,10,20,47,49] but also since a very low level of PRA makes RVH unlikely and should direct the clinician to pursue the possibility of mineralocorticoid excess syndromes before further investigation for RVH is conducted.[10,16] However, not all cases of RVH will demonstrate elevated peripheral renin levels, a dilemma addressed subsequently. Thus the absence of a markedly elevated peripheral renin level is not helpful in eliminating the possibility of RVH. Further, the influence of all antihypertensive agents on renin release confounds the interpretation of peripheral PRA values obtained during treatment with such agents.

The diagnosis of RVH should be considered in every hypertensive patient, but certain subgroups are more likely to be afflicted than others. These include hypertensives under the age of 40 (particularly females), those with hypertension of sudden onset or severe hypertension with funduscopic hemorrhages and exudates, and those hypertensives who are refractory to antihypertensive therapy. Fortunately over 90 percent of these patients can be easily detected by routine use of three readily available, outpatient tests:[17] listening for a systolic-diastolic (S-D) epigastric bruit, measuring peripheral PRA and performing a rapid sequence intravenous pyelogram (RSIVP).[4] The relative value of these screening tests is important to consider and is defined in Table 4-1. If one listens carefully for an epigastric bruit with a systolic *and* diastolic component about one-third of patients with RVH within a hypertensive population will be identified. An abdominal bruit heard only during systole does not have such specific implications. Similarly, more than 40 percent of the patients with RVH will have a peripheral PRA level that is markedly elevated. However, the routine test that will detect the greatest proportion (75 percent) of patients with RVH is the RSIVP. The criteria for an abnormal RSIVP include disparity in renal size, delay in the nephrogram phase, and the appearance of dye in the collecting systems and, delayed excretion of dye. Over 90 percent of the patients with RVH will be detected if one performs all three screening tests. Furthermore, in our experience this three-test panel will have only an 8 percent false positive response making the screening profile highly specific (Table 4-1). Since all three tests can be done on an outpatient basis, the expense of hospitalization can be avoided at the screening level.

In the future, the detection of renal artery stenosis may be greatly simplified by the development and widespread application of a new technique termed *digital subtraction intravenous arteriography* (DSIA).[7,21] This new outpatient procedure allows reasonable visualization of the renal arteries by computer-assisted enhancement of contrast injected via a venous catheter as it appears in the renal arteries. Although DSIA may make other procedures obsolete the false positive and false negative rates of DSIA have not yet been defined. Indeed two reports[7,42] have suggested that the sensitivity (true positive rate) is about 85 percent and the false positive rate is 20 percent which is no better than the bruit, renin measurement and RSIVP (Table 4-1). The potential utility of new procedures, such as nuclear magnetic resonance (NMR), has not been evaluated.

With the development of pharmacologic agents which interfere with the formation of angiotensin II (the converting enzyme inhibitor, captopril) or with its re-

**Table 4-1.** Sensitivity and Specificity of Diagnostic Tests

| Diagnostic Test | No. of positive tests in renal vascular patients[a] | True Positive Sensitivity (%) | No. of Negative Tests in Patients Without Renal Vascular Hypertension[b] | True Negative (Specificity) (%) |
|---|---|---|---|---|
| PRA>30[c] | 14/54 | 26(15–40)[a,d] | 176/185 | 95 (91–98) |
| S-D Bruit | 37/94 | 39 (29–50) | 197/199 | 99 (97.2–99.9) |
| S-D Bruit or PRA>30 | 35/54 | 65 (51–77) | 166/177 | 94 (89.2–96.9) |
| Urogram | 74/94 | 79 (69–86) | 174/177 | 98 (95.2–99.6) |
| Urogram or PRA>30 | 43/54 | 80 (66–89) | 165/177 | 93 (89.1–96.9) |
| S-D Bruit or Urogram | 83/94 | 88 (80–94) | 172/177 | 97 (93.6–99.1) |
| S-D Bruit or Urogram or PRA>30 | 49/54 | 91 (80–97) | 163/177 | 92 (87.3–95.7) |

[a]Patients cured or improved by surgery.
[b]Patients with normal renal arteriogram.
[c]ng/ml/3hr.
[d]Numbers in parentheses indicate 95% confidence limits for the estimate based on the sample studied.

ceptors (saralasin)[22] it was hoped that highly specific pharmacologic tests would be available to detect patients with RVH. However, these acute tests have yielded about the same results as a careful measurement of PRA.[2,22] The major problem with these tests is that of poor specificity because a significant number of patients with essential hypertension also have an angiotensin-dependent process and thus may have a decrease in blood pressure with captopril or saralasin testing.

The ability to measure kidney size and blood flow by nuclear medicine techniques seemed likely to be a simple method to detect RVH. However, these techniques have proven to be no more sensitive or specific than a carefully performed RSIVP. Thus despite the myriad technological advances of the past decade, the anatomic and functional information provided by the RSIVP and the other screening tests continue to provide the most sensitive and specific tools for the identification of patients with RVH.

In some patients in whom surgery or PTA are not deemed advisable, medical therapy should be initiated without invasive testing. If blood pressure cannot be controlled after multiple drug therapy or if renal function deteriorates, reevaluation of the patient and consideration of further investigation for the possibility of RVH

would be appropriate. In rare patients with accelerated hypertension arteriography may be indicated regardless of the outcome of screening tests. If the patient's condition is so demanding of intervention that negative screening tests will not be accepted, arteriography may be used as the initial diagnostic test.

# IS THE RENAL ARTERY STENOSIS CAUSING THE HYPERTENSION?

As early as 1938 animal experiments had shown that an ischemic kidney released a blood pressure-raising substance, subsequently identified as renin. In 1948 Wakerlin[47] demonstrated that the renin content of an ischemic dog kidney was increased while that of the unclipped kidney was reduced. The increased renin content appears in the involved kidney first and then the content of the contralateral kidney decreases.[38] It has also been recently demonstrated that blocking angiotensin II formation with captopril will prevent the development of RVH in the rat.[13] However, in man it was not until 1960 that Helmer and Judson[20] first reported the presence of renin in renal vein blood of patients with hypertension. Indeed in 1959 Peart[35] had concluded that there was not enough pressor activity in renal venous plasma to possibly cause hypertension. Surgical removal of a unilaterally diseased kidney to treat hypertension was widely practiced after Goldblatt's initial report in which he produced experimental hypertension by constricting the renal artery. However, a review of this approach by Smith in 1956 revealed that only 25 percent of patients benefitted from such therapy.[42]

Since renal artery stenosis causes hypertension as a result of increased renin release from the ischemic kidney, the best way to detect this disease is to measure renin in the venous blood of the kidneys. However, since renin release from the kidney in RVH is influenced by the state of sodium balance, by posture and by many antihypertensive agents, these factors must be rigidly controlled in order to insure for the test to accurately reflect the pathophysiology. We believe that failure to control these factors has been a major cause of false negative renal vein renin tests in patients with RVH. We believe this is responsible for the reports of the inconsistent predictive value of renal vein renin measurements by a few investigators in patients with RVH.

With the development of a sensitive and specific radioimmunoassay for angiotensin I, renin activity could be reliably estimated even in samples of blood from patients with conditions associated with very low levels of PRA. During the 1960s the importance of rigidly controlling factors that affect PRA became evident. Cohen et al.[10] reported that most patients with RVH had a normal level of peripheral PRA when measured in the supine position but, when renin release was stimulated by the upright position, the increase in PRA was striking in RVH. Weinberger et al.[49] showed that suppression of PRA by dietary sodium loading was sometimes necessary to demonstrate the increased peripheral renin levels in RVH

by reducing normal values to expose the increased levels in RVH. Michelakis et al.[31,32] demonstrated the importance of simultaneous sampling and the use of a passive tilting to stimulate PRA. Similar conclusions were drawn by Horvath.[23] Simultaneous sampling of blood from both renal veins by bilateral catheters eliminated episodic surges of renin secretion, and tilting provided a greater stimulus to renin release by the ischemic than by the contralateral kidney. In 1971 Strong et al.[46] clearly demonstrated that sodium depletion was necessary to stimulate renin release in order to detect significant differences that were not demonstrable on a normal sodium diet. Finally, our group[30] reported that sodium depletion alone may not always be a sufficient stimulus to identify significant renal vein renin differences in some patients with RVH and that only after using a 45° passive headup tilt for 20 minutes would those patients be found to have an abnormal renal vein renin ratio. These results are summarized on Table 4-2. Indeed, our most recent data suggest that one-third of patients with RVH may have a normal renal vein renin ratio (even though salt depleted) if

**Table 4-2.** Salt Depletion and Tilting Enhance Renin Release from the Ischemic Kidney

| | RENAL VEIN RENIN RATIO: Ischemic Side/Nonischemic Side | | | |
|---|---|---|---|---|
| | Salt Depletion[a] | | Tilting[b] | |
| Patient | Before | After | Before | After |
| 1 | 1.4 | 4.0 | 1.3 | 3.0 |
| 2 | 1.1 | 3.0 | 1.2 | 5.0 |
| 3 | 1.1 | 2.3 | 1.2 | 1.8 |
| 4 | 1.1 | 1.7 | 1.0 | 5.0 |
| 5 | 1.0 | 1.6 | 1.0 | 2.4 |
| 6 | 1.0 | 1.6 | 1.0 | 2.0 |
| 7 | | | 1.0 | 1.9 |
| 8 | | | 1.0 | 1.8 |
| 9 | | | 1.0 | 1.6 |
| 10 | | | 1.0 | 1.5 |
| 11 | | | 0.7 | 4.0 |

[a]Salt depletion: one of 10 mEq/day sodium diet plus ingestion of 40mg of furosemide three times daily on the day before renal vein sampling.
[b]Tilting: Subject maintained at a 45° angle for 20 minutes prior to testing.

they are not tilted to stimulate renin release.

The availability of angiotensin-converting enzyme inhibitors may prove to be another good method for stimulating renin release.[39] It has also become evident that most antihypertensive medications, especially those that act on the sympathetic nervous system (reserpine, alpha-methyldopa, clonidine, guanethidene, guanabenz and all beta blockers), can lower renin release to such an extent that a positive renal vein renin test will become negative. For that reason it is prudent to discontinue such agents for several days before performing renal vein renin studies.

Most authors report that when one finds an abnormal renal vein renin ratio (≥1.5) the patient will usually be cured or improved by renal artery repair, percutaneous dilatation, or nephrectomy. However, the course to be taken when a patient has a renal artery stenosis but does not have an abnormal renal vein renin ratio forms the center of the current debate. It has been our experience that a patient with true RVH will have a significantly increased renal vein renin ratio (involved/uninvolved >1.5:1) if sodium depletion, tilting, simultaneous sampling, and withdrawal of renin-suppressing drugs have been utilized. Most "false negative" renal vein renin ratios reported by other investigators have occurred in the presence of low (suppressed) renin concentration, indicative of failure to stimulate renin effectively.

The absolute level of renal vein renin activity has an important influence on the variability of the radioimmunoassay. With very low or very high levels of renal vein PRA, Morlin et al.[34] found that the chance of observing a false positive renal vein renin ratio of >1.5 increased markedly. One should be especially suspicious of positive renal vein renin ratios when the renal vein renin level is low. This is an ad-ditional reason to stimulate renin release before performing renal vein renin measurements. In patients with no evidence of renal artery stenosis an abnormal renal vein renin ratio of >1.5 was estimated to occur by laboratory error only once in 1000 cases.[27] There is little disagreement among investigators about the predictive value of a positive renal vein renin study. Thus, we believe it is important to ensure that the study will be meaningful by following the criteria provided above to maximize detection of a functionally significant difference.

When the renal venous renins are not different there is more divided opinion about the subsequent course. Since most investigators are reluctant to intervene (i.e., perform surgery) in the absence of significantly elevated renal vein renin ratios, the false negative rate of the procedure is not well defined. Most published reports of patients benefitting from intervention who were said not to manifest a significant renal vein renin difference, had those measurements made under conditions which did not ensure stimulation of the renin system and/or removal of renin-suppressing drugs. Unlike some investigators, we do not advocate arteriographic and venous studies on the same day because of the increased risk of complications. Furthermore we do not agree with many radiologists who advocate transluminal dilatation at the time of arteriography if a lesion of the renal artery is found. There are insufficient reports of the benefit of such indiscriminant behavior and ample reports of the risks, including the loss of kidneys. Furthermore the evaluation of the benefits of such an approach is often limited by the very short or nonexistent follow-up information regarding the change in blood pressure and renal function after the procedure when it is performed in the absence of evidence for functional significance of the lesion.

What should the clinician then do if

he believes the patient has RVH but the renal vein renin ratio is not abnormal? We believe the following approach should be conducted.[16,30]

Ideal patient preparation requires the withdrawal of all antihypertensive agents for 2 weeks. When this is not possible the patient may be maintained on diuretics and hydralazine while renin-suppressing drugs such as beta-blocking agents, alpha-methyldopa, clonidine, reserpine, guanethidine, guanabenz or other antisympathetic agents are withdrawn for 7 to 10 days. If this is not possible the renal vein renin samples can still be obtained, but if they are not significantly different the dilemma is that either the patient has renal artery stenosis unrelated to the hypertension, that the significant renal vein renin ratio was obscured by pharmacological agents or that errors occurred at the time of renal vein blood sampling or assay. In such cases we have readmitted the patient to the hospital in order to carefully withdraw renin-suppressing drugs and repeat the renal vein renin sampling.

The next step of patient preparation that we utilize is to induce sodium depletion the day before renal vein renin sampling in order to enhance the renal vein renin ratio.[30,46] This is done by giving oral furosemide 40 mg at 10 A.M., 2 P.M., and 6 P.M. and limiting sodium intake on this day to 10 mEq and fluid to 25 ml/kg body weight.[16] The following day the patient remains recumbent until the renal vein renin procedure can be performed. Failure to induce sodium depletion prior to renal vein renin sampling is, we believe, a major cause of false negative renal vein renin studies reported by others.[6,9,28,37] We and others have demonstrated that sodium depletion the day prior to renal vein sampling increases the sensitivity of the renal vein renin ratio in RVH.[30,46]

Renal vein renin samples are obtained in both the recumbent and upright positions. At our institution we utilize an X-ray suite with a tilt table because we sample renal vein blood for renin in the recumbent position *and* after 20 minutes of 45° head-up tilt in order to increase the sensitivity of the procedure.[30,31,32] In the last 36 patients that we have studied with RVH, tilting further increased our yield of positive renal vein renin studies by 36 percent (i.e., these RVH patients had a "normal" renal vein renin ratio in the recumbent position before being stimulated with the 45° upright tilt). False negative renal vein renin results may result if the patients are not sodium depleted or tilted.

Technical and anatomical factors may also influence the ability to detect significant renal vein renin differences in RVH. The radiologist must keep in mind that the anatomy of the renal veins is more variable than the renal arteries and many patients will have more than one renal vein on each side. This is particularly important in patients with a branch renal artery stenosis in which segmental sampling of the vein draining the stenotic area must be obtained. The recognition of a segmental or branch stenosis may be justification for performing arteriography before renal vein renin sampling so that particular efforts can be made to sample venous blood from the segment of the kidney involved. In addition, on the left side blood from the gonadal vein may be inadvertently sampled thereby diluting the true renin concentration of renal vein blood. Further, renal renin secretion can vary from minute to minute[34,50] and therefore we use two catheters (one in each renal vein) to insure simultaneous sampling from both sides.

Vaughn et al.[47] have proposed a complex scoring system that evaluates the peripheral and renal vein renin data for absolute and relative levels of renin. A major point of the scoring system is that it gives added weight to the presence of contralateral suppression of renal venous

PRA. However, since the interpretation of these studies requires a normal sodium intake this approach can be expected to mask many cases of significant RVH. Indeed Maxwell et al.[27,28] found that this scoring system misclassified many patients and Christlieb[9] confirmed this by demonstrating a 36 percent false-negative and a 4 percent false-positive result. We have previously reported that the calculation of V-A/A advocated by Vaughn et al. was less accurate in identifying those patients with RVH subsequently cured by surgery than the RVR ratio of 1.5 or greater.[30]

There are many approaches for the use of renal vein renin sampling in the investigation of RVH. Some investigators use renal vein renin levels as the initial screen for RVH. However, knowledge of the location of a renal artery stenosis is often needed in order to be certain one is sampling from the correct site, thus patients with segmental stenosis may be missed if renal vein renin samples are obtained before arteriography. Since sodium depletion and tilting increase the accuracy of renal vein measurements it is important to perform these tests under conditions that maximize the information de-

rived from the study. With the advent of PTA our placement of the renal vein renin studies in the diagnostic algorithm (Fig. 4-1) is determined by what we know of the patient when first seen, in order to avoid an unnecessary second renal arteriogram. If the patient has a systolic-diastolic epigastric bruit, an elevated peripheral PRA, an abnormal RSIVP or an abnormal DSIA we perform renal vein renin studies next under the stimulated conditions previously described and await these results before performing renal arteriography. Thus, when renal arteriography is performed we can decide about concomitant PTA on the basis of available renal vein renin results. There is one other circumstance in which renal vein renin sampling may be informative in the absence of arteriographic evidence of renal vascular disease. This is in the rare case of a renin-secreting tumor where the arteriogram may not demonstrate the small neoplasm. Thus hypertension and elevated PRA, particularly in a young person, may prompt a search for renal vein renin differences as a clue to such a lesion despite a normal arteriogram.

A tabulation of 20 major series of patients with RVH reporting renal vein re-

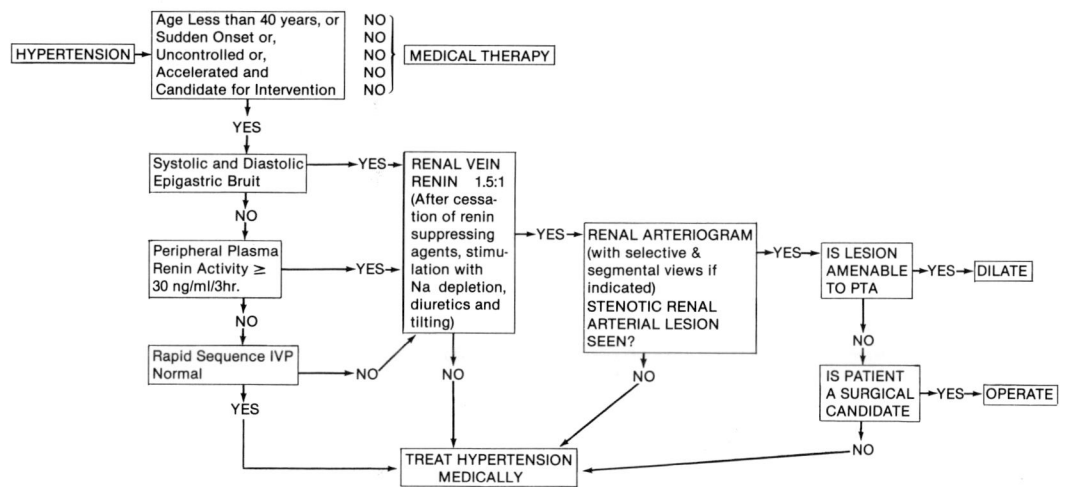

**Fig. 4-1** Algorithm for the evaluation and treatment of hypertension.

**Table 4-3.** Renal Vein Renin Results In Surgically Responsive and Nonresponsive Renal Artery Stenosis

| Author | Sensitivity RVR Test + Disease + | (%) | Specificity RVR Test − Disease − | (%) | Probability of Improving Blood Pressure if RVR Test Negative — Number Improved Test − | (%) | Condition of Study — Low Na Diet | Tilt | 2 Catheters |
|---|---|---|---|---|---|---|---|---|---|
| Stanley[44] | 71/85 | (84%) | | | 14/14 | (100%) | Y | N | N |
| Juncos[26] | 62/68 | (91%) | 3/7 | (43%) | 6/9 | (67%) | N | N | N |
| Melman[30] | 41/44 | (93%) | 9/9 | (100%) | 3/3 | (100%) | Y | Y | Y |
| Messerli[33] | 14/18 | (78%) | 9/9 | (100%) | 4/13 | (31%) | Y | N | N |
| Pawsey[35] | 11/13 | (85%) | 1/2 | (50%) | 2/3 | (67%) | Y | Y | Y |
| Schaeffer[40] | 12/17 | (71%) | | | 5/5 | (100%) | NC | N | N |
| Maxwell[28] | 37/58 | (64%) | 5/9 | (56%) | 21/26 | (81%) | NC | N | N |
| Buda[6] | 48/55 | (87%) | 5/14 | (36%) | 7/12 | (58%) | N | N | N |
| McNair[29] | 22/26 | (85%) | 2/6 | (33%) | 4/6 | (67%) | N | N | Y |
| Gunnells[19] | 15/16 | (94%) | 5/6 | (56%) | 1/5 | (20%) | N | N | Y |
| Stockigt[45] | 21/25 | (84%) | 4/7 | (57%) | 4/8 | (50%) | N | NC | N |
| Vaughn[47] | 18/21 | (86%) | 2/8 | (25%) | 3/5 | (60%) | N | N | N |
| Simmons[41] | 17/18 | (94%) | 2/3 | (67%) | 1/2 | (50%) | N | N | N |
| Fournier[15] | 7/11 | (64%) | 9/9 | (100%) | 4/11 | (36%) | N | N | N |
| Judson[25] | 14/16 | (88%) | 16/16 | (100%) | 2/8 | (11%) | N | N | N |
| Fitz[14] | 10/12 | (83%) | 7/7 | (100%) | 2/9 | (22%) | N | N | N |
| Poutasse[37] | 8/16 | (50%) | 1/2 | (50%) | 8/9 | (89%) | N | N | N |
| Bourgoignie[5] | 8/8 | (100%) | 3/4 | (75%) | 1/4 | (25%) | N | N | N |
| Amsterdam[1] | 7/8 | (88%) | 4/6 | (67%) | 2/7 | (29%) | N | N | N |
| Weiner[50] | 7/9 | (78%) | 4/6 | (67%) | 2/9 | (22%) | N | N | N |
| Totals | 450/544 | (83%) | 82/124 | (66%) | 96/178 | (54%) | | | |

Notes. Test +, the RVR test was abnormal as defined by the author; Test −, the RVR test as normal as defined by the author; Disease +, renovascular hypertension present since patient was either cured or improved by surgery; Disease −, renovascular hypertension not present since patient blood pressure was not changed by surgery. Most authors excluded technical failures (graft thrombosis, etc.) from this group.
Y = Conditions met; N = Not met; NC = done inconsistently.

118

nin results is shown in Table 4-3. A total of 668 patients are summarized who had renal vein renin studies and then underwent surgery. Of these patients 544 were cured or improved and therefore clearly had RVH. A total of 450 of these patients (83 percent) had abnormal renal vein renin ratios as defined by each author. Of the 124 patients who did not respond to surgery 82 (66 percent) had a normal renal vein renin study. Among the 176 patients with a negative renal vein renin study only 94 or 53 percent had an improvement in blood pressure. Thus, in patients with renal artery stenosis having normal renal vein renin studies the probability of cure or improvement of blood pressure decreases significantly (p. <.0001). We believe that the risk of surgery is only justified in patients with renal vein ratios of less than 1.5 if the blood pressure cannot be adequately controlled with medical therapy.

In reviewing these studies several difficulties emerge. In general most studies since 1970 have utilized renal vein renin studies as a major selection criteria for surgery; that is, there are few studies in which patients have been operated with negative renal vein renin results. Most of these studies that report patients with normal renal vein renin studies are hampered by the fact that techniques known to stimulate plasma renin levels and increase the likelihood of detection of an abnormal ratio were not consistently used. Thus these patients may have had false negative renal vein renin studies. Indeed, as indicated in Table 4-3, only studies 1 through 5 consistently used some form of sodium depletion prior to renal vein renin studies and only studies 3 and 5 used tilting as an additional stimulus to renin secretion. Finally, in some (but not all) patients with bilateral RVH, the renin ratio may not be abnormal since there may be hypersecretion of renin from both kidneys. In such instances it may be possible to document the hemodynamic significance of the stenosis at the time of arteriography by direct pressure measurements proximal and distal to the stenotic lesion(s). We find that a drop in pressure across a stenosis of greater than 40 mm Hg is consistently associated with functional significance. One must be certain not to occlude the narrow lumen with the pressure transducer thereby producing an artifactual pressure gradient.

In summary, experimental and clinical data strongly implicate the RAAS in the pathophysiology of RVH. The best way to demonstrate the abnormal physiology is to perform renal vein renin measurements. These must be done under controlled conditions to insure adequate stimulation of renin production. When the renal vein renin values are abnormal the physician and patient can be 90 percent certain that successful correction of the stenosis will alleviate the hypertension. Attempting to correct a stenosis in the absence of abnormal renal vein renin tests does not make good physiologic sense if blood pressure can be adequately controlled with medication and renal function is frequently and carefully evaluated. Furthermore the risks of intervention, whether by surgery or PTA, in the absence of a significant renal venous renin difference do not appear to be justifiable on the basis of the paucity of published data demonstrating the benefit of such an approach.

# REFERENCES

1. Amsterdam EA, Couch NP, Christlieb AR: Renal vein renin activity in the prognosis for renovascular hypertension. Am J Med 47:860, 1969.
2. Atkinson AB, Brown JJ, Cumming AM, et al: Captopril in the management of hypertension with renal artery stenosis: Its long-term effect as a predictor of surgical outcome. Am J Cardiol 49:1460, 1982.

3. Bath NM, Gunnells JC, Robinson RR: Plasma renin activity in renovascular hypertension. Am J Med 45:381, 1968.

4. Bookstein JJ, Abrams HL, Buenger RE: Radiologic aspects of the study, Part 2. The role of urography in unilateral renovascular disease. JAMA 220:1225, 1972.

5. Bourgoignie J, Kunz S, Catanzaro FJ: Renal venous renin in hypertension. Am J Med 48:332, 1970.

6. Buda JA, Baer L, Parra-Carrillo JZ: Predictability of surgical response in renovascular hypertension. Arch Surg 111:1243, 1976.

7. Buonocore E, Meaney TF, Borkowski et al: Digital subtraction angiography of the abdominal aorta and renal arteries. Radiology 139:281, 1981.

8. Case DB, Atlas SA, Marion RM, et al: Long term efficacy of captopril in renovascular and essential hypertension. Am J Cardiol 49:1440, 1982.

9. Christlieb AR: Divided renal vein renins. In Breslin DJ, Swinton NW, Libertin JA, et al, Eds: Renovascular Hypertension. Baltimore, Williams and Wilkins, 1982, p 101.

10. Cohen EL, Rovner DR, Conn JW: Postural augmentation of plasma renin activity. JAMA 197:973, 1966.

11. Couch NP, Sullivan J, Crane C: The predictive accuracy of renal vein renin activity in the surgery of renovascular hypertension. Surgery 79:70, 1976.

12. Dean RH, Kietter RW, Smith BM, et al: Renovascular hypertension anatomic and renal function changes during drug therapy. Arch Surg 116:1408, 1981.

13. Deforrest JM, Knappenberger RC, Antonaccio MJ, et al: Angiotensin II is a necessary component for the development of hypertension in the two kidney, one clip rat. Am J Cardiol 49:1515, 1982.

14. Fitz A: Renal venous renin determinations in the diagnosis of surgically correctable hypertension. Circulation 36:942, 1967.

15. Fournier A, Romeder JM, Salmon D: Predictive criteria of surgical curability of renovascular hypertension. Acta Med Scand 189:391, 1971.

16. Grim CE, Weinberger MH, Higgins JT, Kramer NJ: Diagnosis secondary forms of hypertension: a comprehensive protocol. JAMA 237:1331, 1977.

17. Grim CE, Luft FC, Weinberger MH, Grim, CM: Sensitivity and specificity of screening tests for renal vascular hypertension. Ann Intern Med 91:617, 1979.

18. Grim CE, Weinberger MH: Renal artery stenosis and hypertension. In Seminars in Nephrology, 3:52, 1983.

19. Gunnells JC, McGuffin WL, Johnsrude I, Robinson RR: Peripheral and renal venous plasma renin activity in hypertension. Ann Intern Med 71:555, 1969.

20. Helmer OM, Judson WE: The presence of vasoconstriction and vasopressor activity in renal vein plasma of patients with arterial hypertension. Hypertension 8:38, 1960.

21. Hillman BJ, Ovitt TW, Nudelman S, et al: Digital videosubtraction angiography of renal vascular abnormalities. Radiology 139:277, 1981.

22. Horn ML, Conklin VM, Keenan RE, et al: Angiotensin profiling with saralasin: Summary of the Eaton Collaborative Study. Kid Int 15:S-115, 1979.

23. Horvath JS, Baxter CR, Sherbon K: An analysis of errors found in renal vein sampling for plasma renin activity. Kid Int 11:136, 1977.

24. Hunt JC, Strong CG: Renovascular hypertension: Mechanisms, natural history and management. Am J Cardiol 32:562, 1973.

25. Judson WE, Helmer OM: Diagnostic and prognostic values of renin activity in renal venous plasma in renovascular hypertension. Hypertension 13:79, 1965.

26. Juncos LI, Stong CG, Hunt JC: Prediction of results of surgery for renal and renovascular hypertension. Arch Int Med 134:655, 1974.

27. Maxwell MH, Marks LS, Varady PP: Renal vein renin in essential hypertension. J Lab Clin Med 86:901, 1975.

28. Maxwell MH, Marks LS, Lupu AN: Predictive value of renin determinations in renal artery stenosis. JAMA 238:2617, 1977.

29. McNair A, Neilsen D, Gammelgaard PA, et al: A follow up study of hypertensive patients after operative treatment of unilateral renovascular or renal disease. Acta Med Scand 205:569, 1979.

30. Melman A, Donohue JP, Weinberger MH, Grim CE: Improved diagnostic accuracy of

renal venous ratios with stimulation of renin release. J Urol 117:145, 1977.

31. Michelakis AM, Foster JH, Liddle GW: Measurement of renin in both renal veins. Arch Intern Med 120:444, 1967.

32. Michelakis AM, Woods JW, Liddle GW: A predictable error in use of renal vein renins in diagnosing hypertension. Arch Intern Med 123:359, 1969.

33. Messerli FH, Genest J, Nowaczynski W: Hypertension with renal arterial stenosis: humoral, hemodynamic and histopathologic features. Am J Cardiol 36:702, 1975.

34. Morlin C, Loreliurs L, Wide L: Spontaneous variations in renal vein renin activity in man. Clin Chim Acta 119:31, 1982.

35. Pawsey CGK, Vandongen R, Gordon RD: Renal venous renin ratio in the diagnosis of renovascular hypertension: measurement during active secretion of renin. Med J Aust 1:121, 1971.

36. Peart WS: Hypertension and the kidney II. Experimental basis of renal hypertension. Br Med J 2:1421, 1959.

37. Poutasse EF, Marks LS, Wisoff CP, et al: Renal vein renin determinations in hypertension: falsely negative tests. J Urol 110:371, 1973.

38. Regoli D, Hess R, Brunner H: Interrelationship of renin content in kidneys and blood pressure in renal hypertensive rats. Arch Int Pharm 140:416, 1962.

39. Re R, Novellini R, Escourru M: Inhibition of angiotensin-converting enzyme for the diagnosis of renal-artery stenosis. N Engl J Med 298:582, 1978.

40. Schaeffer AJ, Fair WR: Comparison of split function ratios with renal vein renin ratios in patients with curable hypertension caused by unilateral renal artery stenosis. J Urol 112:697, 1974.

41. Simmons JL, Michelakis AM: Renovascular hypertension: the diagnostic value of renal vein renin ratios. J Urol 104:497, 1970.

42. Smith CW, Winfield AC, Price RR, et al: Evaluation of digital venous angiography for the diagnosis of renovascular hypertension. Radiology, 144:51, 1982.

43. Smith H: Unilateral nephrectomy in hypertensive disease. J Urol 76:685, 1956.

44. Stanley JC, Gewertz BL, Fry WJ: Renal: systemic renin indices and renal vein renin ratios as prognostic indicators in remedial renovascular hypertension. J Surg Res 20:149, 1976.

45. Stockigt JR, Collins RD, Noakes CA, et al: Renal vein renin in various forms of renal hypertension. Lancet 1:1194, 1972.

46. Strong CE, Hunt JC, Sheps SG: Renal venous renin activity enhancement of sensitivity of lateralization by sodium depletion. Am J Cardiol 27:602, 1971.

47. Vaughan ED, Buhler FR, Laragh JH, et al: Renovascular hypertension: renin measurements to indicate hypersecretion and contralateral suppression, estimate renal plasma flow, and score for surgical curability. Am J Med 55:402, 1973.

48. Wakerlin GE, Marshall J, Minatoya H: Renin concentration of the kidney in experimental renal hypertension. In Zweifach BW, Shorr E, Eds: Factors Regulating Blood Pressure. J. Macy Foundation, New York, 1948.

49. Weinberger MH, Dowdy AJ, Nokes GW, et al: Plasma renin activity and aldosterone secretion in hypertensive patients during high and low sodium intake and administration of diuretic. J Clin Endocrinol 28:359, 1968.

50. Winer BM, Lubbe WF, Simon M, et al: Renin in the diagnosis of renovascular hypertension. JAMA 202:121, 1967.

51. Whelton PK, Harrington DP, Russell RP: Renal vein renin activity: a prospective study of sampling techniques and methods of interpretation. Johns Hopkins Med J 141:112, 1977.

# Limitations of Renin Assays

Michael R. Rudnick, M.D.
Morton H. Maxwell, M.D.

In 1934, Goldblatt showed that renal artery stenosis (RAS) induced by a vascular clip in dogs resulted in an ischemic kidney that was responsible for sustained but reversible hypertension.[77] This observation was followed by demonstrations that surgical removal or vascular correction of kidneys associated with RAS in hypertensive patients resulted in normal blood pressures.[18,30,49,98,124,159] The initial enthusiasm generated by this curable form of hypertension was subsequently tempered by reports of hypertensive patients with RAS (35 to 48 percent) whose hypertension failed to resolve despite technically adequate surgery.[112,149,156] Coupled with these reports were the findings from angiographic[55,62] and postmortem[95,171] studies which demonstrated that significant RAS could be present in normotensive individuals. Dustan et al. in a review of translumbar aortograms performed for peripheral vascular disease reported that 50 percent of patients with angiographic evidence of RAS were normotensive.[55] Holley et al. in a postmortem study of 256 patients who had no history of hypertension found moderate or severe renal artery stenosis in 64 percent of the group over the age of 50.[95] Together these observations clearly demonstrated that besides the anatomical presence of RAS, additional "functional" factors must be present for hypertension to result.

Tests currently employed to prospectively determine "functional" significance have centered primarily on those that are dependent on the renin-angiotensin system. It is the purpose of this chapter to review the diagnostic capabilities of these tests and their role in the evaluation of patients with suspected renovascular hypertension (RVHT). It is our belief that these diagnostic tests are of minimal benefit in patients in whom the pretest clinical assessment for likelihood of RVHT is either high or low. These tests may be of some benefit in patients in whom the pretest likelihood for RVHT is intermediate in nature.

## PATHOGENESIS OF RVHT: THE BASIS FOR INTERPRETING RENIN ASSAYS

The application and interpretation of diagnostic tests which attempt to identify those patients with true RVHT, that is, patients with "functionally" significant RAS whose hypertension will be improved by definitive treatment (e.g., surgery), requires an understanding of the pathophysiologic mechanisms responsible for RVHT.

Initial efforts to determine the mechanism for the hypertension in the Goldblatt experiment resulted in the conclusion that the ischemic clamped kidney was releasing a pressor substance into the blood. This conclusion arose in part from the observation that ligation of the renal vein of the partially clamped kidney would prevent the expected hypertension.[76] It was soon appreciated that this renal pressor substance was renin which had previously been discovered by Tigerstedt and Bergman in 1898.[194] The research efforts that followed these reports led to the discovery of the renin-angiotensin system in 1939 by Page and Helmer[150] and Braun-Menendez and colleagues.[19]

The Goldblatt model of hypertension or variations of it has now been reproduced in a wide variety of animal species. These experimental studies have resulted in an assortment of conflicting data both in terms of the blood pressure response to RAS and of the exact pathophysiologic role of the renin-angiotensin system.[21,46] The application of an analysis of vasoconstriction and volume factors responsible for RVHT has significantly helped in the understanding of these various experimental and clinical observations.[122]

In the vasoconstriction-volume analysis there are two separate experimental models of RVHT with each model having its own pathophysiology and clinical counterpart. The first experimental model is known as the "two kidney" Goldblatt preparation and consists of partial clamping of one renal artery with the contralateral kidney remaining intact. The clinical counterpart of this model is unilateral RVHT. A large number of experimental and clinical observations support the concept that this form of hypertension is mediated by an ischemia induced increase in renin secretion that increases angiotensin II production which in turn raises blood pressure by direct arterial vasoconstriction. In support of this mechanism has been the findings of increased peripheral

and renal vein plasma renin activity (PRA), prevention or reversal of the hypertension by administration of either renin or angiotensin II inhibitors, and correction of hypertension by nephrectomy or reversal of the RAS.[122]

The second experimental model of RVHT is the "one-kidney" Goldblatt preparation. In this model, there is again partial clamping of one renal artery but the contralateral kidney is removed by nephrectomy. The clinical counterparts of this model are hypertension resulting from unilateral RAS with renal parenchymal disease of the contralateral kidney or from bilateral RAS. The initial events that lead to hypertension in this model are similar to those in the "two-kidney" model: ischemia → increased renin → increased angiotensin II → vasoconstriction. Angiotensin II in addition to its pressor effect also stimulates aldosterone production with resultant salt and water retention. In the "two-kidney" model, this excess salt and water is excreted by the normal contralateral kidney. In the "one-kidney" model, lack of contralateral natriuresis causes volume expansion to result. This volume expansion suppresses the increased renin secretion but at the same time maintains the hypertension. Therefore, in this experimental model or its clinical counterparts there is an inability to detect an increase in peripheral or renal vein PRA nor will the infusion of renin or angiotensin II inhibitors decrease the blood pressure. Maneuvers that deplete the salt and water content of the animal or patient will however make the hypertension angiotensin dependent.[122]

Although this vasoconstriction–volume analysis is helpful in understanding many of the seemingly disparate experimental and clinical observations in RVHT, there appear to be additional pathophysiologic mechanisms. Observations demonstrating a transition of phases in experimental RVHT could explain why nephrectomy may sometimes fail to cure the hypertension seen in the "two-kidney" experimental model or its clinical counterpart of unilateral RVHT.[26] In the initial phase in the "two-kidney" dog model there is the expected hypertension which at this time is totally dependent on the pressor effects of angiotensin II as described above. Several days later, however, renin levels fall and vascular volume increases. During this second phase, the hypertension is still strongly dependent on the renin-angiotensin system which although reduced, is inappropriately elevated for the degree of volume expansion. Up to this point, removal of the clip or nephrectomy will normalize the blood pressure. However, if the hypertension is allowed to persist longer, a third phase may develop in which correction of the RAS or nephrectomy will be without hemodynamic effect. The explanation offered for this observation is that the initial hypertension, if present for a sufficient period, results in nephrosclerosis in the contralateral kidney which is then able to maintain the hypertension despite correction of the initial RAS. This observation is consistent with the clinical finding that RVHT is more frequently cured when it has been present for only a short duration.[100]

Although the renin-angiotensin system with resultant vasoconstriction and volume expansion mechanisms appears to be the primary factor in the pathogenesis of RVHT, additional factors have been described in experimental RVHT, some of which may have clinical relevance.[133] These other factors include the renal elaboration of other pressor substances, prostaglandins, bradykinin, arteriolar autoregulation, and neurogenic factors.[46] The reader is referred to several excellent reviews for a more detailed description of the pathophysiology of RVHT.[21,32,46,109]

# DIAGNOSTIC TESTS INVOLVING ABNORMALITIES OF THE RENIN-ANGIOTENSIN SYSTEM

In view of the above considerations regarding anatomy, response to surgery, and pathogenesis, several diagnostic tests involving the renin-angiotensin system have been proposed for the *prospective* diagnosis of RVHT. These tests are the measurement of: (a) peripheral plasma renin activity (PRA), (b) renal vein renin ratio (RVRR), and (c) vasodepressor response to saralasin.

In the sections to follow we have critically reviewed the published literature for each test in terms of its accuracy (i.e., sensitivity and specificity) both in the basal state and after a variety of stimulatory maneuvers and the mechanisms responsible for false negative and false positive results. Sensitivity is defined as the probability that the test will be positive when the disease is present and the false negative rate is the probability that the test will be negative when the disease is present. Specificity is defined as the probability that the test will be negative when the disease is absent and the false positive rate is the probability that the test will be positive when the disease is absent. Only those series describing the blood pressure responses following technically successful surgery were included in these analyses. For this review, we have defined RVHT as either a cure or improvement in hypertension following surgery.

In interpreting the results of Tables 4-4 to 4-6, one must keep in mind several limitations inherent in this type of data analysis. The individual series varied in terms of the criteria employed for a positive or negative test result or a beneficial

**Table 4-4.** Peripheral Plasma Renin Activity (PRA) in Renal Vascular Hypertension (RVHT)

| Reference | Sensitivity | Specificity | Surgical Improvement | | Study Conditions | | |
|---|---|---|---|---|---|---|---|
| | | | PRA Negative | PRA Positive | Sodium Depletion | Upright Posture | Renal Vascular Lesion |
| Cohen[42] | 6/6 | — | — | 6/6 | N.G. | + | N.G. |
| Meyer[140] | 12/31 | 18/21 | 19/37 | 12/15 | — | N.G. | Unilateral |
| Bath[10] | 24/25 | 7/7 | 1/8 | 24/24 | — | — | Unilateral |
| Amsterdam[1] | 6/10 | 7/11 | 4/11 | 6/10 | — | — | Unilateral |
| Gunnells[88] | 11/16 | 6/9 | 5/11 | 11/14 | — | + | N.G. |
| Bourgoigne[16] | 11/12 | 1/3 | 1/2 | 11/13 | N.G. | N.G. | Unilateral |
| Bourgoigne[16] | 0/1 | 1/4 | 1/2 | 0/3 | N.G. | N.G. | Bilateral |
| Kirkendall[116] | 7/12 | 1/2 | 5/6 | 7/8 | + | + | N.G. |
| Fournier[69] | 9/25 | 12/18 | 16/28 | 9/15 | — | — | N.G. |
| Strong[190] | 10/62 | 4/5 | 52/56 | 10/11 | + | N.G. | Mixed |
| Stockigt[181] | 12/16 | 1/2 | 4/5 | 12/13 | — | — | Unilateral |
| Poutasse[161] | 5/13 | 2/2 | 8/10 | 5/5 | — | — | Mixed |
| Hussain[103] | 6/17 | 5/7 | 11/16 | 6/8 | — | — | Unilateral |
| Vaughan[203] | 13/18 | 5/6 | 5/10 | 13/14 | — | N.G. | Mixed |
| Messerli[139] | 17/29 | 10/11 | 12/22 | 17/18 | — | + | Unilateral |
| Buda[31] | 42/49 | 5/11 | 7/12 | 42/48 | N.G. | N.G. | Mixed |
| Melman[138] | 3/13 | 2/3 | 10/12 | 3/4 | + | + | Mixed |
| Maxwell[135] | 16/20 | 0/2 | 4/4 | 16/18 | + | + | Unilateral |
| Tucker[199] | 10/15 | 1/1 | 5/6 | 10/10 | N.G. | + | N.G. |
| Streeten[186] | 22/34 | — | 12/12 | 22/22 | + | + | Mixed |
| Grim[81] | 11/41 | — | 30/30 | 11/11 | N.G. | + | N.G. |
| Hansson[90] | 32/35 | 5/12 | 3/8 | 32/39 | N.G. | + | Unilateral |
| Hansson[90] | 9/12 | 3/9 | 3/6 | 9/15 | N.G. | + | Bilateral |
| Chiarini[38] | 16/28 | — | 12/12 | 16/16 | — | — | Unilateral |
| Total | 310/540 (57%) | 96/146 (66%) | 230/326 (71%) | 310/360 (86%) | | | |

Abbreviations: N.G.—Specific information not given in methods section of reference.

response to surgery, the proportion of patients with unilateral, bilateral, or segmental lesions, conditions of sodium balance, and the application of specific stimulatory maneuvers. When possible, these factors were specified for each series in Tables 4-4 to 4-6. In addition, variation also existed between the series for the presence or absence of antihypertensive agents known to affect renin secretion (usually antihypertensive agents were withheld prior to testing), the type of renin assay used and the presence or absence of a control population. Nonspecific factors known to affect surgical outcome[130] such as etiologic type of lesion (atherosclerotic or fibromuscular), age, and duration of hypertension were also variable. Finally, many of the series were biased insofar as only those patients with a positive diagnostic test result underwent surgery. Thus, patients who may or may not have benefited from surgery despite a negative test result may have been missed. Despite these limitations, we feel the collective data (Tables 4-4 to 4-6) is sufficient to permit general statements regarding the sensitivity and specificity of these diagnostic tests.

## Peripheral Plasma Renin Activity (PRA)

Appreciating that increased renin secretion was responsible for the hypertension in experimental RVHT, initial investigative efforts attempted to demonstrate a similar mechanism in patients with this disease. These initial efforts were successful in demonstrating increases in pressor activity in renal vein effluent[78,105,145] and in peripheral vein plasma renin concentration[9,24,25] or activity.[74,197] However, in many of these patients, normal levels for these renin determinants were found. With the availability of a widely accepted reliable method for determining PRA,[15] investigators were hopeful that this test would now have a better diagnostic capability.

Table 4-4 lists the published series which have evaluated the sensitivity and specificity of the PRA as a prognostic test for RVHT. Series in which exact sensitivity and specificity data could not be determined were excluded.[68,115,154,168] Several of these latter series however did conclude that while an elevated PRA is highly suggestive of RVHT, a normal value by no means excludes the diagnosis.[68,115,154,168] The results of the analysis in Table 4-4 reveal that the sensitivity and specificity of an elevated PRA in the diagnosis of RVHT is 57 percent and 66 percent, respectively. Thus, the false negative and positive rates for this test are 43 percent and 34 percent, respectively. In these series, 71 percent of patients with a normal PRA and 86 percent of patients with an elevated PRA benefited from surgery.

There are a variety of possible explanations for the relatively low sensitivity and specificity of the PRA in RVHT and various maneuvers have been suggested to improve the test's diagnostic accuracy. It has been suggested that the physiologic consequences of RAS on renin secretion may not permit an elevated PRA.[50,84,203] Although the stenotic kidney is secreting renin at an increased rate, renin secretion from the contralateral kidney is inhibited. The net effect of these two processes could be a normal PRA.[50,84,203] It is also well known that renin secretion is markedly dependent on sodium balance. A more accurate interpretation of the PRA can be made if the result is related to the 24 hour urinary sodium excretion.[121] However, even when this type of analysis was done in patients with RVHT, the sensitivity of the PRA was still only 72 percent in one series[203] and not significantly improved in others.[165,186] The expanded volume responsible for hypertension in bilateral RVHT or unilateral RVHT with contralateral renal parenchymal disease could also account for a reduced PRA.[122] Segmental lesions resulting in RVHT may not demonstrate an increased PRA due to a dilutional effect from blood draining nonischemic areas of the kidney.[170] Schambelan found a normal PRA in 8 of 9 hypertensive patients with segmental lesions of whom 5 had surgery and were improved.[170]

Posture has also been demonstrated to affect the sensitivity of the PRA. Cohen et al. demonstrated that the normal response of upright posture to increase PRA is greatly exaggerated in RVHT.[42] In the supine position, four of nine patients with proven RVHT had normal PRA while after 4 hours of ambulation six of nine (including the four with normal values) had increased PRA compared to controls. However, other investigators have not been able to document an improvement in sensitivity with upright posture.[81,138,139] False negative PRA values may also occur if the circadian rhythm of renin secretion in RVHT is not taken into account. Grim et al. measured PRA over the course of 24 hours in both the supine and upright positions in patients with proven RVHT.[80] PRA values were significantly greater at noon, 4 P.M., and 8 P.M. in RVHT patients compared to normal controls (regardless of position). In four of seven RVHT patients, supine 8 A.M. values did not discriminate these patients from controls while values measured at 8 P.M. were discriminatory. The authors concluded that the diagnostic ability of the PRA would be improved if measured after 12 hours of upright posture on a high sodium diet.[80]

Saline loading (2 liters NSS) has been

**Table 4-5.** Renal Vein Renin Ratio in Renovascular Hypertension

| Reference | Critical Ratio | Sensitivity | Specificity | Surgical Improvement | | Study Conditions[a] | | | Renal Vascular Lesion[c] |
|---|---|---|---|---|---|---|---|---|---|
| | | | | RVRR Negative | RVRR Positive | Na Depletion, Drugs | Upright Posture | Simultaneous Sampling | |
| Judson[106] | 2 | 16/16 | 15/15 | 0/15 | 16/16 | – | – | – | Unilateral |
| Fitz[64] | 2 | 7/7 | 4/6 | 0/4 | 7/9 | – | – | – | Unilateral |
| Kirkendall[115] | 2 | 6/6 | 2/2 | 0/2 | 6/6 | – | – | – | Mixed |
| Winer[211] | 1.5 | 9/9 | 2/2 | 0/2 | 9/9 | – | – | – | Unilateral |
| Michelakis[141] | 1.5 | 17/18 | 2/3 | 1/3 | 17/18 | – | – | – | Unilateral |
| Bath[10] | 2 | 5/6 | 0/5 | 1/1 | 5/10 | – | – | – | Unilateral |
| Bath[10] | | – | 5/5 | 0/5 | – | – | – | – | Bilateral |
| Amsterdam[1] | 2.5 | 5/8 | 6/6 | 3/9 | 5/5 | – | – | – | Unilateral |
| Shapiro[174] | N.G. | 5/8 | 1/1 | 3/4 | 5/5 | – | – | – | Mixed |
| Mannick[131] | N.G. | 14/15 | 1/1 | 1/2 | 14/14 | + | – | – | Unilateral |
| Gunnels[88] | 2 | 15/16 | 2/5 | 1/3 | 15/18 | – | – | – | Unilateral |
| Bourgoigne[16] | 1.6 | 8/9 | 3/3 | 1/4 | 8/8 | – | – | – | Unilateral |
| Bourgoigne[16] | 1.6 | 1/1 | 1/4 | 0/1 | 1/4 | – | – | – | Bilateral |
| Simmons[175] | 1.5 | 17/18 | 2/3 | 1/3 | 17/18 | – | – | – | Unilateral |
| Chapman[37] | 1.5 | 8/10 | 1/2 | 2/3 | 8/9 | – | – | – | Mixed |
| Kirkendall[116] | 1.5 | 6/9 | 1/1 | 3/4 | 6/6 | + | – | – | Unilateral |
| Bozovic[17] | 1.5 | 4/5 | 4/4 | 1/5 | 4/4 | – | – | – | Unilateral |
| Klatte[117] | 1.5 | 6/8 | – | 2/2 | 6/6 | – | – | – | Bilateral |
| Fournier[69] | 1.5 | 7/11 | 9/14 | 4/13 | 7/12 | – | – | – | Mixed |
| Pawsey[154] | 1.5 | 10/12 | 1/2 | 2/3 | 10/11 | + | + | + | Unilateral |
| Strong[190] | 1.5 | 5/11 | – | 6/6 | 5/5 | – | – | – | Unilateral |
| Strong[190] | 1.5 | 2/7 | 1/1 | 5/6 | 2/2 | – | – | – | Bilateral |
| Strong[190] | 1.5 | 21/23 | 3/3 | 2/5 | 21/21 | + | – | – | Unilateral |
| Strong[190] | 1.5 | 11/13 | 1/1 | 2/3 | 11/11 | + | – | – | Bilateral |
| Ernst[58] | 1.5 | 30/37 | – | 7/7 | 30/30 | + | + | – | Unilateral |
| Guedon[87] | 1.5 | 7/13 | 0/2 | 6/6 | 7/9 | – | – | – | Unilateral |
| Stockigt[181] | 1.5 | 18/20 | 1/2 | 2/3 | 18/19 | – | – | – | Unilateral |
| Stockigt[181] | 1.5 | 3/5 | 0/2 | 2/2 | 3/5 | – | – | – | Bilateral |
| Dean[47] | 1.5 | 31/39 | – | 8/8 | 31/31 | – | – | – | Unilateral |
| Hussain[103] | 1.5 | 13/19 | 8/10 | 6/14 | 13/15 | – | – | – | Unilateral |
| Poutasse[161] | 1.5 | 5/9 | 0/1 | 4/4 | 5/6 | – | – | – | Unilateral |
| Poutasse[161] | 1.5 | 2/3 | 1/1 | 1/1 | 2/2 | – | – | – | Bilateral |
| Vaughan[203] | 1.5[b] | 15/16 | 4/7 | 1/5 | 15/18 | + | – | – | Unilateral |
| Schaeffer[169] | 1.5 | 6/10 | – | 4/4 | 6/6 | + | – | + | Unilateral |
| Schaeffer[169] | 1.5 | 1/7 | – | 6/6 | 1/1 | + | – | + | Segmental |
| Gittes[75] | 1.5 | 6/6 | – | – | 6/6 | + | – | – | Bilateral |
| Grim[80] | 1.5 | 7/7 | – | – | 7/7 | + | + | + | Unilateral |
| Juncos[107] | 1.5 | 62/68 | 3/7 | 6/9 | 62/66 | + | – | – | Mixed |

| | Tesla | | | | | | | | |
|---|---|---|---|---|---|---|---|---|---|
| Messerli[139] | 2.0 | 14/18 | 9/9 | 4/13 | 14/14 | + | − | + | Unilateral |
| Stanley[179] | N.G. | 71/85 | — | 14/14 | 71/71 | + | − | − | Mixed |
| Couch[45] | 1.5 | 15/20 | 0/3 | 5/5 | 15/18 | ± | − | − | Unilateral |
| Buda[31] | 1.5 | 48/55 | 5/14 | 7/12 | 48/57 | − | − | − | Mixed |
| De Quattro[52] | N.G. | 9/12 | 0/1 | 3/3 | 9/10 | − | − | − | N.G. |
| Maxwell[135] | 1.5 | 34/57 | 5/9 | 23/28 | 34/38 | ± | − | + | Unilateral |
| Dean[48] | 1.5 | 18/26 | — | 8/8 | 18/18 | + | − | − | Bilateral |
| Tucker[199] | N.G. | 9/14 | 1/1 | 5/6 | 9/9 | + | − | − | Mixed |
| D'Souza[54] | 1.5 | 13/13 | — | — | 13/13 | + | − | − | Unilateral |
| Hansson[90] | 1.5 | 30/33 | 3/10 | 3/6 | 30/37 | + | + | + | Unilateral |
| Aurell[6] | N.G. | 35/41 | — | 6/6 | 35/35 | + | − | + | Mixed |
| Hughes[100] | 1.4 | 21/26 | 5/10 | 5/10 | 21/26 | ± | − | − | Mixed |
| Luscher[125] | 1.5 | 20/24 | 0/3 | 4/4 | 20/23 | + | − | + | Unilateral |
| Rosenthal[165] | 1.5 | 35/44 | 0/1 | 9/9 | 35/36 | + | + | + | Unilateral |
| Rosenthal[165] | 1.5 | 12/20 | 2/2 | 8/10 | 12/12 | + | + | + | Bilateral |
| Chiarini[38] | 1.5 | 22/26 | 1/1 | 4/5 | 22/22 | + | + | + | Unilateral |
| Sinaiko[176] | 1.4 | 8/9 | 3/3 | 1/4 | 8/8 | + | − | + | N.G. |
| Keith[114] | 1.5 | 14/22 | 1/1 | 8/9 | 14/14 | + | − | + | Mixed |
| Bergrem[12] | 1.5 | 23/29 | 0/2 | 6/6 | 23/25 | + | − | + | Unilateral |
| Novick[146] | 1.5 | 13/18 | 2/3 | 5/7 | 13/14 | − | − | − | Mixed |
| Total—all series | | 875/1097 (80%) | 120/193 (62%) | 222/342 (65%) | 875/948 (92%) | | | | |
| Total—bilateral | | 61/89 (68%) | 10/15 (67%) | 28/38 (74%) | 61/66 (92%) | | | | |
| Total—unilateral stimulated | | 300/377 (80%) | 24/45 (53%) | 77/101 (76%) | 300/321 (93%) | | | | |

[a]Test conditions (stimulation, posture, simultaneous sampling) were assumed not to have been performed if not specified by the author.
[b]Arbitrarily assigned.
[c]Mixed lesions indicate those series in which patients with unilateral and bilateral RAS were reported together.
[d]Only portion of study group stimulated.
Note: N.G.: not given in methods.

**Table 4-6.** Saralasin Test in Renovascular Hypertension

| Investigator | Criteria for Positive Response | Sensitivity | Positive Test in EHT | Sodium Depletion | Saralasin Dose |
|---|---|---|---|---|---|
| | | | | Test Conditions[a] | |
| Donker[53] | Normalization of blood pressure | 0/2 | — | — | Constant infusion, 5–100 μg/kg/min |
| Buda[31] | N.G. | 5/5 | — | N.G. | Constant infusion, 2–10 μg/kg/min |
| Streeten[187] | Fall in b.p. by ≥ 10/8 mm Hg | 7/7 | — | + | Constant infusion, 0.05-5 μg/kg/min |
| Anderson[2] | N.G. | — | 0/34 | + | Constant infusion, 0.25 and 5 μg/kg/min |
| Wilson[210] | | | | | |
|  Unliteral | | 5/5 | 2/15 | + | Constant infusion, 1.3 |
|  Bilateral | Fall in b.p. ≥ 10/6 mm Hg | 6/6 | | + | mg/min |
| Thomas[193] | N.G. | 0/2 | — | + (only 1 case) | Constant infusion, 0.25– 16 μg/kg/min |
| Marks[134] | | | | | |
|  Unilateral | Fall in b.p. ≥ 10/8 mm Hg | 7/8 | 4/15 | + | 10 mg IV bolus followed in 30 min by infusion |
|  Bilateral | | 5/5 | | + | of 10 or 50 μg/kg/min |
| Trainin[196] | N.G. | 0/1 | — | + | Constant infusion, 10 μg/kg/min |
| Tucker[199] | Fall in diastolic b.p. ≥ 8% control | 9/15 | — | + | Constant infusion, 40 mg over 30 min |
| Stokes[183] | Fall in b.p. >10/7 mm Hg | 1/3 | — | + | Constant infusion, 0.1– 10 μg/kg/min |
| Horne[96] | Fall in diastolic b.p. ≥ 8% control | — | 27/118 | + | Constant infusion, 0.8 mg/min |
| Poutasse[160] | | | | | |
|  Unilateral | Fall in b.p. > 10/8 | 12/13 | — | + | 9 mg IV bolus |
|  Bilateral | mm Hg | 1/3 | | + | |
| Grim[81] | Fall in b.p. ≥ 10/8 mm Hg | 12/23 | 2/13 | + | Constant infusion, 0.8 mg/min |
| Hollenberg[94] | Fall in diastolic b.p. ≥ 10 mm Hg | 3/3 | 12/95 | + | Constant infusion, 0.3– 30 μg/kg/min |
| Krakoff[118] | Fall in diastolic b.p. ≥ 5 mm Hg | 15/20 | 4/34 | + | Constant infusion, 18 mg over 30 min |
| Streeten[188] | | | | | |
|  Unilateral | Fall in b.p. by > 10/8 mm Hg | 27/30 | — | + | Constant infusion, 0.05– 5 μg/kg/min |
| Novick[146] | Fall in mean arterial pressure of ≥ 10% control | 11/19 | — | N.G. | Constant infusion[b], 0.3– 10 μg/kg/min |
| Total | | 26/170 (74%) | 51/324 (15.7%) | | |

[a]Position for all series was supine.

[b]Used sarcosine -1, threonine-8, angiotensin II.

Note. Abbreviations: EHT, essential hypertension; NG: specific information not given in methods of section of reference.

proposed as a method to increase the sensitivity of PRA in RHVT.[138] Melman et al. demonstrated a failure of saline loading to suppress PRA in 10 of 14 patients with RVHT.[138] In contrast, only 3 of 13 of these patients had levels of PRA exceeding controls after furosemide stimulation. Others, however, have not found saline loading to be helpful in diagnosing RVHT.[81]

The high incidence of false positive PRA levels also limits the usefullness of this test in RVHT. Other hypertensive conditions associated with an elevated PRA include malignant hypertension,[65] hypertension treated with diuretics or vasodilators, congestive heart failure,[23] or essential hypertension. About 15 percent of patients with essential hypertension have been shown to have elevated PRA levels.[121,108]

In conclusion, it would appear that the low sensitivity and specificity of the PRA severely limits the value of this test in predicting which patients with RAS and hypertension have RVHT. It is doubtful that the various stimulatory or inhibitory maneuvers proposed can sufficiently alter the discriminatory ability of the PRA to make this test diagnostically useful by itself.

## Renal Vein Renin Ratio (RVRR) and Other Measurements of Renal Vein Renin

Previous observations in patients with RVHT, showing that renal vein renin activity was increased in kidneys with RAS compared to contralateral normal kidneys, [92,105,197] led Judson and Helmer in 1965 to suggest that "functional" RAS could be predicted by demonstrating an elevated ratio of renin activity from the stenotic side as compared with the contralateral kidney.[106] In their initial report, the RVRR was greater than 2 (authors' critera for abnormal) in all 16 patients with proven RVHT and was less than 2 in all 16 hypertensive patients who failed to improve after surgery. Since then the RVRR has become a widely accepted test for detection of "functional" RAS. The reasons for this wide acceptance are as follows. First, most series have confirmed that the large majority of patients with abnormal RVRR will benefit from surgery. Second, the test is based on experimental observations in RVHT which support a pathogenetic role for increased renin activity in the venous plasma of the affected kidney. Third, differences between centers for the absolute value of renal vein PRA which is

considered abnormal is obviated with the use of a ratio. Fourth, the ratio also normalizes for conditions (e.g., malignant hypertension) known to increase the absolute values of PRA in both renal veins. Finally, previous reports on the value of the peripheral vein PRA to detect RVHT were disappointing.

Table 4-5 is a summary of reported series evaluating the RVRR as a diagnostic test for RVHT. As in Table 4-4, series evaluating the RVRR in which exact sensitivity or specificity data could not be determined were excluded from the analysis.[120,137,138,158,168] The overall results for all series in Table 4-5 demonstrate that the RVRR has a sensitivity of 80 percent and a false negative rate of 20 percent. The specificity of the test is 62 percent with a false positive rate of 38 percent.

**Pathophysiologic and Technical Reasons for False Negative and False Positive RVRR Results.** A number of pathophysiologic and technical factors have been proposed as possible causes for the significant number of false negative and false positive results associated with the RVRR (Table 4-6).

**Pathophysiologic Factors.** As discussed, it has been proposed that hypertension caused by *bilateral RAS* (or unilateral RAS with contralateral renal parenchymal disease) is volume dependent and is analogous to the "one-kidney" Goldblatt experimental model.[122] Bilateral RAS is not uncommon in patients with suspected RVHT. In the Cooperative Study on RVHT, 25 percent of all patients had bilateral RAS.[14] Because of volume-mediated supresion of renin secretion (and the dependency of a positive RVRR on increased renin secretion in the stenotic kidney), it would not be surprising to find a significant number of false negative results for the RVRR in patients with bilateral RVHT. An analysis of only those series[10,16,48,75,117,161,165,182,190] (Table 4-5) in which RVRR data are provided for bilateral lesions reveals the sensitivity of the RVRR to be 68 percent with a false negative rate of 32 percent. As shown in Table 4-5, this false negative rate is higher than that of both the entire population (20 percent) or only those patients with unilateral RVHT (20 percent). However, this high false negative rate suggesting a volume-related mechanism may be more apparent than real. In the series by Dean et al., 44 of 86 patients (51 percent) with angiographically documented bilateral RAS had improvement in their blood pressure following unilateral renal artery repair.[48] The actual number of patients with bilateral disease who would have benefited from unilateral surgery is probably higher since there were an additional 18 patients who underwent bilateral repair despite having lateralizing RVRR.[48] Similarly, in the series by Strong et al., nine patients with bilateral disease and with lateralizing RVRR benefited from unilateral surgical repair.[190] There were an additional six patients with bilateral disease without lateralizing RVRR who also benefited from unilateral surgery. These data would suggest that many patients with bilateral RAS have a pathophysiologic mechanism responsible for hypertension similar to patients with unilateral RVHT. Thus, despite anatomic evidence of bilateral RAS, it would appear that in many cases, only one of the lesions is "functionally" significant.[117] In patients with bilateral RAS but with lateralizing RVRR, surgery should be performed only on the kidney which lateralizes. In patients with bilateral RAS but without lateralizing RVRR, surgery should also be unilateral and directed to the side with the greater stenosis since (a) a significant number of such patients will benefit by this limited approach[48,190] and (b) bilateral repair is associated with a much higher operative mortality than in unilateral repair.[70] The improvement in blood pressure from unilateral surgery in patients with bilateral disease but without lateralizing RVRR probably results from improvement in the excretion of excess sodium and water.

*Segmental ischemic lesions* due to either stenosis of a branch of the main renal artery, focal infarction, segmental hypoplasia, or a juxtaglomerular cell tumor may also result in a false negative RVRR. The frequency of segmental ischemic lesions causing RVHT has been reported to be 13 percent.[14] In this setting, increased renin content of venous blood draining the segmental area may be significantly diluted by venous blood from the remainder of the kidney with the net result that the renin concentration in the main renal vein is not significantly elevated. Based on earlier observations of false negative RVRR in patients with RVHT due to segmental lesions[181,182] Schambelan et al. systematically evaluated a group of patients with this abnormality.[170] The RVRR was diagnostic in only two of five patients when renin was sampled from the main renal vein of the affected kidney. However, when renin sampling was selectively performed from the intrarenal veins draining the segmental lesion and compared to renin concentration of the main renal vein of the contralateral kidney, the RVRR was now diagnostic in all five patients. These observations provide a strong argument for performing arteriography before renal vein renin sampling.

It is commonly proposed that renin secretion may not be significantly active or increased at the time of renal vein sampling thus resulting in false negative ratios. Possible mechanisms for this include varying sodium balance and ECF volume,[29] posture, and antihypertensive medication, all of which can affect renin secretion in patients with RVHT. In this regard, a variety of *stimulatory maneuvers* designed to maximize renin secretion have been suggested. The success of these maneuvers results in part from experimental and clinical observations which demonstrate that a stenotic ischemic kidney has a greater magnitude of response in terms of renin secretion to stimulatory maneuvers than do the kidneys of normotensive controls or patients with essential hypertension.[110,200] This increased response may be due to the fact that stimulatory maneuvers which reduce perfusion to the kidney will have a greater effect in kidneys with stenotic lesions and already reduced perfusion.[110] Thus for a given stimulatory maneuver, there will be a greater degree of hypoperfusion in a kidney with RAS compared to a kidney with a normal renal artery.[110,200] The failure of a stimulatory maneuver to increase secretion in the contralateral kidney to the same degree as the stenotic kidney maximizes the disparity between the two kidneys in terms of renal vein renin concentration, thus further raising the RVRR.[104,110,131,161,200] There are additional mechanisms which may account for the failure of the contralateral kidney to respond as actively as the stenotic kidney to a given stimulus. In experimental and clinical RVHT, the renin content of the contralateral kidney has been shown to be markedly reduced.[85,89] It is thus possible that stimulation of such a depleted kidney will not result in any additional renin release. Furthermore, the failure of the contralateral kidney to respond to stimulation in RVHT may be due to the high levels of angiotensin II which through a negative feedback mechanism, inhibit secretion of renin from that kidney.[51,201] Such inhibition is supported by the observation that the renal vein renin activity in the contralateral kidney equals the renin activity in the inferior vena cava (the latter is equal to arterial renin concentration) in RVHT.[161] Thus for several reasons, the use of stimulatory maneuvers in patients with suspected RVHT would appear to be attractive in increasing the sensitivity of the RVRR.

A state of *low sodium balance*, induced by diuretics, a diet bereft of sodium, or both will increase renin secretion in both normotensive controls[41,79] and patients with essential hypertension.[207] The application of similar maneuvers to patients with RVHT has been shown in several series to increase both renin secretion and the sensitivity of the RVRR.[6,102,125,190,204] For example, Strong et al. demonstrated a positive RVRR in 8 of 25 patients with RVHT under conditions of sodium repletion compared to a positive RVRR in 33 of 37 patients under conditions of sodium depletion.[190] A few series have not found sodium depletion to be as helpful. Couch et al. had only one positive RVRR test in four patients with proven RVHT despite collection under low sodium stimulation.[45] Similarly, Whelton et al. in a brief report were unable to improve the sensitivity of the RVRR when collected immediately following furosemide.[209] On the whole, however, the majority of the data supports the use of sodium depletion to increase the sensitivity of the RVRR.

Renin secretion can also be increased in normotensive controls and patients with essential hypertension by *upright posture*.[43] Several investigators have demonstrated that 20 to 30 minutes of upright posture or tilting can significantly reduce the likelihood of a false negative RVRR in patients with proven RVHT.[6,42,80,138,142,143] On occassion however, upright posture may decrease the sensitivity of the RVRR. Michelakis et al. demonstrated the occurrence of false negative RVRR if renal vein renins were collected too soon after the patient changed from an upright to a supine position.[143] The explanation given for this observation is that upright posture resulted in large increases in the level of circulating renin. With assumption of the supine position for renin sampling the stimulus for increased secretion is removed. However due to the long half-life of renin, the blood remains renin-rich and now passes through the arteries of both the contralateral and stenotic kidneys. Any small but significant disparity in renin secretion which may have existed between the two kidneys in the recumbent position and which would have resulted in a positive RVRR, could now be obscured by the renin-rich blood. This observation has been confirmed by other investigators.[154] Thus, to avoid this problem, we recommend that patients should be in the supine position for several hours prior to renal vein renin collections. Stimulation that takes advantage of upright posture can be achieved with tilting during the collection of the renal vein renins.

Another technique for stimulating renin secretion has been proposed by D'Souza et al.[54] *Blood pressure cuffs* are applied to all four extremities of the patient with suspected RVHT and inflated to 20 mm Hg above the systolic pressure. After five minutes, the cuffs are deflated to 60 to 80 mm Hg and renal vein renins are collected. Stimulation of renin secretion results from the induction of a reactive hyperemia with subsequent trapping of a large amount of blood in the extremities. Mean renin values rose by 100 percent in renal venous plasma from the stenotic kidneys compared to a mean increase of 53 percent for the contralateral kidneys. The sensitivity of the RVRR with this maneuver increased from 46 percent to 100 percent. The advantages of the cuff maneuver were its technical simplicity, the absence of any precipitous or variable falls in blood pressure as may occur with tilting or pharmacologic stimulation, and any hypotension which might occur could easily be controlled by deflating one or two cuffs.[54]

Nondiuretic *pharmacologic agents* have also been demonstrated to stimulate renin secretion in RVHT.[6,12,104,110,116,131,176,200] Parenteral hydralazine (20 mg) has been reported to preferentially increase renin secretion from the stenotic ischemic kidney compared to the contralateral kidney,[104] to decrease the number of false negative RVRR in patients with proven RVHT,[12,116,131,176] and to raise PRA to a greater extent in RVHT compared to normotensive controls or patients with essential hypertension.[200] For example, Mannick et al. increased the number of positive RVRR from 9 of 15 to 14 of 15 in their patients with RVHT.[131] Possible mechanisms for the renin stimulatory ability of hydralazine include an acute reduction in renal perfusion pressure, increased sympathetic discharge, or altered intrarenal hemodynamics.[200] The first mechanism, although the most attractive, is somewhat weakened due to the failure of several studies to demonstrate a correlation between the fall in blood pressure and the increase in renin activity.[104,131,200] Other vasodilators (e.g., nitroprusside and diazoxide), have also been shown to improve the sensitivity of the RVRR in RVHT.[110,184] Stimulation with any of these agents, however, is not without risk. Adverse effects of flushing, palpitations, chest pain, and nausea have been reported and thus caution must be taken especially in patients with underlying coronary artery disease.[200]

Finally, Re et al. have used a *converting enzyme inhibitor* (CEI) to stimulate renin secretion and improve the sensitivity of the RVRR.[162] Postulated mechanisms for the ability of a CEI to increase renin secretion include an elimination of the inhibition of renin secretion by angiotensin II and hypoperfusion from the reduction in blood pressure caused by the CEI. After giving 0.25 mg/kg of CEI parenterally to six patients with proven RVHT, the sensitivity of the RVRR increased from 50 percent to 100 percent.[162]

Assuming that these various stimulatory maneuvers (low sodium diet, upright posture, and pharmacologic agents) increase the sensitivity of the RVRR in RVHT, we have recalculated the combined sensitivity of the RVRR using only those series in Table 4-5 which studied patients with unilateral RVHT under stimulatory conditions.[12,38,54,58,90,125,133,135,139,154,165,169,190] The sensitivity of this selected cases was still only 80 percent with a false negative rate of 20 percent despite stimulation. It is interesting to note that the false positive rate was greater in the stimulated group (47 percent) compared to the entire population as a whole (38 percent). Thus these tests may result in a decreased specificity of the RVRR while being of questionable benefit in terms of improving sensitivity.

Extensive *collateral circulation* resulting from a stenosis of the main renal artery has been suggested as indicative of a hemodynamically significant lesion. However, extensive collateral vessels have also been reported to cause false negative RVRR.[38,58,178] Ernst et al. arteriographically evaluated 37 patients with proven unilateral RVHT.[58] Collateral vessels were present in 68 percent of the patients. The mean RVRR values for the patients with and without collateral vessels were 1.8 and 3.1 (p<.05), respectively although there was significant overlap between the two groups. However, all of the patients with RVHT and a RVRR<1.4 had collateral vessels compared to a prevalance of 60 percent for collateral vessels in those patients with RVRR>1.4.[58] These clinical observations are supported by experimental studies of RVHT in dogs. In these studies, as the number of collateral vessels increased with time there was an associated progressive fall in the RVRR.[59] Although the ischemic stimulus for renin secretion decreased with development of collateral vessels, it was suggested the mild abnormalities of the renin-angiotensin system remained inappropriately high for the degree of sodium balance and still played a role in the pathogenesis of the hypertension.[59]

Although the majority of studies support the renin-angiotensin system as the primary pathogenetic mechanism in RVHT, evidence for a *non-renin-mediated form of RVHT* in man has been suggested by Marks et al.[133] These investigators described two patients studied under low sodium conditions who demonstrated low PVPRA and plasma aldosterone levels, nonlateralizing RVRR, and an absent vasodepressor response to saralasin infusion. The hypertension of both patients was reduced with surgery. These observations raise the possibility that factors other than the renin-angiotensin system may cause RVHT.[127,128] Others have suggested that the inability to demonstrate renin-angiotensin dependency in these two patients may have been due to a failure to stimulate the system sufficiently by not using vasodilators.[126,177]

## TECHNICAL FACTORS

A variety of *technical factors* related to performance of the test itself have been reported to cause false negative or positive RVRR in patients with RVHT. Careful attention must be paid to catheter placement in the renal vein prior to sampling of blood for renin activity. In sampling the left renal vein, the catheter should be placed beyond the orifices of the adrenal and gonadal veins which empty into this vessel. Failure to properly place the catheter may result in the *admixture* of renal venous blood with blood from nonrenal sites which could dilute the concentration of renin in the renal vein and thus falsely lower the RVRR.[87,148,153,161,211] With the right renal vein, because it is shorter than the left, aspiration of vena caval blood may result if the catheter is not placed far enough into the vessel.[148] Too *vigorous aspiration* of blood from either vein again carries with it the risk of admixture of renal venous blood with blood from the vena cava.[153] Another catheter placement error may occur when *multiple renal veins* exist. In this setting, the catheter may be introduced into a vein not draining the area(s) of the kidney which is (are) most ischemic.[154,161] The frequency of multiple renal veins has been reported to be up to 20 to 28 percent on the right side and 1 to 3 percent on the left side.[161] Finally, a theoretical possibility for a falsely negative RVRR could occur if renin sampling is performed while the patient is straining and raising his intraabdominal pressure. It has been shown that the *Valsalva maneuver* will cause hemodilution which could transiently decrease the renin concentration in the renal vein.[148]

A false negative RVRR from interference with the renin assay by contrast media used to locate catheter position has been proposed,[211] although others have not found this.[208] Similarly, heparin (>100 U/ml) in the collection tubes has been claimed to interfere with the renin assay (bioassay)[110,111] although lower concentrations (< 40 U/ml) seem to have no effect on the renin values.[110]

Spontaneous and rapid variations in renal vein renin activity may occur and are most likely due to alterations in volume, posture, sodium balance, and perfusion pressure.[143] *Nonsimultaneous sampling* of the renal veins for plasma renin activity may result in a false negative or positive RVRR.[161] Several investigators have demonstrated that in patients with and without RVHT serial determinations of renal vein renin activity using simultaneous sampling with two catheters resulted in significant variations in the PRA results.[97,144] These variations could not be explained by variations in the assay method and appeared predominantly due to spontaneous variations in renin secretion from the stenotic kidney.[144] In contrast, Whelton et al. sampled renal vein renin activity both simultaneously and sequentially in hypertensive patients with and without RAS.[208] Mean renal vein renin values collected under both conditions were

not significantly different. Although mean values may not differ, others have shown significant individual variations.[97]

Errors in the measurement of plasma renin activity may also give rise to false negative or positive results.[148,165,173] However, using the radioimmunoassay method, the likelihood of this occurring is very small.[97,144] Stockigt found that the probability of their within assay variation resulting in a RVRR greater than 1.4 was less than 0.004.[181] If renin values are either very large or small, the probability for incorrect data from the assay increases.[144] Potential errors due to assay variation can be minimized by collecting at least two samples from each renal vein.[97]

False negative and false positive RVRR results will also occur if the *critical ratio* chosen is either too high or too low, respectively. Maxwell et al. analyzed the RVRR in 101 of their own patients and 126 patients reported in the literature.[136] All of the patients had essential hypertension with normal renal vasculature (proven by arteriography in the majority). Renal vein renin collections were performed without simultaneous sampling or acute stimulation. These data revealed that the RVRR was ≤1.96 in 96 percent, ≤1.68 in 90 percent, and ≤1.5 in 81 percent of the population. Thus, the probability of a RVRR >1.96 in a patient with essential hypertension was less than 5 percent. However, RVRR >1.5 could be found in 19 percent of patients with essential hypertension. Therefore, the choice of a critical ratio ≥2 would result in a high specificity for the RVRR but would result in a decreased sensitivity. The choice of a ratio of ≥1.5 would significantly improve the sensitivity but would decrease the test's specificity. By altering the criteria for a positive test, the RVRR can be used to exclude or confirm the presence of RVHT, according to the physician's purpose for the test. These findings are consistent with the significant false positive rate of the RVRR noted in Table 4-5 since most of these series used a critical ratio of 1.5.

Explanations for RVRR greater than unity in patients with essential hypertension could be due to spontaneous variations in renin secretion not corrected for by simultaneous sampling and/or disparities in the degree of nephrosclerosis between the two kidneys.[136] The existence of such disparities in patients with essential hypertension has been suggested by renal biopsy studies.[167] Ideally, studies using the RVRR to diagnose RVHT should utilize methods to minimize technical errors (e.g., simultaneous collection, multiple samples, etc.) and have a control group of patients with essential hypertension in which renal vein renin activity was determined in the same manner as performed for the patients with suspected RVHT.

Since the RVRR reflects the measurement of the concentration of renin in the renal veins, an elevation could result from simply a *reduction in renal blood flow* rather than from increased secretion stimulated by ischemia.[155,212] Thus, if renal blood flow were halved and secretion remained constant, the concentration of renin activity in that renal vein would double. This occurrence could result in a RVRR which was falsely positive.[212] Data supporting an increased secretion and not simply a reduction in renal blood flow as the mechanism for the increased RVRR in RVHT has been presented by several groups.[17, 93,110,116,202,212] Woods et al. measured effective renal plasma flow and renal vein PRA in patients with unilateral RAS and hypertension.[212] Renal vein renin effluent for each kidney was obtained by multiplying the renal vein PRA by the effective renal plasma flow for that kidney. Although renin determinations and effective renal plasma flow for a given individual were not measured on the same day, both were determined under identical condi-

tions of posture, diet, and hydration. In patients proved to have RVHT, the RVRR was always ≥1,8. In 10 of these 13 patients, the renal vein renin effluent was also significantly increased on the affected side supporting increased secretion as the mechanism for the increased renal vein PRA.

Finally, a false positive result may occur if there is an unrecognized *technical failure* of the bypass graft surgery. In the Cooperative Study, the anatomic failure rate for primary vascular reconstructive surgery varied from 18 percent to 45 percent.[67] However, this incidence is based on an analysis of only those patients who had postoperative arteriograms. The true incidence of anatomic failures is probably much lower. For example, in one series in which all patients had postoperative arteriograms, the thrombosis rate was only 8 percent.[60]

**Alternative or Supplemental Methods in Analyzing Renal Vein Renin Activity.** Several groups have suggested additional methods of analyzing renal vein renin data to further improve the diagnostic sensitivity and specificity of the RVRR. The method most commonly employed is an assessment of the degree of suppression of renin secretion by the contralateral kidney. In experimental unilateral RVHT, both a suppression of renin secretion[110] and a depletion of renal renin[163,195] have been demonstrated in the contralateral kidney. Lack of such suppression may indicate abnormal blood flow or intrarenal ischemia, either of which could stimulate renin secretion, thus maintaining the hypertension despite adequate surgical correction of the stenotic kidney.[181]

In 1972, Stockigt et al. suggested that a ratio of contralateral renal vein plasma renin activity (Rc) to PRA less than 1.3 demonstrated inhibition of renin secretion by the contralateral kidney.[181] It had been previously shown that the PRA (from a peripheral vein proper or the inferior vena cava below the renal veins) was essentially equal to simultaneously measured arterial plasma renin activity.[172,181] Stockigt proposed that both RVRR ≥1.5 and Rc/PRA ratio <1.3 were needed to predict a beneficial result from surgery.[181] In this series, 15 or 16 patients with surgically proven unilateral RVHT met the requirements for both ratios. In patients who failed to suppress renin secretion from the contralateral kidney (Rc/PRA>1.3), surgical benefit was less likely. Additional investigators have also claimed that suppression of contralateral renin secretion is important for predicting surgical benefit.[168,169,179,203,211] The test has also been helpful in patients with segmental lesions causing RVHT, many of whom have a negative RVRR.[170]

There are, however, some investigators who have not found the demonstration of contralateral suppression to be as helpful.[125,135,165] Maxwell et al. demonstrated that 16 of 57 patients benefited by surgery despite Rc/Inferior vena cava ratios of >1.3.[135] In nine patients who failed to improve with surgery, only six had no evidence for contralateral suppression. Similarly, Luscher et al. found that in 17 patients with suspected renal hypertension (majority RVHT) and no evidence of contralateral suppression, 82 percent still benefited from surgery.[125]

Another approach to improve the diagnostic accuracy of renal renin measurements in RVHT has been suggested by Vaughan et al.[203] These investigators developed a weighted scoring system combining three criteria which are indicative of RVHT: (1) increased PRA when related to urine sodium excretion, (2) suppression of renin from the contralateral kidney, and (3) a significantly increased renal vein renin concentration relative to the arterial renin (peripheral vein or inferior vena cava) in the stenotic kidney. Using their scoring method, the authors predicted a favorable outcome in all 13 patients who eventually did benefit from surgery and a poor outcome in all 5 patients who failed to benefit by surgery. Although the results in the original report appeared excellent, more recent studies are not as encouraging. Rosenthal et al. using the Vaughan scoring method were only able to demonstrate a 66 percent sensitivity for 44 patients evaluated with unilateral lesions.[165] In fact, when the renal vein renin determinations in these same patients were recalculated as the RVRR, the sensitivity of this latter test was 80 percent. A similar sensitivity using this method of scoring has also been reported by Maxwell et al.[135] It would appear that despite its physiologic attractiveness, the weighted scoring method of Vaughan may not offer any diagnostic advantages over the RVRR. The reader is referred to the original publication for additional details regarding scoring, analysis, and technical requirements of this method.[203]

In summary, the RVRR in RVHT has a diagnostic sensitivity of 80 percent and a specificity of 62 percent. In addition, the data in Table 4-5 demonstrates that in those patients suspected of RVHT who underwent corrective surgery and had a RVRR which lateralized, 92 percent benefited from the operation. When surgery was performed in the patients with nonlateralizing RVRR, 65 percent still benefited from the procedure. The diagnostic limitations (20 percent false negative and 38 percent false positive rate) of the RVRR appears to be due to multiple physiologic and technical factors. The cumulative effect of these limitations would appear to prevent total reliance on the RVRR as a means of identifying RVHT.[165] Stimulatory maneuvers as well as additional methods of interpretation such as contralateral suppression or weighted scoring systems are unable to obviate the limitations of this diagnostic test.

## Saralasin

The most recent diagnostic tests for RVHT utilize pharmacologic agents which interfere with the renin-angiotensin system directly. In this regard, the majority of the experience has been with octapeptide, saralasin (sar-1-ala-8-angiotensin II), which is a parenteral competitive inhibitor of the natural hormone angiotensin II.[152] The substitution of alanine for phenylalanine at position 8 results in a markedly diminished vasoconstrictive effect when saralasin (compared to angiotensin II) interacts with vessel receptors.[164] In vivo, saralasin will block the pressor effect of infused angiotensin II in both experimental animals[151] or man.[189] This property has obvious pathophysiologic and diagnostic implications in the evaluation of both experimental and clinical forms of angiotensin dependent hypertension.

Not suprisingly, saralasin has been shown to cause a reduction in blood pressure in experimental "two-kidney" Goldblatt hypertension.[7,28,151] In contrast, blood pressure was not affected by saralasin in experimental "one-kidney" Goldblatt hypertension unless the animals were salt-depleted beforehand.[73] The specificity of saralasin for angiotensinogenic hypertension is further supported by its failure to reduce both experimental and clinical hypertension induced by norepinephrine[152,189] or mineralocorticoids.[152,187] In addition, several studies have shown a strong correlation between the degree of vasodepression with saralasin and the basal level of plasma renin activity.[134,189]

These observations support the clinical application of saralasin as a diagnostic test for RVHT. Table 4-7 lists the diagnostic sensitivity and specificity of saralasin in patients with RAS and hypertension who have been treated surgically. Other studies evaluating saralasin as a screening test to identify hypertensive patients with RAS but who have not been operated on, are not included.[8,94,96,187,198,210] However, some of these studies were used in the analysis (Table 4-7) of patients with essential hypertension who responded to saralasin.

The cumulative results from Table 4-7 demonstrate that 126 of 170 patients with proven RVHT had a positive saralasin test preoperatively. Thus, this test has a sensi-

**Table 4-7.** Renal Vein Renin Ratios: Pathophysiologic and Technical Causes for False-Negative and False-Positive Results

| Pathophysiologic Causes | Technical Causes |
|---|---|
| Equivalent bilateral disease | Catheter malposition with admixture of blood |
| Segmental lesions | |
| Renin suppression by volume posture, or antihypertensive drugs | Vigorous aspiration of blood causing admixture |
| Extensive collateral circulation | Multiple renal veins |
| Non-renin-mediated RVHT (?) | Valsalva maneuver (?) |
| | Contrast media interference with renin assay |
| | Heparin interference with renin assay |
| | Nonsimultaneous sampling |
| | Choice of a critical RVRR which is too high or too low |
| | Errors in renin assay |
| | Reduction in renal blood flow without increased renin secretion |
| | Inadequate surgical repair |

tivity of 74 percent and a false negative rate of 26 percent. The small number of reported patients who have had both a negative saralasin test preoperatively and a negative response to surgery precluded us from calculating the specificity in the usual manner. Another approach to determine the specificity and the false positive rate of saralasin in RVHT is to analyze the response to saralasin in patients with known essential hypertension. Of 324 patients with essential hypertension, 51 had a positive saralasin test for a specificity of 84 percent and a false positive rate of 16 percent. A positive saralasin test in this population presumably is identifying those patients with high renin essential hypertension since the false positive rate of 16 percent is similar to the reported 15 to 20 percent incidence of essential hypertensives with high renin.[29,187]

The limited sensitivity of the saralasin test is due to many of the same pathophysiologic factors previously discussed with the PRA and RVRR. Like these diagnostic tests, a positive or negative vasodepressor response to saralasin is markedly dependent on sodium balance. In healthy volunteers on a customary diet, saralasin produced no change in blood pressure, but after 3 days of a 10 mmol sodium diet, these same individuals responded to saralasin (10 µg/kg/min) with a fall in mean blood pressure from 80.1 ± 3.1 to 74.9 ± 1.8 mm Hg.[187] A similar relationship of an increased vasodepressor response to saralasin resulting from a negative sodium balance has been demonstrated in patients with essential hypertension.[2,35] Thus, it is not surprising that the sensitivity of the saralasin test is enhanced with negative[53,134] and blunted by positive sodium balance.[187] For example, Marks et al. increased the sensitivity of the saralasin test in their patients with RVHT from 46 percent to 92 percent by sodium depletion.[134] Because of these observations, most of the studies in Table 4-7 do include

sodium depletion in preparation of their patients. Another technique suggested to increase sensitivity is to perform the saralasin test in the sitting as opposed to the customary supine position.[198]

Additional factors which may account for a false negative saralasin test include the presence of antihypertensive medications which inhibit renin secretion,[160] inadequate amounts of saralasin employed,[94] bilateral RAS with predominantly volume-dependent hypertension, and the possibility of non-renin-mediated RVHT.[133,199]

One approach to improve the diagnostic sensitivity of saralasin has been suggested by Case and Laragh.[34] These investigators measured the reactive rise in PRA following saralasin (10 µg/kg/min × 30 minutes) in patients with either essential hypertension (both high and normal renin) or RVHT. All patients were in the seated position and on a normal sodium intake. The rise in PRA after 30 minutes of saralasin was equal to or exceeded 14 ng angiotensin I/ml/hour in 11 of 12 patients with RVHT in contrast to 1 of 34 patients with essential hypertension. In addition, a ratio of the reactive to the control PRA exceeding 2.2 was equally discriminative. Similar results were also obtained with the converting enzyme inhibitor SQ 20881 (teprotide) which was given by slow intravenous bolus at a dose of 1 mg/kg. The marked rise in PRA following saralasin or SQ 20881 in the patients with RVHT may be due to the increased sensitivity of the ischemic kidney to any given vasodepressor response as previously shown[42,110] and/or to an interruption of a negative feedback of angiotensin II on renin secretion.[201]

It has been suggested that the weakly agonistic and catecholamine stimulating properties of saralasin may result in an underestimation of the degree of participation of the renin-angiotensin system in a given patient's hypertension. In this regard, patients with RVHT have been evaluated with sarcosine-1, threonine-8, angiotensin II, an angiotensin antagonist which compared to saralasin has even weaker pressor properties and does not stimulate catecholamine release.[68] The infusion of 0.3, 1, or 10 μg/kg/min of this angiotensin II antagonist produced a fall in the mean arterial pressure of 10 percent in 8 of 10 patients with proven RVHT.[68] In three patients not benefited by technically successful surgery, a positive vasodepressor response was also elicited. Thus, despite its pharmacologic differences the initial data with sarcosine-1, threonine-8, angiotensin II fails to suggest any advantage over saralasin.

In general, the saralasin test has been safely performed in large numbers of patients with suspected angiotensin-dependent hypertension.[71,187] However, there have been several reports of significant hypotension (sometimes with syncope) induced by saralasin especially in patients who have received antihypertensive medication at the time of the infusion or have undergone severe salt depletion before hand.[11,96,157,160,187,193,198] An opposite problem is saralasin-induced hypertension which may occur in patients with low renin essential hypertension.[187,206] In this setting, saralasin is able to immediately occupy a large number of vacant angiotensin II vascular receptors allowing the drug's otherwise weak agonistic properties to produce hypertension which is not offset by any antagonistic effect.[206] Another potential danger with saralasin is that of rebound hypertension, which can occur after the infusion of saralasin is stopped. This problem is most likely to occur in those patients in whom the greatest vasodepressor responses were elicited.[113] In addition, there has been a report of saralasin precipitating a catecholamine discharge with a hypertensive crisis in a patient with pheochromocytoma.[56]

In summary, the saralasin test does not appear to have any greater sensitivity or specificity than the RVRR in the diagnosis of RVHT. However, in patients with suspected RVHT but with a non-lateralizing RVRR, a positive saralasin test would be highly suggestive of a favorable surgical outcome.[134,160,210]

# DIAGNOSIS OF RENOVASCULAR HYPERTENSION: A PRACTICAL APPROACH

Due to inherent imperfections in all available tests there exists considerable debate on their role in the evaluation of patients with suspected RVHT. The issue is further complicated by the recent introduction of less invasive or more specific therapies for RVHT such as percutaneous transluminal angioplasty (PTA) or captopril. On one side are those who argue that patients should never undergo operative therapy (with its risk of death) or angioplasty unless diagnostic testing performed beforehand demonstrates "functional" significance and a high probability of success from the procedure. The other side argues that because of the significant number of patients who improve following surgery despite a negative RVRR or saralasin test, the results do not ultimately influence the therapeutic decision and thus the tests need not be performed. In addition, less invasive therapies such as PTA are now available and their relative safety further weakens the clinical value of these diagnostic tests.

In our opinion a uniform recommendation to either use or discard these diagnostic tests in determining whether a hypertensive patient with RAS should undergo definitive treatment is not warranted. The various clinical presentations of RVHT, limitations of currently available diagnostic tests, and new nonsurgical therapies all suggest instead that diagnostic evaluation must be individualized. The approach ultimately chosen is determined by the individual patient's clinical circumstances. Inherent in our approach is an attempt to avoid the seductive but inexcusable practice of doing invasive and potentially dangerous tests when it is clear from the beginning that the results will not influence the therapy ultimately chosen. In order to better appreciate the rationale for our recommendations, we feel it would be beneficial to both briefly review the current status of the various therapeutic modalities presently available and discuss the predictive advantages and limitations of these tests using formal clinical decision analysis techniques.

## Current Therapies for RVHT

*Surgical correction* still remains as the traditional therapy for RVHT. Several series attest to a beneficial effect on blood pressure during follow-up periods lasting 10 to 20 years.[101,123,180,185] The morbidity and mortality of this therapeutic approach, which in the past has limited its application to patients with suspected RVHT, has improved significantly over the past 10 to 15 years. In the Cooperative Study, 502 patients underwent a total of 577 operative procedures.[70] There were 104 major complications (13.1 percent) and 34 deaths (5.9 percent). Closer analysis revealed an operative mortality of 9.3 percent for patients with atherosclerotic RVHT (this group accounted for 28 of the 34 deaths) compared to a mortality of 3.4 percent for patients whose RVHT was due to fibromuscular hyperplasia. Risk factors associated with the highest operative mortalities were clinical evidence (angina or infarction) of coronary artery disease (22.4 percent) and preoperative azotemia (22.5 percent). Simultaneous surgery on both kidneys for bilateral disease (16.2 percent) had a higher operative

mortality than unilateral surgery alone (3.2 percent). Renovascular surgery with simultaneous extrarenal surgery also was associated with a high mortality (25 percent).

The results of operative mortality in more recent surgical series are considerably better, especially for those patients with generalized atherosclerotic RVHT. Overall, surgical mortality in series comprised both of atherosclerotic and fibromuscular RVHT now ranges from 0 to 3.6 percent.[39,124,158,165] The mortality for patients with fibromuscular or focal atherosclerosis (atherosclerotic disease limited to renal artery only) is close to zero.[22,61,178,185] Brewster reported a operative mortality of only 3 percent in patients with generalized atherosclerosis.[22] Appropriate intra- and postoperative care, selection of patients, and type of surgical repair chosen were cited as factors influencing the low operative mortality. Novick et al. had only 2 operative deaths out of 83 patients (2.4 percent mortality) with generalized atherosclerosis operated on for either RVHT or preservation of renal function.[147] The authors attribute their low mortality to preoperative angiographic screening of coronary or carotid arteries in their patients who had a history of cardiac or cerebrovascular disease. Those patients with severe but correctable lesions of these vessels had corrective surgery prior to repair of their RAS. In addition, the authors employed a variety of surgical procedures other than the standard aortorenal bypass to correct the RAS in those patients with severe diffuse atherosclerotic disease of the aorta, thus obviating more dangerous surgery involving the aorta. Finally, on the basis of the Cooperative Study's findings, bilateral simultaneous repair was avoided. Finally, Fry and Fry and no operative deaths in their series of 22 patients of whom 16 had manifestations of extrarenal atherosclerosis.[72] These excellent results were attributed to careful pre and perioperative monitoring using Swan-Ganz, arterial, and urethral catheters to precisely control left-sided cardiac filling pressures, cardiac output, fluid requirements, and blood pressure with afterload reduction using nitroprusside if required.

*Percutaneous transluminal angioplasty* of the main renal artery has become increasingly popular as an alternative therapy to surgery for the treatment of RVHT since the initial report by Grüntzig in 1978 of the first successful application of this technique for correction of RVHT.[86] Reasons for the current popularity of PTA are that it is relatively simple to perform, preserves renal function, avoids major surgery and general anesthesia, is inexpensive, decreases hospital stay, can be repeated on several occasions, does not preclude future surgery if needed, and is associated with a low complication rate. The mechanism of how compression of a stenotic lesion by an inflatable baloon results in a patent artery has only recently been ellucidated.[13,36,191] It appears that angioplasty results in intimal disruption and splitting of the atherosclerotic plaque. This injury allows the media to dehisce from atherosclerotic intima with subsequent expansion of the media. In time, the damaged intima heals and a neointima is formed.

The results of PTA in the treatment of RVHT appear to depend on the type of lesion causing the stenosis. In RVHT due to fibromuscular hyperplasia, the initial results of PTA appear encouraging. Tegtmeyer et al. recently reported their results of PTA in 21 patients with fibromuscular hyperplasia, all of whom had technically successful dilatations.[192] The mean follow-up period was 11.5 months (range 1 to 30 months) during which time only 1 patient experienced restenosis and was successfully redilated. The blood pressure response in these 21 patients was excellent, 13 have been cured and 8 have been

significantly improved. There were no failures nor any major complications. Other centers, although reporting smaller populations and shorter follow-up periods have experienced similar excellent results in their patients with fibromuscular hyperplasia.[44,82,119,166]

The initial findings of PTA in the treatment of RVHT caused by atherosclerotic lesions have been less encouraging. Grim et al. reported recurrence of stenosis in 11 of 16 patients with atherosclerotic lesions (in 4 repeat angiography was refused or was pending at the time of the report) despite a brief follow-up period.[82] Flechner et al. performed PTA in 27 patients with atherosclerotic lesions.[66] In 13, PTA was successful as manifested by a decrease in blood pressure and/or an improvement in renal function (follow-up period 2 to 14 months). In 4 PTA was not technically possible and in 10 other patients, PTA was unsuccessful: 4 required emergency surgery due to complications of the procedure while in 6 there was no change in the degree of stenosis on a post PTA angiogram. Lower recurrence rates have been reported by Kuhlmann et al.[119] and Madias et al.[129] These reported variations in the incidence of restenosis in patients with atherosclerotic lesions may be due to the location of the atherosclerotic plaque. Atherosclerotic lesions located well within the renal artery do not appear to have a high rate of restenosis while lesions at the ostium which arise from aortic plaques extending into the renal artery are more difficult to successfully dilate and are prone to recur.[40] Atherosclerotic lesions which do restenose usually do so within the first 12 months following PTA.[44] Despite the restenosis of some atherosclerotic lesions, redilatation has been successfully performed several times without any obvious adverse consequences.

Although there is no appreciable mortality with PTA, complications have been reported in 5 to 15 percent of patients. These include intimal tears with intramural dissection, arterial thrombosis or perforation, cholesterol embolization, segmental renal infarction, soft-tissue hematoma, contrast media induced acute renal failure, and post-PTA hypotension. Since some of these complications may necessitate emergency surgery, it is important to have a qualified surgeon available at the time the procedure is performed.

At this time the results of PTA in the treatment of RVHT are encouraging especially in patients whose disease is due to fibromuscular hyperplasia and non-ostial atherosclerotic disease. However, it should be pointed out that compared to surgical therapy, the number of patients studied is small and that long-term follow-up is not yet available. As additional experience is gathered, the ultimate role of PTA in the management of RVHT should become more defined.

*Medical management* remains as an alternative treatment for RVHT especially in patients in whom more definitive therapy (surgery or PTA) is either technically not possible, refused, or prohibitively dangerous. In addition, the superiority of either surgery, PTA, or medical management in the treatment of RVHT has not yet been determined by long-term randomized prospective studies. Recently, specific medical therapy for angiotensin-mediated hypertensive states such as RVHT has become available. Captopril is an orally active inhibitor of angiotensin converting enzyme which prevents the conversion of angiotensin I to the pressor molecule angiotensin II.[205] Experimental and clinical studies with captopril demonstrate a decrease in plasma angiotensin II levels, a decrease in plasma and urinary aldosterone levels, an increase in PRA, and blockade of the pressor effects of infused angiotensin I but not angiotensin II.[5,20,63] The initial blood pressure lowering response to captopril correlates with the pretreatment renin level, although for reasons which are not clear this correlation is lost with chronic therapy.[205] Although the drug's primary antihypertensive mechanism of action would appear to be through inhibition of the formation of angiotensin II, other possible mechanisms have been suggested. These include a decrease in the degradation of bradykinin,[57] increased prostaglandin formation,[91] and inhibition of vasconstrictive responses to sympathetic nerve stimulation.[3]

As expected, captopril exhibits a high degree of efficacy in the control of blood pressure in RVHT. Brunner et al. lowered blood pressure with captopril in 8 patients with RVHT from 184/110 ± 10/2 to 137/89 ± 7/4 mm Hg.[27] Case et al. reduced blood pressure to <140/90 mm Hg in all 21 of their patients with RVHT.[33] However, two-thirds of this group (which included 14 patients with bilateral RAS) required additional treatment with diuretics and/or beta-blockers. No drug tolerance was observed. Atkinson et al. demonstrated a good correlation between the individual blood pressures on long term captopril therapy and the postoperative blood pressure off all medication in 10 patients with unilateral RAS who came to surgery.[4] In contrast, postoperative blood pressures did not correlate with the blood pressure which was recorded 2 hours after the first dose of captopril. The authors suggest that this observation portends a poor success rate in predicting surgical outcome for other renin-angiotensin antagonists or inhibitors given only for a short time.[4]

Although captopril appears efficacious in RVHT and is well tolerated by the majority of patients, side effects have been reported.[91] In many of these instances despite a suggestive association, a definite casual relationship remains to be demonstrated for these untoward effects. Reported side effects include neutropenia, proteinuria (1 percent) and rarely nephrotic syndrome, skin rash (8 to 10 percent), loss or alterations in taste (metallic or salty) (6 percent), postural hypotension (with severe sodium depletion at the time of the first dose), and tongue ulcers. Recently, acute renal failure following captopril has been reported in patients with bilateral RAS or RAS in a solitary kidney.[99] The cause of the acute renal failure appears to be functional, possibly resulting from blockade of angiotensin II mediated compensatory mechanisms to maintain glomerular filtration rate (GFR). Mechanisms to maintain GFR are required because of reduced perfusion from the stenosis. It has been proposed that maintenance of GFR is achieved by angiotensin II mediated efferent arteriolar vasoconstriction which raises glomerular capillary hydrostatic pressures. Loss of efferent vasoconstriction in the presence of reduced perfusion would result in a decreased GFR. This outcome would be most pronounced in those patients whose total renal function depends on these compensatory mechanisms. Although these patients appear to recover from acute renal failure following discontinuation of captopril, the data would suggest that captopril be used with extreme caution in patients with bilateral RAS, RAS in a solitary kidney, or unilateral RAS with severe parenchymal disease in the contralateral kidney.

## Clinical Decision Analysis Techniques

The application of formal clinical decision analysis techniques for the appropriate selection and interpretation of a given diagnostic test has become increasingly more popular in the practice of medicine.[83] These techniques allow the physician to more precisely determine the probability that the test result either confirms or excludes the presence of a specific disease. In this section, we will apply

these techniques to the RVRR as a diagnostic test for RVHT. A similar application could also be performed for the saralasin and PRA tests based on the operating characteristics of these tests summarized in Tables 4-4 and 4-5.

The operating characteristics of a test provide us with information about its accuracy in patients in whom the disease is known to be present or absent. Specifically, these characteristics refer to the sensitivity, specificity, false negative rate, and false positive rate of the test. *Sensitivity* is defined as the probability that the test will be positive when the disease is present. The *false negative rate* is the probability that the test will be negative when the disease is present and can be calculated by substracting the sensitivity (percent) from 100. *Specificity* is defined as the probability that the test will be negative when the disease is absent. The *false positive rate* is the probability that the test will be positive when the disease is absent and is calculated by subtracting the specificity (percent) from 100. These operating characteristics are commonly presented with the use of a simple binary table (Fig. 4-2).

From the data summarized in Table 4-5, we have calculated the operating characteristics of the RVRR in patients in whom RVHT was proven by surgical results to be either present or absent. These operating characteristics for the RVRR are displayed using the binary table presentation in Fig. 4-2. The data reveal the sensitivity and specificity for the RVRR in RVHT to be 80 percent and 62 percent, respectively. Thus, the false negative and positive rates for this diagnostic test are 20 percent and 38 percent, respectively.

Once defined, the operating characteristics of a test remain constant and are applicable to the study of any individual patient providing that the criteria and methods for performing the test remain the same as those initially used to define

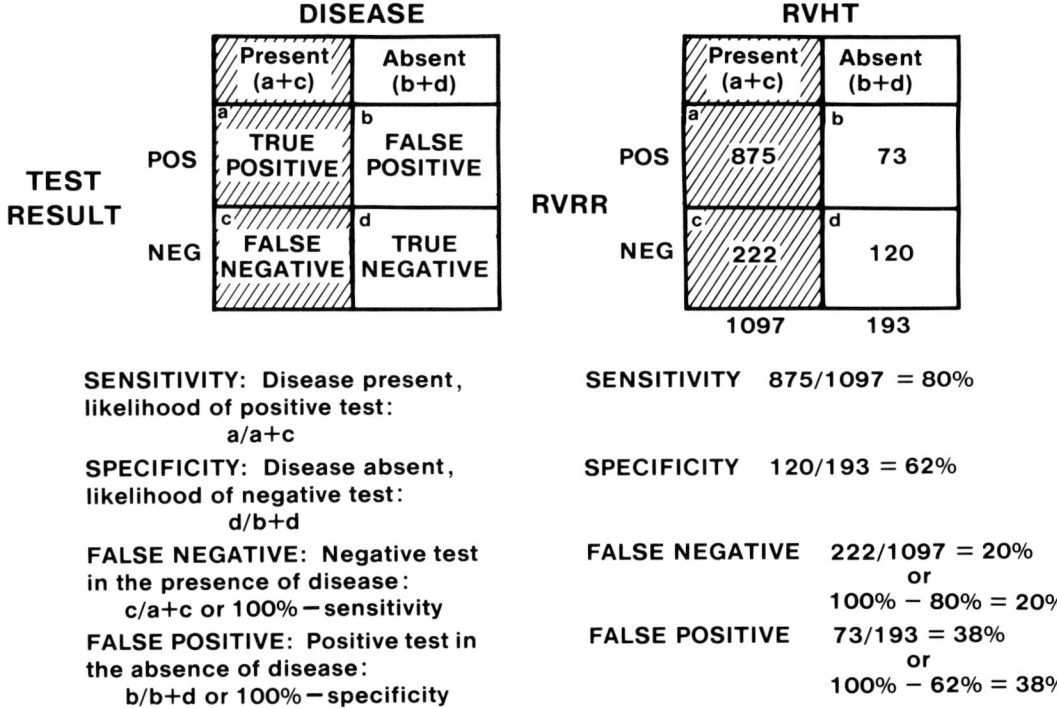

**Fig. 4-2.** Statistical evaluation of renal vein renin ratios: Left panel: Describes the four possible results between a given test and a disease for which the test is used. Hatched area (a and c) indicates the test results in only those patients with the disease, while the clear boxes illustrate test results in those subjects known not to have the disease. Right panel: Results of renal vein renin ratios (RVRR) in 1190 patients with renovascular hypertension (RVHT) culled from the literature. See text for how true and false definition positives and negatives were defined. (Modified with permission from Griner PF, Mayewski RJ, Mushlin AI, Greenland P: Selection and interpretation of diagnostic tests and procedures. Principles and applications. Ann Intern Med 94 (part 2):453, 1981.)

the test's characteristics.[83] Unfortunately, the nature of the information available for constructing Table 4-5 precludes these criteria from being exactly met. However, there exists enough similarity between the individual series in Table 4-5 (in terms of sensitivity and specificity) to allow us to group the data despite variations in the methods and critical ratio.

A common mistake is to make predictions about the probability of the disease being present or absent based solely on the operating characteristics (sensitivity and specificity) of the test. The probability of the disease being present or absent if the test is either positive or negative can only be determined by *coupling* the operating characteristics of the test with the physician's estimate of the probability of the disease being present *before* the diagnostic test is performed.[83] In this regard, the *positive predictive value* is the term used to define the probability that the disease is present if the test is positive. The *negative predictive value* is the term used to define the probability that the disease is absent if the test is negative. The probability that the disease is present if the test is negative is 100 minus the negative predictive value. The positive and negative predictive values can be calculated using the same binary table method used to calculate the test's operating characteristics, as shown in Fig. 4-3. It is important to appreciate that the calculation of these posttest probabilities can be made only if the physician's pretest probability for disease is combined with the known operating characteristics of the test.[83]

Using these principles we have calculated the predictive value of a positive or negative RVRR test result based on the data in Table 4-5. As examples, we have selected three patients in which our pretest clinical estimate of the likelihood of RVHT being present is 90 percent, 50 percent, and 10 percent. These examples are displayed by the binary table method in Fig. 4-3. The first example is an 18-year-old white female with hypertension, abdominal bruits, and an arteriogram demonstrating bilateral fibromuscular dysplasia. Our pre-RVRR estimate of the likelihood of RVHT being present is 90 percent. As shown in Fig. 4-2 for this patient the positive predictive value, that is, the probability that a positive RVRR test indicates that RVHT is present is 95 percent. The negative predictive value, that is, the probability that a negative RVRR test indicates that RVHT is absent is only 26 percent or conversely that the probability of RVHT being present despite a negative test is 74 percent! In this setting performing the RVRR was of no clinical diagnostic help. If the test was positive, the predictive gain from our pretest estimation for RVHT was only 5 percent (pretest 90 percent probability; posttest 95 percent probability). Although the predictive gain from a negative test result was 16 percent (pretest 10 percent probability; posttest probability 26 percent), the patient still had a 74 percent probability of RVHT being present, a value too high to be clinically helpful in excluding the patient from surgery or angioplasty.

Our second example is a 45-year-old

man with a 5-year history of stable hypertension whose arteriogram shows a 50 percent stenosis of the right renal artery due to an atherosclerotic plaque. Our estimated pretest probability for this patient having RVHT is 50 percent. As shown in Fig. 4-3, the calculated positive predictive value is 68 percent and the negative predictive value is 76 percent. In this setting, knowledge of the RVRR result would be more helpful in devising our clinical management. A positive RVRR test result would increase our pretest estimate for RVHT being present from 50 percent to 68 percent, a gain of 18 percent. Similarily, a negative RVRR test result increased our pretest estimated prediction of the absence of disease from 50 to 76 percent, a gain of 26 percent. This latter finding can be restated as a negative RVRR allowed us to predict that the patient has only a 24 percent chance of having RVHT. Thus, having performed the test, we might now feel clinically more comfortable in subjecting this patient to surgery or angioplasty if the RVRR is positive or denying him these potentially dangerous therapies if the RVRR is negative.

Our final example is that of a 55-year-old black female with a 20-year history of stable mild hypertension who during an arteriogram for peripheral vascular disease was noted to have a 20 percent ostial stenosis of the left renal artery from atherosclerosis. For this patient our pretest estimate of the likelihood of RVHT being present is only 10 percent. As shown in Fig. 4-3, the positive predictive value is 19 percent and the negative predictive value is 97 percent. As in our first example, the RVRR test would be essentially of no diagnostic value in this patient. A positive test increased our pretest estimate of likelihood of RVHT being present from 10 percent to only 19 percent, a gain of 9 percent. A 19 percent likelihood that this patient has RVHT probably would not justify surgery or angioplasty especially in

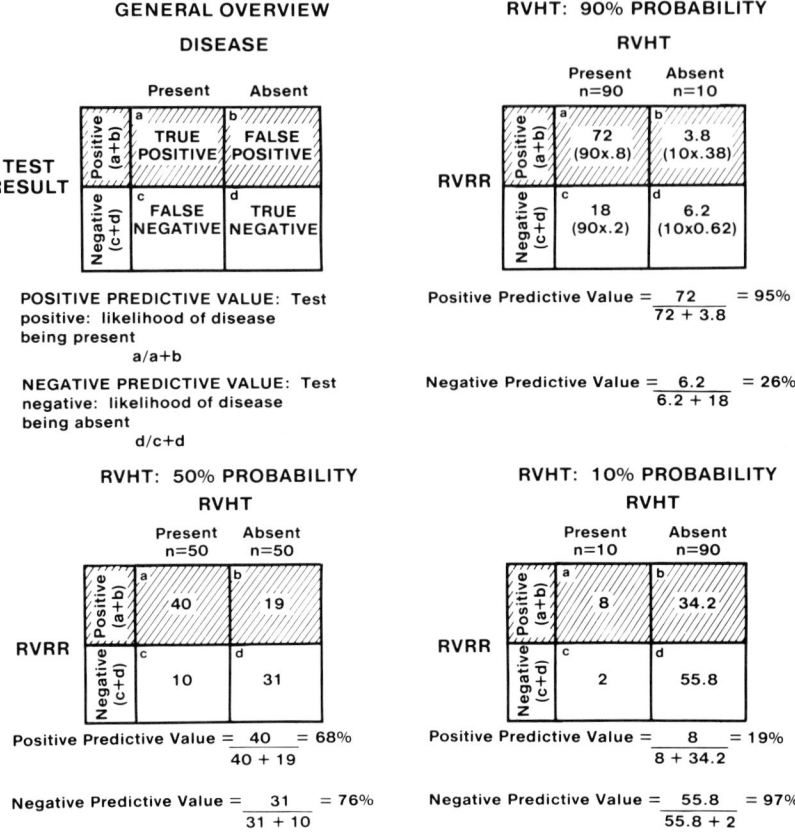

**Fig. 4-3.** Predictive value of RVRR in renovascular hypertension (RVHT): The predictive value of RVRR is based upon the inherent operating characteristics of the test and upon the pretest probability for the presence of RVHT. Probability is expressed in absolute numbers rather than percentages. Thus, a 90% probability means that of 100 patients with similar clinical and laboratory characteristics, 90 will have a pretest probability for RVHT and 10 will not. True Positives (square a): The number of true positives is the product of the test's sensitivity (80%, see Fig. 4-2) and total number presumed to have RVHT (i.e., 90 patients). False Positives (square b): The number of false positives is the product of the test's known false positive rate (38%) and the total number presumed *not* to have RVHT (10 patients). True Negatives (square d): The total number of subjects is the product of the specificity (62%, see Fig. 4-2) and the total number presumed *not* to have RVHT (10 patients). False Negatives (square c): The total number of subjects is the product of the test's known false negative rate (20%, see Fig. 4-2) and the total number of patients presumed to have the disease (90 patients). These numbers were developed in a similar fashion for pretest probabilities of 50% and 10%. Hatched areas (a + b) indicate positive tests in the presence or absence of disease. (Modified with permission from Griner PF, Mayewski RJ, Mushlin AI, Greenland P: Selection and interpretation of diagnostic tests and procedures. Principles and applications. Ann Intern Med 94 (part 2):453, 1981.)

view of the patient's stable mild hypertension. A negative test result increased the likelihood of disease not being present from 90 percent to 97 percent, a gain of only 7 percent. Again the clinical decision to not intervene in this patient (with a pretest probability of 90 percent for RVHT not being present) would not be significantly strengthened with this additional information.

This type of predictive analysis of the RVRR can be performed for any given pretest estimate of the likelihood of RVHT being present. As shown in Table 4-8, the predictive gain from a RVRR test result is greatest when the pretest likelihood for RVHT being present is intermediate in nature. As demonstrated by our examples, the test is least helpful when our clinical suspicion for RVHT being present is either very high or very low. It is interesting to note that in Table 4-5 that the percentage of patients who responded to surgery despite a negative RVRR was 65 percent. This value is not surprising when we look at the prevalence of RVHT for the total population comprising Table 4-5. Of 1290 patients subjected to a RVRR test, 1097 proved to have RVHT, for a prevalence of 85 percent. Thus with this high pretest prevalence for the disease, it was predictable that a negative RVRR test would not be clinically helpful in excluding RVHT (Fig. 4-2). The high prevalance for RVHT in Table 4-5 also demonstrates that the clinical criteria (other than the RVRR) used by the separate authors to determine those patients with suspected RVHT who should undergo surgery, were highly effective in preselecting patients who proved to have the disease. This observation strongly supports our position of the limited value of the RVRR in patients with a high clinical suspicion for RVHT.

In making a final decision regarding the need for definitive therapy, information gained from these formal clinical decision analysis techniques is most helpful when integrated with information already obtained from a careful history and physical examination and a consideration of the risks versus benefit of the particular therapy. This combined approach was employed by us in formulating our recommendations (below) for diagnostic testing in patients with suspected RVHT.

## Recommendations for Evaluation of Patients for Suspected RVHT (Table 4-9)

Having reviewed the relative limitations of the diagnostic tests for suspected

**Table 4-8.** Predictive Gain Expected from RVRR in Confirming or Excluding RVHT According to Prior Estimates of Likelihood of Disease

| Prior Estimate Of Likelihood Of Disease (%) | RVRR Positive | | RVRR Negative | |
| --- | --- | --- | --- | --- |
| | Positive Predictive Value (%) | Incremental Gain (%) | Negative Predictive Value (%) | Incremental Gain (%) |
| 90 | 95 | 5 | 26 | 16 |
| 80 | 89 | 9 | 44 | 24 |
| 70 | 83 | 13 | 57 | 27 |
| 60 | 76 | 16 | 67 | 27 |
| 50 | 68 | 18 | 76 | 26 |
| 40 | 58 | 18 | 82 | 22 |
| 30 | 47 | 17 | 88 | 18 |
| 20 | 34 | 14 | 93 | 13 |
| 10 | 19 | 9 | 97 | 7 |

(Modified with permission from Griner PF, Mayewski RJ, Mushlin AI, Greenland P. Selection and interpretation of diagnostic tests and procedures. Principles and applications. Ann Intern Med 94 (part 2): 453, 1981.)

**Table 4.9** Clinical Syndromes, the Probablity of RVHT, and Renal Vein Renin Ratios

---

I. Clinical Syndromes in Which Demonstrated RAS Would Be Corrected Regardless of Results of RVRR
   - Young patient; abdominal bruit present; fibromuscular dysplasia demonstrated.
   - Elderly patient with recent, unexplained acceleration of hypertension that is poorly controlled.
   - Noncompliant hypertensive with worsening end-organ damage.
   - Drug therapy ineffective or rife with unacceptable side effects.

Rationale: In the first two settings, the high clinical probability for RVHT being present is not significantly altered by a negative RVRR result. In the last two settings, the compelling nature of the illness demands correction of the RAS regardless of the RVRR result. In either case, a negative RVRR will not influence therapy and therefore the test should not be performed.

II. Clinical Syndromes in Which an Invasive Procedure Is Not Indicated:
   - Typical EHT, medically well controlled without side effects or end-organ damage.
   - Patient deemed too ill to undergo PTA or surgery.

Rationale: In the first setting, the benign course and low probability for RVHT (even with a positive RVRR) do not justify risks and costs of diagnostic tests or treatment. Severe illness in the second setting precludes invasive treatment regardless of test result.

III. Clinical Syndromes in Which Correction of RAS Would Be Influenced by the Result of RVRR
   - Clinical features not typical of but consistent with RVHT, BP control and side effects acceptable but not ideal.

Rationale: Clinical probability of RVHT judged to be intermediate, thereby increasing diagnostic gain of RVRR. Physician's pretest decision therefore, is that positive or negative results will influence patient management, unlike in syndromes I and II.

---

RVHT, the application of formal decision analysis in interpreting the results, and the current status of the various treatment modalities presently available, we present our approach for evaluating hypertensive patients for potential RVHT. These recommendations most likely will require modification in the future as additional information is gained regarding current or new diagnostic tests, treatment, and natural history of the disease.

There are several clinical presentations of RVHT which demand definitive action by the physician. It is our position that in these settings diagnostic tests to determine "functional" significance of stenotic lesions need not be done since negative results will not in most cases preclude doing angioplasty or surgery. Included in this group are young adults with angiographic evidence of fibromuscular hyperplasia, elderly patients with a recent onset of hypertension which is severe and diffi-

cult to manage, noncompliant patients who show evidence of progressive end-organ damage, patients whose hypertension is refractory to medical therapy or in whom various antihypertensive agents are unacceptable due to limiting side effects, and patients who demonstrate progressive renal insufficiency, most likely resulting from ischemia. In each of these settings, once the presence of RAS is established, the physician is often compelled to offer corrective definitive therapy either because the consequences of the hypertensive process is so potentially threatening or the clinical presentation alone is associated with a very high probability that "functional" RVHT is present. As shown, the application of formal decision analysis techniques demonstrates minimal diagnostic gain from a positive or negative RVRR result when the pretest likelihood of RVHT being present is high. In addition, the recent ability to perform angioplasty with its almost nonexistent risk of death, further weakens the clinical position to withhold such therapy because of a negative result from a grossly imperfect test.

Patients whose clinical course is typical of essential hypertension and whose blood pressure is mild and well controlled on antihypertensive medication with minimal or no side effects, do not require screening tests for anatomical demonstration of RAS or diagnostic tests for "functional" significance. The results of such tests as shown by decision analysis do not appreciably change the unlikely pretest likelihood of RVHT being present in these clinical settings. In view of the minimal gain, it is difficult to justify both the risks and costs of these diagnostic tests.

There are clinical situations that fall between these two extremes. Included in this group are patients whose clinical features although not highly suggestive of RVHT are nonetheless consistent with such a diagnosis and whose blood pressure control and side effects with medication is acceptable but not ideal. Since definitive vascular procedures in this group of patients may be associated with a high rate of failure and are not critical based on the clinical presentation, then the performance of diagnostic tests for "functional" significance would be appropriate since negative results would be an acceptable stop point. This statement is supported by clinical decision analysis which demonstrates that the diagnostic predictive gain from these tests is greatest when the pretest likelihood for RVHT is intermediate in nature. Another possible clinical situation which would justify the performance of these diagnostic tests would be in those patients whose clinical presentation requires definitive therapy but who will only consent to surgery or angioplasty if the probability of a beneficial result is very high. In this setting, a positive result could provide the extra assurance

needed to convince the patient that surgery or angioplasty is indicated.

In summary, in a patient with hypertension for whom RVHT is a diagnostic possibility, the physician must first decide on the basis of a careful history and physical examination if the likelihood for RVHT warrants tests to demonstrate the presence or absence of RAS. If these tests demonstrate an anatomical lesion, the decision to perform a RVRR or other diagnostic tests for "functional" significance depends on the physicians' initial pretest assessment for the likelihood of RVHT being present. If the likelihood for RVHT being present or absent is very high, then the performance of RVRR or other diagnostic tests should not be done since they will not influence the pretest therapeutic plan. If the likelihood for RVHT is intermediate, the physician can calculate the diagnostic gain of a positive or negative RVRR as demonstrated in Table 4-8. If the calculated negative predictive value is such that the probability of RVHT being present despite a negative test is still too high to accept the negative test result as a stop point, then the RVRR should not be performed in the first place. If on the other hand a negative test result is an acceptable stop point, then the performance of the RVRR or other diagnostic test would be warranted.

The relative infrequency of RVHT and the nonuniformity of published studies dealing with diagnosis and treatment have made it difficult to develop specific clinical guidelines upon which all physicians would agree. However, it is our opinion that the current data is sufficient to provide a thoughtful and appropriate clinical approach for this form of secondary hypertension.

# REFERENCES

1. Amsterdam EA, Couch NP, Christlieb AR, et al: Renal vein renin activity in the

prognosis of surgery for renovascular hypertension. Am J Med 47:860, 1969.

2. Anderson GH, Dalakos TG, Elias A, et al: Diuretic therapy and response of essential hypertension to saralasin. Ann Intern Med 87:183, 1977.

3. Antonaccio MH, Kerwin L: Pre and postjunctional inhibition of vascular sympathetic function in SHR: Implication of vascular angiotensin II in hypertension and antihypertensive actions of captopril. Hypertension 3:I-54 1981.

4. Atkinson AB, Brown JJ, Cumming AMM, et al: Captopril in the management of hypertension with renal artery stenosis: Its long-term effect as a predictor of surgical outcome. Am J Cardiol 49:1460, 1982.

5. Atkinson AB, Brown JJ, Fraser R, et al: Captopril in hypertension with renal artery stenosis and in intractable hypertension; acute and chronic changes in circulating concentrations of renin, angiotensin I and II and aldosterone and in body composition. Clin Sci 57: 139S, 1979.

6. Aurell M, Delin K, Granerus G: Measures to increase the reliability in the diagnostics of renin dependent hypertension. Acta Med Scand [Suppl.] 646:58, 1981.

7. Ayers CR, Vaughan ED Jr, Yancey MR, et al: Effect of 1-sarcosine-8-alanine angiotensin II and converting enzyme inhibitor on renin release in dog acute renovascular hypertension. Circ. Res 34 [Suppl 1]:27, 1974.

8. Baer L, Parra-Garrillo JZ, Radichevich I, et al. G.S.: Detection of renovascular hypertension with angiotensin II blockade. Ann Intern Med 86:257, 1977.

9. Barraclough MA, Bacchus B, Brown JJ, et al: Plasma renin and aldosterone secretion in hypertensive patients with renal or renal artery lesions. Lancet 2:1310, 1965.

10. Bath NM, Gunnells JC, Robinson RR: Plasma renin activity in renovascular hypertension. Am J Med 45:381, 1968.

11. Beckerhoff R, Furrer J, Vetter W, et al: Hypotension during angiotensin blockade with saralasin. Br Med J 2:849, 1976.

12. Bergrem H, Jervell J, Solheim DM, et al: Prognostic value of renal vein renin determination in suspected renovascular hypertension. Acta Med Scand 211:387, 1982.

13. Block PC, Fallon JT, Elmer D: Experimental angioplasty: lessons from the laboratory. AJR 135:907, 1980.

14. Bookstein JJ, Abrams HL, Buenger RE, et al: Radiologic aspects of renovascular hypertension. Part 3. Appraisal of arteriography. JAMA 221:368, 1972.

15. Boucher R, Veyrat R, deChamplain J, et al: New procedures for measurement of human plasma angiotensin and renin activity levels. Canad Med Assoc J 90:194, 1964.

16. Bourgoignie J, Kurz S, Catanzaro FJ, et al: Renal venous renin in hypertension. Am J Med 48:332, 1970.

17. Bozovic L, Castenfors J, Delin A, et al: Pre- and peroperative evaluation and follow-up of hypertensive patients with renal artery stenosis. Scand J Urol Nephrol 5:162, 1971.

18. Braasch WF: The surgical kidney as an etiological factor in hypertension. Can Med Assoc J 46:9, 1942.

19. Braun-Menendez E, Fasciolo JC, Keloir LF, Munonoz, JM: La substancia hypertensinora de la sangre del rinon isquemiado (Astr.). Rev Soc Argent Biol 15:420, 1939.

20. Bravo EL, Tarazi RC: Converting enzyme inhibition with an orally active compound in hypertensive man. Hypertension 1:39, 1979.

21. Breslin DJ: Pathophysiology of renovascular hypertension: An overview. In Breslin DJ, Swinton NW, Jr, Libertino JA, Eds: Renovascular Hypertension. Williams and Wilkins, Baltimore, 1982.

22. Brewster DC: Surgical management of renovascular disease. AJR 135:963, 1980.

23. Brown JJ, Davies DL, Johnson VW, et al: Renin relationships in congestive cardiac failure; treated and untreated. Am Heart J 80:329, 1970.

24. Brown JJ, Davies DL, Lever AF, et al: Variations in plasma renin concentration in several physiological and pathological states. Can Med Assoc J 90:201, 1964.

25. Brown JJ, Davies DL, Lever AF, et al: Plasma renin concentration in human

hypertension. II: Renin in relation to aetiology. Br Med J 2:1215, 1965.

26. Brown JJ, Davies DL, Morton JJ, et al: Mechanism of renal hypertension. Lancet 1:1219, 1976.

27. Brunner HR, Gavras H, Waeber B, et al: Oral angiotensin-converting enzyme inhibitor in long-term treatment of hypertensive patients. Ann Intern Med 90:19, 1979.

28. Brunner HR, Kirshman JD, Sealey JE, et al: Hypertension of renal origin. Evidence for two different mechanisms. Science 174:1344, 1971.

29. Brunner HR, Laragh JH, Baer L, et al: Essential hypertension: renin and aldosterone, heart attack, and stroke. N Engl J Med 286:441, 1972.

30. Brust AA, Ferris EB: The diagnostic approach to hypertension due to unilateral kidney disease. Ann Intern Med 47:549, 1952.

31. Buda JA, Baer L, Parra-Carrillo JZ, et al: Predictability of surgical response in renovascular hypertension. Arch Surg 111:1243, 1976.

32. Bumpus FM, Khosla MC: Pathogenetic factors involved in renovascular hypertension. State of the art. Mayo Clin Proc 52:417, 1977.

33. Case DB, Atlas SA, Marion RM, et al: Long-term efficacy of captopril in renovascular and essential hypertension. Am J Cardiol 49:1440, 1982.

34. Case DB, Laragh JH: Reactive hyperreninemia in renovascular hypertension after angiotensin blockade with saralasin or converting enzyme inhibitor. Ann Intern Med 91:153, 1979.

35. Case DB, Wallace JM, Keim HJ, et al: Usefulness and limitations of saralasin, a partial competitive agonist of angiotensin II, for evaluating the renin and sodium factors in hypertensive patients. Am J Med 60:825, 1976.

36. Castaneda-Zuniga WR, Formanek A, Tadavarthy M, et al: Mechanism of balloon angioplasty. Radiology 135:565, 1980.

37. Chapman WH, O'Brien DJ, McRoberts JW, et al: Diagnosis of renal hypertension using renal activity and renal vein pressor assay. J Urol 103:549, 1970.

38. Chiarini C, Esposti ED, Losinno F, et al: Renal scintigraphy versus renal vein renin activity for identifying and treating renovascular hypertension. Nephron 32:8, 1982.

39. Chung WB, Salvian AJ: Surgical treatment of renovascular hypertension. Am J Surg 138:143, 1979.

40. Cicuto KP, McClean GK, Oleaga JA, et al: Renal artery stenosis: anatomic classification for percutaneous transluminal angioplasty. AJR 139:727,1982.

41. Cohen EL, Conn JW, Rovner DR: Postural augmentation of plasma renin activity and aldosterone excretion in normal people. J Clin Invest 46:418, 1967.

42. Cohen EL, Rovner DR, Conn JW: Postural augmentation of plasma renin activity. Importance in diagnosis of renovascular hypertension. JAMA 197:973, 1966.

43. Cohen EL, Rovner DR, Conn JW, et al: The effects of position, exercise and sodium intake on plasma renin activity in normal people. Clin Res 12:362A, 1964.

44. Collapinto RF, Stronell RD, Harries-Jones EP, et al: Percutaneous transluminal dilitation of the renal artery: Follow-up studies on renovascular hypertension. AJR 139:727, 1982.

45. Couch NP, Sullivan J, Crane C: The predictive accuracy of renal vein renin activity in the surgery of renovascular hypertension. Surgery 79:70, 1976.

46. Davis JO: The pathogenesis of chronic renovascular hypertension. Cir Res 40:439, 1977.

47. Dean RH, Foster JH: Criteria for the diagnosis of renovascular hypertension. Surgery 74:926, 1973.

48. Dean RH, Oates JA, Wilson JP, et al: Bilateral renal artery stenosis and renovascular hypertension. JAMA 197:973, 1966.

49. DeCamp PT, Birchall R: Recognition and treatment of renal arterial stenosis associated with hypertension. Surgery 43:134, 1958.

50. DeChamplain J, Genest J, Veyrat R, et al: Factors controlling renin in man. Trans Assoc Am Physicians 78:135, 1965.

51. DeChamplain J, Genest J, Veyrat R, et al: Factors controlling renin in man. Arch Intern Med 117:355, 1966.

52. DeQuattro V: Renovascular disease and saralasin test. Ann Intern Med 87:790, 1977.

53. Donker AJM, Leenen FHH: Infusion of angiotensin-II analogue in two patients with unilateral renovascular hypertension. Lancet 2:1535, 1974.

54. D'Souza VJ, Tobian L, Formanek A, et al: A new simple test for renin sampling. Radiology 129:351, 1978.

55. Dustan HP, Humphries AW, deWolfe VG, et al: Normal arterial pressure in patients with renal arterial stenosis. JAMA 187:138, 1964.

56. Dunn FG, DeCarvalho JGR, Kem DC, et al: Pheochromocytoma crisis induced by saralasin: Relationship of angiotensin analogue to catechcholamine release. N Engl J Med 295:605, 1976.

57. Erdös EG: Angiotensin I converting enzyme. Circ Res 36:247, 1975.

58. Ernst CB, Bookstein JJ, Montie J, et al: Renal vein rein ratios and collateral vessels in renovascular hypertension. Arch Surg 104:496, 1972.

59. Ernst CB, Dagherty ME, Kotchen TA: Relationship between collateral development and renin in experimental renal arterial stenosis. Surgery 80:252, 1976.

60. Ernst CB, Stanley JC, Marshall FF, et al: Autogenous saphenous vein aortorenal grafts. A ten-year experience. Arch Surg 105:855, 1972.

61. Ernst CB, Stanley JC, Marshall FF, et al: Renal revascularization for arteriosclerotic renovascular hypertension: Prognostic implications of focal renal arterial vs. overt generalized arteriosclerosis. Surgery 73:859, 1973.

62. Eyler WR, Clark MD, Garman JE, et al: Angiography of the renal areas including a comparative study of renal arterial stenoses in patients with and without hypertension. Radiology 78:879, 1962.

63. Ferguson RK, Brunner HR, Turini GA, et al: A specific orally active inhibitor of angiotensin-converting enzyme in men. Lancet 1:775, 1977.

64. Fitz A: Renal venous renin determinations in the diagnosis of surgically correctable hypertension. Circulation 36:942, 1967.

65. Fitz AE, Armstrong ML: Plasma vasoconstrictor activity in patients with renal, malignant and primary hypertension. Circulation 29:409, 1964.

66. Flechner S, Novick AC, Vidt D,: The use of percutaneous transluminal angioplasty for renal artery stenosis in patients with generalized atherosclerosis. J Urol 127:1072, 1982.

67. Foster JH, Maxwell MH, Franklin SS, et al: Renovascular occlusive disease. Results of operative treatment. JAMA 231:1043, 1975.

68. Fouad FM, Gifford RW, Jr, Fighali S, et al: Predictive value of angiotensin II antagonists in renovascular hypertension. JAMA 249:368, 1983.

69. Fournier A, Romeder JM, Salmon D, et al: Predictive criteria of surgical curability of renovascular hypertension. Acta Med Scand 189:391, 1971.

70. Franklin SS, Young JD, Jr, Maxwell MH, et al: Operative morbidity and mortality in renovascular disease. JAMA 231:1148, 1975.

71. Frohlich ED, Maxwell MH, Baer L, et al: Editorial. Use of saralasin as a diagnostic test in hypertension. Report of a consensus committee. Arch Intern Med 142:1437, 1982.

72. Fry RE, Fry WJ: Renovascular hypertension in the patient with severe atherosclerosis. Arch Surg 117:938, 1982.

73. Gavras H, Brunner HR, Vaughan ED, Jr, et al: Angiotensin-sodium interaction in blood pressure maintenance of renal hypertensive and normotensive rats. Science 180:1369, 1973.

74. Genest J: Studies on the renin-angiotensin system in hypertensive patients. Canad Med Assoc J 90:263, 1964.

75. Gittes RF, McLaughlin AP: Unilateral operation for bilateral renovascular disease. J Urol 111:292, 1974.

76. Goldblatt H: The Renal Origin of Hypertension. Charles C. Thomas. Springfield, Ill., 1948.

77. Goldblatt H, Lynch J, Hanzal RF, et al: Studies on experimental hypertension. I Production of persistent elevation of systolic blood pressure by means of renal ischemia. J Exp Med 59:347, 1934.

78. Goorno WE, Kaplan NM: Renal pressor material in various hypertensive diseases. Ann Intern Med 63:745, 1965.
79. Gordon RD, Wolfe LK, Island DP, et al: A diurnal rhythm in plasma renin activity in man. J Clin Invest 45:1587, 1966.
80. Grim CE, Keitzer WF: Circadian rhythm of renin and aldosterone in unilateral renovascular hypertension. Pre-and postoperative studies. Ann Intern Med 80: 298, 1974.
81. Grim CE, Luft FC, Weinberger MH, et al: Sensitivity and specificity of screening tests for renal vascular hypertension. Ann Intern Med 91:617, 1979
82. Grim CE, Luft FC, Yone HY, et al: Percutaneous transluminal dilatation in the treatment of renal vascular hypertension. Ann Intern Med 95:439, 1981.
83. Griner PF, Mayewski RJ, Mushlin AI, et al: Selection and interpretation of diagnostic tests and procedures. Principles and applications. Ann Intern Med 94 (Part 2):557, 1981.
84. Gross F, Brunner H, Ziegler M: Renin-angiotensin system, aldosterone and sodium balance. Recent Prog Horm Res 21:119, 1965.
85. Gross F, Lichtlen P: Pressor substances in kidneys of renal hypertensive rats with and without adrenals. Proc Soc Exp Biol 98:341, 1958.
86. Grüntzig A, Vettler W, Meier B, et al: Treatment of renovascular hypertension with percutaneous transluminal dilitation of a renal-artery stenosis. Lancet 1:801, 1978.
87. Guedon J, Safar M, Fournier A, et al: Prognostic value of simultaneous renal venous renin and split function studies in unilateral renal hypertension. Rev Eur Étud Clin Et Biol 17:757, 1972.
88. Gunnells JC, McGuffin WL, Johnsrude I, et al: Peripheral and renal venous plasma renin activity in hypertension. Ann Intern Med 71:555, 1969.
89. Haas E, Goldblatt H: Studies on renin. Biochem Z 338:164, 1963.
90. Hansson BG, Bergentz SE, Dymling JF, et al: Pre- and post-operative studies in 72 hypertensive patients with renal artery stenosis, with special reference to renin activity and aldosterone. Acta Med Scand 210:249, 1981.
91. Heel RC, Brogden RN, Speight TM, et al: Captopril: A preliminary review of its pharmacological properties and therapeutic efficacy. Drugs 20:490, 1980.
90. Helmer OM: Renin activity in blood from patients with hypertension. Canad Med Assoc J 90:221, 1964.
93. Hollenberg NK, Epstein M, Basch RI, et al: Renin secretion in the patient with hypertension. Relationship to intrarenal blood flow distribution. Circ Res 24, 25:Suppl 1: 113, 1969.
94. Hollenberg NK, Williams GH, Adams DF, et al: Response to saralasin and angiotensin's role in essential and renal hypertension. Medicine 58:115, 1979.
95. Holley KE, Hunt JC, Brown AL, Jr, et al: Renal artery stenosis. A clinical-pathologic study in normotensive and hypertensive patients. Am J Med 37:14, 1964.
96. Horne ML, Conklin VM, Keenan RE, et al: Angiotensin II profiling with saralasin: Summary of eaton collaborative study. Kidney Int 15 [Suppl 9]: S115, 1979.
97. Horvath JS, Baxter CR, Sherbon K, et al: An analysis of errors found in renal vein sampling for plasma renin activity. Kidney Int 11:136, 1977.
98. Howard JE, Berthrong M, Guld DM, et al: Hypertension resulting from unilateral renal vascular disease and its relief by nephrectomy. Bull Hopkins Hosp 94:51, 1954.
99. Hricik DE, Browning PJ, Kopelman R, et al: Captopril-induced functional renal insufficiency in patients with bilateral renal-artery stenoses or renal-artery stenosis in a solitary kidney. N Engl J Med 308:373, 1983.
100. Hughes JS, Dove HG, Gifford RW Jr, et al: Duration of blood pressure elevation in accurately predicting surgical cure of renovascular hypertension. Am Heart J 101:408, 1981.
101. Hunt JD, Sheps SG, Harrison EG Jr, et al: Renal and renovascular hypertension. A reasoned approach to diagnosis and management. Arch Intern Med 133:988, 1974.
102. Hunt JC, Strong CG, Sheps SG, et al: Di-

agnosis and management of renovascular hypertension. Am J Cardiol 23:434, 1969.

103. Hussain RA, Gifford RW, Stewart BH, et al: Differential renal venous renin activity in diagnosis of renovascular hypertension. Am J Cardiol 32:707, 1973.

104. Huvos A, Yagi S, Mannick JA, et al: Stimulation of renin secretion by hydralazine: II. Studies in renovascular hypertension. Circulation 36, 37 (suppl. II): 118, 1965.

105. Judson WE, Helmer OM: Determination of constrictor substances in plasma by means of strips of rabbit aorta as done in the differential diagnosis of renal vascular occlusive disease. J Lab Clin Med 56:828, 1960.

106. Judson WE, Helmer OM: Diagnostic and prognostic values of renin activity in renal venous plasma in renovascular hypertension. Hypertension 13:79, 1965.

107. Juncos LI, Strong CG, Hunt JC: Prediction of results of surgery for renal and renovascular hypertension. Arch Intern Med 134:655, 1974.

108. Kaplan NM: Renin profiles. The unfulfilled promises. JAMA 238:611, 1977.

109. Kaplan NM: Renovascular hypertension. In Clinical Hypertension. 3rd Ed. Williams and Wilkins, Baltimore, 1982.

110. Kaneko Y, Ikeda T, Takeda T, et al: Renin release during acute reduction of arterial pressure in normotensive subjects and patients with renovascular hypertension. J Clin Invest 46:705, 1967.

111. Kaufman JJ, Lupu AN, Franklinss, et al: Diagnostic and predictive value of renal vein renin activity in renovascular hypertension. J Urol 103:702, 1970.

112. Kaufman JJ, Maxwell MH: Surgery for renovascular hypertension. Analysis of 67 cases. JAMA 190:709, 1964.

113. Keim HJ, Drayer JIM, Case DB, et al: A role for renin in rebound hypertension and encephalopathy after infusion of sar-1-ala-8-angiotensin II. N Engl J Med 295: 1175, 1976.

114. Keith TA III: Renovascular hypertension in black patients. Hypertension 4:438, 1982.

115. Kirkendall WM, Fitz AE, Lawrence MS: Renal hypertension. Diagnosis and surgical treatment. N Engl J Med 276:479, 1967.

116. Kirkendall WM, Kioschos JM: Studies on patients with renal artery stenosis. Trans Am Clin Chematol Assoc 82:101, 1970.

117. Klatte EC, Worrell JA, Forster JH, et al: Diagnostic criteria of bilateral renovascular hypertension. Radiology 101:301, 1971.

118. Krakoff LR, Ribeiro AB, Gorkin JU, et al: Saralasin infusion in screening patients for renovascular hypertension. Am J Cardiol 45:609, 1980.

119. Kuhlmann U, Vetter W, Grüntzig A, et al: Percutaneous transluminal dilatation of renal artery stenosis: 2 years' experience. Clin Sci 61:481S, 1981.

120. Lagneau P, Michel JB: Arterial reconstructive surgery for renovascular hypertension. Arch Surg 116:999, 1981.

121. Laragh JH, Baer L, Brunner HR, et al: Renin, angiotensin and aldosterone in pathogenesis and management of hypertensive vascular disease. Am J Med 52:633, 1972.

122. Laragh JH, Sealey JE, Bühler FR, et al: The renin axis and vasoconstriction volume analysis for understanding and treating renovascular and renal hypertension. Am J Med 58:4, 1975.

123. Lawrie GM, Morris GC, Jr, Soussou ID, et al: Late results of reconstructive surgery for renovascular disease. Ann Surg 191:528, 1980.

124. Leadbetter WF, Burkland CE: Hypertension in unilateral renal disease. J Urol 39:611, 1938.

125. Lüscher TF, Vetter A, Studer A, et al: Renal venous renin activity in various forms of curable renal hypertension. Clin Nephrol 15:314, 1981.

126. MacCarthy P, Stokes G: Non-renin-mediated renovascular hypertension. Lancet 1: 1312, 1977.

127. Macdonald GJ, Boyd GW, Peart WS: Effect of the angiostensin II blocker 1-sar-8-ala-angiotensin II on renal artery clip hypertension in the rat. Circ Res 37:640, 1975.

128. Macdonald GJ, Louis WJ, Renzini V, et al: Renal clip hypertension in rabbits immunized against angiotensin II. Circ Res 27:197, 1970.

129. Madias NE, Ball JT, Millan VG: Percutaneous transluminal renal angioplasty in

the treatment of unilateral atherosclerotic renovascular hypertension. Am J Med 70:1078, 1981.

130. Maiz HB, Safar M, Ayed HB, et al: Renovascular hypertension: The role of nonspecific factors in the antihypertensive effect of surgery. Clin Nephrol 7:26, 1977.

131. Mannick JA, Huvos A, Hollander WE: Post-hydralizine renin release in the diagnosis of renovascular hypertension. Ann Surg 170:409, 1969.

132. Marks LS, Maxwell MH: Renal vein renin. Value and limitations in the prediction of operative results. Urol Clinic North Am 2:311, 1975.

133. Marks LS, Maxwell MH, Kaufman JJ: Non-renin-mediated renovascular hypertension: A new syndrome? Lancet 1:615, 1977.

134. Marks LS, Maxwell MH, Kaufman JJ: Renin, sodium and vasodepressor response to saralasin in renovascular and essential hypetension. Ann Intern Med 87:176, 1977.

135. Maxwell MH, Marks LS, Lupu AN, et al: Predictive value of renin determinations in renal artery stenosis. JAMA 283:2617, 1977.

136. Maxwell MH, Marks LS, Varady PD, et al: Renal vein renin in essential hypertension. J Lab Clin Med 86:901, 1975.

137. McNair A, Nielsen MD, Gammelegaard PA, et al: A follow-up study of hypertensive patients after operative treatment of unilateral renovascular or renal disease. Acta Med Scand 205:569, 1979.

138. Melman A, Donohue JP, Weinberger MH, Grim CE: Improved diagnostic accuracy of renal venous renin ratios with stimulation of renin release. J Urol 117:145, 1977.

139. Messerli FH, Genest J, Nowaczynski W, et al: Hypertension with renal arterial stenosis: humoral, hemodynamic, and histopathologic factors. Amer J Cardiol 36:702, 1975.

140. Meyer P, Ecoiffier J, Alexandre JM, et al: Prognostic value of plasma renin activity in renovascular hypertension. Circulation 36:570, 1976.

141. Michelakis, A.M., Foster, J.H., Liddle, G.W., et al: Measurement of renin in both renal veins. Its use in diagnosis of renovascular hypertension. Arch Intern Med 120:444, 1967.

142. Michelakis AM, Simmons J: Effect of posture on renal vein renin activity in hypertension. Its implications in the management of patients with renovascular hypertension. JAMA 208:659, 1969.

143. Michelakis AM, Woods JW, Liddle GW, et al: A predictable error in use of renal vein renin in diagnosing hypertension. Arch Intern Med 123:359, 1969.

144. Mörlin C, Lörelius L-E, Wide L: Spontaneous variations in renal vein renin activity in man. Clinica Chimica Acta 119:31, 1982.

145. Morris RE, Ransom PA, Howard JH: Studies on the relationship of angiotensin to hypertension of renal origin. J Clin Invest 41:1386, 1962.

146. Novick AC, Fouad FM, Textor SC, et al: Predictive value of angiotensin II blockade with (sarcosine-1, threonine-8) angiotensin II in renovascular hypertension. J Urol 129:7, 1983.

147. Novick AC, Straffon RA, Stewart BH, et al: Diminished operative morbidity and mortality in renal revascularization. JAMA 246:749, 1981.

148. Ofstad J, Willassen Y: Physiological aspects on the diagnosis of renal artery stenosis. Acta Med Scand Suppl 603:47, 1977.

149. Page IH, Dustan HP, Poutasse EF: Mechanisms, diagnosis and treatment of hypertension of renal vascular origin. Ann Intern Med 51:196, 1959.

150. Page IH, Helmer OM: A crystalline pressor substance, angiotonin, resulting from the reaction between renin and renin activator (Abstr.). Proc Soc Clin Invest 12:17, 1939.

151. Pals DT, Fulton RW: Mechanism of the antihypertensive effect of 1-sar-8-ala-angiotensin II during the acute phase of experimental renal hypertension. Arch Int Pharmacodyn Ther 204:20, 1973.

152. Pals DT, Masucci FD, Denning, GS, Jr, et al: Role of the pressor action of angiotensin II in experimental hypertension. Circ Res 29:673, 1971.

153. Paster SB, Adams DF, Abrams HL: Errors in renal vein renin collections. Am J

Roentgenol Rad Ther Nucl Med 122:804, 1974.

154. Pawsey CGK, Vandongen R, Gordon RD: Renal venous renin ratio in the diagnosis of renovascular hypertension: Measurement during active secretion of renin. Med J Austr 1:121, 1971.

155. Peart WS: Pressor assays in the evaluation of renal hypertension. In Proceedings of the Third International Congress on Nephrology: Karger, Basel, Vol. 3:140, 1967.

156. Perloff D, Sokolow M, Wylie EJ, et al: Renal vascular hypertension, further experiences. Am Heart J 74:614, 1967.

157. Pettinger WA, Keeton K: Hypotension during angiotensin blockade with saralasin. Lancet 1: 1387, 1975.

158. Pinkerton JA, Crouch TT, Sharma JN: Surgical treatment of renovascular hypertension. Am J Surg 138:759, 1979.

159. Poutasse EF, Dustan HP: Arteriosclerosis and renal hypertension. Indications for aortography in hypertensive patients and results of surgical treatment of obstructive lesions of the renal artery. JAMA 165:1521, 1957.

160. Poutasse EF, Gonzales-Serva L, Wendelken JR, et al: Saralasin test as a diagnostic and prognostic aid in renovascular hypertensive patients subjected to renal operation. Trans Am Assoc Genit -Urinary Surg. 71:96, 1979.

161. Poutasse EF, Marks LS, Wisoff CP, et al: Renal vein renin determinations in hypertension: falsely negative tests. J Urol 110:371, 1973.

162. Re R, Novelline R, Escourrou MT, et al: Inhibition of angiotensin-converting enzyme for diagnosis of renal-artery stenosis. N Engl J Med 298:582, 1978.

163. Regoli D, Brunner H, Peters G, et al: Changes in renin content in kidneys of renal hypertensive rats. Proc Soc Exp Biol Med 109:142, 1962.

164. Regoli D, Park WK, Rioux F: Pharmacology of angiotensin. Pharmacol Rev 26:69, 1974.

165. Rosenthal JT, Libertino JA, Zinman LN, et al: Predictability of surgical cure of renovascular hypertension. Ann Surg 193:448, 1981.

166. Saddekni S, Sniderman KW, Hilton S, et al: Percutaneous transluminal angioplasty of nonatherosclerotic lesions. AJR 135: 975, 1980.

167. Saltz M, Sommers SC, Smithwick RH: Clinicopathologic correlations of renal biopsies from essential hypertensive patients. Circulation 16:207, 1957.

168. Salvetti A, Arzilli F, Sassano P, et al: Clinical significance of plasma renin activity in human renovascular hypertension. Clin Sci Mol Med 51:239S, 1976.

169. Schaeffer AJ, Fair WR: Comparison of split function ratios with renal vein renin ratios in patients with curable hypertension caused by unilateral renal artery stenosis. J Urol 112:697, 1974.

170. Schambelan M, Glickman M, Stockigt JR, et al: Selective renal-vein renin sampling in hypertensive patients with segmental renal lesions. N Engl J Med 290:1153, 1974.

171. Schwartz CJ, White TA: Stenosis of renal artery: An unselected necropsy study. Br Med J 2:1415, 1964.

172. Sealey JE, Bühler FR, Laragh JH, et al: The physiology of renin secretion in essential hypertension: Estimation of renin secretion rate and renal plasma flow from peripheral and renal vein renin levels. Am J Med 55:391, 1973.

173. Sealey JE, Gerten-Barnes J, Laragh JH: The renin system: variations in man measured by radioimmunoassay or bioassay. Kidney Int 1:240, 1972.

174. Shapiro AP, Perez-Stable E, Scheib ET, et al: Renal artery stenosis and hypertension. Observations on current status of therapy from a study of 115 patients. Am J Med 47:175, 1969.

175. Simmons JL, Michelakis AM: Renovascular hypertension: the diagnostic value of renal vein renin ratios. J Urol 104:497, 1970.

176. Sinako AR, Mirkin BL: Influence of salt depletion and hydralizine-induced vasodilatation on accuracy of selective renal vein sampling in patients with essential hypertension and renal artery stenosis. Am J Nephrol 2:261, 1982.

177. Skrabal F: Non-renin-mediated renovascular hypertension. Lancet 1:1103, 1977.

178. Stanley JC, Fry WJ: Renovascular hypertension secondary to arterial fibrodysplasia in adults. Criteria for operation and results of surgical therapy. Arch Surg 110: 922, 1975.

179. Stanley JC, Gewertz BL, Fry WJ: Renal:systemic renin indices and renal vein renin ratios as prognostic indicators in remedial renovascular hypertension. J Surg Res 20:149, 1976.

180. Starr DS, Lawrie GM, Morris GC Jr: Surgical treatment of renovascular hypertension. Long-term follow-up of 216 patients up to 20 years. Arch Surg 115:494, 1980.

181. Stockigt JR, Collins RD, Noakes CA, et al: Renal vein renin in various forms of renal hypertension. Lancet 1:1194, 1972.

182. Stockigt JR, Hertz P, Schambelan M, Biglieri EG, et al: Segmental renal-vein renin sampling for segmental renal infarction. Ann Intern Med 79:67, 1973.

183. Stokes GS, MacCarthy EP, Frost GW, et al: False negative saralasin responses in renovascular hypertension. Br J Urol 51: 92, 1979.

184. Stokes GS, Weber MA, Gain J, et al: Diazoxide-induced renin release in diagnosis of remediable renovascular hypertension. Austral New Zeal J Med 6:26, 1976.

185. Stoney RJ, Dehuccia ND, Ehrenfeld WK, et al: Aortorenal arterial autografts. Long term assessment. Arch Surg 116:1416, 1981.

186. Streeten DHP, Anderson GH Jr. Bredenberg CE, et al: The diagnosis and treatment of renovascular hypertension. Clin Invest Med 1:155, 1978.

187. Streeten DHP, Anderson GH, Dalakos TG: Angiotensin blockade: its clinical significance. Am J Med 60:817, 1976.

188. Streeten DHP, Anderson GH Jr, Sunderlin FS Jr, et al.: Identifying renin participation in hypertensive patients. In, Laragh JH, Buhler FR, Seldin DW, Eds: Frontiers In Hypertension Research. Springer-Verlag, New York, 1981.

189. Streeten DHP, Phil D, Anderson GH, et al: Use of an angiotensin II antagonist (saralasin) in the recognition of "angiotensinogenic" hypertension. N Engl J Med 292:657, 1975.

190. Strong CG, Hunt JC, Sheps SG, et al: Renal venous renin activity. Enhancement of sensitivity of lateralization by sodium depletion. Am J Cardiol 27:602, 1971.

191. Tegtmeyer CJ Editorial: Percutaneous transluminal renal angioplasty. The evolution of a procedure. Arch Intern Med 142:1085, 1982.

192. Tegtmeyer CJ, Elson J, Glass TA, et al: Percutaneous transluminal angioplasty: The treatment of choice for renovascular hypertension due to fibromuscular dysplasia. Radiology 143:631, 1982.

193. Thomas RD, Ball SG, Lee MR: Failure of saralasin to predict a response to surgery in renovascular hypertension. Lancet 1:724, 1977.

194. Tigerstedt R, Bergman PG: Niere und kreislauf. Scand Arch Physiology 8:223, 1898.

195. Tobian L: Interrelationship of electrolytes, juxtaglomerular cells and hypertension. Physiol Rev 40:280, 1960.

196. Trainin, EB, Lala VR, Gomez-Leon G, et al: Negative saralasin response in correctable renovascular hypertension. J Pediatr 93:460, 1978.

197. Tremblay GY, Veyrat R, deChamplain J, et al: Criteria for success of surgery in renovascular hypertension. Trans Assoc Amer Physicians 77:201, 1964.

198. Tucker RM, Sheps SG, Brennan LA: Saralasin infusion in renovascular hypertension. Increased response rate in seated patients. Mayo Clin Proc 55:99, 1980.

199. Tucker RM, Strong CG, Brennan LA, Jr: Renovascular hypertension: Relationship of surgical curability to renin-angiotensin activity. Mayo Clin Proc 53:373, 1978.

200. Ueda H, Yagi S, Kaneko Y: Hydralazine and plasma renin activity. Arch Intern Med 122:387, 1968.

201. Vander AJ, Geelhoed GW: Inhibition of renin secretion by angiotensin II. Proc Soc Exp Biol 120:399, 1965.

202. Vander AJ, Miller R: Control of renin secretion in anesthetized dog. Am J Physiol 207:537, 1964.

203. Vaughan ED, Jr, Bühler ER, Laragh JH, et al.: Renovascular hypertension: renin measurements to indicate hypersecretion and contralateral suppression, estimate renal plasma flow, and score for

surgical curability. Am J Med 55:402, 1973.

204. Vermillion SE, Sheps SG, Strong CG, et al: Effect of sodium depletion on renin activity of renal venous plasma in renovascular hypertension. JAMA 208:2302, 1969.

205. Vidt DG, Bravo EL, Fouad FM: Captopril. N Engl J Med 306:214, 1982.

206. Weber MA: Saralasin testing for renin-dependent hypertension. Arch Intern Med 139:93, 1979.

207. Weinberger MH, Dowdy AJ, Nokes GW, et al: Plasma renin activity and aldosterone secretion in hypertensive patients during high and low sodium intake and administration of diuretic. J Clin Endocrinol 28:359, 1968.

208. Whelton PK, Harrington DP, Russell RP, et al: Renal vein renin activity: a prospective study of sampling techniques and methods of interpretation. Johns Hopkins Med J 141:112, 1977.

209. Whelton PK, Russell RP, Harrington DP, et al: Renal venous renin sampling: Physiological variation and pharmacological stimulation. Kidney Int 8:445, 1976.

210. Wilson HM, Wilson JP, Slaton PE, et al: Saralasin infusion in the recognition of renovascular hypertension. Ann Intern Med 87:36, 1977.

211. Winer BM, Lubbe WF, Simon M, et al: Renin in the diagnosis of renovascular hypertension. Activity in renal and peripheral vein plasma. JAMA 202:139, 1967.

212. Woods JW, Michelakis AM: Renal vein renin in renovascular hypertension. Arch Intern Med 122:392, 1968.

# 5

# Treatment of Renovascular Hypertension

# The Case for Percutaneous Angioplasty

## Donald E. Schwarten, M.D.

The value of revascularization of ischemic kidneys in patients with renovascular hypertension (RVH) has been clearly documented. Hunt[13] demonstrated that patients with RVH managed surgically fared better than a comparable population managed with the medical therapy. The surgically managed group did better despite the fact that similar blood pressure control was obtained with medication. The role of more potent and specific antihypertensive agents made available since Hunt's study may yet improve the long-term outlook for the medically managed patient.

Surgical revascularization is no longer the only alternative to pharmacologic therapy of RVH. Grüntzig modified his balloon catheter system, which was initially used only for the percutaneous management of small vessel stenoses[10] for treating renal arterial disease.[11] This therapeutic breakthrough has provided the skilled angiographer with a nonoperative means of correcting RVH. During the past five years, numerous reports of relatively large numbers of patients have appeared, documenting the value of percutaneous transluminal angioplasty (PTA) in the management of RVH.[18,19,25,26]

Dilatation of stenotic renal arteries as a therapy for RVH is not a new development made available only because of Grüntzig's balloon catheter. Intraoperative renal vascular dilatation has been used for years and is of proven benefit in treating RVH.[22] Indeed, there is no a priori reason to doubt that dilatation of a stenotic renal artery with a catheter similar to that developed by Grüntzig would be as effective as the intraoperative procedure. In fact, since the design of the balloon catheter is such that only a radial dilating force is applied to the stenosis, one might expect better results than those obtained by using rigid dilators as is done intraoperatively. This method introduces an abrading shear force which may ultimately damage the vessel. It is a well described experimental observation that if a shear force is applied to the vascular intima and the animal is then placed on a high-cholesterol diet, extensive atherosclerosis develops at the site of trauma. Furthermore, the obvious advantage to balloon catheter therapy of renal artery stenosis is that it can be performed under local anesthesia without the attendant risks of surgery.

It is difficult to evaluate and compare different surgical series reporting results of renal artery revascularization because of the wide variety of operations used and because of certain differences in reporting methods. For purposes of discussion I have, therefore, elected to compare the PTA studies with the ongoing surgical series from the University of Michigan.[23] Using this single, representative study, coming from one center encompassing a large number of patients, and where one operative technique (vein graft bypassing) is used, provides a certain consistency to our interpretations.

To assess the value of treating RVH by PTA and to compare the procedure to surgical therapy, it is of value to consider the following modifying factors:

**1. Patient Selection:** Are the criteria for doing PTA the same as those used in selecting patients for surgical revascularization? As Stanley[23] did in his assessment of the operative results in 264 patients exhibiting renal artery occlusive disease, I will separately evaluate PTA in the following four groups of patients.

a. Pediatric patients.

b. Adult patients with fibromuscular disease.

c. Atherosclerotic renal artery stenosis and renovascular hypertension. (1) Adults with only renal arterial atherosclerotic disease (2) Adults with renal and extrarenal terial atherosclerotic disease.

d. Adults with renal and extrarenal atherosclerotic disease.

Reports of treating RVH with surgery and those using PTA, have included patients with and without hyperreninemia. Because of the known incidence of false negative renin studies (see Chapter 4), most surgical and angioplasty series will include patients who were revascularized when clinical and arteriographic findings strongly suggested a high probability of RVH, regardless of renin levels.[15,17] It is probable that when all series are counted, little, if any, difference in patient selection based on proof of renin dependency, will be apparent.

2. Primary success rate of balloon dilatation.

3. How long are the beneficial effects of PTA sustained?

4. The incidence and nature of procedural-related complications.

5. Cost.

## PEDIATRIC PATIENTS

Stanley's surgical series included 27 patients in the pediatric age group.[23] The most common operation employed was autogenousvein graft. Twenty-four of the 27 patients (89 percent) were classified as cured by surgery. Two (7 percent) were improved and only one (4 percent) was considered a failure. Three secondary nephrectomies were required. Eighteen of the patients were considered to have fibromuscular disease as the etiology of the renal artery stenosis.

I am unable to find reports of sufficient numbers of pediatric patients with RVH treated by PTA and followed for a reasonable period. However, since the majority of those reported had fibromuscular disease, it may be reasonable to consider these patients in the following discussion of adults with similar renal arterial lesions.

## ADULT PATIENTS WITH FIBROMUSCULAR DISEASE

It is well known that one of the most important determinants of success or failure of the revascularization procedure for RVH is the etiology of the renal artery stenosis. Cure or improvement of hypertension with little to no operative mortality may be expected in more than 90 percent of patients with fibromuscular disease.[2] In Stanley's series of 113 adult patients operated on for hypertension secondary to fibromuscular disease, 62 patients were cured (55 percent), 45 were improved (40 percent) and six were surgical failures (5 percent). There were no operative deaths. In this series, age did not influence the rate of cure or improvement (Table 5-1).

Reports of PTA therapy of fibromuscular disease all include far fewer patients than Stanley's surgical series. However, several representative series reported at a recent international symposium on PTA therapy will provide a basis for discussion.[1]

Tegtmeyer[27] recently reported a series

**Table 5-1.** Surgical Treatment of Fibromuscular Disease

| Author | Patients (number) | Cure plus Improvement | Secondary Operations | Secondary Nephrectomies[a] |
|---|---|---|---|---|
| Stanley (23) | 113 | 107 (95%) (107 patients) | 29 | 11 |

[a]Included as part of the 29 secondary operations.

of 21 patients with 23 stenoses caused by fibromuscular dysplasia. All stenoses were successfully dilated without a major complication. Thirteen of the 21 patients (62 percent) were considered cured, that is, the average diastolic pressure was less than 90 mm Hg with at least a 10 mm Hg decrease in predilatation level. Eight patients (38 percent) were considered improved, giving an overall cure–improvement rate of 100 percent. The median follow-up period was 12 months. One patient in Tegtmeyer's series developed a recurrent stenosis at the site of angioplasty and was successfully retreated.

We have recently presented a series of patients who were restudied by digital subtraction angiography to obtain anatomic information about the angioplasty site after a minimum of two years had elapsed.[20] Seven patients treated for medial fibroplasia did not develop restenoses and as judged by criteria used by Tegtmeyer,[27] all patients remained cured or improved from their hypertension. Since 1978, we have attempted 173 angioplasty procedures with 161 anatomic successes (93 percent primary sucess). Thirty-seven of these procedures were performed in patients with fibromuscular disease and their primary success rate was 97 percent. The functional success rate, according to

the aforementioned criteria, was 89 percent cured or improved of their hypertension, with a mean follow-up of 24 months. No complications requiring surgical intervention occurred in the patients with fibromuscular disease.

Katzen[14] reported a series of 28 patients treated with PTA for RVH caused by fibromuscular disease. Primary success was achieved in all cases (one patient required two procedures). At one year, the hypertension was either cured or improved in all patients. Two complications were encountered; one vessel perforated which did not require surgical intervention, and one patient sustained a segmental renal infarction.

Table 5-2 summarizes the results of the angioplasty series reviewed for the treatment of fibromuscular disease. Clearly, fibromuscular disease is amenable to dilatation (Fig. 5-1). Short-term and long-term results are excellent whether the dilatation is done in the operating room under direct vision or in the angiography suite under fluoroscopic guidance. Not all patients with fibromuscular disease are candidates for PTA, however. Patients with medial fibroplasia with large aneurysms should be managed surgically with a bypass graft procedure. But, short of this finding, when dilatation is possi-

**Table 5-2.** Percutaneous Transluminal Angioplasty Treatment of Fibromuscular Disease

| Author (ref) | Number of Patients | Primary Success (%) | Cure plus Improvement (%) | Follow-up Time (mean) | Complications |
|---|---|---|---|---|---|
| Tegtmeyer (27) | 23 | 100 | 100 | 12 months | 0 |
| Schwarten (20) | 37 | 97 | 89 | 24 months | 0 |
| Katzen (14) | 28 | 100 | 100 | 12 months | 2 (nonsurgical) |

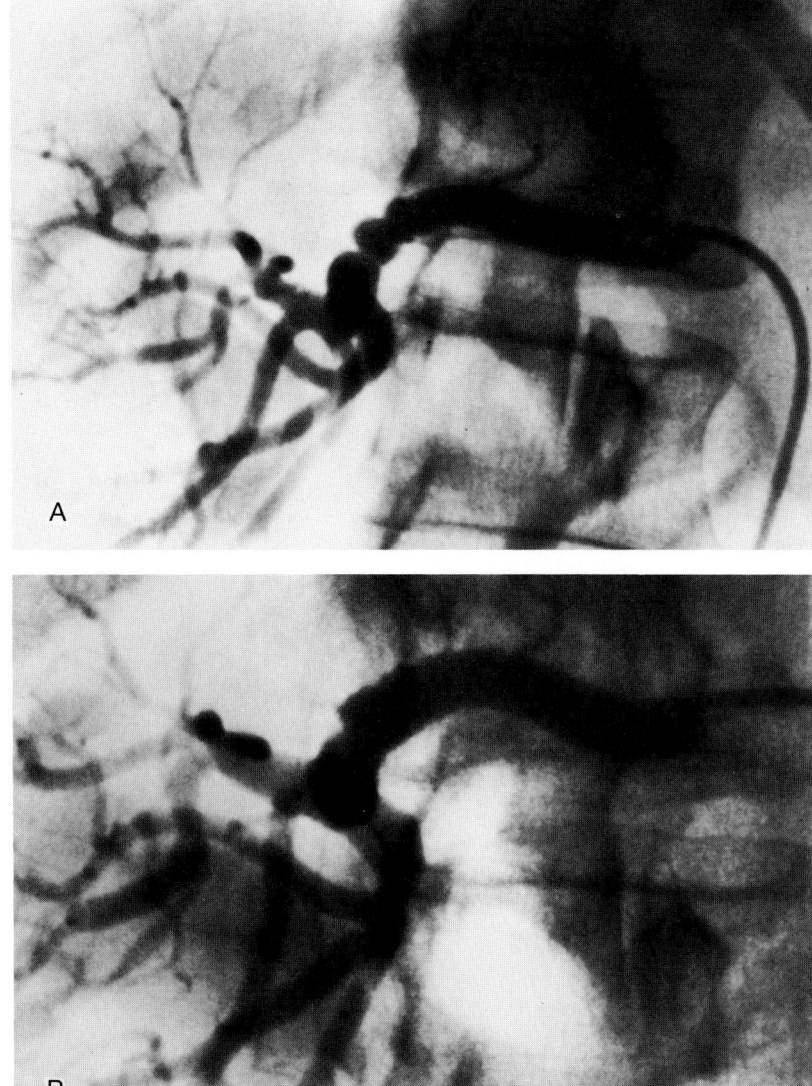

**Fig. 5-1** (A) Preangioplasty arteriogram showing medical fibroplasia with aneurysms. (B) Postangioplasty arteriogram.

ble, it seems unnecessary to perform a major operative procedure to effect dilatation. As Tegtmeyer has aptly pointed out, even small branch vessel lesions can be successfully managed percutaneously without undue risk[27] (Fig. 5-2).

In all series where patients with RVH secondary to fibromuscular disease have been managed by PTA, the primary success rate of the balloon dilatation has been very high, averaging well over 90 percent. The available clinical and angiographic data suggest that the procedure is long-lasting with restenosis occurring in less than five percent of patients with fibromuscular disease. The incidence of significant complications related to the procedure is extremely low. The cost of the procedure compares favorably with the cost of medical therapy and certainly com-

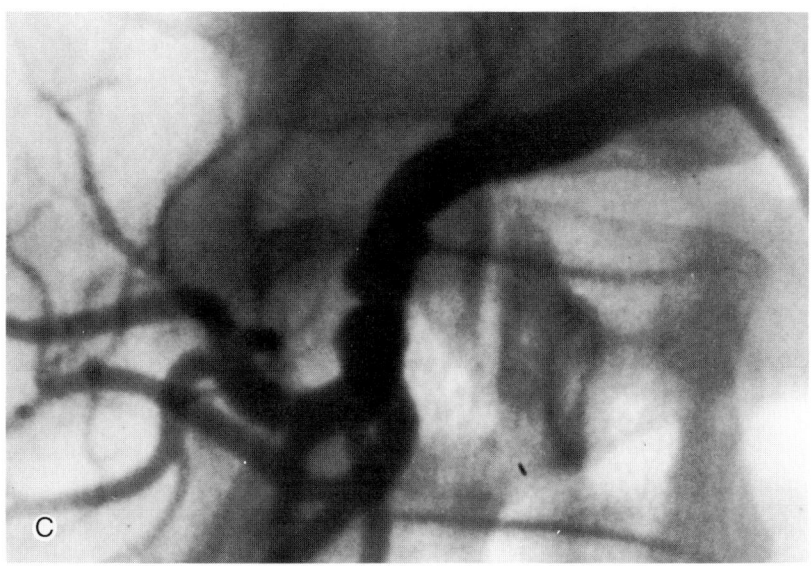

**Fig. 5-1 (Cont.)** (C) Arteriogram three years postangioplasty.

pares more than favorably with the cost of operative management. For example, to treat a patient with 100 mg of metoprolol daily as the only antihypertensive agent for 10 years, would cost $1173.50. The average cost of a single angioplasty procedure, including a 2-day hospital stay in the midwest, is approximately $875.00. These data compare most favorably with reported operative results[23] (Table 5-1). Of the 113 patients being treated surgically, 29 required secondary operations, including 11 nephrectomies. Late aneurysmal dilatation was demonstrated in four saphenous vein grafts, and significant stenotic lesions were found in four additional grafts. These findings support Tegtmyer's contention that PTA is the treatment of choice for RVH due to fibromuscular dysplasia.[27]

Fibromuscular disease is progressive in some cases. In Stanley's series, approximately 12 percent of patients had verified progression of their fibromuscular lesion. A more recent study suggested that the rate of progression of fibromuscular disease is unpredictable, highly variable, and may lead to renal infarction, particularly in the case of sub-adventitial fibromuscu-

lar dysplasia.[17] Katzen's series[14] included a patient with bilateral fibromuscular disease in whom unilateral balloon dilatation was performed as guided by differential renal vein renin values (see Chapter 4). The patient initially experienced a favorable therapeutic result but had a recurrence of hypertension, and at angiography there was demonstration of progression of the fibromuscular disease on the nondilated side, while the dilated artery maintained an essentially normal postangioplasty appearance. These angiographic follow-up data suggest that progression of fibromuscular disease does not occur after the involved vessel has been subjected to angioplasty.

## ATHEROSCLEROTIC RENAL ARTERY STENOSIS AND RENOVASCULAR HYPERTENSION

### General Comments

When atherosclerosis is the etiology of RVH, formidable problems may be pre-

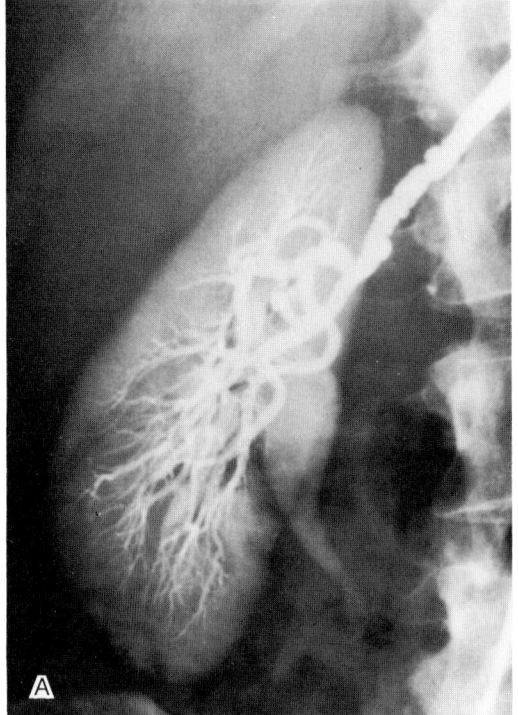

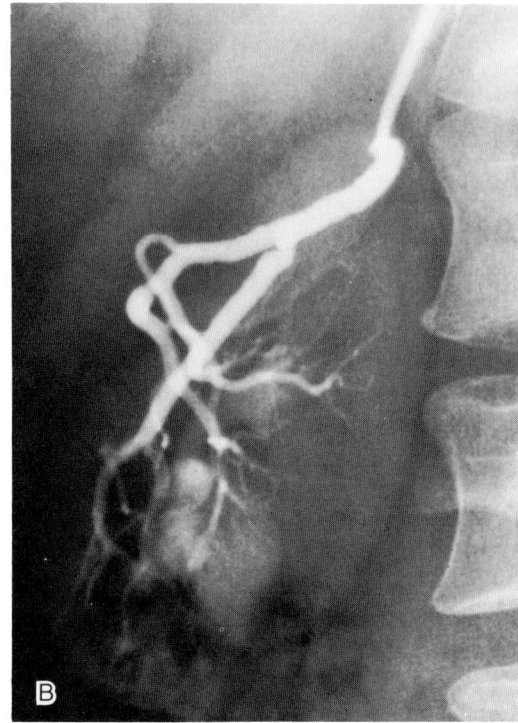

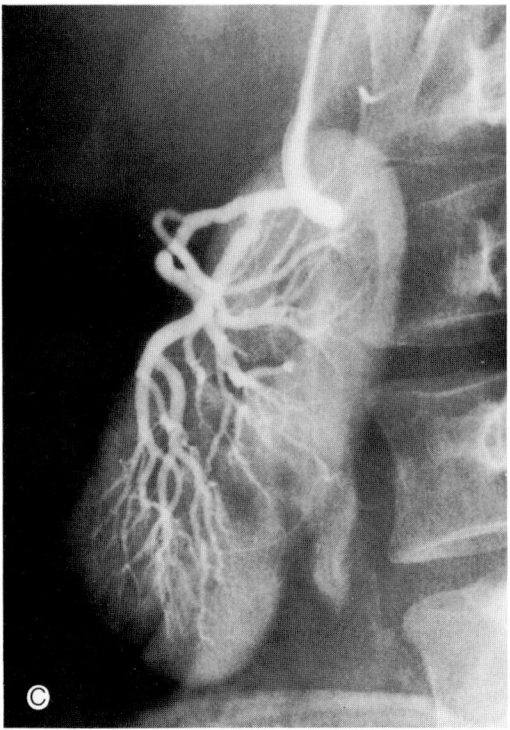

**Fig. 5-2.** (A) Preangioplasty arteriogram showing medial fibroplasia with aneurysms. (B) Oblique arteriogram obtained after angioplasty of the main renal artery. (C) Oblique arteriogram after angioplasty of the branch stenoses.

sented to the surgeon and the angiographer. Whether the atherosclerosis is essentially localized to the renal artery or is part of a diffuse process, has a profound effect upon the results of operative revascularization and an equally profound effect on the results of PTA. If the angiographer is to avoid results such as those presented by Grim et al.,[9] careful consideration must be given to the angiographic anatomy as outlined by Cicuto et al.[3] It appears that the most important determinant in the primary success or failure of an attempted renal angioplasty procedure in an atherosclerotic patient is the angiographic appearance of the renal artery stenosis and the immediate adjacent abdominal aorta (Fig. 5-3). This critical point was not generally recognized among angiographers when renal angioplasty was first made available, therefore, most series with reasonably long follow-up periods did not differentiate between patients with generalized atherosclerosis, patients with abnormalities of the orifice of the renal artery and immediately adjacent abdominal aorta, and patients with focal renal artery atherosclerosis located well inside the ostium of the renal artery. Most angioplasty series merely categorize patients into atherosclerotic and nonatherosclerotic categories. Of necessity, therefore, I shall review a representative series to provide general information about the results of renal angioplasty in the presence of atherosclerosis without defining the extent of the atherosclerotic process. There does appear to be sufficient information to also permit a reasonably close comparison between surgical and PTA series of focal atherosclerotic disease and similarly with generalized atherosclerotic disease.

Colapinto et al.[4] recently reported their results of PTA in 68 patients with renal artery stenoses requiring 80 procedures. Fifty-one of these patients were classified as having atherosclerotic disease and 44 (86 percent) had a successful result from PTA. The hypertension of the successfully dilated patients was cured or improved in 84 percent with follow-up periods ranging from 1 to 36 months. Three restenoses occurred, all within the first 12 months following the original dilatation, and each was uneventfully redilated. One of the 51 atherosclerotic patients required a heminephrecomy after attempted dilatation of a accessory polar renal artery. One patient sustained a subendocardial infarction and one patient thrombosed an iliac artery and developed acute tubular necrosis from which she recovered. No other major complications were encountered in this series (Table 5-3).

## Adults with Only Renal Atherosclerotic Disease

Large atherosclerotic plaques localized to the ostia of the renal artery offer major mechanical impediments to the balloon catheter. To make valid comparisons between PTA and surgical therapy of atherosclerosis-induced renal arterial stenosis, I shall only report angioplasty series in which nonostial atherosclerotic lesions were subjected to dilatation, whether or not clinically significant generalized atherosclerotic disease was present. These reports will be compared to Stanley's surgically treated subgroup in which atherosclerotic disease was considered to be essentially limited to the renal arteries.[23]

Stanley (Table 5-4) reported that 31 percent of these patients were considered cured of their hypertension following operative intervention.[23] Sixty percent were improved and 9 percent were considered treatment failures. No deaths related to the operative procedures occurred. However, there were three primary nephrectomies and two secondary nephrectomies in this group of 54 patients for a nephrectomy rate of more than 9 percent. We consider a nephrectomy a *primary* ne-

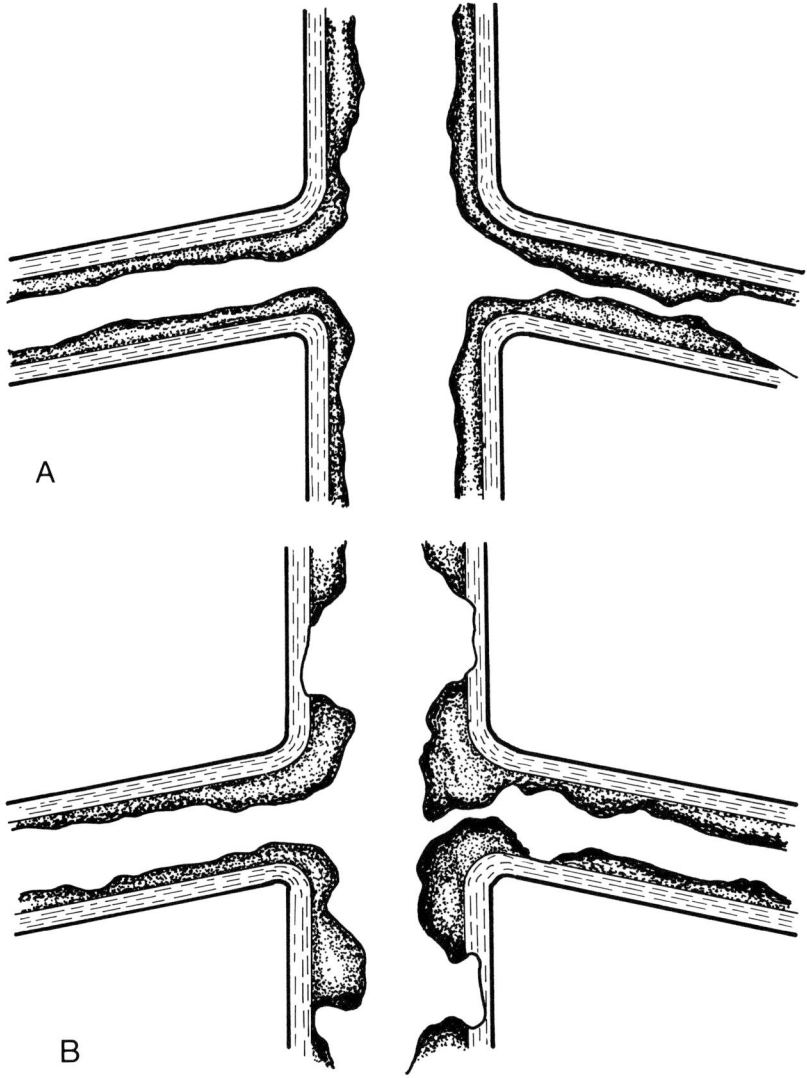

**Fig. 5-3** (A) Drawing of the ideal anatomy for angioplasty in atherosclerosis. (B) Diagram of an aortic plaque encroaching on the renal arterial ostium. Angioplasty is unlikely to succeed in this setting.

phrectomy when it is the initial therapy and treatment of choice for renovascular hypertension. A nephrectomy is considered secondary when it is a second operation to remove a kidney after failure of a bypass graft or other vascular reconstructive procedure. Again, the most common operation employed in this series was autogenous vein graft. In a separate study, Stanley[21] analyzed the late angiographic

appearances of 74 consecutive grafts obtained 8 to 109 months after revascularization. Twenty-nine of the 74 grafts appeared normal when restudied some 40 months (average) postoperatively. Thirty-three of the grafts were dilated, manifesting a mean increase in graft diameter of 18 percent. Six of the vein grafts exhibited aneurysmal dilatation with an average increase in diameter of 114 percent, and

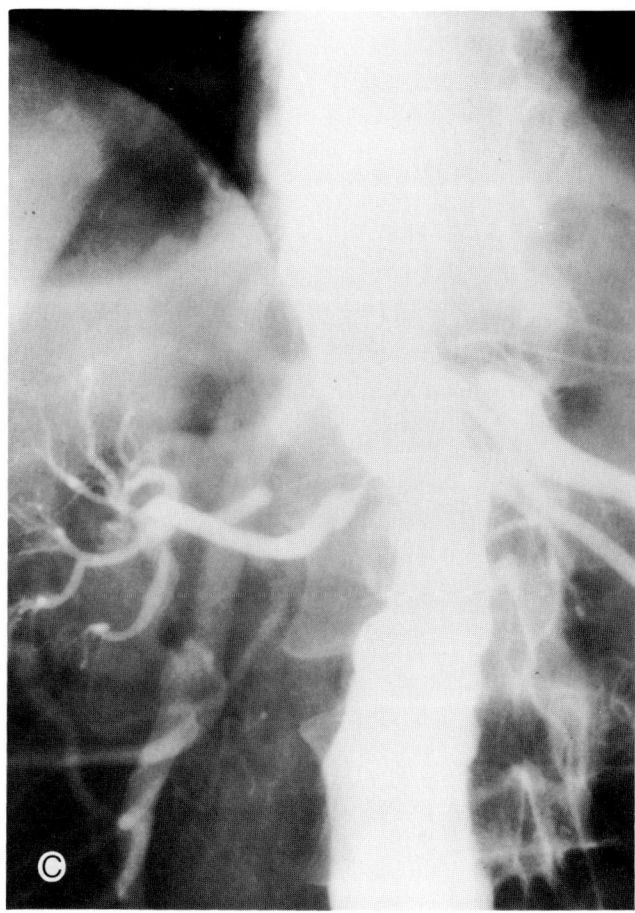

**Fig. 5-3 (cont.)**   (c) Arteriogram in a setting comparable to (B).

seven of the vein grafts developed significant stenotic lesions. Stanley noted that vein graft stenoses posed difficult problems for the surgeon, reoperation, in general, is difficult at best.

Grim et al.[8] report a vein graft failure rate of 20 percent. This figure, along with that of Stanley and the diverse nature of the atherosclerotic process are perhaps responsible for the wide variety of operative procedures advocated by different surgeons for managing arteriosclerotic RVH. This variability contributes to the difficulty in making precise therapeutic comparisons.

The surgeon with extensive experience in the management of RVH is likely to have better results than the surgeon who only occasionally operates upon the renal artery. In a similar fashion, PTA should not be performed by the occasional angiographer. The potential problems that one may encounter in attempting renal angioplasty are formidable and require the skills of an experienced angiographer as well as the availability and cooperation of an experienced renovascular surgeon. The angiographer has a limited number of approaches and materials with which to effect dilatation of a stenotic renal artery. Prior to selecting a patient for renal angioplasty, arteriography must be performed. The anatomic information obtained predicts the success or failure of renal angioplasty in the atherosclerotic patient. When the atherosclero-

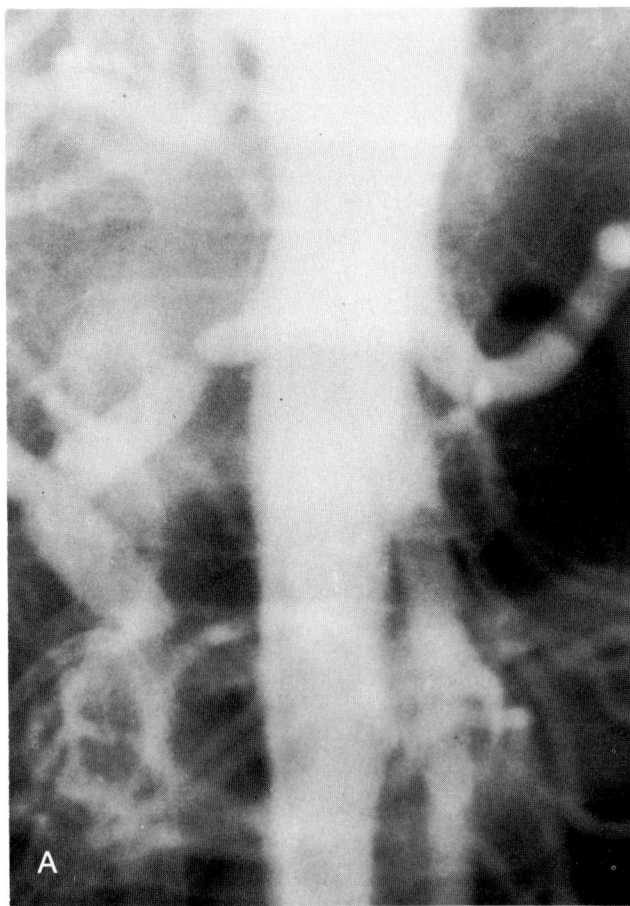

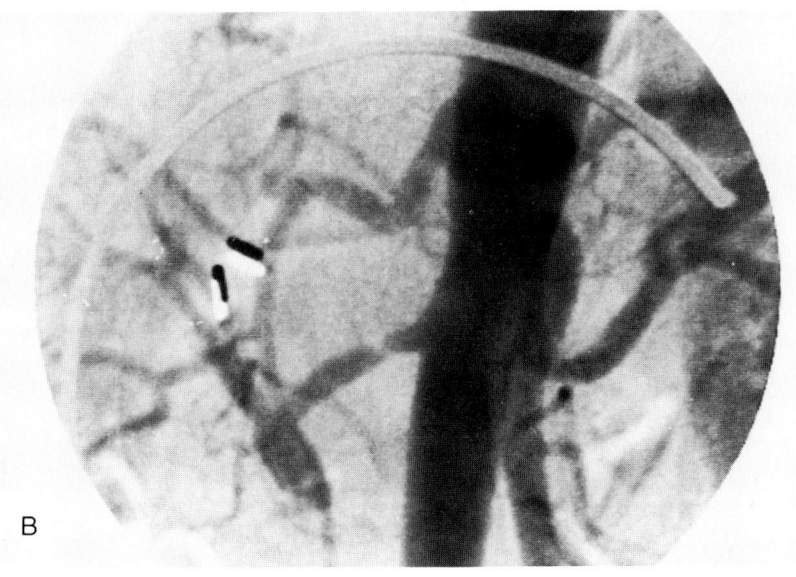

**Fig. 5-4.** (A) Arteriogram obtained after bypass surgery demonstrating an occluded graft and stenosis of the native renal artery. (B) Digital subtraction angiogram of (A).

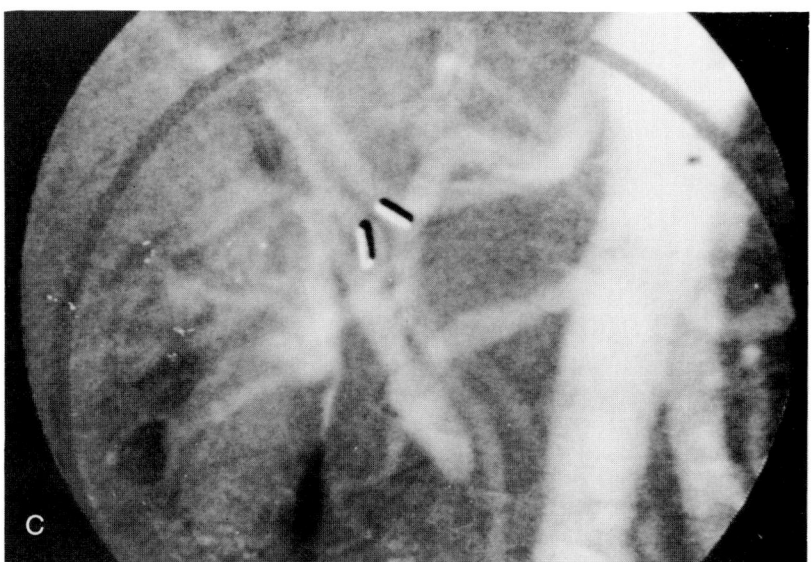

**Fig. 5-4 (cont.)**    (C) Digital subtraction angiogram following successful percutaneous angioplasty.

tic lesion is located well within the renal artery, that is, 3.0 to 4.0 mm distal to the ostium, Cicuto et al.[3] found that regardless of the presence or absence of disease in the aorta, he and his coworkers were able to achieve an excellent or good result from angioplasty in 83 percent of their patients (Figs. 5-4,5-5).

In our own recent follow-up series, 33 of the 40 patients with satisfactory digital angiograms who were more than two years postangioplasty, were found to be cured or improved of their hypertension according to National Cooperative Study Guidelines. The digital subtraction angiography studies revealed, however, that within this group of clinically cured or improved patients, there were three recurrent stenoses (Fig. 5-6). Conversely, among the 18 percent with recurrent hypertension, considered to be treatment failures, the digital subtraction angiogram demonstrated a widely patent renal artery in only one patient. It is important to note that this study was carried out on consecutive patients, all of whom were two or more years postangioplasty. As noted by Colapinto et al.[4] and by Grüntzig,[12] it is extremely uncommon for recurrent stenoses to develop after 12 months have elapsed following the angioplasty procedure. It is also important to point out that none of the patients included in these follow-up studies had extensive disease in the abdominal aorta immediately adjacent to and compromising the orifice of the renal artery. This, in essence, is the angiographer's counterpart to the surgeon's focal renal artery atherosclerosis. This group of patients, in whom strict arteriographic, pathologic anatomical criteria were adhered to, angioplasty was primar-

**Table 5-3.** Percutaneous Transluminal Angioplasty in Atherosclerosis

| Author (ref) | Number Patients | Primary Success | Cure plus Improvement | Follow-up Time (mean) | Complications |
|---|---|---|---|---|---|
| Colapinto (3) | 51 | 86% (44 patients) | 84% | 1–36 months | 3 |

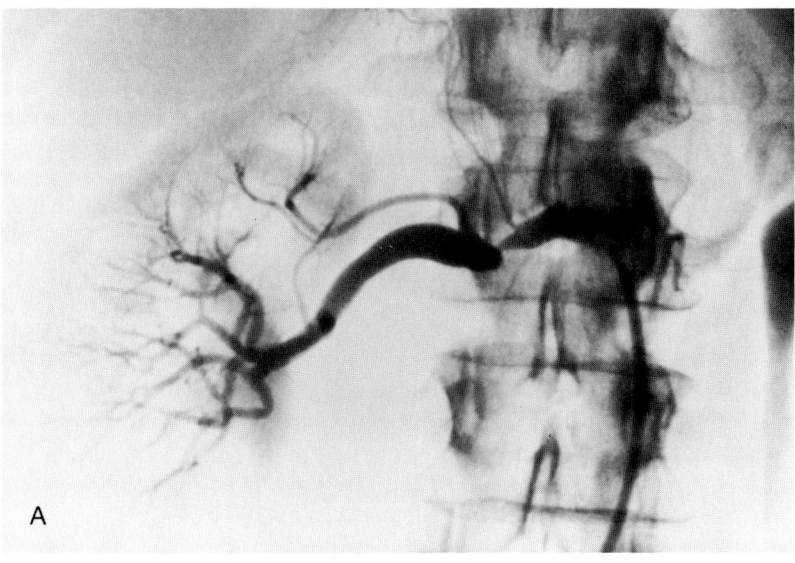

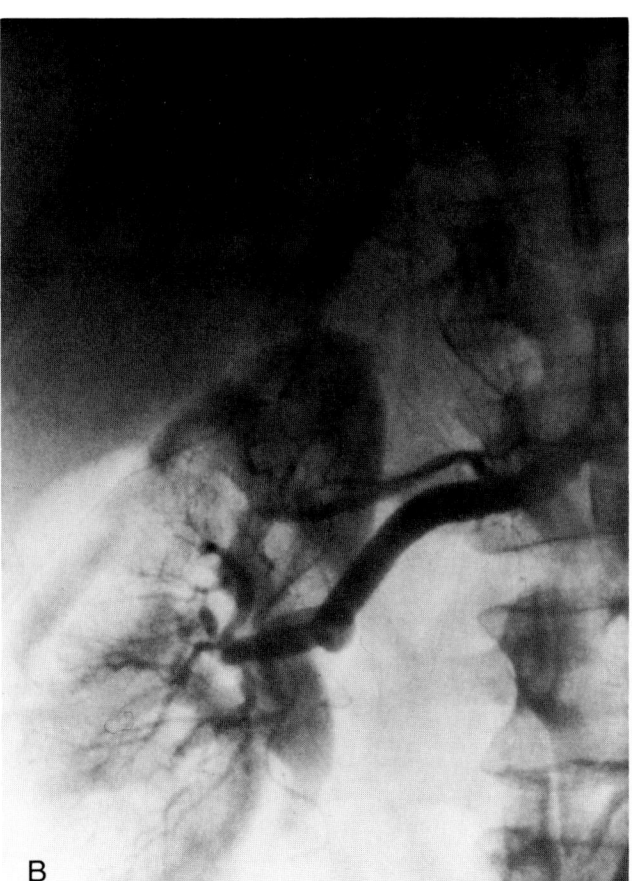

**Fig. 5-5.**  (A) Focal atherosclerotic lesion that is optimal for balloon angioplasty therapy. (B) Postangioplasty study.

**Table 5-4.** Surgical Treatment of Atherosclerosis Localized to the
Renal Artery

| Author (ref) | Number Patients | Cure plus Improvement | Secondary Operations | Secondary Operations |
|---|---|---|---|---|
| Stanley (23) | 54 | 91% (49 patients) | 5 | 2 |

ily successful in 96 percent of original attempts. No significant complications occurred (Table 5-5).

The cure rate of hypertension obtained with balloon dilatation appears to be slightly lower than that resulting from operative revascularization. The 9 percent difference in blood pressure response (82 percent versus 91 percent) may be more than offset by the 9.5 percent nephrectomy rate associated with surgery.

## Adults with Renal and Extrarenal Artery Atherosclerotic Disease (Fig. 5-6)

Wollenweber and associates[28] concluded that no significant difference existed in the 5-year survival rates of patients treated for arteriosclerotic renovascular disease surgically than those treated medically. Should renal revascularization be attempted in patients with diffuse atherosclerotic disease? The question may certainly be debatable, but the issue at hand is a comparison between surgical therapy and PTA. The subcategory of patients with renal and extrarenal atherosclerotic disease reported by Stanley et al,[23] appears to be an extension of an earlier study.[6] Ernst reported on 36 patients having clinically overt extrarenal arteriosclerotic cardiovascular disease in conjunction with RVH.[6] This group underwent a variety of operative procedures and only 53 percent realized a cure or improvement of hypertension following operative intervention. During the 41 months of follow-up, 31 percent of these patients died. There were two operative deaths (5.6 percent). In Stanley's later

communication, 51 patients with diffuse atherosclerotic disease were reported. Twenty-six percent of the patients were classified as cured of hypertension, 47 percent improved and 20 percent were considered failures after operative management. There were five primary nephrectomies and five secondary nephrectomies (19.6 percent nephrectomy rate). There were a total of eight secondary operations and there were three operative deaths, two of these in patients with severely compromised renal function (Table 5-6).

In Cicuto's[3] patients with diffuse disease of the abdominal aorta with atherosclerotic plaques encroaching upon the ostium of the renal artery, good to excellent results were achieved in 24 percent of attempted angioplasty procedures with negligible morbidity.

In our own series, PTA was attempted in 20 patients with stenoses of the renal arterial ostium and severe atherosclerotic involvement of the abdominal aorta especially in the area of the renal arteries. Ten of these patients had high-grade bilateral renal artery stenoses, and 17 had significantly compromised renal function. Technical success was achieved in 14 of the 20 attempts (70 percent). A beneficial, hypotensive response was observed in ten patients (50 percent) with a mean follow-up time of 28 months. Acute renal failure occurred following angioplasty in four patients, all of whom had had significantly compromised renal function. Three of these patients were diabetic and all received more than 80 grams of iodine in contrast medium during the procedure. Since Lang's publica-

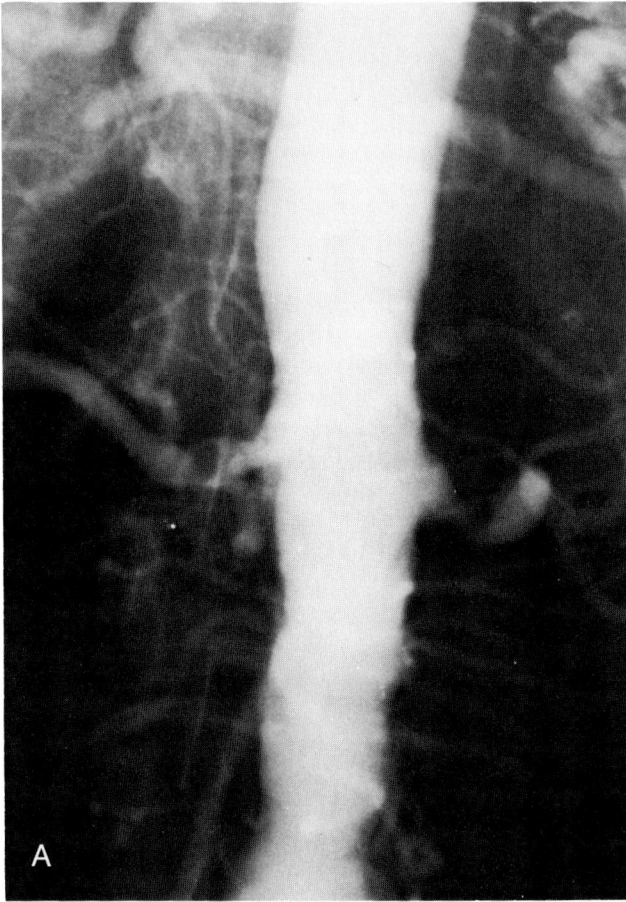

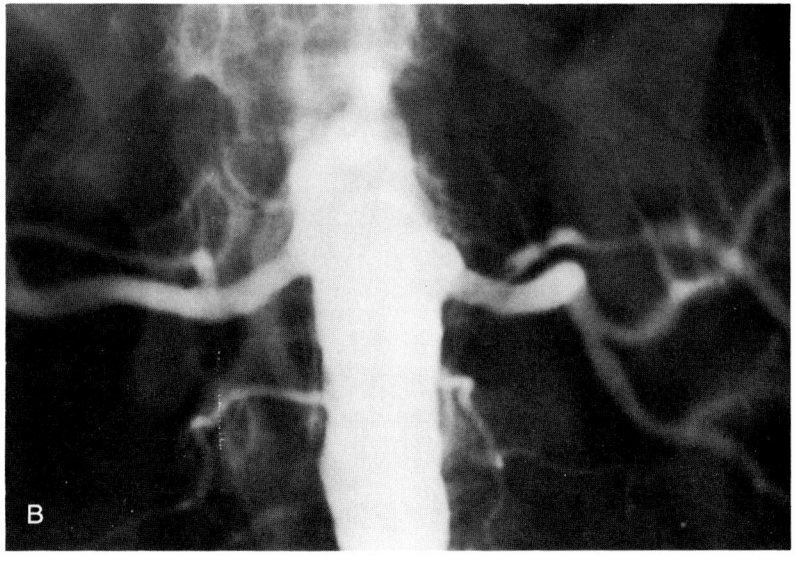

**Fig. 5-6.**   (A) Preangioplasty arteriogram. (B) Immediate Postangioplasty arteriogram.

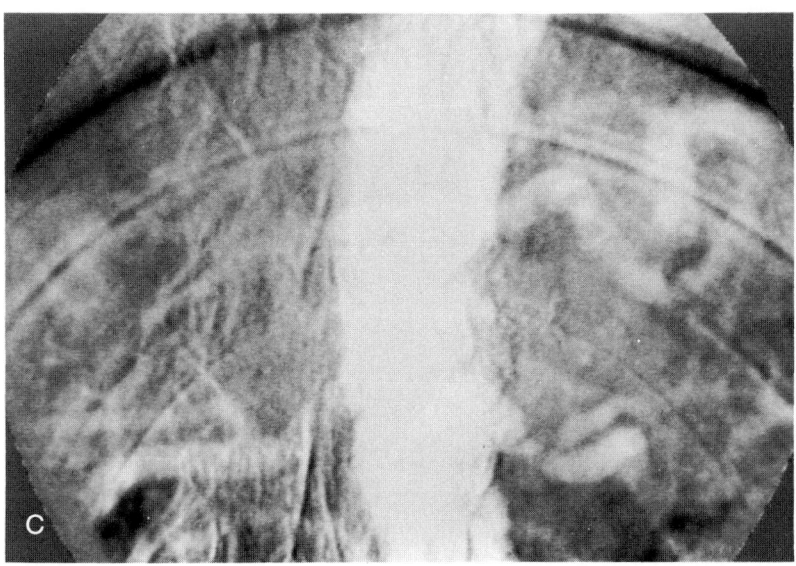

**Fig. 5-6 (cont.)**   (C) Digital subtraction angiogram three years postangio-plasty. Recurrent stenoses are evident despite clinical improvement.

tion[16] decrying the use of excessive amounts of dye, we now arbitrarily limit contrast iodine to 75 grams per procedure and have had no episodes of clinically significant acute renal insufficiency induced by contrast material. The serum creatinine of three of the four patients returned to their preangioplasty levels or less, while one patient required chronic hemodialysis (Table 5-7).

Obviously, patients with clinically significant generalized atherosclerotic disease are at high risk for either operative revascularization of stenotic renal arteries or PTA. However, when contrast volume is rigidly controlled and patients optimally hydrated, the risk of angioplasty becomes minimal. While the hemodynamic effects of surgery were better than with PTA, the absence of secondary ne-

phrectomy makes the latter technique more attractive.

The imminent availability of less hypertonic contrast agents and the probability that they will have less adverse effects on renal function, further enhances the potential attractiveness of balloon angioplasty.

I have not, as yet, addressed the topic of renal revascularization for the *preservation of renal function*, but the loss of renal function is intimately associated with RVH whether it be of atherosclerotic origin or caused by fibromuscular disease. Stewart et al. have shown that atherosclerotic plaques affecting the main renal artery causes progressive arterial narrowing in one-third of nonoperated patients.[24] Dean[5] has shown that renal artery stenoses can progress to occlusion in the ath-

**Table 5-5.** Percutaneous Transluminal Angioplasty in Nonostial Renal Atherosclerosis

| Author (ref) | Number of Patients | Cure plus Improvement | Follow-up Time | Complications |
|---|---|---|---|---|
| Schwarten (5) | 40 | 83% (33 patients) | 24 months | 0 |

**Table 5-6.** Surgical Treatment in the Presence of Generalized Atherosclerosis

| Author (ref) | Number of Patients | Cure plus Improvement | Secondary Operations | Secondary Nephrectomies |
|---|---|---|---|---|
| Stanley (23) | 51 | 73% (27 patients) | 8 | 5 |

erosclerotic patient, ultimately causing loss of functioning renal parenchyma. In our own experience, we have encountered six patients who were referred for balloon angioplasty having undergone diagnostic arteriography and acquisition of renin data two days to four months prior to their referral. These patients had 90 percent narowing of the affected renal artery and normal renal function at the time of diagnosis. These stenoses progressed to occlusion and in each case there was a marked reduction in renal size. These data suggest that in patients with high grade renal artery stenosis, prompt intervention may preserve functioning renal tissue. It may be prudent, in fact, to perform angioplasty at the time of diagnosis of such highgrade lesions if it can be accomplished using reasonable contrast volumes.

# CONCLUSIONS

Percutaneous ballon dilatation of renal artery stenosis is a relatively new therapeutic modality, recently made available to manage the patient with RVH. The procedure has been in use since 1978 and data is rapidly accumulating to support its efficacy. In patients with fibromuscular disease and RVH, the beneficial hemo-dynamic results of PTA are nearly comparable to those obtained with classical operative procedures, but the risk of secondary nephrectomy is greatly reduced. Comparison of angioplasty to operative management in patients with atherosclerotic RVH is more difficult, but it appears that angioplasty effectively reduces blood pressure to levels closely approximating those achieved by experienced surgeons. Again the risk of secondary nephrectomy is much reduced by PTA. Patients with generalized atherosclerosis are more difficult to treat with PTA. However, when contrast volume is minimized, angioplasty can be safely attempted as a first-line procedure and a significant number will obtain beneficial results.

Follow-up studies utilizing digital substraction angiography have demonstrated that patients with fibromuscular disease with an initially successful angioplasty rarely develop recurrent stenosis. It has also been shown that approximately 20 percent of patients who had been successfully treated by PTA for atherosclerotic renal arterial stenosis, will develop a recurrence. If the restenosis does not occur within the first year, it is unlikely to develop later. Should a recurrent stenosis develop at any time, however, a repeat angioplasty procedure can be performed with no greater difficulty than the initial procedure. Recurrent disease or late fail-

**Table 5-7.** Percutaneous Transluminal Angioplasty in Generalized Atherosclerosis (Renal Ostial Stenosis)

| Author Reference | Number of Patients | Cure plus Improvement | Follow-up Time | Complications |
|---|---|---|---|---|
| Schwarten (20) | 20 | 50% (10 patients) | 24 months | 4 (all ATN)[a] |

[a]ATN: acute tubular necrosis.

ures of operative procedures are not so easily retrieved.

# REFERENCES

1. A Cooperative Study: The Second Symposium on Percutaneous Transluminal Angioplasty. Nurenberg, May 1982.
2. Brewster DC: Surgical managment of renovascular disease. Am J Roentgenol 135: 963, 1980.
3. Cicuto KP, McLean GK, Oleaga JA, et al: Renal artery stenosis: anatomic classification for percutaneous transluminal angioplasty. Am J Roentgenol 139:727, 1982.
4. Colapinto RF, Stronell RD, Harries-Jones EP, et al: Percutaneous transluminal dilatation of the renal artery: Follow-up studies on renovascular hypertension. Am J Roentgenol 139:727, 1982.
5. Dean RH: Renovascular hypertension. Combined and aortic procedures. Natural history. Presented at the IV Congress of the Michael E. DeBakey International Cardiovascular Society, Buenos Aires, April 1982.
6. Ernst CB, Stanley JC, Marshall FF, et al: Renal revascularization for arteriosclerotic renovascular hypertension. Prognostic implications of focal renal arterial vs overt generalized arteriosclerosis. Surgery 73:859, 1973.
7. Goncharenko V, Gerlock AJ, Shaff MI, et al: Progression of renal artery fibromuscular dysplasia in 42 patients as seen on angiography. Radiology 139:45, 1981.
8. Grim CE, Yune MY, Weinberger MH, et al: Balloon dilatation for renal artery stenosis causing hypertension. Criteria, concerns and cautions. Ann Intern Med 92:117, 1980.
9. Grim CE, Luft FC, Yune MY, et al: Percutaneous transluminal dilatation in the treatment of renovascular hypertension. Ann Intern Med 95:439, 1981.
10. Grüntzig A: Transluminal dilatation of coronary artery stenosis. Experimental report. In Zeitler E, Grüntzig A, Schoop W, Eds: Percutaneous Vascular Recanalization: Technique, Application, Clinical Results. Springer, Berlin, 1978, pp 57–65,
11. Grüntzig A, Kuhlmann U, Vetter W, et al: Treatment of renovascular hypertension with percutaneous transluminal dilatation of a renal artery steonosis. Lancet 1:801, 1978.
12. Grüntzig A: The incidence of recurrent stenoses in arteries after successful percutaneous transluminal angioplasty. Presented at the Second Symposium on Percutaneous Transluminal Angioplasty. Nurenberg, May 1982.
13. Hunt JC, Strong CG: Renovascular hypertension; mechanisms, natural history and management. Am J Cardiol 32:562, 1973.
14. Katzen BT, Edwards KC, Albert A: Percutaneous transluminal angioplasty for treatment of renovascular hypertension due to fibromuscular dysplasia. Presented at the annual meeting of the Radiological Society of North America, Chicago, November 1982.
15. Kaufman JJ, Marks LS, Maxwell MH: Renovascular hypertension. Ann Surg 11: 313, 1979.
16. Lang EK, Foreman J, Schlegel JU: The incidence of contrast medium induced acute tubular necrosis following arteriography. Radiology 138:203, 1981.
17. Novick AC, Stewart BH: Surgical treatment of renovascular hypertension. Curr Prob Surg 16:1, 1979.
18. Puijlaert CBAJ, Boomsma JMB, Ruijs JMJ, et al: Transluminal renal artery dilatation in hypertension: technique, results and complications in 60 cases. Urol Radiol 2:201, 1981.
19. Schwarten DE: Transluminal angioplasty for renal artery stenosis; 70 experiences. Am J Roentgenol 135:969, 1980.
20. Schwarten DE: The use of digital intravenous subtraction angiography as the principal method in the follow-up of patients who have had successful percutaneous transluminal renal angioplasty. Presented at the annual meeting of the Radiological Society of North America, Chicago, November 1982.
21. Stanley JC, Ernst CB, Fry WJ: Fate of 100 aortorenal vein grafts: characteristics of late graft expansion, aneurysmal dilatation and stenosis. Surgery 74:931, 1973.
22. Stanley JC, Fry WJ: Renovascular hyper-

tension secondary to arterial fibrodysplasia in adults; criteria for operation and results of surgical therapy. Arch Surg 110:922, 1975.

23. Stanley JC, Fry WJ: Surgical treatment of renovascular hypertension. Arch Surg 112:1291, 1977.

24. Stewart BH, Dustan HP, Kiser WS, et al: Correlation of angiography and natural history in evaluation of patients with renovascular hypertension. J Urol 104:231, 1970.

25. Tegtmeyer CJ, Dyer R, Teates CD, et al: Percutaneous transluminal dilatation of the renal arteries. Radiology 135:589, 1980.

26. Tegtmeyer CJ, Teates CD, Crigler N, et al: Percutaneous transluminal angioplasty in patients with renal artery stenosis. Follow-up studies. Radiology 140:323, 1981.

27. Tegtmeyer CJ, Elson J, Glass TA, et al: Percutaneous transluminal angioplasty: The treatment of choice for renovascular hypertension due to fibromuscular dysplasia. Radiology 143:631, 1982.

28. Wollenweber J, Sheps SG, David ED: Clinical course of arteriosclerotic renovascular disease. Am J Cardiol 21:60, 1968.

# The Case for Surgical Therapy

Andrew C. Novick, M.D.

## INTRODUCTION

The first reports of surgically curable hypertension in the late 1930s led to enthusiasm among clinicians for removing kidneys with arterial stenosis in hypertensive patients. The development of vascular surgical techniques in the 1950s made it possible to achieve successful renal revascularization in many of these cases. However, the cause and effect relationship between a stenotic renal artery lesion and hypertension was poorly understood and many patients treated surgically had no improvement of blood pressure postoperatively. Continued experience in this field during the past two decades has significantly improved our understanding of the natural history and functional significance of renovascular disorders. Patients with renovascular hypertension can now be identified with a high degree of accuracy and successful renal revascularization is possible in most cases. Nevertheless, multiple factors must be weighed in determining whether medical or surgical therapy is more appropriate for a given patient. These include the causal relationship of renovascular disease to hypertension, the adequacy of blood pressure control with medical therapy, the natural history of untreated renovascular disease with particular regard for the risk of losing renal function, the medical condition of the patient, the morbidity and results of surgical therapy, and the availability of other therapeutic options such as percutaneous transluminal dilatation.

## CLASSIFICATION AND NATURAL HISTORY OF RENAL VASCULAR DISORDERS (Table 5-8)

### Atherosclerosis

Approximately 60 percent of all renovascular lesions are caused by atherosclerosis.[41] This disease may be limited to the renal artery but, more commonly, is a manifestation of generalized atherosclerosis involving the abdominal aorta, coronary, cerebral, and lower extremity vessels. Atherosclerotic stenosis usually occurs in the proximal two centimeters of the main renal artery and distal arterial or branch involvement is distinctly uncommon. Due to the proximal location of these lesions, oblique aortic views are often needed to adequately visualize the area of stenosis.

There have been relatively few published reports on the natural history of atherosclerotic lesions in patients managed nonoperatively. The available data suggest that progressive arterial stenosis, occasionally eventuating in total occlusion, is a relatively common sequela of this disease. In 1968, Wollenweber reviewed 30 patients with atherosclerotic renovascular disease who had been followed with serial renal angiograms from three to 88 months apart; progressive renal artery stenosis was observed unilaterally in 13 patients (43 percent) and bilaterally in six patients (20 percent).[74] Also in 1968, Meaney et al. reported progression

181

**Table 5-8.** Classification of Atherosclerotic and Fibrous Renal Artery Disease

| Renal Artery Disease | Incidence (%) | Age (Yrs) | Male (M) vs Female (F) Occurrence | Location of Lesion in Renal Artery | Natural History | Angiographic Appearance |
|---|---|---|---|---|---|---|
| Atherosclerosis | 60 | > 50 | M:F 2:1 | Proximal 2 cm, Branch disease rare | Progression in 44%, often to total occlusion | Circumferential stenosis extending from aorta into proximal renal artery |
| Fibrous Dysplasias: | | | | | | |
| Intimal fibroplasia | 4–5 | Children, young adults | M = F | Mid-main renal artery and/or branches | Progression in most cases, dissection and/or thrombosis common | Smooth focal stenosis, abundant collateral vessels, frequent renal atrophy |
| Medial fibroplasia | 30 | 25–50 | F>M | Distal main renal artery and/or branches | Progression in 33%, dissection and/or thrombosis rare | "String of beads," Rare collateral vessels, Renal atrophy uncommon |
| Perimedial fibroplasia | 4–5 | 15–30 | F only | Mid-to-distal main renal artery or branches | Progression in most cases, dissection and/or thrombosis common | Focal stenosis or diffuse beading of a artery, Diameter of beads < normal renal artery; abundant collateral vessels, frequent renal atrophy |
| Fibromuscular hyperplasia | < 1 | Children, young adults | M = F | Mid-renal artery or branches | Progression in most cases | Smooth focal stenosis, radiographically indistinguishable from intimal fibroplasia |

of atherosclerotic renal artery stenosis in 14 of 39 patients (36 per cent) followed with serial angiography during intervals ranging from 6 months to 7 years.[39]

More recently, Schreiber et al. reviewed the outcome of atherosclerotic renovascular disease in 85 patients treated medically and followed with sequential renal angiography during intervals of three to 172 months.[60] The mean angiographic follow-up interval was 52 months and the mean clinical follow-up period in these patients was 87 months. Progressive renal artery obstruction from atherosclerosis was observed in 37 patients (44 percent), including 14 patients (16 percent) wherein complete arterial occlusion developed. Clinical follow-up revealed that serial decreases in both overall renal function (p<.02) and the size of the involved kidney (p <.001) occurred more commonly in patients who developed progressive renovascular disease than in those who did not. However, serial blood pressure control was no different in these two groups, and is not, therefore, useful as a marker for progressive disease. This study indicates not only that atherosclerotic renal artery disease progresses in a large number of patients but also that such progression is commonly associated with clinically detectable loss of functioning renal parenchyma.

### Fibrous Dysplasias

The fibrous dysplasias comprise approximately 40 percent of all renovascular disorders.[41] These lesions are considered to be congenital dysplasias with maldevelopment of the fibrous, muscular, and elastic tissues of the renal artery. They are subcategorized according to the layer of the arterial wall involved.[24] This classification is important since each type of fibrous dysplasia has distinct histologic and angiographic features, and occurs in a different clinical setting.[39]

Primary intimal fibroplasia occurs in children and young adults, and comprises approximately 10 percent of the total number of fibrous lesions. This lesion is characterized by a circumferential accumulation of collagen inside the internal elastic lamina. Angiography generally reveals a smooth, fairly focal stenosis involving the midportion of the vessel or its branches. With nonoperative management, progressive renal artery obstruction and ischemic atrophy of the involved kidney invariably occur. Severe intimal fibroplasia may subsequently develop de novo in the contralateral renal artery. Although primary intimal fibroplasia most commonly affects the renal arteries, this may also occur as a generalized disorder with concomitant involvement of carotid, upper and lower extremity, and mesenteric vessels.[57]

Medial fibroplasia is the most common of the fibrous lesions, comprising 75 to 80 percent of the total number. It tends to occur in women between the ages of 25 and 50 years, and often involves both renal arteries. It may involve other vessels in the body, most notably the carotid, mesenteric, and iliac arteries. Microscopically, there are alternating thickened areas of the media where the muscle is replaced by collagen; in other areas, there is severe thinning of the media with the development of microaneurysms lined by only the external elastica. Angiographically, medial fibroplasia demonstrates a typical "string of beads" appearance involving the distal two-thirds of the main renal artery and branches. Schreiber et al. studied the natural history of renal artery disease due to medial fibroplasia in 66 patients who were followed with serial angiography.[60] Progressive renal artery stenosis occurred in 22 patients (33 percent) and, contrary to an earlier report, this occurrence was no different in patients greater than or less than 40 years of age. Significantly, there were no cases of progression to total arterial occlusion in this group. Also, clinical follow-up revealed that serial decreases in either overall renal function or the size of the involved kidney seldom occurred in patients with progressive medial fibroplasia suggesting that the risk of losing renal function is relatively small in patients with this disease who are managed medically.

Perimedial fibroplasia occurs predominantly in young women between the ages of 15 and 30. It comprises about 10 to 15 percent of the total number of fibrous lesions and occurs only in the renal artery. Microscopically, stenosis is caused by a collar of dense collagen which is present in the outer border of the media for variable lengths and thicknesses. The arteriogram may give the appearance of arterial beading, but careful observation shows that the caliber of the normal segment of the vessel is not exceeded by the "bead." This fact, along with the frequent occurrence of extensive collateral circulation, differentiates this lesion angiographically from that of medial fibroplasia. Perimedial fibroplasia produces severe stenosis and progressive obstruction with ischemic renal atrophy occurs in almost all patients managed nonoperatively.

Fibromuscular hyperplasia is an extremely rare disease, comprising only 2 to 3 percent of fibrous lesions, and tends to occur in children and young adults. This is the only renal arterial disease in which true hyperplasia of the smooth muscle cells is present. Angiographically, fibromuscular hyperplasia presents as a smooth stenosis of the renal artery or its branches and, from a radiographic standpoint, may be indistinguishable from intimal fibroplasia. Most patients with this disease have developed progressive vascular obstruction when followed with serial angiographic studies.

## Renal Artery Aneurysms

Renal artery aneurysms may require surgical treatment when they are the cause of significant hypertension or to obviate the risk of rupture. The latter is of greatest concern with aneurysms that are larger than 2 cm in diameter and noncalcified, particularly when they occur in premenopausal females, because of the predisposition for aneurysmal rupture during pregnancy.[42] Saccular aneurysms are the most common type and comprise about 75 percent of renal artery aneurysms.[53] They generally occur at the bifurcation of the renal artery and branch arterial involvement is therefore common. There are several mechanisms by which saccular aneurysms may be causally related to hypertension. These include compression or displacement of renal artery branches with resulting ischemia, aneurysmal erosion into a renal vein with formation of an arteriovenous fistula, mural thrombus formation within the aneurysm with peripheral renal embolization, and the association of some aneurysms with stenosing fibrous renal artery disease. It is also well appreciated that saccular aneurysms can cause hypertension in the absence of the above sequelae, most likely due to relative renal ischemia caused by the turbulent flow of blood as it passes through the aneurysmally dilated arterial segment. Less commonly encountered types of renal artery aneurysms are fusiform aneurysms, dissecting aneurysms, and intrarenal aneurysms.[53]

## Renal Arteriovenous Fistulas

Renal arteriovenous fistulas are relatively uncommon lesions which are generally discovered during the course of angiographic evaluation for suspected renal or renovascular disease.[42] The most common clinical symptoms, when present, are hematuria, high-output cardiac failure, and diastolic hypertension. Congenital or cirsoid fistulas comprise approximately 25 percent of these lesions, while acquired fistulas account for 70 to 75 percent of such disorders. Acquired fistulas secondary to closed renal biopsy or blunt trauma will generally close spontaneously with simple observation. Surgical therapy may be indicated for fistulas that are the cause of severe hypertension or other symptoms.

## Middle Aortic Syndrome

The middle aortic syndrome is a rare disorder, occurring in children or young adults, characterized by nonspecific stenosing arteritis affecting the aorta and its major branches including the renal arteries.[30] This is thought to be a form of Takayasu's disease, and an autoimmune pathogenesis is suspected. This disease can extensively involve the subdiaphragmatic aorta or, in some cases, may spare the aorta and involve primarily the renal or splanchnic vessels. The inflammatory process generally does not extend to involve the iliac arteries.

## Neurofibromatosis

Neurofibromatosis affecting the renal arteries is a congenital hereditary disorder characterized by café-au-lait cutaneous pigmentation, cutaneous neurofibromas, tumors of the central nervous system, skeletal disorders, and occasional gigantism. Hypertension in patients with neurofibromatosis is most often due to renal artery stenosis;[20,72] less commonly, this may be the result of an associated pheochromocytoma or aortic coarctation. In the kidney, arterial stenosis usually occurs at the origin or in the proximal third of the main renal artery and the angiographic appearance may be indistinguishable from that of intimal fibroplasia.

## Renal Artery Thrombosis or Embolism

Acute occlusion of the renal artery or its branches may result from thrombosis or embolism. Embolic occlusions may occur as a complication of rheumatic heart disease, subacute bacterial endocarditis, cardiac operations, saccular aneurysm of the renal artery, or renal artery catheterization. Thrombosis of the renal artery is somewhat less common and is associated with a variety of diseases such as intimal fibroplasia, segmental arteritis, polycythemia vera, tumors, trauma, or umbilical arterial catheterization. Blunt trauma to the renal artery may result in disruption of the intima with subsequent dissection and thrombotic occlusion.

## Extrinsic Obstruction of the Renal Artery

Extrinsic obstruction of the renal artery has been observed but is extremely rare.[63] Neural tissue, musculocutaneous fibers, and diaphragmatic crura have been suggested as etiologic factors contributing to this process. Other possible causes of extrinsic perivascular fibrosis include inflammation, trauma, tumor, or prior radiation.

## Renal Parenchymal Disease

Renin-mediated hypertension may be secondary to a variety of renal parenchymal diseases.[35,73] The incidence of hypertension in patients with chronic pyelonephritis is approximately 5 to 10 percent. The mechanism of renin-mediated hypertension in such kidneys with segmental scars is ischemia of the relatively normal renal cortex in proximity to areas of interstitial fibrosis, within which are multiple small vessels with intimal thickening.[54] Other renal disorders that may cause hypertension include hydronephrosis,[2,55] congential hypoplasia or dysplasia,[40] segmental hypoplasia (Ask-Upmark kidney),[56] vesicoureteral reflux,[66] renal cell carcinoma, benign cyst, Wilms' tumor, radiation nephritis, or juxtaglomerular-cell tumor.

# DIAGNOSIS OF RENOVASCULAR HYPERTENSION

It is important to differentiate between renovascular disease and renovascular hypertension since occlusive lesions of the renal artery do not always result in hypertension. The diagnosis of renovascular disease depends on angiographic demonstration of a stenotic lesion in the renal artery or its branches, whereas the diagnosis of renovascular hypertension can be confirmed only in retrospect and connotes permanent relief of hypertension after revascularization or removal of the affected kidney. In our experience, the most useful clinical assessments for establishing a diagnosis of renovascular hypertension are the rapid sequence intravenous pyelogram,[18,26] a systolic-diastolic abdominal bruit,[11] a short (< 5 years) duration of hypertension,[27] and the finding on angiography of a high-grade stenotic lesion involving the renal artery. Lateralization to the affected kidney (≥2:1) with differential renal vein plasma renin assays and/or a depressor response to angiotensin II inhibition strongly support the presence of renin-dependent hypertension but these tests must be interpreted with caution when they are negative.[6,25,37,43] The most accurate prediction of the blood pressure response to surgical treatment is obtained by considering all of these factors rather than any single test. A more detailed discussion of methods for establishing a diagnosis of renovascular hypertension is found elsewhere in this book (see Chapter 4).

# SELECTION OF PATIENTS FOR SURGICAL TREATMENT

Factors favoring surgical therapy in patients with suspected renovascular hypertension include: (1) young age, (2) severe associated hypertension, (3) satisfactory medical condition, (4) renal function threatened by progressive vascular disease. Although a randomized, controlled study of medical versus surgical treatment of renovascular hypertension has not been performed, Hunt et al. enrolled 214 patients with this disease in a prospective study.[28] Of these, 100 patients underwent operation and 114 patients were treated medically. After 7 to 14 years of follow-up, 16 percent of the surgically treated patients had died, as compared to 40 percent of those treated medically. Myocardial infarction, cerebrovascular accidents, and end-stage renal failure were more commonly observed in the medical group than in the surgical group. Furthermore, hypertension was cured or improved in more than 90 percent of the surgical survivors. These data would seem to attest the long-term efficacy of surgical therapy in properly selected patients.

In patients with fibrous dysplasia, the approach to treatment is guided by the specific type of fibrous disease based on angiographic findings and the associated natural history. Medical management of hypertension is the initial preferred treatment for patients with medial fibroplasia since loss of renal function from progressive obstruction is uncommon with this disease. Surgical treatment in the latter category is reserved for patients whose blood pressure is difficult to control with multiple drug antihypertensive therapy. Conversely, renal artery stenosis due to intimal fibroplasia, perimedial fibroplasia, or true fibromuscular hyperplasia generally progresses, and ischemic renal strophy is rather common. Furthermore, these lesions generally occur in younger patients and cause hypertension that is extremely difficult to control. Early renal revascularization in these groups is therefore indicated both to preserve renal function and to minimize the need for long-term antihypertensive medication.

In patients with atherosclerotic renovascular hypertension, the distinction between focal renal arterial versus generalized atherosclerosis is important in reaching a decision regarding medical versus surgical therapy. Several studies have shown that blood pressure control and late patient survival are significantly better in patients with isolated renal atherosclerosis than in those with diffuse disease.[13,34] Patients in the former group are generally younger and present with unilateral renovascular disease and a recent onset of hypertension; therefore, they are excellent candidates for operative therapy. In patients with generalized atherosclerosis, the available data would seem to favor more restrictive criteria for surgical treatment. In this group, more vigorous attempts at medical management are warranted and multiple drug regimens which control the blood pressure are often preferable to vascular reconstruction. Operative therapy is best reserved for patients whose hypertension cannot be adequately controlled or where renal function is threatened by advanced vascular disease. The latter designation applies to patients with moderate azotemia and/or bilateral high-grade arterial stenosis or patients with arterial stenosis involving a solitary kidney. In such patients, since the consequences of progressive atherosclerotic renovascular disease are particularly grave, revascularization warrants stronger consideration for the dual purpose of improving blood pressure control and preserving renal parenchyma.

The morbidity and mortality associated with operative therapy must also be considered in making the decision regarding medical versus surgical treatment of renovascular hypertension. Patients with fibrous dysplasia are generally young and otherwise healthy, and the morbidity of revascularization in this group has been minimal. However, several studies have indicated a significant operative risk in patients with atherosclerotic renovascular hypertension. In the National Cooperative Study, operative mortality was 9.3 percent in patients with atherosclerosis.[17] Two large single-center studies have also reported operative mortality rates of 5.1 percent and 7.6 percent in this population.[16,75] In the National Cooperative Study,[17] the major determinants of operative mortality were coronary artery disease, bilateral renovascular disease, azotemia, and the magnitude of the operation performed. Coronary artery disease has been the most important operative risk factor and is also the leading cause of late mortality in patients with renovascular disease treated either medically or surgically.

At the Cleveland Clinic, we have adopted several measures to reduce operative morbidity and mortality in patients undergoing vascular reconstruction for atherosclerotic renal artery disease. These include preliminary screening and correction of existing coronary or cerebrovascular occlusive disease, avoidance of bilateral simultaneous renal operations, and reliance upon methods of revascularization that obviate operation on a badly diseased aorta. The impact of these policies was evaluated in 100 consecutive patients with atherosclerotic renovascular disease who underwent renal revascularization from 1974 to 1980.[44] These patients comprised a high-risk group for surgical therapy in view of the large number with extrarenal atherosclerosis (83 percent), azotemia (31 percent), bilateral renovascular disease (61 percent), or a solitary kidney (24 percent). In this group of 100 patients, there were only two operative deaths (two percent) and eight minor postoperative complications. These data indicate that, when appropriate measures are taken, renal revascularization can be safely performed in older high risk patients with generalized atherosclerosis.

# SURGICAL METHODS OF TREATMENT

## Nephrectomy

Although it is now possible to achieve successful renal revascularization in most cases, total or partial nephrectomy retains a role in the management of renovascular hypertension. These operations are indicated in patients with main or branch renal artery occlusion and infarction, severe arteriolar nephrosclerosis, renal atrophy (<9 cm renal length), segmental renal hypoplasia, and noncorrectable renovascular lesions such as large intrarenal anurysms or arteriovenous malformations. Nephrectomy may also be indicated in the elderly, poor-surgical-risk patient with a normal contralateral kidney or following a failed revascularization procedure where extensive renal hilar fibrosis precludes satisfactory secondary revascularization. In properly selected patients, the results are equal to those obtained following revascularization procedures.

It is also appropriate to emphasize that angiographic demonstration of complete renal artery occlusion does not necessarily imply a nonsalvable kidney. With gradual renal artery occlusion, although renal function may be severely impaired, renal viability can be maintained by the development of collateral arterial supply from ureteral, lumbar, adrenal, capsular, or mesenteric vessels. The most important clinical assessments suggesting a salvable kidney in this setting are angiographic demonstration of retrograde renal artery filling from collateral vascular supply and an intraoperative renal biopsy showing intact glomeruli with minimal

vascular sclerosis. When the latter are present, revascularization can allow both control of hypertension and improvement in overall renal function.[36,58,33]

## Aortorenal Bypass

Although a variety of renal revascularization procedures have been employed to treat renovascular hypertension, aortorenal bypass with autogenous saphenous vein or arterial grafts is now the preferred method in most cases (Fig. 5-7). Although excellent clinical results have been obtained with both types of bypass grafts,[41] long-term studies of aortorenal saphenous vein grafts have shown a large number of patent grafts on follow-up angiography.[7,64] The clinical significance of these observations remains uncertain since most of these patients continue to be normotensive with excellent renal function (see below).[12,15,68] Nevertheless, these findings have led to preferential use of arterial autografts when these are available. The viscoelastic properties of arterial grafts, in contrast to the saphenous vein, match those of the renal artery and postoperative graft patency has not been observed. We have used the hypogastric and splenic arteries as free bypass grafts with cure or improvement of hypertension in 96 percent of patients postoperatively;[45] similar results have been reported by other authors with aortorenal arterial autografts.[67]

Currently, aortorenal bypass with a synthetic material is indicated only when autogenous vascular grafts are not available or when adjunctive aortic replacement is performed. Although the long-term results with Dacron grafts are satisfactory, there has been an increased tendency to thrombosis in the early postoperative period.[31] The recently developed polytetrafluorethylene graft is soft, nonelastic, easy to suture, and allows for inner fibrous healing with minimal tissue reactivity. Excellent results have been re-

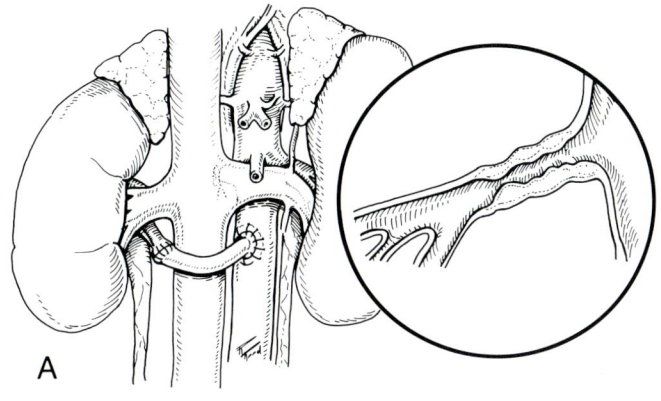

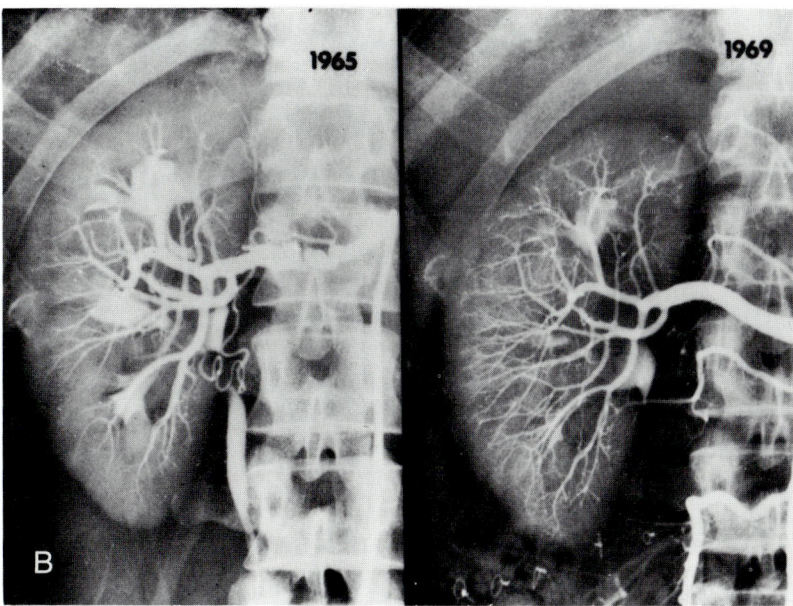

**Fig. 5-7.** (A) Sketch of completed right aortorenal bypass graft with end-to-side anastomosis of the graft to the aorta and end-to-end anastomosis of the graft to the distal renal artery. (Reproduced from Modern Technics in Surgery, edited by Ehrlich, R, Futura Publishing Company, Mount Kisco, New York, 1981.) (B) Preoperative arteriogram (left) shows right renal artery stenosis from medial fibroplasia. Four years following aortorenal bypass with an arterial autograft, the arteriogram (right) demonstrates patent bypass graft. (Reproduced from Vascular Problems in Urologic Surgery, edited by Novick AC and Straffon RA, W.B. Saunders, Philadelphia, 1982.)

ported with such grafts in peripheral arterial reconstruction[23] and they appear to be preferable when renal artery replacement with a synthetic material is indicated.

Revascularization is more complicated when vascular disease extends into the branches of the renal artery or when reconstruction is required for a kidney supplied by multiple renal arteries. Newly developed microvascular techniques now often permit successful revascularization in situ with an aortorenal bypass operation when disease-free distal arterial branches occur outside the renal hilus.[46]

The most useful technique for in situ revascularization of multiple segmental renal arteries is aortorenal bypass with a branched autogenous vascular graft. Either the hypogastric artery is obtained intact with its branches, or if this is unsuitable, a branched saphenous vein graft is fashioned. Such autogenous branched bypass grafts allow separate end-to-end anastomosis of each graft branch to each renal artery branch and overall renal ischemia is thus minimal[69] (Fig. 5-8).

## Techniques in the Surgically Difficult Aorta

In some patients with renal artery disease, severe atherosclerosis or previous operations on the abdominal aorta may preclude safe performance of aortorenal bypass. Complete excision of the aorta and replacement with a prosthesis can be done but, when combined with renal revascularization, has been associated with operative mortality rates of 30 percent, 10.3 percent, and 6 percent.[16,19,62] This approach should therefore be limited to patients with an abdominal aortic aneurysm or symptomatic aortoiliac occlusive disease. Transaortic endarterectomy is also an extensive operation with a significant potential morbidity. In patients with a surgically difficult aorta, we have found that alternate techniques are preferable, such as splenorenal bypass, hepatorenal bypass, ileorenal bypass, renal autotransplantation, and superior mesenterorenal bypass. These methods allow renal revascularization to be accomplished safely and effectively, while obviating operation on a severely diseased aorta[47] (Fig. 5-9).

**Splenorenal bypass** provides an excellent method of performing left renal revascularization when preoperative aortography with selective celiac arteriography demonstrate a healthy splenic artery. The advantages of this procedure are that it can be carried out in untouched vascular tissues at a distance from the aorta, and it involves performance of only a single vascular anastomosis. In 1977, we reviewed the long-term results of splenorenal bypass for left renal revascularization in 32 patients with renovascular hypertension.[48] With follow-up of 1 to 12 years, postoperative hypertension was cured or improved in 26 patients (81 percent) and late graft stenosis developed in only three patients (9.4 percent). Surgical morbidity was minimal and there were no pancreatic complications following the operation (Fig. 5-10).

**Hepatorenal Bypass.** The hepatic circulation is ideally suited for a visceral-right renal arterial bypass operation. The liver receives 28 percent of the cardiac output in resting adults and is unique in having a dual circulation from the portal vein and hepatic artery. The portal vein and hepatic artery contribute 80 percent and 20 percent of hepatic blood flow, respectively. Hepatic oxygenation is equally derived from these two circulations. It has been well demonstrated that hepatic artery flow can be safely interrupted.[49] When this occurs, hepatic function and morphology are maintained by increased extraction of oxygen from portal venous blood and by the rapid development of an extensive collateral arterial flow to the liver.

In patients considered for a hepatorenal bypass operation, preoperative aortography and selective celiac arteriography with lateral views are needed to ensure patent celiac and hepatic arteries. An interposition saphenous vein graft is anastomosed end-to-side to the common hepatic artery and end-to-end to the distal right renal artery. This technique preserves distal hepatic arterial flow, thereby further diminishing the risk of ischemic liver damage. The results of hepatorenal bypass in 36 patients from the Lahey Clinic and Cleveland Clinic were recently

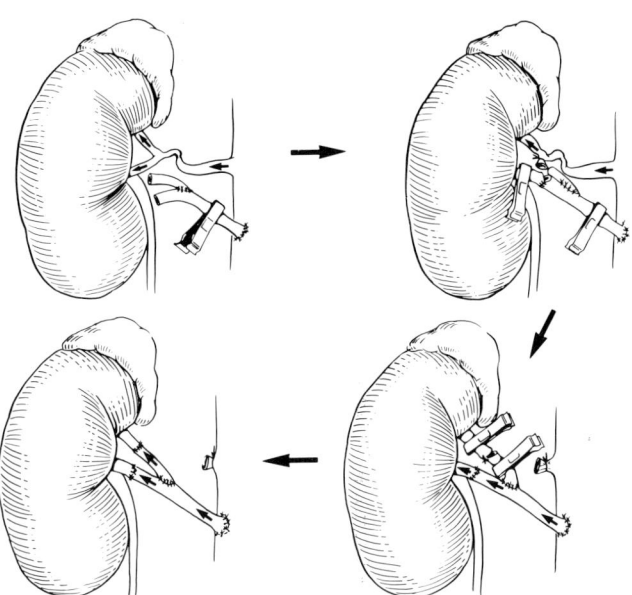

**Fig. 5-8.** Sketch illustrating sequential vascular anastomoses volved in performing aortorenal bypass with a double-armed branched saphenous vein graft for stenosing disease that extends into the renal arterial branches. (Reproduced from Kelalis P, King L, Belman B, Eds: Clinical Pediatric Urology, W.B. Saunders Company, Philadelphia, p. 19.)

reported.[5] Follow-up ranged from 1 to 8 years with a mean of 4 years. No patient developed any permanent hepatic impairment or complication. Renal revascularization was successful in 33 patients (92 percent) with no major operative morbidity (Fig. 5-10).

**Renal autotransplantation** may be used for revascularization of either kidney in patients with severe aortic atherosclerosis, provided there is good flow through the diseased aorta and in the absence of significant iliac disease. Autotransplantation is also indicated in children with re-

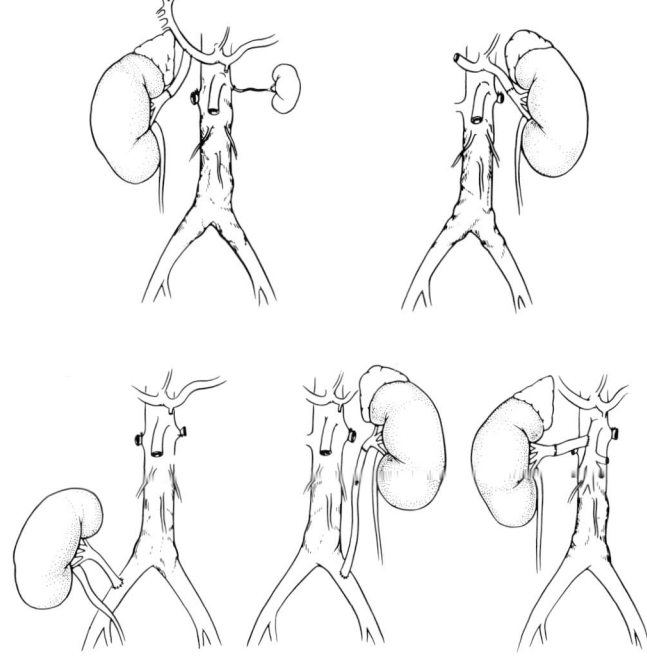

**Fig. 5-9.** Methods of renal revascularization for patients with a surgically difficult aorta. These include hepatorenal bypass (top left), splenorenal bypass (top right), autotransplantation (bottom left), ileorenal bypass (bottom middle), and superior mesenterorenal bypass (bottom right). (Reproduced from Kendall RA, Karafin L, Eds: Practice of Surgery: Urology, Harper and Row Publishers, New York, Philadelphia 1983.)

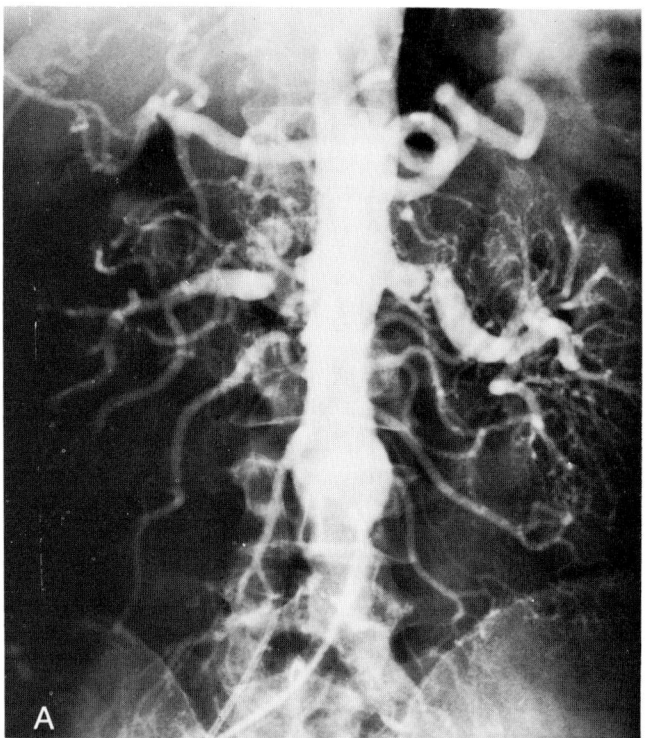

**Fig. 5-10.** (A) Preoperative aortogram of 60-year-old man with severe hypertension demonstrates bilateral high-grade atherosclerotic renal artery stenosis with badly diseased aorta. (B) Patient underwent sequential left splenorenal and right hepatorenal bypass operations. Postoperative selective celiac arteriogram demonstrates patient splenorenal and hepatorenal anastomosis. (Reproduced from Modern Technics in Surgery, edited by Ehrlich, R, Futura Publishing Company, Mount Kisco, New York, 1981.)

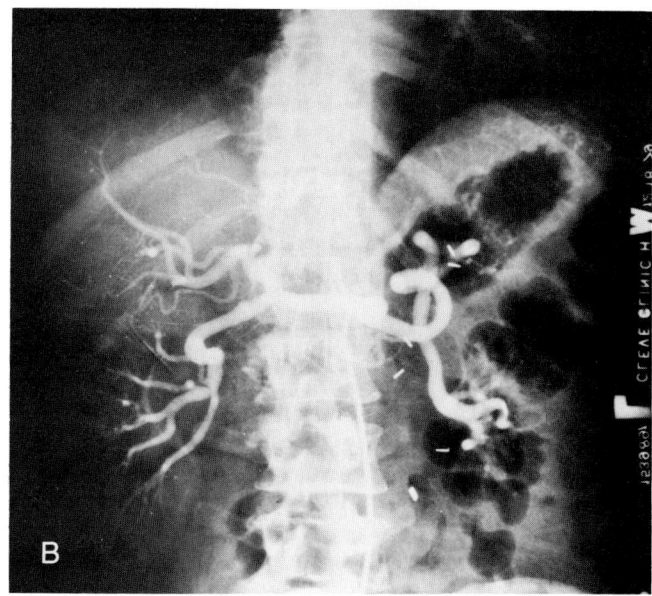

novascular hypertension and the middle aortic syndrome where the iliac vessels are generally free of disease. In these cases, the ureter is left intact and, although it may follow a redundant course to the bladder, normal ureteral peristalsis provides effective drainage of urine from the kidney. From 1976 to 1982, we performed autotransplantation for these indications in 11 patients. Postoperatively, hypertension was cured or improved in all cases and there were no major surgical complications.

**Iliorenal bypass** with a long saphenous vein graft may also be considered in patients with severe aortic atherosclerosis, good flow through the aorta and relatively disease-free iliac arteries.[50] Although both autotransplantation and iliorenal bypass can be used in this setting, the latter has the theoretical advantage of less operative time, a shorter period of renal ischemia, and preservation of collateral renal arterial supply. Iliorenal bypass may also be preferable in patients with significant arteriolar nephrosclerosis, since such kidneys may not flush well for an autotransplant operation. From 1976 to 1982, we have performed iliorenal bypass in 10 patients with severe aortic atherosclerosis. In all cases, the postoperative blood pressure was cured or improved, renal function was stable or improved, and there were no major surgical complications.

**Superior Mesenterorenal Bypass.** In unusual cases, aortography will reveal an enlarged superior mesenteric artery that may then be employed for visceral arterial bypass to either kidney. This situation has most often been observed in patients with total occlusion of the infrarenal aorta. In such cases, when stenosis of the celiac artery has precluded performance of splenorenal or hepatorenal bypass, a mesenterorenal bypass operation has been performed. This is accomplished by anastomosis of an interposition saphenous vein graft end-to-side to the superior mesenteric artery and then end-to-end to the distal renal artery. We have performed this operation in four patients with excellent technical success and no evidence of intestinal ischemia postoperatively (Fig. 5-11).

## Extracorporeal Microvascular Branch Renal Arterial Reconstruction and Autotransplantation

Extracorporeal microvascular repair and autotransplantation are indicated in patients with extensive branch renal artery stenosis, where intrarenal vascular disease precludes a satisfactory in situ repair.[51] Prior to the advent of extracorporeal surgery, such patients would have been considered either inoperable or candidates for nephrectomy. The advantages of performing extracorporeal revascularization include optimum exposure and illumination, a bloodless surgical field, greater protection from prolonged renal ischemia, and more facile employment of microvascular techniques and optical magnification. The removed kidney is flushed with an intracellular electrolyte solution and is then submerged in ice slush saline to maintain hypothermia. Under these conditions, the kidney can safely tolerate periods outside the body far in excess of those required to perform even the most complex arterial repair. Extracorporeal revascularization is accomplished with a branched autogenous vascular graft of the hypogastric artery, saphenous vein, or inferior epigastric artery. The repaired kidney is then autotransplanted to the iliac fossa, using the same technique as in renal allotransplantation (Fig. 5-12).

From 1977 to 1982, we performed extracorporeal revascularization and autotransplantation in 26 patients with severe branch renal artery disease. The pathologic diagnosis was fibrous dysplasia in 17 patients and an arterial aneurysm in nine patients. In these 26 patients, a total of 76 renal artery branches have been repaired (mean 2.9 per patient). There have been no cases of postoperative branch arterial stenosis or thrombosis on follow-up an-

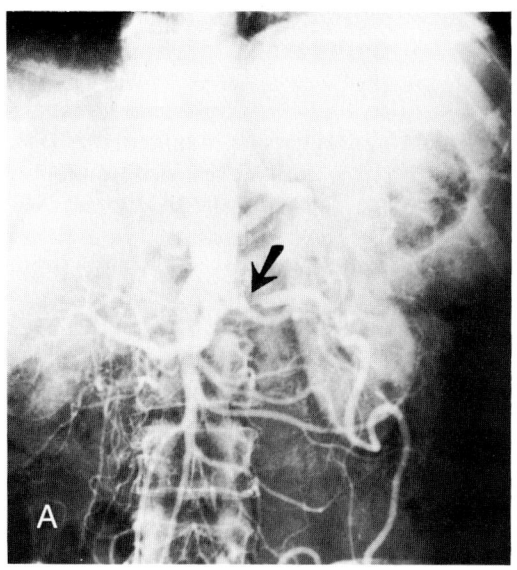

Fig. 5-11. (A) Preoperative arteriogram in 55-year-old man with severe hypertension. The aorta is completely occluded below the superior mesenteric artery, and the left renal artery is involved with high-grade proximal stenosis (arrow). (B) This patient underwent superior mesenterorenal bypass with saphenous vein graft and is currently normotensive. The postoperative arteriogram demonstrates patent mesenterorenal bypass graft to the left kidney (arrow). (Reproduced with permission from Modern Techniques in Surgery, Ehrlich R, ed. Futura Publishing Company, Mount Kisco, New York, 1981.)

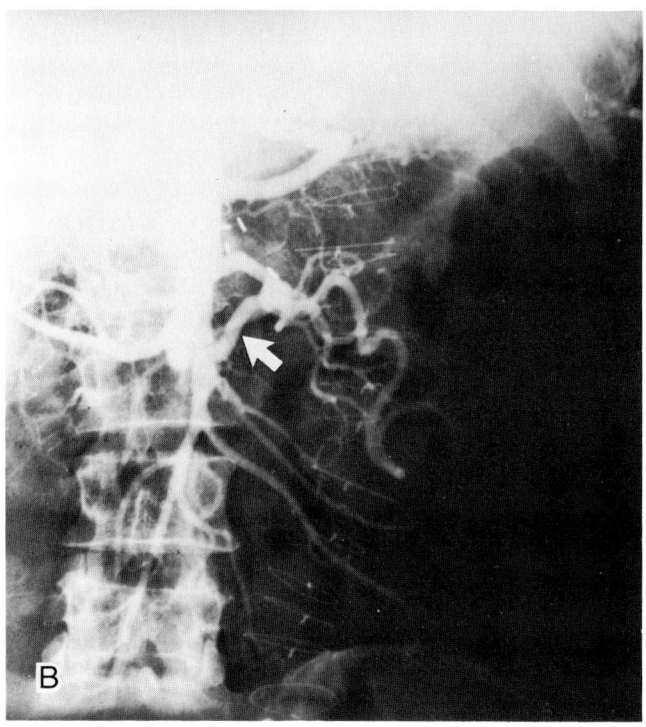

giographic or isotope studies. All of these patients currently have a normal blood pressure with stable or improved renal function.

# RESULTS OF SURGICAL TREATMENT OF RENOVASCULAR HYPERTENSION

In evaluating the results of surgical treatment of renovascular hypertension, patients are considered cured if the blood pressure is 140/90 mm Hg or less without medication, with a minimum follow-up interval of 6 months postoperatively. Patients are considered improved if they have shown a reduction in diastolic pressure of 15 mm Hg or more, or are normotensive on medication. Failures are those who do not qualify for either of the aforementioned categories. Table 5-9 illustrates the results obtained at the Cleveland Clinic with the revascularization procedures described in this chapter. In properly selected patients and employing an appropriate method of vascular reconstruction, the results of surgical therapy have been excellent.

In patients with bilateral renovascular disease, our policy has been to revascularize the kidney with angiographically more severe arterial stenosis or higher renal vein renin levels, or both. Bilateral simultaneous revascularization not only increases the risk of operation but is also unnecessary since most patients with bilateral disease will experience relief of hypertension from unilateral revascularization.[8] Contralateral repair is reserved for patients with persistent hypertension postoperatively and when repeat renal vein renin assays lateralize to the unoperated side.

The results of surgical treatment for renovascular hypertension must also be viewed within the context of the patho-

logic diagnosis. Several major referral centers for patients with this disease have reported long-term cure or improvement of hypertension following renal revascularization in approximately 90 percent of patients with fibrous dysplasia.[12,67,68] Less satisfactory results have traditionally been reported in patients with atherosclerotic renovascular hypertension, particularly those with generalized atherosclerotic vascular disease.[13,15,34] From 1974 to 1980, renal revascularization was performed in 78 patients as treatment for atherosclerotic renovascular hypertension at the Cleveland Clinic.[44] There were 17 patients with focal renal arterial atherosclerosis and 61 patients with generalized atherosclerosis. Postoperatively, the blood pressure was cured in 31 patients (40 percent), improved in 40 patients (51 percent), and there were seven failures (nine percent). This recent experience attests to the efficacy of vascular reconstruction as treatment for renovascular hypertension in patients with atherosclerotic disease (Table 5-10).

Starr et al.[65] reported long-term results of surgical treatment for renovascular hypertension in 216 patients who underwent operation between 1959 and 1979. The cause of renal artery disease was atherosclerosis in 137 patients (63 percent), fibrous dysplasia in 58 patients (27 percent), renal artery aneurysm in eight patients (4 percent), and various other disorders in the remainder. Renal revascularization and nephrectomy were done in 89 percent and 11 percent of the patients, respectively. The postoperative follow-up interval ranged from 1 to 20 years. Actuarial patient survival at 5 years was 93 percent, at 10 years 80 percent, and at 20 years 70 percent. Normal blood pressure was present at 5 years in 81 percent of the survivors, at 10 years in 77 percent, and at 15 years in 74 percent. These results indicate the excellent long-term results of surgical treatment for re-

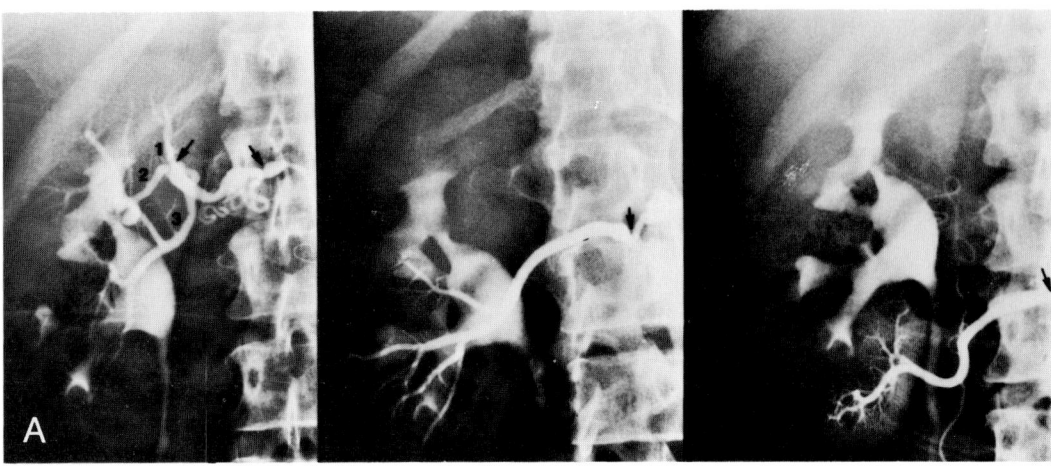

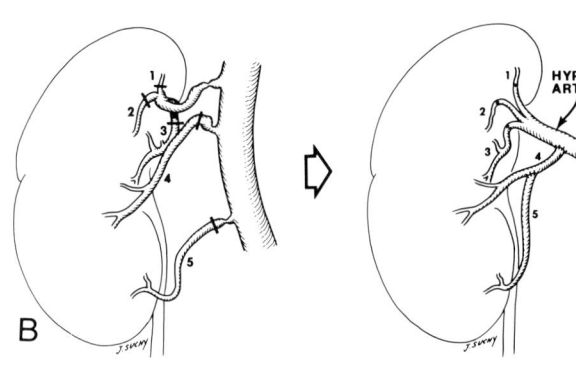

**Fig. 5-12.** (A) Preoperative arteriogram shows that the right kidney is supplied by three renal arteries, each involved with severe proximal stenosis. Vascular disease in the upper artery extends into three distal branches. Arrows indicate sites of stenosis. (B) Sketch illustrating the preoperative extent of renal arterial disease (left) and completed extracorporeal repair with a branched hypogastric arterial graft (right). (C) Operative photograph of a completed extracorporeal revascularization of five segmental branches. The three diseased upper branches were repaired with a branched graft of the hypogastric artery. The middle and lower renal arteries were anastomosed end-to-side into the graft and adjacent branch, respectively.

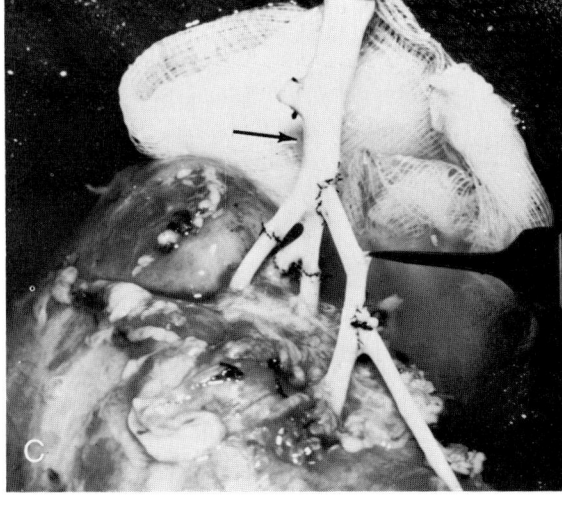

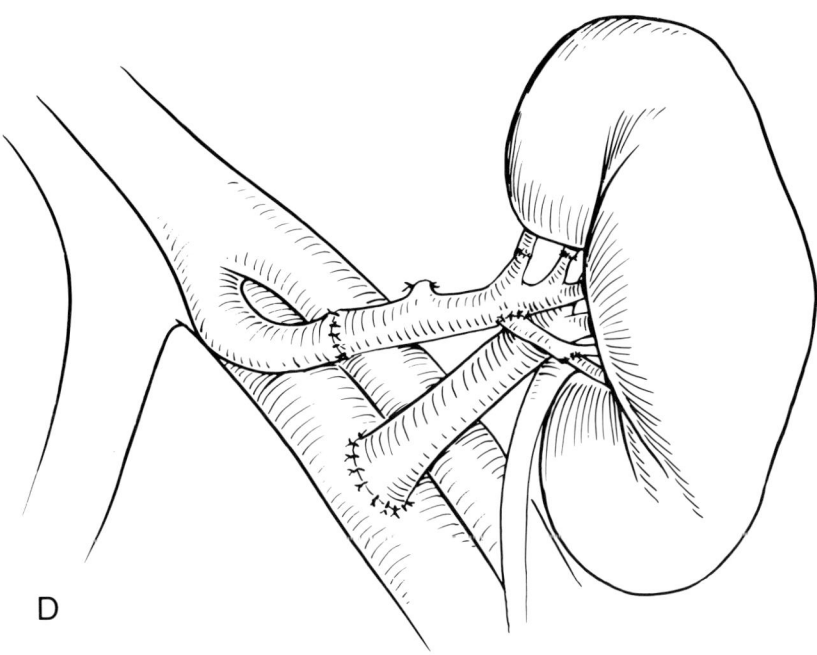

D

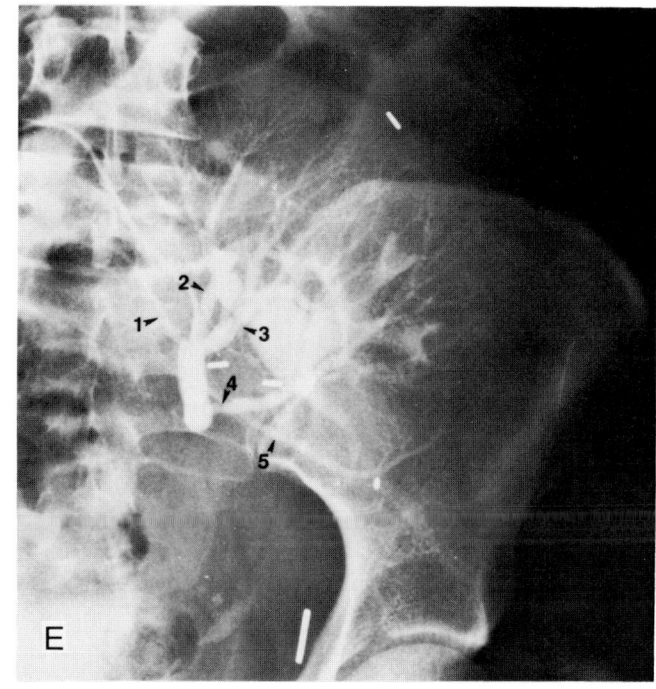

E

**Fig. 5-12 (Continued).** (D) Sketch of a revascularized kidney following autotransplantation into the iliac fossa. (E) Postoperative arteriogram of an autotransplant demonstrating patency of all five revascularized segmental arteries. (Figures A, B, C, E reproduced from Novick AC: Management of intrarenal branch arterial lesions with extracorporeal microvascular reconstruction and autotransplantation. J Urol 126:150. © 1981, The Williams and Wilkins Company, Baltimore.)

**Table 5-9.** Results of Renal Revascularization as Treatment for Renovascular Hypertension

| Operation | No. Patients | Cure or Improved | Failed | Graft Stenosis or Occlusion |
|---|---|---|---|---|
| Aortorenal bypass[68] with saphenous vein (1965–74) | 81 | 71 ( 88%) | 10 (12%) | 9% |
| Aortorenal bypass with arterial autograft (1965–79) | 40 | 39 ( 98%) | 1 ( 2%) | 0 |
| Splenorenal bypass[48] (1965–76) | 32 | 26 ( 81%) | 6 (19%) | 9% |
| Hepatorenal bypass[a] (1974–82) | 36 | 33 ( 92%) | 3 ( 8%) | 8% |
| Iliorenal bypass (1976–82) | 10 | 10 (100%) | 0 | 0 |
| Mesenterorenal bypass (1975–82) | 4 | 4 (100%) | 0 | 0 |
| Autotransplantation (1976–82) | 11 | 11 (100%) | 0 | 0 |
| Ex vivo reconstruction and autotransplantation (1977–82) | 26 | 26 (100%) | 0 | 0 |

[a]Combined Lahey Clinic and Cleveland Clinic Data

novascular hypertension in appropriate patients.

## REVASCULARIZATION TO PRESERVE RENAL FUNCTION

A more recent indication for elective renal revascularization in our program has been to preserve renal function in patients with advanced atherosclerotic renovascular disease. The screening and selection of patients for this approach is based, in part, on an early study by Gifford et al.[18] These investigators found that in 53 of 75 older patients (71 percent) with unilateral renal atrophy, the artery to that kidney was stenotic or occluded, generally from atherosclerotic disease. More-over, unsuspected disease involving the artery to the contralateral normal-sized kidney was present in 22 of these 53 patients (42 percent). More recently, Lawrie et al.[33] reported 40 patients with renal atrophy from total arterial occlusion and observed stenosis of the opposite renal artery in 31 of these patients (78 percent). These observations confirm a high prevalence of renovascular disease, which is often bilateral, in patients with generalized atherosclerosis and evidence of renal atrophy. The associated finding of mild or moderate azotemia in this setting strengthens the indication for angiographic study to define the presence of correctable renovascular occlusive disease.

Following angiographic diagnosis of atherosclerotic renal artery obstruction, and with regard for the natural history of

**Table 5-10.** Results of Revascularization in 78 Patients with Atherosclerotic Renovascular Hypertension (1974–80)

| | No. Patients | No. Cured | No. Improved | No. Failed |
|---|---|---|---|---|
| Focal renal arterial atherosclerosis | 17 | 13 (76%) | 4 (24%) | 0 |
| Diffuse atherosclerosis, unilateral renovascular disease | 20 | 7 (35%) | 12 (60%) | 1 ( 5%) |
| Diffuse atherosclerosis, bilateral renovascular disease | 41 | 11 (27%) | 24 (59%) | 6 (14%) |
| Overall | 78 | 31 (40%) | 40 (51%) | 7 ( 9%) |

(From Novick AC, Straffon RA, Stewart BH, et al: Diminished operative mobidity and mortality following revascularization for atherosclerotic renovascular disease. JAMA 246: 749, 1981. Copyright 1981, American Medical Association.)

this disease as outlined earlier in this chapter, one can identify those patients for whom the risk of renal functional impairment from progressive vascular disease is greatest. This designation includes patients with arterial stenosis involving a solitary kidney, patients with bilateral high-grade arterial stenosis, and patients with moderate azotemia and a small but viable kidney with severe arterial stenosis or, more commonly, chronic total arterial occlusion. Having been identified, such patients are followed closely with serial determinations of renal size and overall renal function; serial decreases in the latter parameters have correlated strongly with progressive atherosclerotic renal artery obstruction (p <.02).[60] In such patients with advanced atherosclerotic renovascular disease, particularly those in whom progressive gradual loss of renal function has been observed, elective surgical revascularization to preserve renal function may be considered.

This approach is generally not rewarding in patients with severe azotemia since advanced underlying renal parenchymal disease is inevitably present and obviates improvement in renal function with restored perfusion. Patients with chronic bilateral total renal artery occlusion represent an exception to the latter admonition. In these patients, renovascular disease has already progressed to the end point of complete bilateral obstruction but, fortuitously, the viability of one or both kidneys is maintained through an abundant collateral supply. Several reports have described the clinical assessments which are most helpful in determining whether the kidney is salvageable in such cases.[33,36,58] The degree of preoperative renal functional impairment is often severe and the improvement following revascularization may be equally dramatic. It is appropriate to emphasize that this clinical presentation is rare and a less favorable outcome of bilateral arterial occlusion on renal viability is unfortunately far more common.

In 1979 Schreiber et al. reported a small series of 14 patients with advanced atherosclerotic renovascular disease who underwent revascularization to preserve renal function at the Cleveland Clinic; 13 of these patients experienced improvement in overall renal function postoperatively.[59] This experience has since been augmented and 51 patients managed in this fashion have now been reported.[52] In this series, postoperative renal function was improved in 34 patients (67 percent), unchanged in 14 patients (27 percent), and deteriorated in three patients (6 percent). The results in specific patient categories are illustrated in Table 5-11. This experience suggests that it is possible to identify a group of patients wherein the risks associated with progressive atherosclerotic vascular disease are greatest in whom functional renal recovery is an attainable goal of vascular reconstruction (Fig. 5-13).

# PERCUTANEOUS TRANSLUMINAL DILATATION

Percutaneous transluminal dilatation (PTD) of arteries obstructed by atherosclerotic disease was first introduced by Dotter and Judkins in 1964.[9] Their original report described the use of a semirigid coaxial cathether, which was best suited for vessels in the lower extremities and pelvis. The introduction and availability of a soft, flexible, double-lumen balloon catheter, described by Grüntzig,[22] has extended the application of PTD to visceral arteries including patients with renal artery stenosis.

In the original description of PTD, the mechanism of action was attributed to compression and redistribution of atheromata within the vessel wall. Early propo-

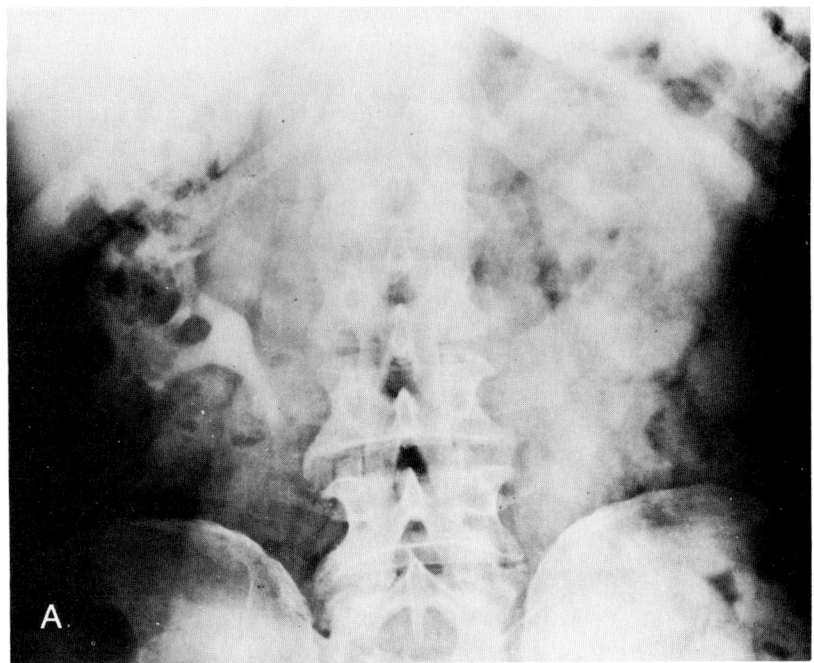

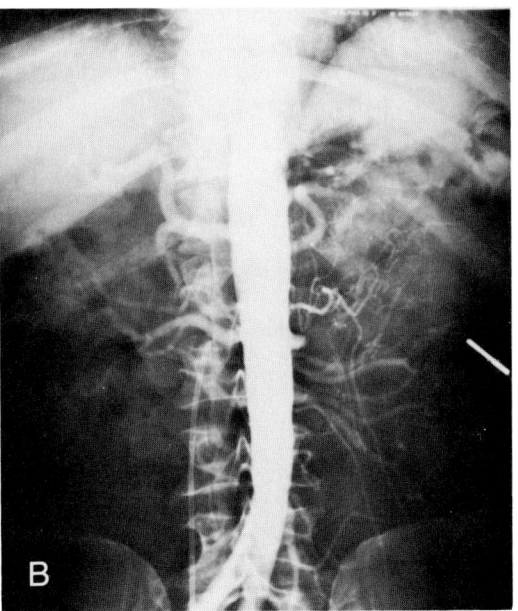
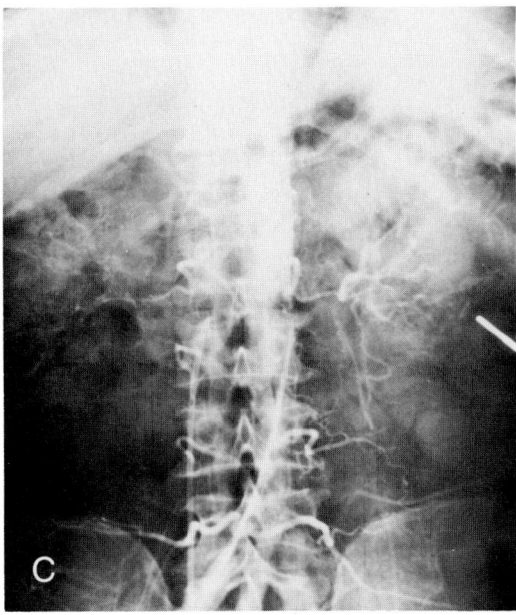

**Fig. 5-13.** (A) A preoperative intravenous pyelogram from a 61-year-old male with a serum creatinine of 3.0 mg/dl, shows no excretion of contrast material by the left kidney at 15 minutes. The left kidney measures 11.4 cm in length. (B) Preoperative aortography reveals complete occlusion of left renal artery. (C) Delayed angiographic films show filling of distal left renal artery branches from collateral vascular supply.

**Fig. 5-13 (continued).** (D) Left renal biopsy at the time of surgical exploration demonstrates well preserved renal histology with intact viable glomeruli. Therefore, a left aortorenal bypass operation was done. (E) Postoperative intravenous pyelogram shows prompt left renal function at five minutes, with kidney now measuring 13.5 cm in length. Five years later, the serum creatinine level remains 1.6 mg/dl. (Figures A, B, C, E reproduced from Novick AC, Pohl MA: Atherosclerotic renal artery occlusion extending into branches: Successful revascularization in situ with a branched saphenous vein graft. J. Urol, 122:240. © 1979, The Williams and Wilkins Company, Baltimore.)

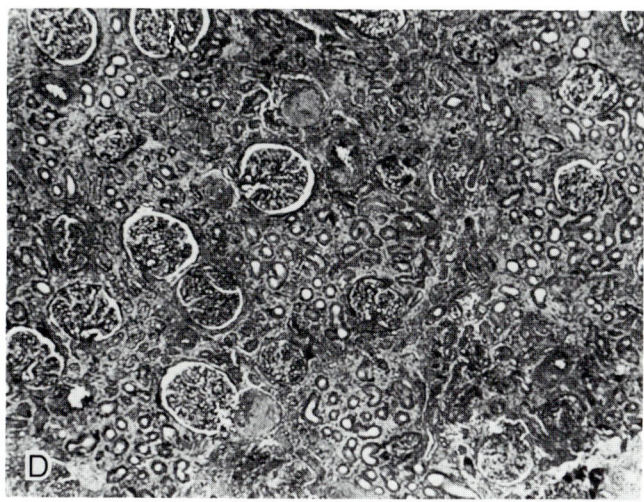

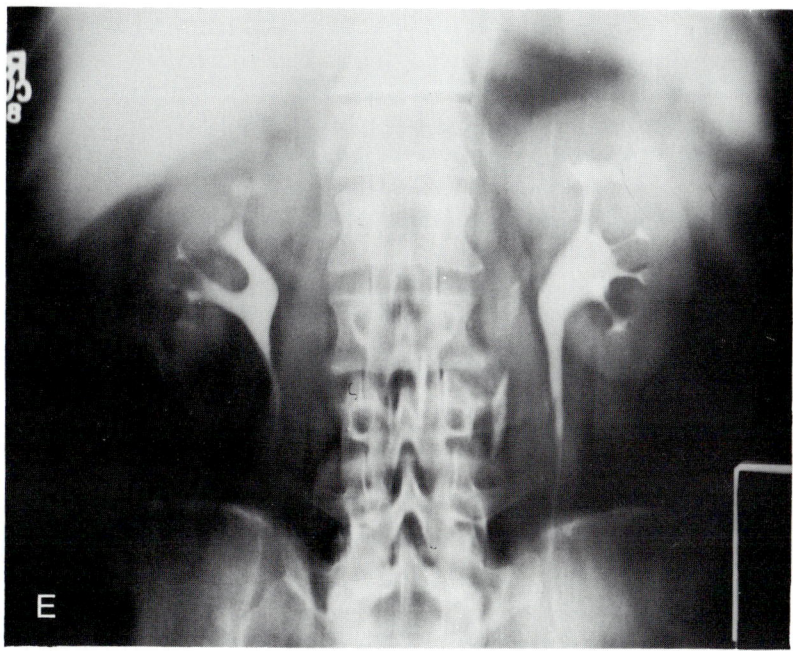

nents of PTD described it as a nonoperative approach requiring "no incision, no wound healing, and no scar."[10] Grüntzig and Hopff have described the procedure as a "controlled injury.[22] However, recent experimental and autopsy studies have clarified the pathophysiology of transluminal dilatation. In fact, compression of atherosclerotic plaques does not occur. Rather, the caliber of the vessel is increased by splitting of the plaque with disruption of the intima and overstretching of the media.[3,4] It has been postulated that healing of the separated

**Table 5-11.** Results of Renal Revascularization to Preserve Renal Function in 51 Patients[52]

| Postoperative Renal Function | Group I | Group 2 | Group 3 | Group 4 | Total No. Patients |
|---|---|---|---|---|---|
| Scr improved | 4 | 7 | 11 | 12 | 34 |
| $\left(\dfrac{\text{mean preop mg/dl}}{\text{mean postop mg/dl}}\right)$ | $\left(\dfrac{7.05}{2.15}\right)$ | $\left(\dfrac{3.20}{2.36}\right)$ | $\left(\dfrac{2.43}{1.67}\right)$ | $\left(\dfrac{2.31}{1.58}\right)$ | $\left(\dfrac{3.01}{1.84}\right)$ |
| Scr unchanged | 1 | 4 | 5 | 4 | 14 |
| $\left(\dfrac{\text{mean preop mg/dl}}{\text{mean postop mg/dl}}\right)$ | $\left(\dfrac{6.8}{7.4}\right)$ | $\left(\dfrac{1.95}{1.85}\right)$ | $\left(\dfrac{1.78}{1.68}\right)$ | $\left(\dfrac{2.03}{1.95}\right)$ | $\left(\dfrac{2.26}{2.21}\right)$ |
| Scr elevated | | 3 | | | 3 |
| $\left(\dfrac{\text{mean preop mg/dl}}{\text{mean postop mg/dl}}\right)$ | 0 | $\left(\dfrac{2.73}{3.30}\right)$ | 0 | 0 | $\left(\dfrac{2.73}{3.30}\right)$ |

Notes: Scr, serum creatinine; group 1, chronic bilateral total renal arterial occlusion; group 2, arterial stenosis in a solitary kidney; group 3, bilateral high-grade renal artery stenosis; group 4, azotemia and unilateral chronic total renal arterial occlusion.

(From Novick AC, Pohl MA, Schreiber M, et al: Renal revascularization for preservation of kidney function in patients with atherosclerotic renovascular disease. J. Urol (in press) © 1984 The Williams and Wikins Co., Baltimore.)

arterial layers then occurs by the formation of a new layer of neointima and fibrous tissue. Unfortunately, subintimal dissection and thrombosis have been less favorable outcomes of this technique in some patients. Indeed, as Beebe and associates have indicated,[1] PTD shares with vascular reconstruction two essential qualities: it is invasive and it alters structure to achieve a change in function.

There has been considerable interest in the use of PTD as a nonsurgical method of treatment for occlusive renovascular disorders. Nevertheless, even the most favorable clinical reports on its use in this regard have provided only short-term data with many patients having been followed for less than one year. This is particularly important since the long-term results following appropriate renal arterial reconstruction are excellent and have stood the test of time. Renal arterial complications following PTD have included intramural dissection, rupture, thrombotic occlusion and distal embolization. The true incidence of such complications following PTD in various types of renal artery disease has yet to be eluci-

dated. We reported our initial experience at the Cleveland Clinic with attempted PTD in 27 patients with atherosclerotic renal artery stenosis.[14] Significant complications following PTD occurred in 10 patients (37 percent). These included total renal arterial occlusion from intramural dissection or thrombosis in five patients (Figs. 5-14, 5-15), large groin hematomas in four patients (Fig. 5-16), and peripheral embolization in one patient. Immediate surgical exploration was undertaken in four of the patients who were noted to have complete renal arterial occlusion following PTD. In three patients, the involved kidney was salvaged with a successful revascularization operation, while in one patient, extension of intramural dissection deep into intrarenal branches precluded vascular reconstruction and necessitated a nephrectomy. We have since encountered a similar experience in a patient with fibrous dysplasia who developed an extensive intramural dissection with thrombosis of the renal artery following PTD and required performance of a nephrectomy (Fig. 5-17).

Most of the initial clinical data with

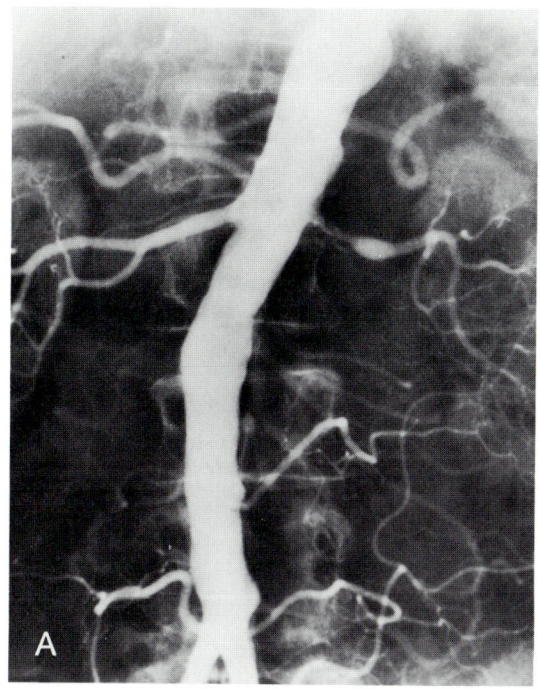

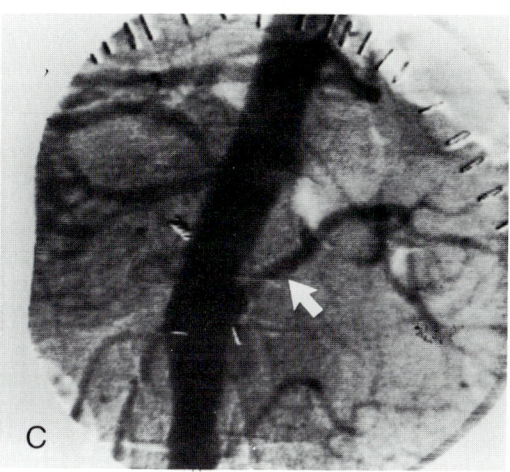

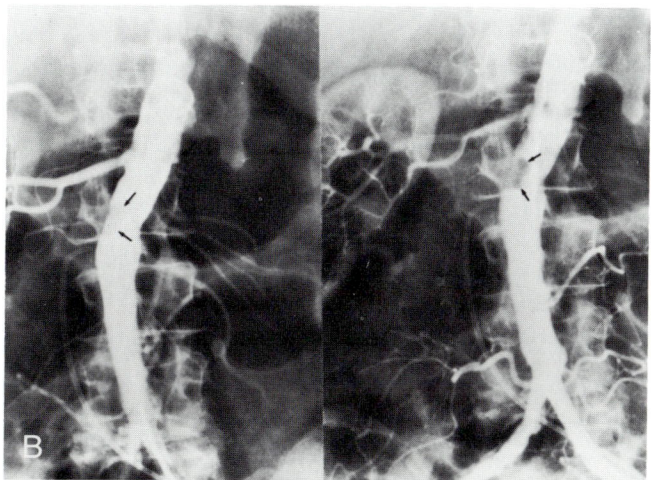

**Fig. 5-14.** (A) Aortogram in a 62-year-old woman shows atherosclerotic stenosis of the left renal artery. (B) Repeat aortography after percutaneous transluminal dilatation of the left renal artery shows thrombosis with complete occlusion. Note aortic filling defect which proved to be clot formation on traumatized aortic surface. (C) An emergency left aortorenal bypass and aortoplasty were performed. Postoperative digital subtraction angiogram shows patent left aortorenal saphenous vein graft (arrow). (Figure A, B, C reproduced from Flechner S, Novick AC, Vidt D, et al: The use of percutaneous transluminal angioplasty for renal artery stenosis in patients with generalized atherosclerosis. J Urol 127:1072. © 1982, The Williams and Wilkins Company, Baltimore.)

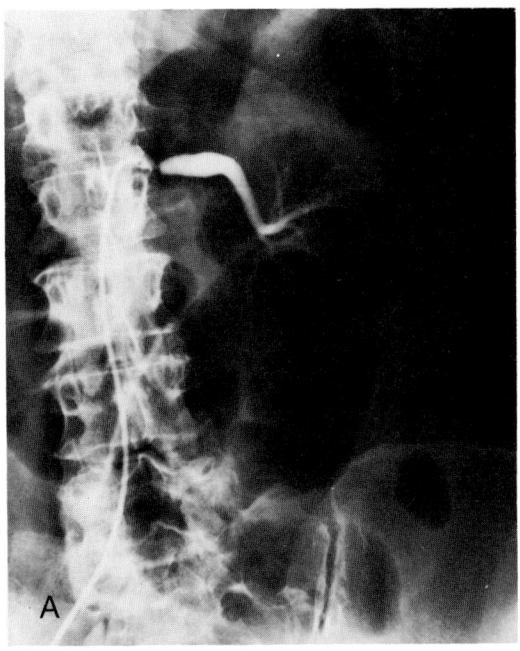

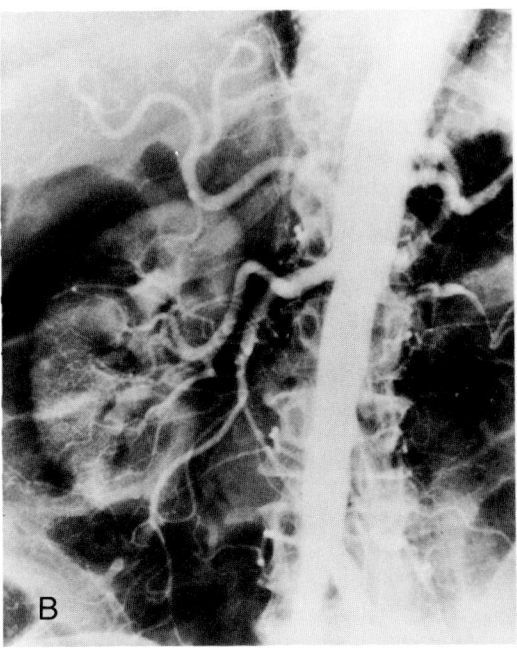

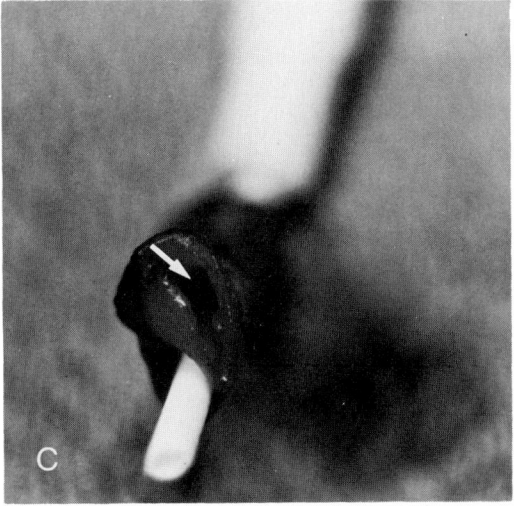

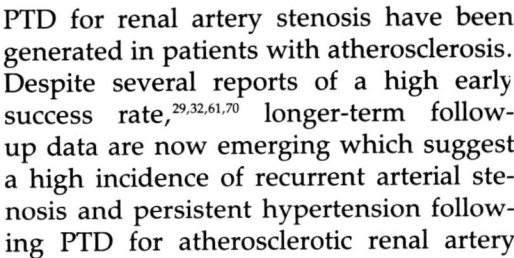

**Fig. 5-15.** (A) Selective left renal arteriogram in a 61-year-old woman shows high-grade stenosis of proximal left renal artery from atherosclerosis. (B) Repeat aortography following percutaneous transluminal dilatation of left renal artery shows intramural dissection (arrow) extending from proximal third of left renal artery into distal intrarenal branches. This precluded vascular reconstruction and a nephrectomy was done. (Reproduced from Flechner, Novick AC, Vidt D, et al.: The use of percutaneous transluminal angioplasty for renal artery stenosis in patients with generalized atherosclerosis. J Urol, 127:1072. © 1982, The Williams and Wilkins Company, Baltimore.) (C) Photograph of excised renal artery shows false lumen created by intramural dissection (containing catheter), and adjacent true arterial lumen (arrow).

PTD for renal artery stenosis have been generated in patients with atherosclerosis. Despite several reports of a high early success rate,[29,32,61,70] longer-term follow-up data are now emerging which suggest a high incidence of recurrent arterial stenosis and persistent hypertension following PTD for atherosclerotic renal artery disease. Grim et al.[21] reported recurrent stenosis in 12 of 12 patients (100 percent) with atherosclerotic disease who underwent repeat angiography ≥12 months following PTD. Grim et al. also evaluated the efficacy of PTD compared to surgical treatment in ameliorating atherosclerotic renovascular hypertension after a mini-

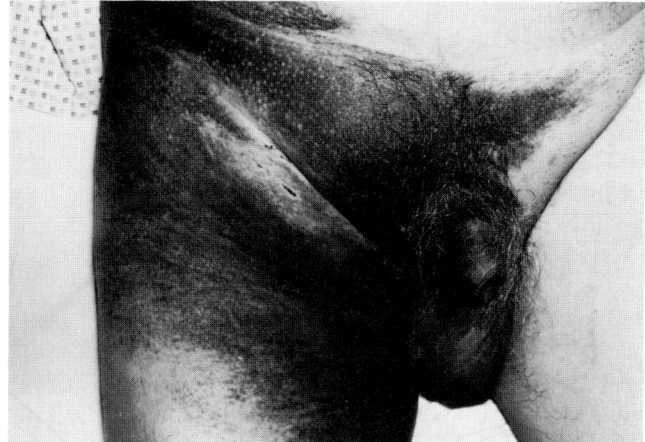

**Fig. 5-16.** Photograph demonstrates large groin hematoma in a patient who underwent percutaneous transluminal dilatation for renal artery stenosis.

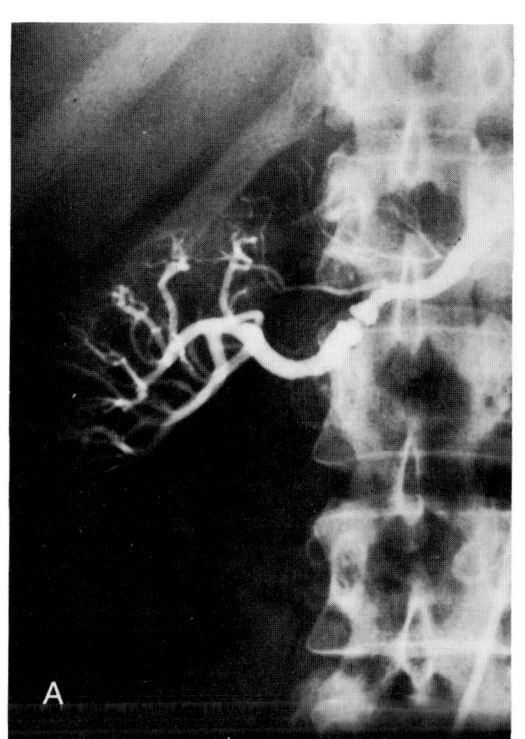

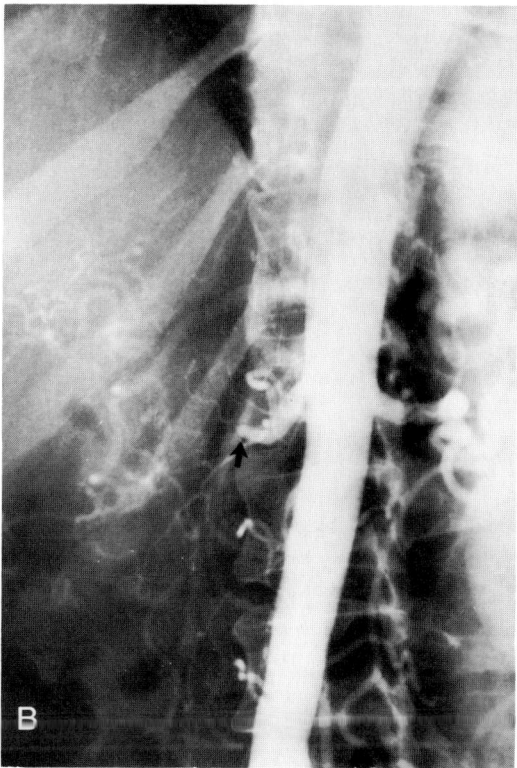

**Fig. 5-17.** (A) Selective right renal arteriogram in a 35-year-old female with hypertension demonstrates focal main arterial stenosis from medial fibroplasia. (B) Repeat aortography after percutaneous transluminal dilatation of right renal artery shows complete occlusion. At surgery, intramural dissection was found extending into renal artery branches and a nephrectomy was done.

mum 1-year follow-up interval; the cure or improvement rate was 89 percent with operative intervention and only 37 percent with PTD (p<.03).

The initial results with PTD for fibrous renal artery disease appear somewhat more promising. Cure or improvement of fibrous renovascular hypertension was achieved in seven of eight patients by Martin et al.,[38] in six of 10 patients by Grim et al.,[21] and in 21 of 21 patients by Tegtmeyer et al.[71] In the majority of patients from these reports, fibrous dysplasia was located either in the main renal artery or in a very proximal branch. Distal and/or multiple branch renal artery involvement is relatively common in the fibrous dysplasias and the efficacy of PTD in this setting is yet to be established. It should also be emphasized that patients with fibrous dysplasia and associated hypertension represent optimal candidates for vascular reconstruction from the standpoints of operative morbidity and long-term cure of hypertension. Once again, the long-term results of PTD will have to match those of surgical revascularization for PTD to be considered a viable therapeutic option in such patients.

# SUMMARY

Vascular reconstruction is the established method of treatment for properly selected patients with renovascular disease, either as therapy for associated hypertension or to preserve renal function. Surgical revascularization can be achieved safely with excellent long-term results in most cases. It is currently impossible to assign PTD a fixed role in the therapeutic armamentarium for renal artery stenosis since the risks and results in various types of renovascular disease are not yet established. The role of PTD is continuing to evolve, however, at present, this technique remains experimental and is unproven as a definitive treatment modality for patients with renovascular disease. Ultimately, the merits of PTD must be weighed against the established long-term efficacy of vascular reconstruction.

# REFERENCES

1. Beebe HG, Stark R, and Freeny PC: Indications for transluminal angioplasty: A surgical view. Am J Surg 140:31, 1980.
2. Belman AB, Kropp KA, Simon NM: Renal-pressor hypertension secondary to unilateral hydronephrosis. N Engl J Med 278: 113, 1968.
3. Block PC, Fallon JT, ElmerD: Experimental angioplasty: Lessons from the laboratory. Am J Radiol 135:907, 1980.
4. Castaneda-Zuniga WR, Formanek A, Tadavarthy M, et al: The mechanism of balloon angioplasty. Diag Radiol 135: 565, 1980.
5. Chibaro EA, Libertino JA, Novick AC: Use of the hepatic circulation for renal revascularization. Ann Surg. (in press).
6. Couch NP, Sullivan J, Crane C: The predictive accuracy of renal vein renin activity in the surgery of renovascular hypertension. Surgery 79:70, 1976.
7. Dean RH, Wilson JP, Burko H, et al: Saphenous vein aortorenal bypass grafts: Serial arteriography study. Ann Surg 180: 469, 1974.
8. Dean RH, Oates JA, Wilson JP, et al: Bilateral renal artery stenosis and renovascular hypertension. Surgery 81:53, 1977.
9. Dotter CT, Judkins MP: Transluminal treatment of arteriosclerotic obstruction. Circulation 30:654, 1964.
10. Dotter CT, Rosch J, Anderson JM, et al: Transluminal iliac artery dilatation: Nonsurgical catheter treatment of atheromatous narrowing. JAMA 230:117, 1974.
11. Eipper DF, Gifford RW, Stewart BH, et al: Abdominal bruits in renovascular hypertension. Am J Cardiol 37:48, 1976.
12. Ernst CB, Stanley JC, Marshall FF, et al: Autogenous saphenous vein aortorenal grafts: A ten-year experience. Arch Surg 105:855, 1972.

13. Ernst CB, Stanley JC, Marshall FF, et al: Renal revascularization for atherosclerotic renovascular hypertension: Prognostic implications of focal renal arterial versus overt generalized atherosclerosis. Surgery 73:859, 1973.

14. Flechner S, Novick AC, Vidt D, et al: The use of percutaneous transluminal angioplasty for renal artery stenosis in patients with generalized atherosclerosis. J Urol 127:1072, 1982.

15. Foster JH, Maxwell MH, Franklin SS, et al: Renovascular occlusive disease: Results of operative treatment. JAMA, 231:1043, 1975.

16. Foster JH, Dean RH, Pinkerton JA, et al: Ten years' experience with the surgical management of renovascular hypertension. Ann Surg 177:755, 1973.

17. Franklin SS, Young JD, Maxwell MH, et al: Operative morbidity and mortality in renovascular disease. JAMA, 231:1148 1975.

18. Franklin SS, Maxwell MH: Clinical workup for renovascular hypertension. Urol Clin N Am 2:301, 1975.

18. Gifford RW, McCormack LJ, Poutasse EF: The Atrophic Kidney: Its Role in Hypertension. Mayo Clin Proc 40:834,1965.

19. Gomes M, Bernatz PE: Aortoiliac occlusive disease: Extension cephalad to origin of renal arteries, with considerations and results. Arch Surg 101:161, 1970.

20. Grad E, Rance CP: Bilateral renal artery stenosis in association with neurofibromatosis (Recklinghausen's disease): Report of two cases. J Pediatr 80:804, 1972.

21. Grim CE, Luft FC, Yune HY, et al: Percutaneous transluminal dilatation in the treatment of renal vascular hypertension. Ann Intern Med 95:439, 1981.

22. Grüntzig A, Hopff H: Perkutane rekanalisation chronoischer arterieller verschulusse mit einem neuen dilatationkatheter. Dtsch Med Wochenschr 99:2502, 1974.

23. Haimon H, Giron F, Jacobson JH: The expanded polytetrafluorethylene graft: Three years' experience with 362 grafts. Arch Surg 114:673, 1972.

24. Harrison HG, McCormack LJ: Pathologic classification of renal artery disease in renovascular hypertension. Mayo Clin Proc 46:161, 1971.

25. Horne ML, Conklin YM, Keenan RE, et al: Angiotensin II profiling with saralasin: Summary of Eaton collaborative study. Kidney Int 15:5, 1979.

26. Hughes JS, Dove HG, Gifford RW, et al: Noninvasive predictors of surgical cure for renovascular hypertension (Abstract). Clin Res 25: 265A, 1977.

27. Hughes JS, Dove HG, Gifford RW, et al: Duration of blood pressure elevation in accurately predicting surgical cure of renovascular hypertension. Am Heart J 101: 408, 1981.

28. Hunt JC, Sheps SG, Harrison EG, et al: Renal and renovascular hypertension. A reasoned approach to diagnosis and management. Arch Intern Med 133:988, 1974.

29. Katzen B, Chang J, Lukowsky G, et al: Percutaneous transluminal angioplasty for treatment of renovascular hypertension. Radiology 131:53, 1979.

30. Kaufman JJ: The middle aortic syndrome: Report of a case treated by renal autotransplantation. J Urol 109:711, 1973.

31. Kaufman JJ: Dacron grafts and splenorenal bypass in the surgical treatment of stenosing lesions of the renal artery. Urol Clin North Am 2:365, 1975.

32. Kuhlman U, Vetter W, Furrer J, et al: Renovascular hypertension: treatment by cutaneous transluminal dilatation. Ann Intern Med 92:1 1980.

33. Lawrie GM, Morris GC, DeBakey ME: Long-term results of treatment of the totally occluded renal artery in 40 pateints with renovascular hypertension. Surgery 88:753, 1980.

34. Lawrie GM, Morris GC, Soussou ID, et al: Late results of reconstructive surgery for renovascular disease. Ann Surg 191:528, 1980.

35. Leadbetter WF, Burkland CE: Hypertension in unilateral renal disease. J Urol 39:611, 1938.

36. Libertino JA, Zinman L, Breslin DJ, et al: Renal artery revascularization: Restoration of renal function. JAMA 244:1340, 1980.

37. Marks LS, Maxwell MH, Varady PD, et al: Renovascular hypertension: Does the renal vein renin ratio predict operative results? J Urol 115:365, 1976.

38. Martin EC, Mattern RF, Baer L, et al: Renal

angioplasty for hypertension: Predictive factors for long-term success. Am J Radiol 137:921, 1981.

39. Meaney TF, Dustan HP, McCormack LJ: Natural history of renal arterial disease. Radiology 91:881, 1968.

40. Meares EM, Gross DM: Hypertension owing to unilateral renal hypoplasia. J Urol 108:197, 1972.

41. Novick AC, Stewart BH: Surgical treatment of renovascular hypertension. Curr Prob Surg 16(8):1,1979.

42. Novick AC: Renal artery aneurysm and arteriovenous malformation. In Novick AC, Straffon RA, Eds: Vascular Problems in Urologic Surgery. Saunders Philadelphia, 1982.

43. Novick AC, Fouad FM, Textor SC, et al: Predictive value of angiotensin II blockade with (SAR¹ THUR⁸)A$_{II}$ in renovascular hypertension. J Urol, 129:7, 1983.

44. Novick AC, Straffon RA, Stewart BH, et al: Diminished operative morbidity and mortality following revascularization for atherosclerotic renovascular disease. JAMA 246:749, 1981.

45. Novick AC, Stewart BH, Straffon RA: Autogenous arterial grafts in the treatment of renal artery stenosis. J Urol 118:919, 1977.

46. Novick AC, Straffon RA, Stewart BH: Surgical management of branch renal artery disease: In situ versus extracorporeal methods of repair. J Urol 123:311, 1980.

47. Novick AC, Stewart BH, Straffon RA, et al: Renal revascularization in patients with atherosclerosis or a previous operation on the abdominal aorta. Surg Gyn Obstet 144:211, 1977.

48. Novick AC, Banowsky LH, Stewart BH, et al: Splenorenal bypass in the treatment of stenosis of the renal artery. Surg Gyn Obstet 144: 891, 1977.

49. Novick AC, Palleschi J, Straffon RA, et al: Experimental and clinical hepatorenal bypass as a means of right renal revascularization. Surg Gyn Obstet 148:557, 1979.

50. Novick AC, Banowsky LH: Iliorenal saphenous vein bypass: Alternative for renal revascularization in patients with surgically difficult aorta. J Urol 122:243, 1979.

51. Novick AC: Management of intrarenal branch arterial lesions with extracorporeal

microvascular reconstruction and autotransplantation. J Urol 126: 150, 1981.

52. Novick AC, Pohl MA, Schreiber M, et al: Renal revascularization for preservation of kidney function in patients with atherosclerotic renovascular disease. J Urol, 129:907, 1983.

53. Poutasse EF: Renal artery aneurysms. J Urol 113:433, 1975.

54. Poutasse EF, Stecker JF, Ladaga LE, et al: Malignant hypertension in children secondary to chronic pyelonephritis. Laboratory and radiologic indications for partial or total nephrectomy. J Urol 119:264, 1978.

55. Riehle RA, Vaughan EJ: Renin participation in hypertension associated with unilateral hydronephrosis. J Urol 126:243, 1981.

56. Rosenfeld JB, Cohen L, Garty I, et al: Unilateral renal hypoplasia with hypertension (Ask-Upmark Kidney). Br Med J 2:217, 1973.

57. Rybka SJ, Novick AC: Concomitant carotid, mesenteric, and renal artery stenosis due to primary intimal fibroplasia. J Urol, 129:798, 1983.

58. Schefft P, Novick AC, Stewart BH, et al: Renal revascularization in patients with total occlusion of the renal artery. J Urol 124:184, 1980.

59. Schreiber MJ, Pohl M, Novick AC: Renal revascularization to preserve kidney function. Presented at the 12th Annual Meeting of the American Society of Nephrology, Boston, 1979.

60. Schreiber MJ, Novick AC, Pohl MA: The natural history of atherosclerotic and fibrous renal artery disease. Presented at the Thirteenth Meeting of the American Society of Nephrology, Washington DC, November, 1980.

61. Schwarten DE: Transluminal angioplasty of renal artery stenosis: 70 experiences. Am J Radiol 135:969, 1980.

62. Shahian DM, Najafi H, Javid H, et al: Simultaneous aortic and renal artery reconstruction. Arch Surg, 115:1491, 1980.

63. Silver D, Clements JB: Renovascular hypertension from renal artery compression by congenital bands. Ann Surg 183:161, 1976.

64. Stanley JC, Ernst CB, Fry WJ: Fate of 100

aortorenal vein grafts: Characteristics of late graft expansion, aneurysmal dilatation, and stenosis. Surgery 75:931, 1973.

65. Starr DS, Lawrie GM, Morris GC: Surgical treatment of renovascular hypertension: Long-term follow-up of 216 patients up to 20 years. Arch Surg 115:497, 1980.

66. Stickler GB, Kelalis PP, Burke E, et al: Primary interstitial nephritis with reflux: A cause of hypertension. Am J Dis Child 122:144, 1971.

67. Stoney RJ, Deluccia N, Ehrenfeld WK, et al: Aortorenal arterial autografts: Long-term assessment. Arch Surg 116:1416, 1981.

68. Straffon RA, Siegel DF: Saphenous vein bypass graft in the treatment of renovascular hypertension. Urol Clin North Am 2:377, 1975.

69. Streem SB, Novick AC: Aortorenal bypass with a branched saphenous vein graft for in situ repair of multiple segmental renal arteries. Surg Gyn Obstet, 155:855, 1982.

70. Tegtmeyer CJ, Dyer R, Teates CD, et al: Percutaneous transluminal dilatation of the renal arteries. Diag Radiol 135:589, 1980.

71. Tegtmeyer CJ, Elson J, Glass TA, et al: Percutaneous transluminal angioplasty: The treatment of choice for renovascular hypertension due to fibromuscular dysplasia. Radiology 143:631, 1982.

72. Tilford DL, Kelsch RC: Renal artery stenosis in childhood neurofibromatosis. Am J Dis Child 126:665, 1973.

73. Vaughan ED, Buhler FR, Laragh JH, et al: Hypertension and unilateral parenchymal renal disease: Evidence for abnormal vasoconstriction-volume interaction. JAMA 233: 1177, 1975.

74. Wollenweber J, Sheps SG, Davis GD: Clinical course of atherosclerotic renovascular disease. Am J Cardiol 21:60, 1968.

75. Wylie EJ: Endarterectomy and autogenous arterial grafts in the surgical treatment of stenosing lesions of the renal artery. Urol Clin North Am 2:351, 1975.

# 6

# Hypertensive Emergencies

# The Case for Gradual Reduction of Blood Pressure

## Howard I. Hurtig, M.D.

It may sound controversial to advocate a gradual reduction of blood pressure in accelerated hypertension, but the rationale for such a position is based on a sound body of scientific evidence that, upon examination, becomes a persuasive brief for an important new concept. In fact, there is probably little disagreement between my own view and that of Dr. Franklin. We both believe that extreme elevations of blood pressure should be promptly brought under control. We both agree that the potent drugs now available for lowering blood pressure should be handled with great caution and respect. We both agree that hypertension is the most important risk factor for stroke and heart disease so far identified in the epidemiologic literature.[40] Therefore, it is perhaps an overstatement to classify our paired statements on this subject as *real* controversy. Let us, instead, say that we are two physicians from different disciplines, engaged in an intelligent discussion of one of medicine's most vital issues. So much data have been gathered in the last 20 years to incriminate hypertension as a major contributor to death and disease in Western society, that it has been appropriately annointed the silent killer.[11] Its importance as a public health problem in developed countries cannot be overestimated.

The case against high blood pressure has become so irrefutable, that obligatory treatment of significant hypertension has become a matter of public policy. Numerous studies,[28,61,76,77] have shown in eloquent detail that treatment of moderate and advanced high blood pressure effectively reduces morbidity and mortality from target organ diseases, namely stroke, heart attack and renal failure. The medical profession has almost unanimously endorsed the wisdom of early detection and continuous treatment of hypertension, although there is, as yet, no clear mandate for treating mild elevation.[1,22,34] It is perhaps because of the growing public understanding of the importance of high blood pressure that mortality from all cardiovascular diseases, especially stroke, has declined dramatically in the last decade. Figure 6-1 graphically illustrates this decline, which has been pronounced for men, women, blacks, and whites.[51] Since black Americans have twice the prevalence of high blood pressure compared with whites, the drop in mortality is perhaps even more striking among this segment of the population.[8]

Progress in research on hypertension in recent time has led to a wider set of therapeutic options. The introduction of more potent and less noxious drugs has improved patient compliance and doctors have begun to realize that treating hypertension requires a long-term commitment. These developing trends have been healthy for everyone, but in our

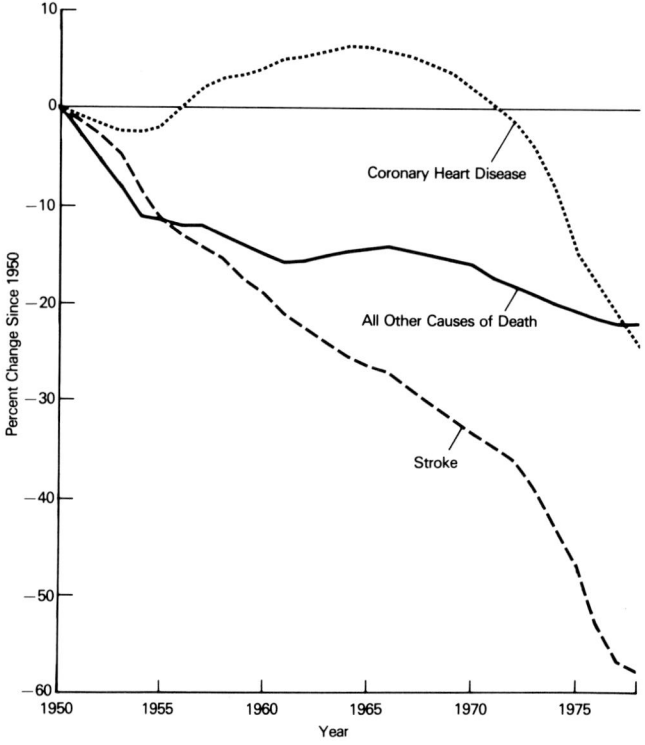

**Fig. 6-1.** Percent change in death rates since 1950 for coronary heart disease, stroke, and all other causes from ages 35–74. United States, 1950–1978. From: Levy RI, Declining mortality in coronary heart disease. Arteriosclerosis 1: 312, 1981 Reprinted with permission of the National Heart, Lung and Blood Institute).

*Age-Averaged.

collective rush to improve the lot of hypertensive mankind, it is easy to ignore the costs of progress. Each new weapon in the arsenal carries with it the potential risk of doing harm. The net result of the impressive advances in the treatment of high blood pressure has been overwhelmingly positive, but the excesses of our good intentions should be underscored to illustrate the need for a cautious and, yes, gradual approach to blood pressure reduction.

The last decade has brought us such effective antihypertensive drugs as diazoxide, nitroprusside, prazosin, and minoxidil. On a parallel frontier, we have learned much during this time about the relationship between blood pressure and the brain. This dual advance has been especially salubrious in light of the interaction between effective drugs and a complex cerebrovascular physiology.

Hypertension usually has an insidi-

ous and persistent pathologic effect on blood vessels throughout the body. It is well-known that arteriosclerosis and hypertension work in negative synergism. High blood pressure interacts with other risk factors, such as diabetes mellitus, hyperlipidemia, cigarette smoking, and genetic predisposition to create a fertile ground for development of serious and life-threatening vascular disease.[39] It is this effect on blood vessels, particularly cerebral arteries and arterioles, that will be the main focus of my exercise in controversy. Much that has been learned is applicable in the day-to-day management of patients with high blood pressure.

## THE CONTROL OF BLOOD PRESSURE

Regulation of blood pressure has three basic, interconnected control mechanisms: (1) neurogenic; (2) myogenic; and (3) hormonal. Each of these regulators will be considered in turn.

1. The neurogenic mechanism is, in itself, complicated. The sympathetic nervous system appears to play an important role in blood pressure control, since sympathetic nerves richly innervate blood vessels throughout the body, and catecholamines—important sympathetic neurotransmitters—seem to play a significant role.[63] Blood pressure is maintained within a "normal" range by feedback systems mediated through the lower diencephalon, brain stem, and spinal cord with outflow through the perivascular sympathetic chain. The carotid and aortic baroreceptors form a link in the feedback system to facilitate automatic adjustment of blood pressure and maintenance of "normal" perfusion to all tissues of the body. Extreme hypertension has been produced[13] by experimental disruption of the feedback loop at various sites, particularly the nucleus tractus solitarius in the floor of the fourth ventricle. Afferent (incoming) neural input from baroreceptor sympathetics probably terminates here.[63] Although the exact nature of the neurogenic influence on blood pressure control is the subject of real controversy,[12,35] there is little doubt that a neurogenic input is important to the system of overall control. Sympathetic nerves probably contribute to vascular tone of arteries and arterioles. The net result is constrictive. Potentiation of vascular resistance with a secondary rise in blood pressure are the major physiological effects of this tonic sympathetic state.

2. The process of constriction and dilatation of arteries and arterioles with muscular walls is, perhaps, the most important intrinsic factor contributing to the regulation of normal blood pressure. Bayliss[2] was one of the earliest observers to take note of the automatic constricting response of an arteriole to intraluminal stretch. Blood vessels throughout the body have this inherent capacity for instantaneous response to changes in tension within their walls—independent of metabolic or neurogenic forces—to determine their steady-state caliber. The myogenic response in probably the fundamental element in cerebral "autoregulation" of blood flow (see below); that is, the homeostatic ability of cerebral and other blood vessels to guarantee a predictable and reasonably "normal" supply of blood, despite potentially flow-altering fluctuations in systemic arterial pressure. A totally pressure-dependent system of flow would have obvious, disastrous effects on an organ such as the brain that has a constant, large need for a dependable supply of blood-borne glucose and oxygen.

3. Finally, the hormonal factor in blood pressure control can be further subdivided into volume and electrolyte systems that influence the kidney's salt and water regulation via the pituitary–adrenal–renal axis. This highly complex network of interlocking feedback loop mechanisms is also responsible for maintaining blood pressure (as well as fluid balance) within a healthy range. Disruption of any of the components of this tripartite system by disease can lead to progressive loss of blood pressure control. Hypertension is a direct consequence of an imbalance of one or more of the controlling factors.

## THE INTERPLAY OF BLOOD PRESSURE AND CEREBRAL BLOOD FLOW

The intimate relationship between blood pressure and cerebral blood flow was established soon after Kety and Schmidt in 1945 introduced the nitrous oxide ($N_2O$) technique for quantifying cerebral circulation. Their methodology was based on the Fick principle (c.1855)* of arteriovenous difference in the quantity of a perfused substance.[44] Cerebral blood flow prior to this technique[50] had been roughly estimated by directly measuring arterial and jugular venous oxygen content (catheter samples), using the formula

$$CBF = \frac{CMRO_2}{A\text{-}VO_2} \tag{1}$$

Where

$$CBF = \text{cerebral blood flow}$$

$$CMRO_2 = \text{cerebral metabolic rate for oxygen}$$

$$A\text{-}VO_2 = \text{arterial-venous oxygen difference}$$

$CMRO_2$ was assumed to be constant, hence the convenient transformation of the formula to:

$$CBF = \frac{1}{A\text{-}VO_2} \tag{2}$$

The nitrous oxide technique offered for the first time the capability of direct measurement of CBF, so that $CMRO_2$ could be accurately derived by solving Equation (1) with measured CBF and $A\text{-}VO_2$ values. Kety and Schmidt's contribution opened the door to a new era in the investigation of brain function. Although cerebral metabolism and blood flow are found to be tightly coupled in many situations,[65] and measured oxygen consumption is usually constant in hypertension,[42] independent quantification of flow and metabolism is clearly essential to the comprehensive assessment of brain pathophysiology.

In 1948, Kety et al.[42] reported a study of 13 patients with hypertension, all of whom had measurements of cerebral blood flow by the nitrous oxide method. Cerebral blood flow was calculated by extrapolating from the basic Fick formula:

$$CBF = \frac{100Qt}{A\text{-}Vt}$$

where

100Qt = quantity of substance in cc/100 g brain being consumed in time,

A-Vt = measured arteriovenous difference of a substance for the same unit of time

The differences between arterial and venous concentrations of $N_2O$ were integrated from zero time when the gas was first inhaled to a later time when venous blood and brain were in equilibrium. Kety et al. made the important observation that cerebral blood flow and cerebral oxygen consumption stayed within a narrow range for the 13 hypertensives, irre-

*Fick Principle:* The quantity of any substance taken up in a given time by an organ from the blood which perfuses it, is equal to the total amount delivered by arterial blood less the amount removed by venous drainage for the same period.

spective of a wide range of mean arterial blood pressures (MAP) among the subjects (124 to 190 mm Hg). The other important finding in this population was a two-fold increase in cerebrovascular resistance (CVR), as measured by the formula:

$$CVR = \frac{MAP}{CBF}.$$

He concluded that essential hypertension might be due to primary vasoconstriction of small arteries and arterioles from 50 to 100 μm in diameter (reflected by increased cerebrovascular resistance), with blood pressure rising secondarily to maintain a steady cerebral blood flow. Furthermore, he also postulated that the inverse relationship could apply with blood pressure rising primarily and cerebrovascular resistance becoming a secondary, homeostatic reaction to protect the brain from hyperperfusion.

This early study of cerebral blood flow and its relationship to high blood pressure bolstered the already prevalent concept of a cerebral circulation that maintained its blood flow automatically within a narrow range, irrespective of wide fluctuations in blood pressure. Lassen in his classic review paper later[47] coined the term "autoregulation" to describe this phenomenon.

It soon became apparent to Kety and others using the nitrous oxide technique that intrinsic control of cerebral blood flow was not without limits. Kety et al.,[43] and later Finnerty,[17] observed that cerebral blood flow tended to fall if blood pressure was reduced below a certain critical lower threshold. Kety[43] lowered blood pressure in hypertensive patients by means of a spinal sympathetic block and Finnerty induced hypotension by using hexamethonium (a ganglionic blocking agent) and controlled tilting. It was especially noteworthy and prescient in Finnerty's report that hypertensive patients began to develop symptoms of cerebral ischemia (dizziness, yawning, faintness) at blood pressures considerably above those that produced the same symptoms of cerebral ischemia in both young and old normotensive controls undergoing the same manipulation. Patients with the most advanced degree of hypertension had the earliest threshold for symptomatology as blood pressure was reduced. Finnerty postulated that chronic, advanced hypertension tended to produce fixed changes in the cerebral resistance vessels, which remained functionally constricted in face of sustained high blood pressure; their natural tendency to dilate as an autoregulatory response to falling blood pressure was thus compromised. It can be inferred in retrospect that Finnerty assumed a structural pathology of the arterial muscular wall to explain the fixed resistance encountered in his patients.

Figure 6-2 illustrates the principle of cerebral autoregulation as described by Lassen.[47] It can be noted that cerebral blood flow is constant despite wide changes in blood pressure until the lower limit is reached at approximately 60 mm Hg. Acute and chronic conditions that influence blood pressure have little effect on cerebral resistance vessels, the structural control center for the autoregulatory process. Lassen speculated that autoregulation might be altered by chronic hypertension because of the increase in cerebrovascular resistance that had been observed. He also hypothesized that if blood pressure were normalized by treatment, the vascular and hemodynamic changes might be reversible. He could not, at the time, have known that his

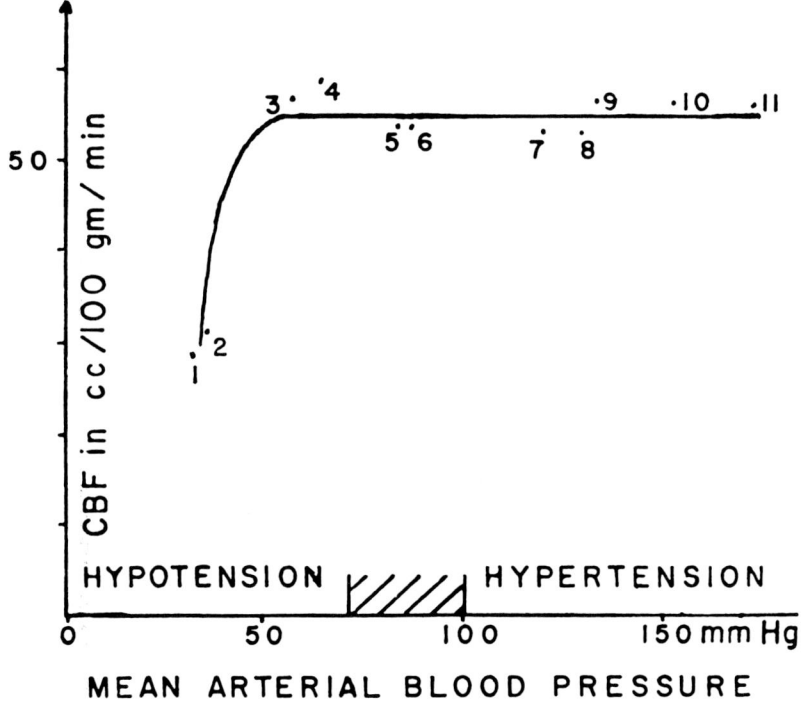

**Fig. 6-2.** Cerebral blood flow and blood pressure. Mean values of 11 groups of subjects reported in 7 studies, have been plotted. Various acute and chronic conditions have been selected and characterized by a change in blood pressure. In all, this figure is based on 376 individual determinations. 1 and 2, Drug-induced severe hypotension; 3 and 4, Drug-induced moderate hypotension; 5 and 6, Normal pregnant women and normal young men; 7, Drug-induced hypertension; 8, Hypertensive toxemic pregnancy; 9, 10, 11, Essential hypertension. (From: Lassen NA, Cerebral blood flow and oxygen consumption in man. Physiol. Rev. 39: 183, 1959.)

conjectures would later be confirmed by experimental evidence in man and animal.

The clinical impact of sustained hypertension was known in the 19th century, but it was Volhard[78] in 1914 who drew attention to the devastating effect of severe hypertension on blood vessels throughout the body. He reported a clinical-pathological case study of a patient whose life was terminated by an accelerated phase of hypertension that produced severe abnormalities of the optic fundus, convulsions, and neurologic death. Oppenheimer and Fishberg[58] in-

troduced the term hypertensive encephalopathy to describe the syndrome of sudden, acute elevation of blood pressure, usually from acute nephritis or pregnancy, in which the affected patient developed a variety of stereotyped symptoms, including convulsive seizures, headache, and confusion in association with a rapid rise in blood pressure. Oppenheimer and Fishberg were concerned mainly with the acutely hypertensive patient from specific causes. They documented clinical improvement in a single patient whose seizures stopped when elevated blood pressure was lowered.

They offered as an explanation that pressure-induced vasospasm and secondary cerebral ischemia were responsible for the neurologic symptoms. Fog's direct experimental observation of pial arteries and arterioles in the hypertensive cat in the 1930s lent some support to this hypothesis, which was greatly strengthened by Byrom's classic work in 1954 on hypertensive rats.[20]

Byrom's elegant and careful experiments,[7] in which he produced extreme renal vascular hypertension, showed that directly visualized small arteries and arterioles on the surface of the brain responded to artificial blood pressure elevations by segmental constriction. He was able to produce and reverse these constrictions by raising and lowering blood pressure, respectively, in his experimental animals. Furthermore, if the elevated blood pressure was sustained, the animals eventually developed convulsions and terminal coma. He discovered that these dying animals, if previously given a protein-bound dye such as Evans Blue, had dye-stained regions in the gray matter of the cerebral cortex, indicating leakage or extravasation of the material through the wall of the blood vessel. This finding, he concluded was due to probable ischemic changes in the wall of the vessel caused by excessive vasoconstriction at the observed narrow points in the arterioles. This so-called "sausage-string" effect was thought to be typical of cerebral vasospasm induced by elevations of blood pressure, particularly if they were rapid. The phenomenon was extrapolated to the human condition with obvious clinical-pathologic correlations for the syndrome of hypertensive encephalopathy. Thus, Byrom hypothesized that hypertension of this sort induced vasospasm and cerebral ischemia, which in turn led to cerebral edema, increased intracranial pressure and, eventually, death from rostro-caudal herniation of the swollen brain. These important findings were not only impressive in their own right, but were entirely concordant with prior experimental, clinical, and pathological observations regarding severe hypertension and the cerebral circulation.

Byrom's observations and conclusions were generally well-received, but some were unable to reproduce his findings and were therefore skeptical of the overall hypothesis.[66] Yet the concept had indirect support from clinicians in the 1950s,[28,45] who were beginning to recognize the poor prognosis of malignantly elevated blood pressures, especially in patients with symptoms of encephalopathy. The funduscopic picture of vasular narrowing, microinfarctions, and papilledema consistently correlated with the clinical severity and aggressiveness of the hypertensive process.

Byrom's experimental results were highly influential, but a major revision in thinking on this subject was about to take place. The first step in this direction occurred in 1964 when Giese[23] reproduced Byrom's "sausage-string" in an experimental mesenteric arterial preparation. He observed that an intravascular dye, colloidal carbon, extravasated into the perivascular tissues of hypertensive experimental animals, exclusively in vascular regions that ocrresponded to the *dilated*, rather than the constricted portions of the "sausage-string." In other words, leakage was taking place not necessarily as a consequence of ischemia, but as an effect of over distention from hyperperfusion. Byrom, himself, took these observations into account when he later admitted that the constricted segments might, in fact, have been the normal, adaptive response, whereas the expanded or dilated vascular segments were pathologic, representing the vessel's failure to adapt.[5,6] A series of experiments ensured in pursuit of this concept of cerebral vasodilatation or failed constriction as a substitute explanation for the pathophysiology of hypertensive encephalopathy.

The new wave of thinking on this subject was centered in Lassen's cerebral blood flow laboratory in Copenhagen with contributions from Jones and Graham from the Laboratory of Neuropathology in Glasgow, Scotland. Until the late 1960s, the focus of study had been on direct observation of pial blood vessels through a bone window in the skulls of animals, and from studies of extravasating dyes that diffuse through blood vessels as evidence for disruption of the natural endothelial barrier between blood and brain. The emphasis was beginning to shift to include cerebral blood flow as a complimentary third mode of study.

The first of two important experiments in this phase of the movement, reported in 1972 by Häggendal and Johansson,[27] showed that acute elevations of blood pressure in a single-step produced extravasation of Evan's Blue dye from cerebral arterioles in cats, whereas a slower, multistep increase in blood pressure to the same height was not associated with extravasation. This finding provided the best evidence to date that an acute, large rise in blood pressure produced vascular overdistention and secondary extravasation; multistep increases permitted vascular accommodation, presumably from an adaptive musculature of the arteriolar wall. The integrity of the endothelial barrier could thus be protected.

The second important experiment from this period demonstrated the combined effect of changing blood pressure and arterial carbon dioxide tension on cerebral blood flow. Using the well-known fact that $CO_2$ is a potent vasodialator,[65] Ekstrom-Jodal et al.[15] found in dogs that cerebral blood flow autoregulated normally with changing blood pressure

when $PCO_2$ was also normal. At higher, vasodilating levels of $PCO_2$, the upper limit of autoregulation was exceeded and CBF increased at levels of blood pressure that had been easily accommodated at a lower $PCO_2$ without any effect on blood flow. These investigators, for the first time, raised the possibility of an *upper* limit of autoregulation: blood pressure, above which the constricting arteriolar myogenic response can no longer resist increasing hydrostatic force; cerebral *hyperperfusion* is the untoward result.

The discovery of an upper limit of autoregulation led the Danish investigators to the next plateau of their evolving investigation of the cerebral circulation in hypertension. Lassen and Agnoli[48] first advanced the concept of cerebral hyperperfusion as the basis of hypertensive encephalopathy in man. They hypothesized a "breakthrough" of autoregulation's upper limit by excessive hypertension as an extension of the work by Ekstrom-Jodal.[15] Thereafter, in a series of experiments organized by Strandgaard et al., this proposed pathogenesis of hypertensive encephalopathy became more firmly grounded on experimental and clinical evidence supporting the concept of "breakthrough."

Strandgaard and his colleagues[75] first investigated cerebral blood flow in ten hypertensive and three normotensive patients, using the method of A-V oxygen differences. They varied blood pressure by using angiotensin and trimethaphan, confirming in three patients the previously hypothetical breakthrough of the upper limit of autoregulation. However, none of these patients had symptoms because of the highly controlled experimental conditions. The investigators also noticed an important correlation between the height of an individual patient's resting mean arterial pressure and the *lower* limit of autoregulation, that is, the higher the resting blood pressure, the higher the lower limit; hence, the more likely that hypoxic symptoms (dizziness, confusion, syncope) would occur as blood pressure was lowered to seemingly "normal" levels in patients with extreme hypertension. As noted by Finnerty 20 years before, the lower limit of autoregulation might be set at a mean arterial pressure of 100 mm Hg in a patient with sustained hypertension, whereas, the lower limit for a normotensive person might be the 60 mm Hg estimated by Lassen. Thus, hypertension in time shifts the autoregulatory curve to the right. Figure 6-3 illustrates the basic differences between the average autoregulatory lower limit among the ten hypertensives (mean arterial pressure approximately 6–100 mm Hg), compared with the three normotensives (mean arterial pressure approximately 60 mm Hg). Figure 6-4 shows the linear relationship between the resting or "habitual" mean arterial pressure of all thirteen subjects and: a) the lower limit of autoregulation; b) the cerebral blood flow level at which hypoxic symptoms appear. These findings led Strandgaard to devise the following scheme to explain the sequence of events leading to the development of encephalopathic symptoms in extreme hypertension:[74] rapid rise in blood pressure → increased arteriolar and capillary dilation → extravasation of plasma through distended blood vessel wall → brain edema → secondary capillary and vascular compression → decreased CBF → acute encephalopathy (combined effects of decreased CBF and increased brain edema).

Strandgaard and Skinhøj elevated the blood pressure in two other patients,[70] using a more direct method of measuring cerebral blood flow ([133]Xenon clearance by intracarotid injection) and found similar breakthrough in the two. A third patient was studied in the rare and fortuitous circumstances of acutely evolving hypertensive encephalopathy at the

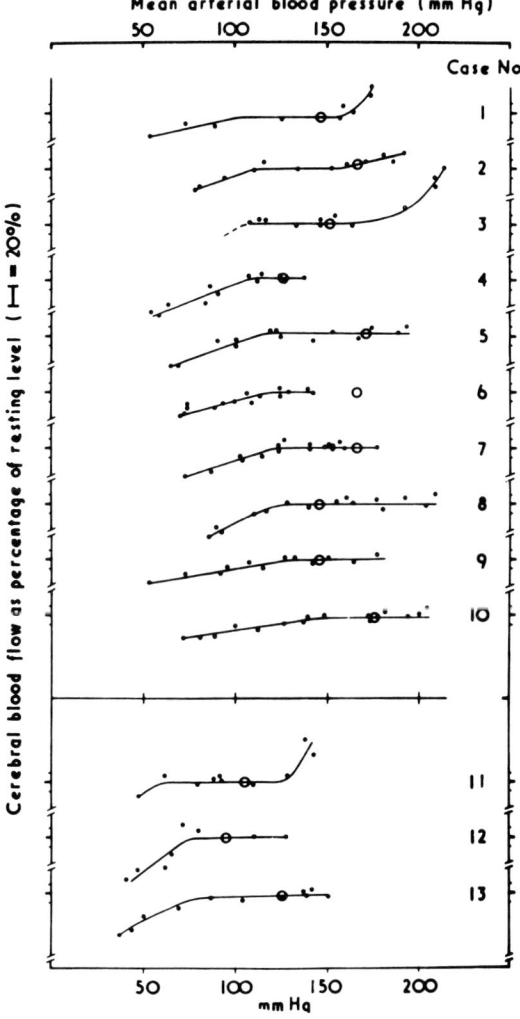

**Fig. 6-3.** Autoregulation of brain circulation in 13 subjects. The ordinate shows cerebral blood flow as a percentage of the resting level. For each curve, drawn by visual interpolation of the points, cerebral blood flow ± 10% is marked. An estimate of the patients' habitual mean arterial pressure is indicated by ○. It is clear how the autoregulation curves of the hypertensive patients (1–10) are shifted upward compared with the controls (11–13). Some of the patients show an upper limit of autoregulation beyond which cerebral blood flow increases. (From: Strandgaard S, et al., Autoregulation of brain circulation in severe hypertension. Br Med J 1: 507, 1978. Reproduced by permission of the Authors and Editors of the British Medical Journal.)

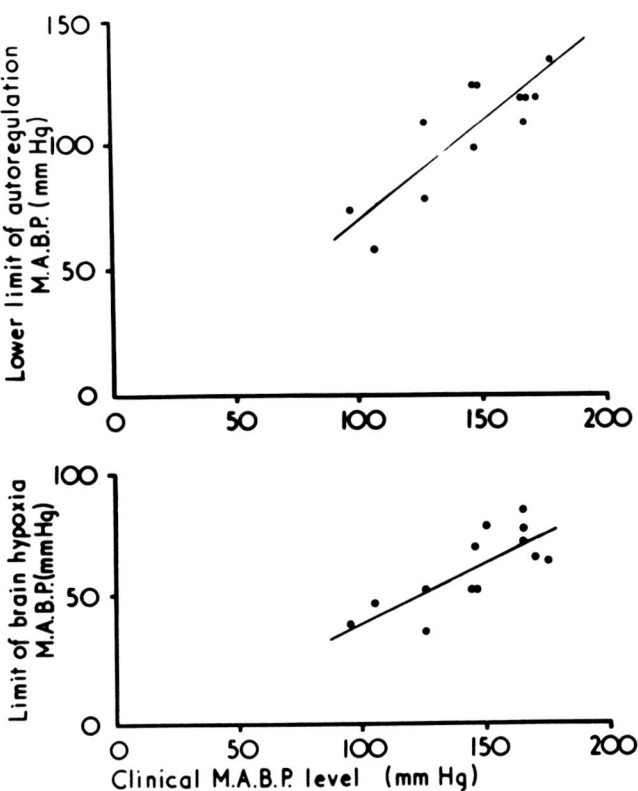

**Fig. 6-4.** (A) Correlation between estimate of habitual mean arterial blood pressure level (M.A.B.P.) and lower limit of autoregulation (r + 0.8470, p<0.001). (B) Correlation between estimate of habitual mean arterial blood pressure and mean arterial blood pressure at which brain hypoxia was elicited (r = 0.7759, p<0.01). (From: Standgaard S, et al., Autoregulation of brain circulation in severe hypertension. Br Med J 1: 507, 1973. Reproduced by permission of the Authors and Editors of the British Medical Journal.)

time of a diagnostic carotid arteriogram. Xenon was injected into the carotid artery and cerebral blood flow measurements were done during the early phase, when the patient had severe headache, confusion, and a blood pressure of 180/120, and later when seizures and coma had developed. Cerebral blood flow was markedly elevated initially (twice normal) and had fallen to half normal at the time of the second study 24 hours later, when the patient was unconscious. This only instance of serial cerebral blood flow measurements obtained in the midst of an evolving acute encephalopathy helped to give real clinical meaning to the above hypothetical chain of events.

Strandgaard's group extended their blood flow evaluations to animals to explore further the upper limit phenomenon, which they confirmed both in the

normo- and hypertensive baboon.[73,74] The upper limit was shifted to the right in the hypertensive animals, implying the same adaptive mechanism of tonic vasoconstriction that prevents symptoms from occurring in some patients with sustained, marked elevation of blood pressure. More recently, Barry et al.,[2] have demonstrated the same rightward shift (20 mm Hg compared with controls) in two different strains of hypertensive rats. Moreover, the hypertensive animals developed ischemic cerebral lesions during hypotension; the normotensive ones did not.

The final phase of this series of experiments focused on the effect of antihypertensive treatment on autoregulation. Strandgaard et al.[71] studied several groups of patients, using the Kety-Schmidt technique. He divided twenty-five hypertensive patients into four sub-

**CEREBRAL BLOOD FLOW** percent of rest

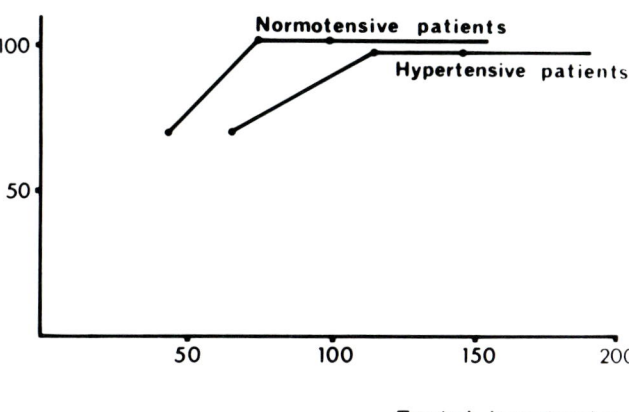

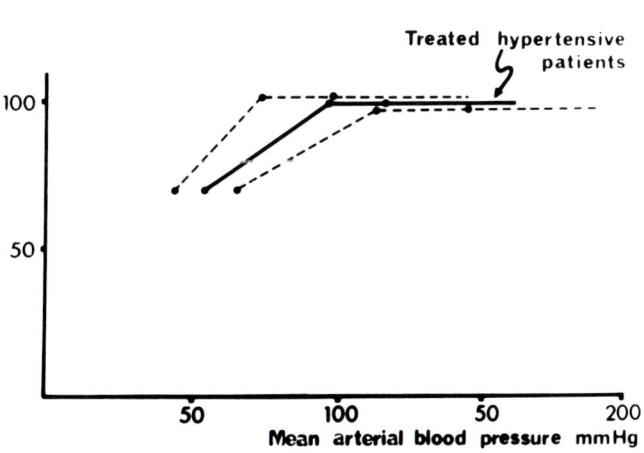

Mean arterial blood pressure mmHg

**Fig. 6-5.** Mean CBF autoregulation curves from normotensive, severely hypertensive and effectively treated hypertensive patients. (From: Standgaard S, Autoregulation of cerebral blood flow in hypertensive patients. Circulation 53: 720, 1976. By permission of the American Heart Association, Inc.)

groups: (1) severe hypertension; (2) formerly hypertensive but now effectively treated; (3) normotensive; and (4) patients twice studied—first when hypertensive and later when blood pressure was controlled. This interesting study showed a shift of the autoregulation curve to the right in the severely hypertensive patients as had been documented in previous animal and clinical studies. Also, hypertensive patients developed hypoxic symptoms at higher levels of blood pressure, as blood pressure was being reduced, in keeping with the observed shift of the curve to the right. Perhaps the most significant finding was that some of the treated hypertensive patients had autoregulation curves that tended to revert to normal, but others

showed no change. Figure 6-5 illustrates both the hypertensive shift and the normalized reversion. Neither age nor level of blood pressure correlated with the tendency for the curve to normalize. The authors concluded from these observations that:

1. Hypertensive patients were vulnerable to cerebral insufficiency if blood pressure was reduced too quickly to "normal" levels during the course of treatment;

2. Some hypertensives, following treatment, will readapt the autoregulatory curve over time to a more nearly normal configuration (Fig. 6-5). Thus, blood pressure might be *slowly* reduced to normal over a period of weeks or

months as the resistance vessels readapt by relaxing hypertrophied muscular walls. The principle of structural readaptation has been shown experimentally[21,52,80] and the occurrence of healing of the classic hypertensive changes, especially fibrinoid necrosis, has been well documented in man.[9]

3. Treatment of extreme elevations of blood pressure should follow the general principle of gradual, rather than aggressive, reduction, except in special circumstances when severe hypertension has produced the critical symptoms of hypertensive encephalopathy.

In summary, most of the studies of direct visualization of pial blood vessels, blood-brain barrier penetration, and cerebral blood flow in man and animal have built an impressively strong argument to support the concept of an autoregulatory breakthrough with cerebral hyperperfusion and the hemodynamic mechanism for the pathogenesis of hypertensive encephalopathy. A hypertensive rightward shift of cerebral autoregulation is induced by reactive narrowing of the caliber of resistance arteries, in part due to pathologic muscular hypertrophy and fibrinoid necrosis.

Although highly persuasive, there is still a gap between the theoretical nature of the experimental observations and direct observation of actual clinical manifestations of the hypertensive syndrome. It is reasonable to postulate that hyperperfusion would be followed by edema and a subsequent fall in cerebral blood flow from increased intracranial pressure, as suggested by Strandgaard. However, patients dying from true hypertensive encephalopathy do not consistently show signs of brain edema at postmortem, such as increased brain weight or herniation grooving.[9] Although pathologic changes, especially fibrinoid necrosis, in the walls of cerebral blood vessels may

correlate with the presumed structural adaptation that accounts for the fixed changes in resistance vessels, a leap of faith is required to assume that we now understand autoregulatory shift in hypertension. The essential truth of these findings must be proved by many additional human observations, especially from laboratories that have the capability of performing noninvasive testing of cerebral blood flow. Unfortunately, acute hypertensive encephalopathy is such a life-threatening illness that the luxury of time-consuming experimental procedures usually cannot be afforded.

# CLINICAL MANIFESTATIONS AND PATHOLOGY

When blood pressure is high enough to produce neurologic symptoms, the effects are dramatic. It is well known that chronic, sustained hypertension causes primary damage to the walls of blood vessels and accelerates the process of arteriosclerosis.[61] The cerebral circulation is one of the prime targets for this insidious process, and stroke, whether ischemic or hemmorrhagic, is the feared clinical culmination of the progressive intravascular events that are associated with hypertension. It is convenient to divide the neurologic complications of hypertension into two large categories: hypertensive stroke and hypertensive encephalopathy.

## Hypertensive Stroke

The clinical syndromes that have been identified as typically associated with chronic hypertension are actually not exclusive to the hypertensive state. However, the following disorders occur frequently in hypertensives and the cerebral localization, both clinically and radiographically, is even more characteristic of hypertensive cerebrovascular disease because of the nature of the underlying vascular pathology.

**Lacunar States.** Lacunes (lakes) are small, variably sized infarctions of brain that were first described by C. Miller Fisher.[18] They are as often silent as they are clinically evident. Lacunes are commonly found at autopsy in hypertensive patients and tend to occur in subcortical arterial territories. The usual diameter of a typical lacune is less than 5 mm. Because of the small size, clinical manifestations also tend to be small and self-limiting.

Table 6-1 lists four lacunar syndromes that have been carefully described and, in some cases, correlated with brain pathology by Fisher.[18] Clinical identification is important because these syndromes are usually relatively benign, although outcome is correlated with the size of the actual lacune on CT scan.[81] The generally good level of spontaneous recovery is a hallmark of most lacunes. Hypertension is an antecedent risk factor in the majority,[54] particularly those with CT lesions smaller than 5 mm. These patients usually do not require angiography or anticoagulation, and are perhaps at greater risk of cerebral hemorrhage if such drugs are used.

**Multiinfarct State.** Patients with uncontrolled hypertension are likely to develop multiple small lacunar strokes, which if distributed widely through the brain, can produce a clinical picture of dementia, dysarthria, difficulty swallowing, emotional lability, sphincter incontinence, and small-stepped gait. It is not uncommon for this picture to evolve slowly and without episodic deterioration, thereby implying that each discrete, small infarction occurs silently and subclinically. It is only in the aggregate that the cumulative impact is noted. These multiple, silent strokes are the neurologic counterpart to the "silent" progression of hypertension in general.

**Hypertensive Intracranial Hemorrhage.** Hypertensive hemorrhage is, perhaps, the clinical disorder most strongly associated with uncontrolled hypertension, although brain infarction is statistically more common. Bleeding into the brain is often hard to distinguish clinically from infarction but, because of the deep location of most hypertensive hemorrhages, consciousness is depressed as a result of involvement of the deep-seated reticular activating system of the brain. Patients typically develop symptoms while awake, in contrast to cerebral infarction, which commonly occurs during sleep. Sudden, severe headache is a common early symptom but is not always present. The severity of the clinical condition is directly proportional to the size of the hemorrhage, which tends to occur in one of the four locations listed in Table 6-2. Therefore, when the intra-

**Table 6-1.** Lacunar Stroke Syndromes

| Name | Site | Pathways Involved | Clinical Signs |
|------|------|-------------------|----------------|
| Pure motor hemiparesis | Internal capsule or pons | Corticobulbar, corticospinal tracts | Weakness of face, arm, and leg |
| Pure sensory stroke | Thalamus | Medial lemniscus and spinothalamic pathways | Numbness and sensory loss over face, arm trunk and leg |
| Homolateral ataxia and crural paresis | Internal capsule or corona radiata | Corticopontine (ataxia) and corticospinal tracts | Weakness of leg, ataxia of arm and leg |
| Dysarthria and clumsy hand | Pons | Corticobulbar, corticospinal tracts | Dysarthria, central facial weakness, deviation of tongue weakness and ataxia of arm |

**Table 6-2.** Signs of Intracerebral Hemorrhage

| Site | Eye movements | Pupils | Visual fields | Motor/sensory |
|------|---------------|--------|---------------|---------------|
| Pons | Impaired lateral eye movements | Pinpoint | Not testable | Quadriplegia |
| Putamen | Eyes deviate to side of lesion | Normal | Homonymous hemianopsia | Hemiplegia most prominent |
| Thalamus | Eyes stare down to tip of nose | Small and sluggish | Normal or transient homonymous hemianopsia | Hemisensory deficit most prominent |

parenchymal hematoma is large, the patient's symptoms may evolve from early headache and mild unilateral weakness to progressive obtundation, hemiplegia, and coma. As the deep hematoma expands, it dissects and compresses brain tissue and, if fatal, causes death by herniation and compressive brain stem ischemia. The various modes of clinical presentation for the different locations are also listed in the Table 6-2.

**Cerebellar Hemorrhage.** Hemorrhage into a cerebellar hemisphere is an especially notable clinical entity because appropriate treatment (in this case surgical) can make the difference between full recovery and death. C. Miller Fisher also contributed to the modern day recognition of this syndrome, when he described its clinical characteristics in great detail in 1965.[19] He emphasized that patients usually develop sudden onset of nausea, vomiting, and inability to stand or walk. Deterioration may proceed rapidly within hours to a state of unconsciousness with paralysis of gaze, to the side of the cerebellar hemorrhage. There is a clear dissociation between the presence of the foregoing signs and the absence of pyramidal tract dysfunction (true weakness). Prompt diagnosis of cerebellar hemorrhage is the most critical first step in management. A CT scan usually localizes the hemorrhage to the cerebellar hemisphere. Surgical decompression is critical to a favorable outcome and is best done early in the course. However, some patients with cerebellar hem-

orrhage have been managed conservatively, particularly if the lesion on CT is small and the symptoms are nonprogressive.[30]

## Hypertensive Encephalopathy

This term was introduced by Oppenheimer and Fishberg in 1928, when they described recurrent seizures in a young patient with acute nephritis and marked hypertension.[58] Their patient, like Volhard's 14 years before, was distinguished from similar patients by the relatively normal renal function; hence, the synonym "false uremia" had a certain descriptive appeal. Most experts agree that true encephalopathy associated with hypertension is uncommon, although the term has been somewhat misused over the years to include all patients with hypertension and neurological symptomatology. Zeigler made an effort to differentiate true hypertensive encephalopathy from various other neurological problems, such as ischemic and hemorrhagic stroke, uremic encephalopathy associated with hypertension, and other neurologic disorders such as meningitis, encephalitis, and so on. He reviewed the records of an unselected series of 43 cases diagnosed as hypertensive encephalopathy and found that only three had features characteristic of the true syndrome. More recently, Healton et al.[29] reviewed 34 patients with accelerated hypertension and were able to subdivide the total number into three distinct groups:

1. Malignant hypertension: Diastolic blood pressure greater than or equal to 130; papilledema, retinal hemorrhages or cotton wool spots; papilledema was not required for entry into this group.

2. Uremic encephalopathy: Decreased mental alertness, confusion, myoclonic jerking or twitching, asterixis and seizures, all associated with severe renal failure and improvement when the renal disease was treated.

3. Hypertensive encephalopathy: Decreased mental alertness, seizures, delirium, cortical blindness, mild focal neurologic signs, all associated with extreme hypertension without significant renal failure.

These authors underscored the importance of differentiating true hypertensive encephalopathy from the other two groups because of the urgent need to bring blood pressure under control immediately in the encephalopathic patients. Patients with *prominent* focal findings such as hemiparesis were considered to have major vascular occlusion in addition to encephalopathy. Such patients are at risk for aggravation of clinical signs if blood pressure is reduced too rapidly. Autoregulation is temporarily "paralyzed" in acute stroke,[79] particularly in large infarcts, and a drop in blood pressure could lead to a corresponding passive fall in cerebral blood flow thereby worsening cerebral ischemia.

It has become axiomatic that an acute, large increase in blood pressure is more likely to be associated with encephalopathic symptoms than a chronic and stepwise increase.[6,69] This well-recognized clinical distinction is supported by experimental evidence cited above showing that rapid, not stepwise elevation of blood pressure causes disruption of the blood-brain barrier. Moreover, the sudden elevation of blood pressure is most often seen in the acute systemic

diseases, such as nephritis and toxemia of pregnancy, both of which occur on a background of normotension. The combined effect of acute elevation and unadapted cerebral resistance vessels is perhaps critical to the occurrence of encephalopathic symptoms. Extreme hypertension is statistically much more common in the form of Healton's category (1) than (3), because malignant hypertension most often evolves as an uncontrolled phase of essential hypertension, wherein cerebral resistance vessels have years to adapt to a chronic, stepwise elevation. In the final analysis, encephalopathy is uncommon in clinical practice because its acute systemic causes are becoming increasingly rare.

The following case illustrates the important features of hypertensive encephalopathy. A 14-year-old girl had been in good health until the day before hospitalization when she complained to her mother of moderate frontal headache. On the following day while standing in her bedroom, she suddenly lost all vision but for light perception and cried out for help. Over the next hour, she became somnolent and began to have twitching of the right side of her face. The mother rushed her to the hospital where upon entering the emergency ward she began having frequent focal seizures involving the right arm, leg, and face. She remained in status epilepticus for 20 minutes until the convulsions could be brought under control. On admission the blood pressure was 220/120; she was comatose, had bilateral Babinski signs, and moderate bilateral papilledema. A lumbar puncture gave an opening pressure of 250 mm $H_2O$ and a protein value of 120 mg/dl. The fluid was clear and contained 100 RBCs per cu mm. The BUN was 85 mg/dl and RBC casts were present in the urinary sediment. Over the next 24 to 48 hours while receiving antihypertensive treatment she recovered

full consciousness and vision, the Babinski signs disappeared and the papilledema regressed. A second lumbar
puncture several days later was completely normal. Subsequently, a renal biopsy yielded a diagnosis of acute proliferative glomerulonephritis.

This case highlights the relatively abrupt rise in blood pressure and the underlying acute systemic illness (nephritis). Consider the sudden blindness and
seizures, increased intracranial pressure
cerebrospinal fluid (CSF) pressure of 250
mm H$_2$O), disrupted blood-brain barrier
(elevated CSF protein), and reversibility
of the syndrome with effective antihypertensive treatment. Children appear to
have a lower threshold of vulnerability to
rapidly rising blood pressure than adults.
Consequently, encephalopathy might become manifest at only moderately hypertensive pressures, as in this 14-year-old.

Disturbance of vision, as described,
has been attributed to ischemia of the oc-
cipital cortex rather than retina or optic
nerve. The only report of this phenomenon[37] also described visual loss prior to
seizures. Whether blindness is merely an
initial phase of the evolving seizures or
actually due to cortical ischemia is unclear. It is also possible that visual symptoms occur as a result of retinal and optic
disc compression from acute vascular distention. Ischemia, however, may be the
final end product of a swift chain reaction, triggered by a rapidly rising intravascular hydrostatic force.

# PATHOGENESIS OF HYPERTENSIVE CEREBROVASCULAR DISEASE

Numerous descriptions of the pathology of hypertensive vascular disease
can be cited from the medical literature.
A representative study by Chester and
colleagues[9] has recently analyzed the
brains of 20 patients dying of malignant
hypertension. All had diastolic blood
pressures in the range of 130 to 165 mm
Hg and all had diffuse encephalopathy
with papilledema during life. The authors also included in their analysis ten
patients with benign hypertension who
died with diastolic blood pressures in the
range of 100 to 110 mm Hg. The latter
group served as a hypertensive "control"
group.

The most important findings in this
study are shown in the authors' own table (Table 6-3). Fibrinoid necrosis of
small arteries and arterioles (resistance
vessels), intraluminal fibrin thrombi and
small infarcts were the hallmark lesions
that separated the two patient groups
(see Fig. 6-6). The table shows that
larger infarcts, including the lacunar
type, and large hemorrhages were
equally represented in both samples. The
other striking observation was the localization of these pathologic vascular
changes to the brainstem, especially the
anterior portion of the pons (basis
pontis). The vascular abnormalities, however, were also well represented in the
diencephalic and basal ganglionic structures. These are sites of both ischemic
and hemorrhagic brain lesions that produce familiar clinical syndromes. The cerebral white matter, cerebral cortex, and
spinal cord were the least affected. In addition, the authors noted that cerebral
edema was not a consistent finding, despite the presence of papilledema in
many patients during life. Brain weight
was not higher in the malignant group
compared to the benign group, and CSF
pressure measurements in some patients
were often not elevated despite the presence of papilledema. It should be pointed
out that most or even all of the cases had
been patients with long-standing hypertension that had become terminally
malignant. Acute hypertensive encephal-

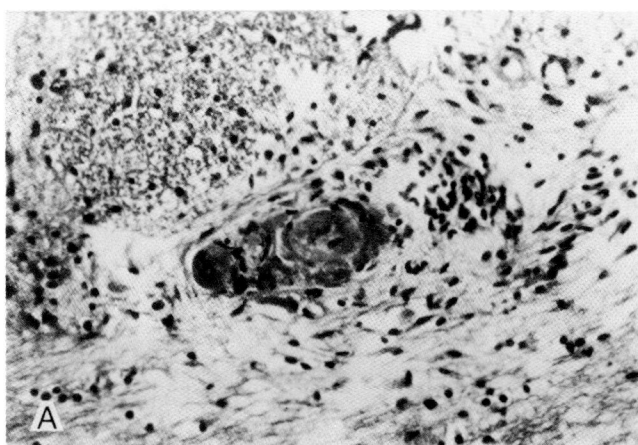

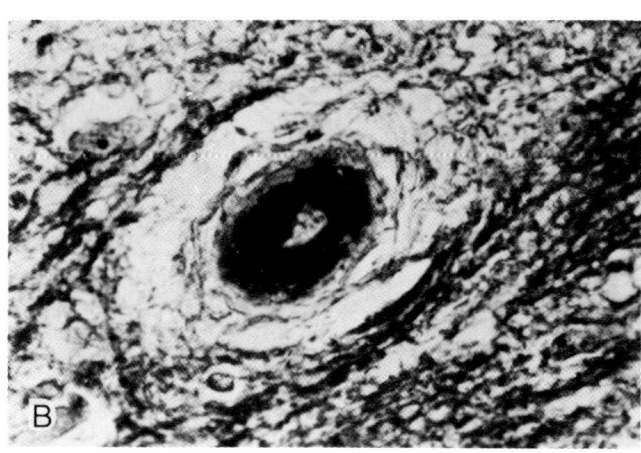

**Fig. 6-6.** (A) Medulla. Arteriole with fibrinoid necrosis and thrombosis surrounded by microinfarct. Hematoxylin and eosin, × 170. (B) Pons. Arteriole with fibrinoid necrosis. PTAH, × 430. (From: Chester EM, Agamanolis DP, Banker BQ, et al.: Hypertensive encephalopathy: a clinicopathologic study of 20 cases. Neurology 28: 928, 1978.)

opathy associated with nephritis or toxemia of pregnancy was not represented. Therefore, since cerebral edema is more likely to occur from acute elevations and the corresponding extravasation from overdistention of unadapted, "naive" arteries, it is not surprising that this population had relatively normal brain weights. Rather, some of the neurological symptoms during life in these patients might have been related to the presence of the severe, widespread occlusive small vessel disease and associated ischemia so prevalent throughout the brain. The authors could neither confirm nor refute the contribution of vasospasm, since a living, pulsating set of arteries would be required for such an assessment.

The progression of hypertensive vascular disease might follow this hypothetical sequence of pathologic events: Accelerated elevation of blood pressure → increased intraluminal hydrostatic pressure → damage to the medial wall of arteries and arterioles → transudation of fluid into the wall of the blood vessel → platelet aggregation and fibrin formation → fibrinoid necrosis, endothelial proliferation → cerebral ischemic symptoms or encephalopathy.

An additional small vessel pathologic change in hypertensive brain known as lipohyalinosis was found by Chester et al.[9] Lipohyalinosis may very well explain the changes in small subcortical arteries and arterioles that ultimately lead to mi-

**Table 6-3.** Neuropathologic findings in patients with hypersensitive encephalopathy and controls with nonmalignant hypertension

|  | Hypertensive encephalopathy (20 patients) | Nonmalignant hypertension (10 patients) |
|---|---|---|
| Brain weight (range) | 1490–990 | 1480–940 |
| Fibrinoid necrosis | 13 | 0 |
| Fibrin thrombi | 12 | 0 |
| Microinfarcts/ microglial nodules | 19 | 0 |
| Petechial hemorrhages | 9 | 0 |
| Lacunar infarcts | 13 | 5 |
| Large infarcts | 2 | 2 |
| Large hemorrhages | 3 | 3 |

(From Chester EM, Agamanolis DP, Banker BQ, et al: Hypersensitive encephalopathy: A clinicopathologic study of 20 cases. Neurology 28: 928, 1978.)

croinfarcts, lacunes, and intraparenchymal brain hemorrhages. Russell[68] has postulated that small arteries and arterioles develop weakened walls from the mechanical distention of sustained high blood pressure. Small microaneurysms materialize and they may thrombose to produce a lacune or rupture into the substance of the brain to cause a deep, expanding hematoma (see Fig. 6-7).

## TREATMENT OF HYPERTENSIVE EMERGENCIES

This section of my remarks has the greatest potential for generating significant heat of controversy. Treatment of hypertension in general is almost unanimously supported by physicians. However, some have cautioned against systematic treatment of mild high blood pressure,[53] since heterogeneity of risk is much greater among the mildly hypertensive than in patients with moderate or severe disease. Thus, the probability of a bad outcome is not high enough to justify the exposure to the possible, cumulative morbidity incurred from years of us-

ing potentially harmful antihypertensive medications.

It is well to restate at this time the cautionary conclusion that Standgaard derived from his many observations on the lower limits of autoregulation in man and animal.[71] From the data gathered by Strandgaard and his associates, it seems clear that patients with chronic hypertension tend to be more vulnerable to rapid and aggressive reduction of blood pressure because their autoregulation curve is generally shifted to the right (see Fig. 6-5). Although many of the experimental observations are theoretical, this resetting of the autoregulatory lower limit to a higher level seems to have real clinical applicability. The practical clinician, however, might contend that the risk of gradual reduction of blood pressure in accelerated hypertension is greatly offset by the opposing risk of serious and even fatal damage to target organs if extremely high levels of blood pressure are not lowered with proper dispatch. I will argue that these theoretical considerations have been substantiated in recent years by a growing number of reported cerebral ischemic complications resulting from overly aggressive antihypertensive treat-

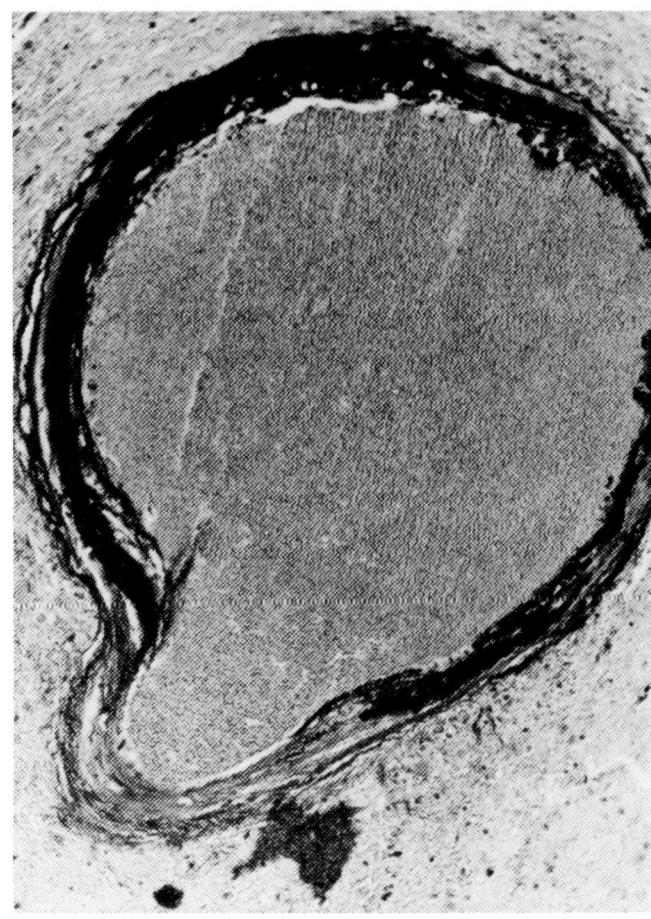

**Fig. 6-7.** Cross-section of micro-aneurysm showing plasma insudation of wall. (PTAH; × 90). (From: Russell RWR: How does blood pressure cause stroke? Lancet 2: 1283, 1975.)

ment. Such reports emphasize several thematic points that can serve as a guide to intelligent management.

First, hypertensive emergencies must be appropriately classified according to the underlying conditions. True *hypertensive encephalopathy*, "malignant" hypertension (extremely elevated blood pressure with papilledema and/or retinal hemorrhages and exudates but no *serious* neurological signs or complaints), and uncomplicated accelerated hypertension (diastolic pressures greater than 130) require treatment of differing urgencies. Hypertensive encephalopathy, like any true emergency, must be treated promptly. Blood pressure should be lowered in a hospital setting that permits

minute-to-minute manipulation of the potent drugs required for instantaneous blood pressure reduction. Malignant and uncomplicated accelerated hypertension also require carefully controlled therapy, but it may be inappropriate to classify these as true emergencies. A more gradual reduction of blood pressure can be justified because such a program of treatment has the best chance of avoiding the autoregulatory precipice. Furthermore, gradual treatment will permit structural readaptation of cerebral resistance vessels, so that cerebral blood flow will not be compromised as blood pressure is eventually brought into the normal range. Since the process of structural readaptation may take weeks or months, it is, therefore, realistic to reach the goal of normalization of blood pressure slowly and deliberately without fear of jeopardizing the patient's welfare.

Second, the various categories of advanced hypertension must also be distinguished from extreme elevations of blood pressure associated with ischemic or hemorrhagic stroke. It is well known that cerebral autoregulation is disrupted by cerebral infarction.[79] Blood flow may be falsely increased as a result of the phenomenon of "luxury" perfusion, secondary to reflex vasodilatation in the region of the infarct.[31,57] This type of reactive vasodilation is probably caused by acidosis of infarcted brain tissue; cerebral perfusion, therefore, becomes completely dependent upon a higher perfusion pressure than would be necessary if autoregulation were intact. Thus, if blood presure is greatly reduced in such a setting, cerebral perfusion will fall dramatically and the ischemic territory may be expanded. Although it is tempting for a concerned physician to reduce blood pressure in such a patient, the therapeutic effort could paradoxically worsen the neurologic condition. This peculiar loss of autoregulation in stroke has led some to propose the use of pressor agents during the acute phase to maintain blood pressure at a higher than usual level.[82] Cerebral perfusion could then be guaranteed at a critical time while the brain repairs itself and autoregulatory control is restored. However, pressor therapy is for the same reason potentially harmful because of the risk of hyperperfusion and breakthrough hemorrhage into vulnerable, ischemic brain. It is probably best to allow the blood pressure to seek its own level as long as it is not permitted to move significantly into an arbitrarily determined danger zone on either end of the spectrum. In other words, the blood pressure in the setting of an acute stroke should probably be maintained within

the bounds of 150/90 to 180/110. The patient's clinical conditions should serve as the best guide to sensible management, since circumstances vary tremendously.

Third, there is some evidence to show that autoregulation is impaired by the aging process,[4,32,33] and that hypertensive elderly are more likely to suffer the complications of overtreatment because of the combined effects of aging and sustained high blood pressure on the cerebral circulation.[33] Patients over 60 should probably be viewed as a specific therapeutic group. Many of the reports of cerebral ischemia complicating antihypertensive treatment pertain to the elderly.[36] A spate or two of such reports in the last few years has spawned editorial caution[14] specifically relating to the wisdom of blood pressure reduction in elderly patients, whose tolerance for the side effects of medication is notoriously poor. Some select people, particularly the very old, may do better left completely alone despite considerable hypertension. The rightward shift of the autoregulation curve may go further to the right in old people compared to the young.[4] Hoffman et al.[32,33] have shown that a similar aging shift probably occurs in old hypertensive rats subjected to Strandgaard type CBF-blood pressure manipulation. The vasodilating effect of $CO_2$ on cerebral blood vessels is also blunted by aging.[4] Sclerotic arteries are therefore less resilient in responding to variations in blood pressure. All of these factors may contribute to the increased risk of complications in the treated hypertensive elderly.

It is important to keep the scope of this argument in rational proportion. The overwhelming majority of patients treated for all categories of hypertensive disease with potent drugs respond favorably without serious adverse effects, especially if there is no overt indication that target organs have already been damaged by the hypertensive process. Although this record of achievement may be impressive, there is a continuing need to be vigilant against the possibility of *any* iatrogenic complication. Graham[25] and Jones and Graham[38] have shown in two illustrative cases that casual use of antihypertensives can plunge extremely high blood pressures to low or unrecordable levels. Their two patients, both elderly, died as a result of the extreme hypotension and irreversible cerebral ischemia. The ischemic changes in those two brains are shown in Figure 6-8. The damage is localized to the so-called boundary zones of greatest vulnerability situated at the end of the supply lines for each of the three major branches of cerebral arteries that deliver blood to the brain (anterior cerebral, middle cerebral, and posterior cerebral arteries). These authors, like Strandgaard et al., emphasized the changes in autoregulation that occur in chronic hypertension and the need for special caution in using aggressive antihypertensive therapy.

Numerous and scattered case reports have appeared over the last six years, documenting the occurrence of blindness from optic nerve ischemia,[11] myocardial infarction,[46] stroke, and coma[49] as a result of antihypertensive treatment. Leddingham and Rajogopalan collected ten patients at the Radcliffe Infirmary, Oxford, all of whom experienced cerebral complications from overzealous treatment of hypertension. Most of their patients had an exaggerated response to diazoxide (Hyperstat) or to a combination of diazoxide and other drugs, such as chlorpromazine, hydralazine, prochlorperazine. Some of their patients had true hypertensive encephalopathy, but others had malignant and uncomplicated accelerated hypertension. Most complications seemed to occur from drug combinations, but in some, diazoxide alone was responsible for the exaggerated hypotensive re-

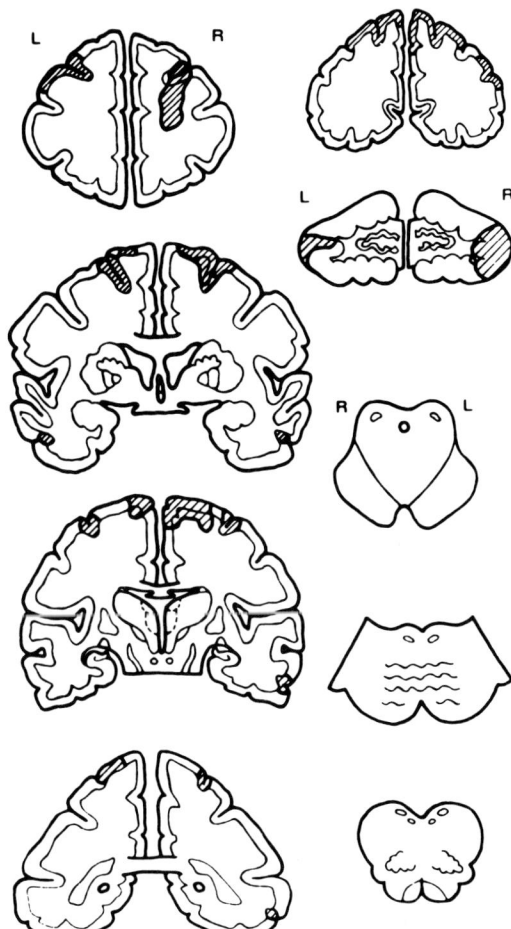

**Fig. 6-8.** Distribution of infarction in the boundary zones between the major arterial territories of the cerebral and cerebellar hemispheres (hatched). (From Graham DI: Ischemic brain damage of cerebral perfusion failure type after treatment of severe hypotension. Br Med J 2: 735, 1975. Reproduced by permission of the Authors and Editors of the British Medical Journal.)

sponse. The dose of diazoxide in these cases was not excessively high. The authors cautioned against too rapid reduction of blood pressure, even under emergency conditions. They, like others, emphasized the increased vulnerability of older people, in whom preexisting arteriosclerotic stenosis or occlusion of one or more major arteries to the brain might set the stage for catastrophe in the course of antihypertensive treatment.

Diazoxide was introduced as an effective and convenient antihypertensive drug for use in hypertensive emergencies in 1973. Its ease of administration has made it extremely popular and relatively safe. Finnerty[16] strongly endorsed diazoxide as the drug of choice, reporting that he had used it in over a thousand patients without complication. Ninety-five percent of these patients responded to the initial bolus dose of 300 mg. He observed "no sign of postural hypotension, cerebral ischemia or collapse." He also recommended the combined use of furosemide with diazoxide to prevent sodium retention and azotemia, although he admitted that the potential for postural hypotension might be increased if these two medications were used together.

Others have advocated a more deliberate use of diazoxide. Ram and Kaplan[63] proposed the use of several mini-bolus injections, rather than a single large dose of the drug. In their series of 20 severely hypertensive patients treated with small, multiple doses of diazoxide (150 mg initially and every five minutes to a maximum of 600 mg), all patients responded satisfactorily and without complications. At the time of their report, 40 major morbid events had been attributed to diazoxide after standard injections, including five deaths, two strokes, and four myocardial infarctions. The authors concluded that gradual reduction of blood pressure, particularly in patients with a history of unstable coronary insufficiency, was preferable to immediate reduction, even in a so-called hypertensive emergency. This point of view, favoring the multiple dose application (minibolus) of diazoxide, has been endorsed by others,[55] and is now the official method recommended by Schering, the drug's manufacturer.[60,75]

Nitroprusside (Nipride) has been used to lower blood pressure since the late 1920's, but has only been generally available to clinicians for the last eight to ten years. It, along with diazoxide, is the most popular agent used in lowering blood pressure acutely under controlled, in-hospital conditions. Unlike diazoxide, nitroprusside must be titrated in every case. It requires constant monitoring and observation in an intensive care setting. Nitroprusside is an arteriolar and venodilator, whereas diazoxide only produces dilatation of the arterioles. Nitroprusside is more difficult to use because of the additional controls required, compared with diazoxide. It is also light-sensitive and is not as chemically stable.

Table 6-4 shows the important features of drugs used in the treatment of hypertensive emergencies. Modes of pharmacologic action differ. There are certain theoretical considerations regarding the effects of these agents on cerebral blood flow that could have clinical import. For example, several studies of cerebral blood flow in patients receiving nitroprusside and hydralazine indicate that under certain conditions, cerebral blood flow and intracranial pressure might be increased by these drugs, separate from the effect they have on the blood pressure-autoregulation coupling mechanism. However, it is probable that these effects are not clinically important in hypertensive patients undergoing emergency treatment.

One recent study of the effect of alpha-methyldopa in hypertensive patients suggested that Aldomet might disrupt autoregulation in high doses and in people older than 60.[24] This study, however, contained few subjects and the results can only be construed as a tentative caveat against the use of high doses of

**Table 6-4.** Drugs for Treatment of Hypersensitive Emergencies

| Drug | Course of action | | | Dose (IV) | Mechanism of Action | Effect on Cerebral Hemodynamics | Comment |
|---|---|---|---|---|---|---|---|
| | Onset | Max | Duration | | | | |
| **A. Sympatho reducers** | | | | | | | |
| Methyldopa | 2 hr | 4 hr | 6–12 hr | 500–1000 mg | Decreased central sympathetic output | High doses in elderly may cause loss of autoregulation[24] | Onset too slow and uncontrollable for extreme emergencies |
| Trimethaphan | 2 min. | 5 min. | 10 min. | 0.5–5mg/min. | Ganglionic blockade | None[56] | Especially useful in dissecting aortic aneurysm; tachphylaxis & enteric paralysis occur later. |
| **B. Vasodilators** | | | | | | | |
| Diazoxide | 2 min. | 3 min. | 4–12 hr | 75 mg STAT 150 mg q5' Max. of 675 mg | Arteriolar dilation | — | Ease of administration makes this an attractive drug. Reflex increase in sympathetic activity may precipitate coronary insufficiency; hypotensive response to rapid 300 mg bolus can cause cerebral ischemia |
| Hydralazine | 15 min. | 30 min. | 4–8 hr | 10–50 mg | Arteriolar dilatation (?venodilation) | ↑ICP, ↓PP ↑CBF[58,69] | Onset too slow for extreme emergency; reflex ↑ cardiac output and coronary insufficiency may occur. |
| Nitroprusside | 1 min. | 1–2 min. | 3–5 min. | 0.2mg/min. (Avg.) | Arteriolar & venodilation | ↑ICP[10] No effect[26] | Patients with disruption of BBB might be at risk from effect on ICP. Good drug in presence of severe myocardial disease. |

CBF, cerebral blood flow; PP, perfusion pressure; ICP, intracranial pressure; BBB, blood-brain barrier.

235

Aldomet in older people, pending further investigation.

I have tried, in this essay, to formulate a balanced view of the treatment of severe hypertension. Balance between too much and too little intervention is a worthy objective in all of medicine. This hoary principle clearly applies to the effective management of patients with high blood pressure. The single most important summary statement that might be made on this subject is that there is nothing casual about treating any phase of hypertension, from minimal to extreme. One might say casual begets casualty. The important, new hemodynamic findings that have come to light in the last decade have illuminated a previously muddled set of concepts regarding blood pressure and the cerebral circulation. The sequential experimental observations by Strandgaard and his group have a compelling internal logic. Their work and the valiant efforts of other investigators should be incorporated into our programs of clinical decision-making. Although the scientific advances of the last 20 years have been impressive, they still need vigorous scrutiny in the laboratory of the acute care hospital. They also must be tested by the two great yardsticks of scientific durability, experience and time.

# REFERENCES

1. Alderman MA, Madhaven S: Management of the hypertensive patient: A continuing dilemma. Hypertension 3:192, 1981.
2. Barry DI, Strandgaard S, Graham DI, et al: Cerebral blood flow in rats with renal and spontaneous hypertension: Resetting of the lower limit of autoregulation. J Cereb Blood Flow Metab 2:347, 1982.
3. Bayliss WM: On the local reactions of the arterial wall to changes of internal pressure. J Physiol 28:220, 1902.
4. Bessman A, Alman RW:, Fazekas JF: Ef-

fects of acute hypotension on cerebral hemodynamics and metabolism of elderly patients. Arch Intern Med 89:893, 1952.
5. Byrom FB: Hypertensive encephalopathy. Lancet 1:766, 1973.
6. Byrom FB: The Hypertensive Vascular Crisis: An Experimental Study. Grune & Stratton, New York, 1969.
7. Byrom FB: Pathogenesis of hypertensive encephalopathy and its relation to the malignant phase of hypertension: Experimental evidence in the hypertensive rat. Lancet 2:201, 1954.
8. Cerebrovascular Diseases: 13th Princeton Conference. Reivich M, Hurtig HI, eds: New York, Raven, 1983.
9. Chester EM, Agamanolis DP, Banker BQ, Victor M: Hypertensive encephalopathy: A clinicopathologic study of 20 cases. Neurology 28:928, 1978.
10. Cottrell JE, Patel K, Turndorf H, Ranshoff J: Intracranial pressure changes induced by sodium nitroprosside in patients with intracranial mass lesions. J Neurosurg 48:329, 1978.
11. Cove DH, Seddon M, et al: Blindness after treatm for malignant hypertension. Br Med J 2: 245, 1979.
12. Cowley AV, & Scher AM: Comment and Reply: Postscript to Ito CS and Scher AM Circ Res 48:576, 1981.
13. Doba N, Reis DJ: Acute fulminating neurogenic hypertension produced by brainstem lesions in Pat. Circ Res 32:584, 1973.
14. Editorial: Hypertension in the elderly. Lancet 1:684, 1977.
15. Ekstrom-Jodal B, Haggendal E, Linder LE, Nilsson NJ: Cerebral blood flow autoregulation at high arterial pressures and different levels of $CO_2$ tension in dogs. Europ Neurol 6:6, 1972.
16. Finnerty FA: Hypertensive emergencies. In Hypertension Manual. New York, Yorke, 1974.
17. Finnerty FA, Witkin L, Fazekas JF: Cerebral hemodynamics during cerebral ischemia induced by acute hypotension. J Clin Invest 33:1227, 1954.
18. Fisher CM: Lacunes: Small, deep cerebral infarcts. Neurology 15:774, 1965.
19. Fisher CM, Piacard EH, Polak A, et al:

Acute hypertensive cerebellar hemorrhage: diagnosis and surgical treatment. J Nerv Ment Dis 140:38, 1965.

20. Fog M: Cerebral Circulation: Reaction of pial arteries to increases in blood pressure. Arch Neurol Psychiatr 41:260, 1939.

21. Folkow B, Hallback M, Lundgren Y, Weiss L: Effects of intense treatment with hypotensive drugs on structural design of resistance vessels in spontaneously hypertensive rats. Acta Physiol Scand 83:280, 1971.

22. Freis ED: Should mild hypertension be treated? N Engl J Med 307:306, 1982.

23. Giese J: Acute hypertensive vascular disease: II. Studies on vascular reaction patterns and permeability changes by means of vital microscopy and colloidal tracer technique. Acta Pathol Microbiol Scand 62:497, 1964.

24. Goldberg H, Weinberger J: Effect of methyldopa on cerebral blood flow in hypertension. In Proceedings of the IX International Symposium on Cerebral Blood Flow and Metabolism. Acta Neurol Scand Suppl. 72, Vol. 60, ed. Gotoh, E. & Nagai, H. 1979, pp. 144–145.

25. Graham DI: Ischemic brain damage of cerebrce perfusion failure type after treatmtre of severe hypertension. Br Med J 4: 739, 1975.

26. Griffiths DPG, Cummins BH, Greenbaum R, et al: Cerebral blood flow and metabolism during hypotension induced with sodium nitroprusside. Br J Anesth 46:671, 1974.

27. Haggendal E, Johansson B: On the pathophysiology of the increased cerebrovascular permeability in acute arterial hypertension in cats. Acta Neurol Scand 48:265, 1972.

28. Harrington M, Kincaid-Smith P, McMichael J: Results of treatment in malignant hypertension. Br Med J 2:969, 1959.

29. Healton EB, Brust JC, Feinfeld DA, Thomson GE. Hypertensive encephalopathy and the neurologic manifestations of malignant hypertension. Neurology 32:127, 1982.

30. Heiman TD Satya-Murti S: Benign cerebellar hemorrhages. Ann Neurol 3:366, 1978.

31. Hoedt-Rasmussen K, Skinhoj E, Paulson OB, et al: Regional Cerebral blood flow in acute apoplexy. Arch Neurol 17:271, 1967.

32. Hoffman WE, Albrecht RF, Miletich DJ: The influence of aging and hypertension on cerebral autoregulation. Brain Res 214:196, 1981.

33. Hoffman WE, Miletich DJ, Albrecht RF: Influence of antihypertensive therapy on cerebral autoregulation in aged hypertensive rats. Stroke 13:701, 1982.

34. Hypertension Detection and Follow-up Program Cooperative Group. The effect of treatment on mortality in mild hypertension. N Engl J Med 307:976, 1982.

35. Ito CS, Scher AM: Hypertension following arterial baroceptor denervation in the unanestheitzed dog. Circ Res 48:576, 1981.

36. Jackson G, Mahon W, Pierscianowski TA, Condon J: Inappropriate antihypertensive therapy in the elderly. Lancet 2.1317, 1976.

37. Jellinek EH, Painter M, Prineas J, et al: Hypertensive encephalopathy with cortical disorders of vision. Quart J Med 33:239, 1964.

38. Jones JV, Graham DI: Hypertension and the cerebral circulation: its relevance to the elderly. Am Heart J 96:270, 1978.

39. Kannel WB Current status of the epidemiology of brain infarction associated with occlusive arterial disease. Stroke 2:295, 1971.

40. Kannel WB, Wolf PA, Verter J, et al: Epidemiological assessment of the role of blood pressure in stroke: The Framingham Study. JAMA. 214:301, 1970.

41. Kaplan NM: Clinical Hypertension. New York, Medcom, 1973.

42. Kety SS, Hafkenschiel JH, Jeffers, WA, et al: Blood flow, vascular resistance and oxygen consumption of the brain in essential hypertension. J Clin Invest 27:511, 1948.

43. Kety SS, King BD, Hovath SM, et al: The effects of an acute reduction in blood pressure by means of differential spinal sympathetic block on the cerebral circulation of hypertensive patients. J Clin Invest 29:402, 1950.

44. Kety SS, Schmidt CF: The determination of cerebral blood flow in man by use of

nitrous oxide in low concentrations. Am J Physiol 143:53, 1945.

45. Kincaid-Smith P, McMichael J, Murphy EA: Clinical course and pathology of hypertension with papilledema. Quart J Med 27:117, 1958.

46. Kumar GK, Dastoor FC, Robayo JR, Razzaque MA: Side effects of diazoxide. JAMA 235:275, 1976.

47. Lassen NA: Cerebral blood flow and oxygen consumption in man. Physiol Rev 39:183, 1959.

48. Lassen NA, Agnoli A: The upper limit of autoregulation of cerebral blood flow on the pathogenesis of hypertensive encephalopathy. Scand J Clin Lab Invest 30:113, 1972.

49. Ledingham JGC, Rajagopalan B: Cerebral complications in the treatment of accelerated hypertension. Quart J Med 48:25, 1979.

50. Lennox WG Gibbs EL: The blood flow in the brain and the leg of man and the changes induced by alterations of blood gases. J Clin Invest 11:1155, 1932.

51. Levy RI: Declining mortality in coronary heart disease. Arteriosclerosis 1:312, 1981.

52. Lundgren Y: Regression of structural cardiovascular changes after reversal of experimental renal hypertension in rats. Acta Physiol Scand 91:275, 1974.

53. Madhaven S, Alderman MH: Potential effect of blood pressure reduction on cardiovascular disease: A cautionary note. Arch Intern Med 141:1583, 1981.

54. Miller VT: Lacunar stroke: A reassessment. Arch Neurol 40:129, 1983.

55. Nies AS: Clinical pharmacology of antihypertensive drugs. Med Clin North Am 61:675, 1977.

56. Olesen J: Quantitative evaluation of normal and pathologic cerebral blood flow regulation to perfusion pressure changes in man. Arch Neurol 28:143, 1973.

57. Olsen TS, Larsen B, Skriver EB, et al: Focal cerebral hyperemia in acute stroke. Stroke 12:598, 1981.

58. Oppenheimer BS, Fishberg AM: Hypertensive encephalopathy. Arch Intern Med 41:264, 1928.

59. Overgaard J, Skinhoj E: A paradoxical ce-

rebral hemodynamic effect of hydralazine. Stroke 6:402, 1975.

60. Physicians Desk Reference. Med. Econ. Co. Oradell, NJ, 1983. p. 1812.

61. Pickering, G.W. High Blood Pressure. 2nd Edition. Churchill-London 1968.

62. Ram, C.V.S. & Kaplan, N. Individual titration of diazoxide dosage in the treatment of severe hypertension. Am. J. Card. 43:627, 1979.

63. Reis, D.J. The brain and arterial hypertension: evidence for a neural-imbalance hypothesis. In Abbound FM, Reis D, eds: Disturbances in Neurogenic Control of the Circulation. American Physiolical Society, Bethesda, Md., 1981, pp 87–104.

64. Reivich MR: Arterial $pCO_2$ and cerebral hemodynamics. Am J Physiol 206:25, 1964.

65. Reivich MR: The use of cerebral blood flow and metabolic studies in cerebral localization. In Thompson RA, Green JR New Perspectives in Cerebral Localizations, New York, Raven, 1982, pp 115–143.

66. Rosenblum WI, Donnenfeld H, Alev F: Effects of increased blood pressure on cerebral vessels in mice. Arch Neurol 14:631, 1966.

67. Rowe GG, Maxwell GM, Crumpton CW: The cerebral hemodynamic response to administration of hydralazine. Circulation 25:970, 1962.

68. Russell RWR: How does blood-pressure cause stroke? Lancet 2:1283, 1975.

69. Skinhoj E, Strandgaard S: Pathogenesis of hypertensive encephalopathy. Lancet 1:461, 1973.

70. Strandgaard S: Autoregulation of cerebral blood flow in hypertensive patients. Circulation 53:720, 1976.

71. Strandgaard S: Autoregulation of cerebral circulation in hypertension. Acta Neurol Scand [Suppl] 66:1, 1978.

72. Strandgaard S, Jones JV, McKenzie ET, Harper AM: Upper limit of cerebral blood autoregulation in experimental renovascular hypertension in the baboon. Circ Res 37:164, 1975.

73. Strandgaard S, McKenzie ET, Sengupta D, et al: Upper limit of autoregulation of

cerebral blood flow in the baboon. Circ Res 34:435, 1974.

74. Strandgaard S, Olesen J, Skinhøj E, Lassen NA: Autoregulation of brain circulation in severe hypertension. Br Med J 1:507, 1973.

75. Tezzoni R: personal communication.

76. VA Cooperative Study Group on Antihypertensive Agents: Effects of treatment on morbidity in hypertension. Results in patients with diastolic blood pressure averaging 115 through 129 mm Hg. JAMA 202:1028, 1967.

77. VA Cooperative Study Group on Antihypertensive Agents: II: Results in patients with diastolic blood pressure averaging 90 through 114 mm Hg. 213: 1143, 1970.

78. Volhard F, Fahr T: Die Brightsche Nierenkrankheit. Vol. 2, Berlin, Springer, 1914, p 232.

79. Waltz AG: Effect of blood pressure on blood flow in ischemic and non-ischemic cerebral cortex. Neurology 18:613, 1968.

80. Warshaw DM, Root DT, Halpern W: Effects of antihypertenisve drug therapy on the morphology and mechanics of resistance arteries from spontaneously hypertensive rats. Blood Ves 17:257, 1980.

81. Weisberg LA: Lacunar infarcts. Arch Neurol 39:37, 1982.

82. Wise G, Sutter R, Burkholder J: Treatment of brain ischemia with vasopressor drugs. Stroke 3:135, 1972.

# The Case for More Rapid Lowering of Blood Pressure

## Stanley S. Franklin, M.D.

## INTRODUCTION

High blood pressure rarely constitutes a medical emergency, despite the large number of patients with chronic hypertension. Indeed, the hypertensive crises probably occur in less than 1 percent of the hypertensive population. In the majority of cases, accelerated, malignant hypertension, or hypertensive emergencies, represent a failure of early diagnosis and inadequate drug therapy.

Not all patients who present with severe hypertension have true hypertensive emergencies. A hypertensive emergency is not only defined by the severity of blood pressure, but also by the immediate potential for vascular damage. Therefore, a physician's first task is to accurately diagnose if a patient's severe hypertension represents (1) a true hypertensive emergency; (2) urgent hypertension; or (3) labile hypertension without evidence of an immediate threat to the vasculature or vital organs.

If, indeed, a true hypertensive emergency exists, the physician must choose the proper antihypertensive agent or agents, and make a decision in regard to how rapidly blood pressure should be lowered and to what extent. The question of the desirability of rapid lowering of blood pressure must, of course, take into account the risk of excessive delay in lowering blood pressure versus the risk of neurologic damage brought about by excessive reduction in blood pressure. There is no question that physicians in the past have made errors in both directions. The general theme of this presentation is that accurate diagnosis of the hypertensive state will determine how rapidly blood pressure should be lowered; the ultimate therapeutic goal is to maximize benefit and minimize risk.

## DIFFERENTIAL DIAGNOSIS OF HYPERTENSIVE EMERGENCIES

A true hypertensive crisis is a life-threatening condition that requires immediate lowering of blood pressure.[3,7,10,12,16,17,28,33,34,36] Both idiopathic and secondary hypertension can lead to a hypertensive crisis. The diagnosis is not based on any specific level of blood pressure, but depends on numerous factors including the rapidity in rise of blood pressure, the duration of hypertension, and a clinical determination of the immediate direct threat to the patient. For example, a young woman with eclampsia could develop a hypertensive emergency with a blood pressure of only 170/110 mm Hg, while a patient with long-standing hypertension may not be in a crisis situation with a blood pressure level of 250/150 mm Hg.

Conditions which require immediate

**Table 6-5.** Classification of Severe Hypertension

A. Severe hypertension constituting a true crisis or emergency for BP reduction
   Hypertensive encephalopathy
   Toxemic crises
   Pheochromocytoma crises
   Drug-induced catecholamine excess syndrome
   Accelerated malignant hypertension with:
      Decreasing vision
      Acute renal failure
      Mesenteric insufficiency
      Acute GI hemorrhage
      Acute pancreatitis
B. Moderate to severe hypertension constituting a true crisis when complicated by
   Refractory pulmonary edema
   Refractory crescendo angina or myocardial infarction
   Dissecting aneurysm or leaking abdominal aortic aneurysm
   Intracranial hemorrhage
   Postoperative bleeding at vascular suture lines
C. Urgent hypertension requiring slower reduction in BP
   Diastolic BP greater than 130 mm Hg without evidence of acceleration
   Accelerated, malignant hypertension without complications
   Moderate to severe hypertension (diastolic BP 105–129 mm Hg) with:
      TIA's
      Evolving cerebral thrombosis
      Congestive heart failure

reduction in blood pressure are listed in Table 6-5, A and B. Hypertensive encephalopathy represents an emergency characterized by markedly elevated blood pressure with symptoms and signs of increased intracranial pressure or cerebral edema. The hypertensive crises of toxemia of pregnancy, pheochromocytoma, or drug-induced catecholamine excess syndromes frequently is associated with a very rapid rise in blood pressure to crisis level, which can cause an acute intracranial bleed even in the absence of hypertensive encephalopathy. In contrast, malignant hypertension, defined as severe hypertension with hemorrhages, exudates, and papilledema of the optic fundi, may not represent a true hypertensive emergency unless also associated with encephalopathy. Other threatening presentations that demand immediate lowering of malignant hypertension are decreasing visual acuity, the onset of acute renal failure, mesenteric insufficiency, acute gastrointestinal hemorrhage, or acute pancreatitis. Moderate to severe elevations in blood pressure, without features of accelerated, malignant hy-

pertension, may constitute a true crisis situation when complicated by refractory pulmonary edema, crescendo angina, or recent myocardial infarction, dissecting or leaking aneurysm, intracranial hemorrhage, or postoperative bleeding at vascular suture lines.

In contrast to the true hypertensive emergencies listed in Table 6-5, A and B, Table 6-5 C lists urgent hypertension requiring a slower reduction in blood pressure over a period of hours to several days. A review of the clinical manifestations and the differential diagnostic features of each of the entities listed in Table 6-5 is clearly beyond the scope of this presentation. However, accurate clinical diagnosis represents the keystone to successful therapeutic management of these high-risk patients.

# DANGERS OF RAPID LOWERING OF BLOOD PRESSURE

Whenever arterial blood pressure rises to high or falls to low values, the cerebral arteries constrict or dilate, respectively, to ensure a constant cerebral blood flow. This phenomenon, referred to as *autoregulation*, occurs primarily in the small resistance arterioles of the cerebral arteries. The range of blood pressure over which autoregulatory control of cerebral blood flow occurs has been studied in animals and man.[14,19,29,30,31] In normotensive subjects, cerebral blood flow is autoregulated down to a mean blood pressure of 60 mm Hg.[30] As the blood pressure falls below this critical level, no further dilation of the vascular bed of the brain can compensate for the decreased perfusion pressure, and thus, cerebral blood flow decreases. Early symptoms of hypoxia follow, such as light-headedness, confusion, and dimming of vision.[30] If mean blood pressure falls below 35 to 40 mm Hg, somnolence and loss of consciousness ensue. On the other hand, if blood pressure exceeds the upper limit of autoregulation (150 to 200 mm Hg of mean blood pressure), cerebral blood flow increases and hypertensive encephalopathy may develop.[14,29]

In both chronically hypertensive patients and animals, the lower limit of blood pressure for maintaining autoregulation of cerebral blood flow is higher than in normotensive controls. Standgaard et al. found that cerebral blood flow began to decrease when mean arterial pressure was rapidly lowered to approximately 120 mm Hg in 10 severely hypertensive patients.[30] Moreover, the shift of the lower end of the cerebral autoregulatory curve to higher blood pressure levels suggests that the upper end of the curve is also shifted to the right; this would imply a chronically hypertensive patient has a greater resistance to autoregulatory breakthrough of cerebral blood flow than does his normotensive counterpart. A shift in the autoregulatory curve to the right is thought to result from chronic hypertension with gradual development of hypertrophy in

the media of the cerebral arterial wall.[31] Finally, effectively treated hypertensive patients show a readaptation of the cerebral blood flow toward normal autoregulation in some, but not all, cases studied.[31]

Hypertensive encephalopathy is best explained as a severe hypertensive state in which there is a decompensation of the normal cerebral autoregulation of blood flow resulting in breakthrough hyperperfusion with focal damage to arterioles, increased permeability, petechial hemorrhage, infarctions, and necrosis.[14,29] Thus, hypertensive encephalopathy may develop in a previously normotensive individual at a blood pressure as low as 110 mm Hg diastolic, while it may not be observed in the chronically hypertensive patient until diastolic blood pressure exceeds 160 mm Hg. A possible explanation for the early morning headache of hypertensive encephalopathy is earlier breakthrough of increased cerebral blood flow brought about by the shift of the autoregulatory curve to the left in association with hypercapnia of sleep.[19]

The upper and lower limits of the autoregulatory blood pressure curve are also affected by the pH of the local perivascular space. A low pH is associated with vasodilatation and a shift of the curve to the left, whereas, a high pH produces vasoconstriction and a shift of the curve to the right.[19]

Furthermore, the autoregulation of cerebral blood flow may be lost in the presence of cerebral ischemia or edema, as well as from local tissue acidosis resulting from an acute stroke, brain trauma, or status epilepticus.[2,6,23,32] In the presence of a completed cerebral thrombosis, minimal reduction in systemic arterial blood pressure may lead to further ischemia to the compromised area of the brain; this may cause an enlargement of the original infarct with worsening of neurologic symptoms. Deterioration in cerebral blood flow during reduction in systemic blood pressure may result in part from a steal syndrome, by which the normal surrounding areas of the brain maintain normal cerebral blood flow at the expense of the injured area.[32] Disturbed autoregulation of cerebral blood flow has recently been observed in patients with accelerated malignant hypertension who develop acute neurologic signs and symptoms in association with rapid lowering of blood pressure. A review of the literature has disclosed 19 such patients;[9,11,13,18,20,27] individual patient profiles are summarized in Table 6-6, and a general summary of clinical characteristics is found in Table 6-7. The average age of these patients was 36 years (4 children and 15 adults) with an almost equal number of males and females. These patients had evidence of severe antecedent hypertension as evidenced by mean blood pressure of 188 ± 19 mm Hg. Seventy-nine percent had malignant hypertension with Grade IV optic fundi, and 53 percent had symptoms compatible with hypertensive encephalopathy. Anti hypertensive drug therapy reduced mean blood pressure to 84 ± 18 mm Hg, which represented a 56 percent mean decrease in blood pressure level, clearly well below the autoregulatory range of patients with chronic, severe hypertension. The rapidity of blood pressure lowering occurred in minutes in 26 percent, and over a period of many hours in 74 percent of the patients. Perhaps a critical factor in the development of neurologic deterioration was the long duration of induced low blood pressure. This varied from many hours to up to a day or longer in all 19 patients.

Neurologic complications consisted of permanent blindness in 47 percent of the subjects, especially evident in the very young patients. In addition, 32 percent of the patients developed coma, 32 percent pyramidal tract signs, 58 percent with residual neurologic deficits, and 3 patients (16 percent) died.

A review of the antihypertensive therapy given these 19 patients revealed that 15 out of 19 patients (79 percent) received diazoxide in the form of an intravenous bolus administration. Eighty-seven percent of the patients who received diazoxide were also receiving other antihypertensive therapy. On the other hand, there were two patients (13 percent) who received diazoxide alone. In addition, three patients (16 percent) received multiple oral antihypertensive agents in the absence of any parenteral therapy. The last patient in this series had an intravenous ganglionic blocking agent.

In summary, patients who sustain neurologic damage in association with antihypertensive therapy most frequently had malignant hypertension, often with symptoms of hypertensive encephalopathy and extremely high systolic and diastolic blood pressure values. Blood pressures were reduced well below the accepted autoregulatory range for patients with chronic hypertension, and once having been lowered, remained at extremely low levels for many hours or longer. The main reason for the long duration of low blood pressure in these patients was the selection of antihypertensive agents with a long duration of action.

## CLINICAL STRATEGIES: DIAGNOSTIC AND THERAPEUTIC

### Proper Assessment of Risk from Severe Hypertension and Risk from Abrupt Lowering of Blood Pressure

During the initial evaluation of the severely hypertensive patient, an effort should be made to triage the patient into one of several categories: A pseudohypertensive crisis patient can be treated with sedation and reassurance, and sent home; a true hypertensive emergency state frequently requires parenteral therapy and intensive care unit observation; and finally, the intermediate state of urgent hypertension can be treated with oral antihypertensive agents. A brief but concise history and physical examination are necessary to establish an accurate etiologic diagnosis and to determine if a completed stroke has occurred; this has an important clinical bearing on the safety of subsequent reduction of blood pressure values. Clinical assessment, often accompanied by screening laboratory tests, electrocardiogram, and chest x-ray, are of paramount importance in answering the following questions: How rapidly should the blood pressure be lowered? What is the first endpoint in blood pressure reduction? What agent or agents should be used? What should be the route of administration? And finally: Is there a need for intensive care unit monitoring?

## Strategy for Proper Drug Selection

The ideal medication for hypertensive emergencies should have a rapid onset and offset of action, be easy to administer and monitor, not adversely affect critical organs such as the brain, heart, or kidneys, and have few side effects. Such an ideal drug is not available.

**Trimethaphan camsylate (Arfonad)** is a short-acting ganglionic blocking drug which has long been in use.[5] The advantages of trimethaphan are that it is potent, acts rapidly, and its hypotensive action can be reversed rapidly by stopping the infusion and placing the patient in a Trendelenburg position. However, its adverse effects are many and result from its ganglionic blockade action. These include paralytic ileus, urinary retention, and the development of tachy-

phylaxis. Because of the availability of newer drugs with fewer side effects, trimethaphan is seldom used today.

**Diazoxide (Hyperstat)** is a benzothiadiazine derivative that is closely related chemically to thiazide diuretics.[22,24] Diazoxide exerts its hypotensive effect by reducing arteriolar vascular resistance through direct relaxation of arteriolar smooth muscle. It has little effect on capacitance vessels and no direct effect on the heart or autonomic reflexes. Consequently, when the drug decreases arterial pressure, baroreceptor reflexes are activated, leading to an increase in heart rate, myocardial contractility, stroke volume, and cardiac output. In addition to reflex increased sympathetic activity, diazoxide has several other recognized disadvantages. With the bolus administration of 300 mg of diazoxide, blood pressure may rapidly decrease to normal or even subnormal levels. An alternate method of multiple small intravenous injections of 50 to 100 mg of diazoxide at 10 minute intervals would appear to produce a more controlled reduction in blood pressure.[37] However, the duration of action of diazoxide is from 2 to 12 hours or more, thereby preventing rapid return of blood pressure to baseline levels in the presence of any deterioration in neurologic or cardiac function. It should be noted that diazoxide was used in 79 percent of the reported cases of patients developing neurologic damage in association with reduction of severe hypertension. This occurred commonly in the presence of multiple drug administration, but it was also reported in two patients who had not received any additional antihypertensive therapy. Undoubtedly, the longer duration of action, which caused hypotension to be present for many hours before recovery, played an important role in the neurologic damage sustained by these patients. It would appear, therefore, that diazoxide is not the drug of choice in treating (1) hyperten-

**Table 6-6.** Neurologic Damage Resulting from Acute Lowering of Blood Pressure in Patients with Severe

| Case | Reference | BP on Admission | | Lowest BP after Treatment | | Time to Reach BP Nadir |
| | | Syst/Diast | Mean | Syst/Diast | Mean | |
|---|---|---|---|---|---|---|
| 1. 60 M | Graham[11] | 240/140 | 173 | 120/85 | 97 | 2 Hrs. |
| 2. 35 F | Graham[11] | 240/170 | 193 | Unobtainable | | 1–2 Min. |
| 3. 63 M | Kumar[18] | 290/160 | 203 | Unobtainable | | 15 Min. |
| 4. 11 M | Hulse[13] | 280/190 | 220 | 90/50 | 63 | 24 Hrs. |
| 5. 12 F | Hulse[13] | 270/180 | 220 | 90/60 | 70 | Hrs. |
| 6. 11 M | Hulse[13] | 190/110 | 137 | Not recorded | | ? |
| 7. 30 F | Cove[9] | 270/175 | 207 | 90/50 | 63 | Many Hrs. |
| 8. 32 F | Cove[9] | 250/170 | 197 | 90/70 | 77 | 10 Min. |
| 9. 14 M | Pryor[27] | 240/190 | 207 | 110/10 | 77 | Hrs. |
| 10. 60 M | Ledingham[20] | 240/190 | 207 | 130/90 | 133 | 12 Hrs. |
| 11. 57 M | Ledingham[20] | 220/155 | 179 | 130/80 | 97 | Hrs. |
| 12. 30 M | Ledingham[20] | 220/145 | 170 | 70/40 | 50 | Mins. |
| 13. 56 M | Ledingham[20] | 230/130 | 163 | 120/80 | 93 | 1 Min. |

Hypertension: A Review of the Literature

| Duration of Time at or Near BP Nadir | Presenting Symptoms | K-W Optic Fundi | Treatment | Neurologic Symptoms After Treatment |
|---|---|---|---|---|
| Hrs. | ? | III | Methyldopa<br>Bethadine | Coma; recovered 4 hours later. |
| ?Hrs. | ? | IV | IV pentolineum | |
| ?Min. to Hrs. | Headache, syncope, dizziness | ? | Diazoxide<br>300 mg<br>300 mg | Coma; bilateral Babinski. Recovered with mental impairment<br>Coma; R. hemiparesis—persistent. Gradually regained consciousness. |
| Few Hrs. | Lethargic, headaches, vomiting | IV | Diazoxide<br>Propranolol<br>Hydralazine<br>Furosemide | Coma; pupils dilated and fixed. Within few hours conscious, but with complete loss of vision. |
| 24 Hrs. | Failing vision, drowsy | IV | Diazoxide<br>Methyldopa<br>Thiazide | Restless. Both pupils dilated and fixed. Became completely blind. Flaccid paralysis with gradual recovery. |
| Hrs. | Headaches, vomiting, semiconscious | IV | Diazoxide<br>Propranolol<br>Hydralazine | Blindness, L. homonymous hemianopsia. |
| Many Hrs. | Blurred vision | IV | Methyldopa<br>Propranolol<br>Moduretic® | Confused & drowsy, hallucinations. Complete loss of vision. |
| 3 days | Blurred vision | IV | Diazoxide<br>Atenolol<br>Furosemide | Dilated, fixed pupils. Complete loss of vision. |
| Hrs. | Headache, vomiting, blurred vision | IV | Diazoxide<br>Propranolol<br>Hydralazine | Complete loss of vision. |
| Many Hrs. | Headaches, giddiness, depression | III | Diazoxide<br>Propranolol<br>Furosemide | Confused, disoriented. R. pyramidal signs, eye blind. Recovery over 4 days. |
| Hrs. | Confused, disoriented | IV | Diazoxide<br>Hydralazine<br>Chlorpromazine | Seizure during diazoxide. Residual vision loss & mental impairment. |
| 24 Hrs. | Vomiting, confused and drowsy | IV | Diazoxide<br>Primozine | Seizure, anuria. Died 4 days later of cardiac arrest. |
| Hours | Conscious | IV | Diazoxide<br>300 mg<br>600 mg | Respiratory arrest. Recovered, but with neurological signs refereable to basal ganglia & cerebellum. |

*(continued)*

**Table 6-6.** Neurologic Damage Resulting from Acute Lowering of Blood Pressure in Patients with Severe

| Case | Reference | BP on Admission | | Lowest BP after Treatment | | Time to Reach BP Nadir |
|------|-----------|-----------------|------|---------------------------|------|------------------------|
|      |           | Syst/Diast | Mean | Syst/Diast | Mean | |
| 14. 64 F | Ledingham[20] | 240/130 | 167 | 150/90 | 10 | Days |
| 15. 48 F | Ledingham[20] | 300/190 | 207 | 140/80 | Hrs. | Hrs. |
| 16. 33 M | Ledingham[20] | 250/150 | 183 | 80/60 | 67 | Hrs. |
| 17. 56 M | Ledingham[20] | 210/150 | 170 | 130/80 | 98 | Hrs. |
| 18. 50 M | Ledingham[20] | 210/170 | 183 | 120/75 | 94 | 24 Hrs. |
| 19. 34 F | Ledingham[20] | 250/140 | 177 | 100/70 | 80 | 8 Hrs. |

sive encephalopathy, (2) toxemic crisis, (3) dissecting or leaking aneurysm, (4) refractory hypertension in association with angina or myocardial infarction, evolving cerebral thrombosis, or transient ischemic attacks.[15,25]

**Sodium nitroprusside (Nipride)** is predictably the most effective drug for the treatment of hypertensive emergencies.[8,26] The mechanism of action of sodium nitroprusside is a direct peripheral vasodilatation with a balanced effect on both the capacitance and resistance blood vessels. When administered by intravenous infusion, the antihypertensive effect of nitroprusside is apparent within seconds and is highly dose-dependent. After discontinuation of therapy, blood pressure rises rapidly to previous levels within 1 to 5 minutes. In many centers, nitroprusside has become the drug of choice for maintaining hypotension during surgery because of its ease of admin-

istration and its sparing of sympathetic reflexes. Serious toxicity and death from cyanide accumulation have rarely occurred, and only with a total dose that exceeds 300 mg/hour. Safe maximum doses recommended for short-term use have ranged from 0.5 to 1.5 mg/kg/hour. Since nitroprusside reduces both venous return and afterload, it can be used safely and effectively in the presence of cardiac failure. It can be used in dissecting aneurysms, but should be combined with intravenous propranolol in order to effectively reduce myocardial contractility. It may even be the drug of choice in the treatment of pheochromocytoma in patients who have become refractory to phentolamine.[21]

The following suggested protocol for nitroprusside use appears efficacious.[12] Sodium nitroprusside is supplied as a 50 mg lyophilized powder which can be dissolved in 500 ml of 5 percent dextrose in

Hypertension: A Review of the Literature (continued)

| Duration of Time at or Near BP Nadir | Presenting Symptoms | K-W Optic Fundi | Treatment | Neurologic Symptoms After Treatment |
|---|---|---|---|---|
| Days | "Blackouts," conscious | IV | Diazoxide Reserpine | Coma, pupils dilated & fixed. Bilateral Babinski. Died 36 hours later with progressive hypotension. |
| Hrs. | Irrational, drowsy | IV | Diazoxide IM chlorpromazine | Seizure, oliguria. Bilateral flaccid paralysis. Coma. Arrested 4 days later. |
| Hrs. | Chest pain | III | Diazoxide Hydralazine IV trimethophan | Coma. R. hemiplegia. Left with hemiplegia & mental impairment. |
| Hrs. | Chest pain, dyspnea | IV | Propranolol Hydralazine Moduretic® | Disoriented. L. facial weakness, later dysphagia. Later conscious state improved considerably. |
| 24 Hrs. | Chest pain, drowsiness, confusion | IV | Diazoxide Propranolol Hydralazine | Unrousable. Bilateral Babinksi. Recovered slowly. |
| Hrs. | Headache | IV | Diazoxide Hydralazine Prochlorperazine | Drowsy and disoriented. Signs of meningismus. |

water, yielding a final concentration of 100 μg/ml. Infusions are started at a rate of approximately 0.5 μg/kg body weight/min, using an infusion pump (IVAC, Holter or Harvard pump). There are three phases to nitroprusside administration:

1. Initial titration phase: infusion rates are doubled every 3 to 5 minutes, until blood pressure falls. When this occurs, the infusion can be turned off until the blood pressure begins to turn upward once again.

2. Stabilization phase: The nitroprusside infusion is restarted at rates halfway between the last two values of the titration phase. If there is a fluctuation in blood pressure, the rate is adjusted until the pressure is stabilized.

3. Discontinuation phase: Oral antihypertensive agents are used concurrently with nitroprusside. The nitroprus-

side infusion can be discontinued at 4 to 6 hour intervals to determine new baseline blood pressures and to assess need for continuation of parenteral therapy.

The use of nitroprusside requires careful monitoring of the patient in an intensive care unit and use of an arterial line to accurately monitor blood pressure. Experienced nursing care for assessment of blood pressure and cardiac and neurologic status is necessary to ensure safe management.

Many other drugs have been used to treat hypertensive emergencies in the past, but they do not appear to be ideal agents. Parenteral reserpine was one of the first drugs used in treating hypertensive emergencies. Its slow onset of action, excessive lowering of blood pressure to shocklike levels, prolonged duration of action, and marked sedation and somnolence are strong contraindica-

**Table 6-7.** Summary of Characteristics in Patients Developing Neurological Damage after Acute Lowering of Severe Hypertension

| |
| --- |
| Severe antecedent hypertension |
|   Mean BP 188 ± 19 mm Hg; systolic BP 244 ± 28 mm Hg; diastolic BP 156 ± 21 mm Hg. |
|   Grade IV K-W optic fundi 79% (15/19 Pts.) |
|   Hypertensive encephalopathy 53% (10/19 Pts.) |
| Excessive reduction of BP |
|   Mean BP 84 ± 18 mm Hg, systolic BP 110 ± 23 mm Hg; diastolic BP 70 ± 15 mm Hg. |
|   Mean BP reduction: 56 ± 12%. |
| Speed of lowering BP |
|   Rapid (minutes) 26% (15/19 Pts.) |
|   Slow (many hours) 74% (14/19 Pts.) |
| Duration of low BP |
|   Many hours to days 100% (19/19 Pts.) |
| Neurologic complications |
|   Blindness 47% (9/19 Pts.) |
|   Coma 32% (6/19 Pts.) |
|   Pyramidal tract signs 32% (6/19 Pts.) |
|   Residual neurologic signs 58% (11/19 Pts.) |
|   Death 16% (3/19 Pts.) |
| Type of therapy |
|   IV bolus diazoxide 79% (15/19 Pts.) |
|     with other anihypertensive therapy 87% (13/15 Pts.) |
|     no other antihypertensive agents 13% (2/15 Pts.) |
|   Oral multiple antihypertensive agents 16% (3/19 Pts.) |

(Data from references 9, 11, 13, 18, 20, 27.)

tions to its use. Angiotensin-blocking agents, both competitive antagonists and converting enzyme inhibitors, have been shown to decrease blood pressure dramatically in severely hypertensive patients.[17] Similarly, calcium entry blockers are also effective in this regard.[4] However, these agents have the drawbacks of poor control of the rate of blood pressure reduction and long duration of action, which make them less useful than nitroprusside in the final titration of blood pressure to optimal levels in a true hypertensive crises.

For the uregnt hypertensive patient (Table 6-5C) the administration of antihypertensive therapy by intravenous infusion is most often not necessary. At the present time, oral clonidine loading (i.e., 0.2 mg of clonidine given orally, followed by 0.1 mg hourly for several hours, or until blood pressure has reached the desired level) has been used effectively and safely in the management of urgent hypertension.[1] Because clonidine is a central alpha$_2$ agonist, there is no interfer-

ence with normal baroreceptor reflex control of blood pressure. Angiotensin-converting enzyme inhibitors and the oral calcium entry blockers have also been used successfully for urgent hypertension.[14,17] Long-term studies will be necessary to compare the efficacy and safety of these various agents.

## Defining the Level to Which the Blood Pressure Should Be Reduced

From the preceding discussion, it is obvious that blood pressure ought not be reduced to values below the autoregulatory range for cerebral and myocardial blood flow. Studies done by Strandgaard (see above) suggest that cerebral blood flow is maintained in the normal range if hypertensive pressures are not reduced to mean values below 120 mm Hg.[30,31] This value of 120 mm Hg is two standard deviations greater than the mean blood pressure found in patients sustaining iatrogenic neurologic damage (Table 6-7).

Therefore, an initial blood pressure reduction to a mean value of 130 to 120 mm Hg, which translates into a blood pressure of 170/110 to 160/100, respectively, would appear to be a safe level for initial blood pressure reduction. There may be a rare patient who develops deteriorating neurologic symptoms at this level, especially if there is an unrecognized completed stroke in association with accelerated malignant hypertension; the discontinuation of a nitroprusside infusion would then allow rapid return of blood pressure to previous baseline levels, hopefully thereby, preventing irreversible neurologic damage.

# SUMMARY

When antihypertensive therapy induces neurologic deterioration in patients with severe hypertension, the problem is not only one of excessive lowering of blood pressure, but also of inaccurate diagnosis and improper drug selection and use. The physician must use clinical judgment in deciding which patient has a true hypertensive emergency, and which patient has less severe, urgent hypertension, which can be lowered more slowly and with oral agents. Thus, accurate diagnosis determines: (1) selection of the route of administration, (2) selection of a specific agent, (3) the need for special monitoring, and (4) determination of how rapid the initial lowering of blood pressure should be.

In the true hypertensive emergency, blood pressure should be lowered in a controlled manner to intermediate blood pressure levels below the danger level of hypertensive catastrophe, but above the level of impaired autoregulatory control of cerebral and myocardial blood flow. This is best achieved by using parenteral drugs which can be given via slow infusion in a controlled manner, by using a drug that has a rapid onset and offset of action, and by using it in a setting where optimal monitoring of myocardial and cerebral function can be achieved, that is in an intensive care unit with specially trained nurses in attendance. A review of the literature suggests that parenteral diazoxide does not have the ideal properties for optimal blood pressure control, and indeed, has been associated with a significant number of neurologic complications when used in patients with hypertensive emergencies. In contrast, sodium nitroprusside would appear to be a safer agent and the drug of choice in a variety of hypertensive emergency states.

In the true hypertensive emergency, the rate at which the blood pressure is lowered should be dictated simply by the speed of the nitroprusside titration (see above). It generally takes 20 to 60 minutes to smoothly achieve a mean pressure of 120 mm Hg.

# REFERENCES

1. Anderson RJ, Hart GR, Crumpler CP, et al: Oral clonidine loading in hypertensive urgencies. JAMA 246:848, 1981.
2. Auer L: The role of cerebral perfusion pressure as origin of brain edema in acute arterial hypertension. Eur Neurol 15:153, 1977.
3. Becker CE, Benowitz NL: Hypertensive emergencies. Med Clin North Amer 63:127, 1979.
4. Beer N, Gallegos I, Cohen A, et al: Efficacy of sublingual nifedipine in the acute treatment of systemic hypertension. Chest 79:571, 1981.
5. Bhatia SK, Frohlich ED: Hemodynamic comparison of agents useful in hypertensive emergencies. Am Heart J 85:367, 1973.
6. Britton M, de Faire U, Helmers C: Hazards of therapy for excessive hypertension in acute stroke. Acta Med Scand 207:253, 1980.
7. Chobanian AV: Ten hypertensive crises:

When to lower blood pressure immediately. Mod Med 47:40, 1979.

8. Cohn JN, Burke LP: Nitroprusside. Ann Intern Med 91:752, 1979.

9. Cove DH, Seddon M, Fletcher RF, et al: Blindness after treatment for malignant hypertension. Br Med J 2:246, 1979.

10. deCarvalho JGR, Messerli FH, Frohlich ED: Treatment of hypertensive emergencies. Drug Therapy, March 107, 1979.

11. Graham DI: Ischemic brain damage of cerebral perfusion failure type after treatment of severe hypertension. Br Med J 2:739, 1975.

12. Grim CE: Emergency treatment of severe or malignant hypertension. Geriatrics December 57, 1980.

13. Hulse JA, Taylor DSI, Dillon MJ: Blindness and paraplegia in severe childhood hypertension. Lancet 2:553, 1979.

14. Johannson B, Strandgaard S, Lassen NA: On the pathogenesis of hypertensive encephalopathy—The hypertensive "breakthrough" of autoregulation of cerebral blood flow with forced vasodilatation, flow increase, and blood-brain-barrier damage. Circ Res Suppl 1, 34:1, 1974.

15. Kanada SA, Kanada DJ, Hutchinson RA, et al: Anginalike syndrome with diazoxide therapy for hypertensive crisis. Ann Intern Med 84:696, 1976.

16. Kincaid-Smith P: Malignant hypertension. Cardiovasc Rev 1:42, 1980.

17. Koch-Weser J: Current concepts:Hypertensive emergencies. N Engl J Med 290:211, 1974.

18. Kumar GK, Dastoor FC, Rabayo JR, et al: Side effects of diazoxide. JAMA 235:275, 1976.

19. Lassen NA, Agnoli A: Editorial: The upper limit of autoregulation of cerebral blood flow—On the pathogenesis of hypertensive encephalopathy. Scand J Clin Lab Invest 30:113, 1972.

20. Ledingham JGG, Rajagopalan B: Cerebral complications in the treatment of accererated hypertension. Q J Med 189:25, 1979.

21. Lipson A, Hsu T-H, Sherwin B, et al: Nitroprusside therapy for a patient with pheochromocytoma. JAMA 239:427, 1978.

22. McDonald WJ, Smith G, Woods JW, et al: Intravenous diazoxide therapy in hypertensive crisis. J Cardiol 40:409, 1977.

23. Meyer JS, Teraura T, Marx P, et al: Brain swelling due to experimental cerebral infarction. Brain 95:833, 1972.

24. Miller WE, Gifford RW Jr, Humphrey DV, et al: Management of severe hypertension with intravenous injections of diazoxide. Am J Cardiol 24:870, 1969.

25. O' Brien KP, Grigor RR, Taylor PM: Intravenous diazoxide in treatment of hypertension associated with recent myocardial infarction. Br Med J 4:74, 1975.

26. Palmer RF, Lasseter KS: Drug therapy: Sodium nitroprusside. N Engl J Med 292:294, 1975.

27. Pryor JS, Davies PD, Hamilton DV: Blindness and malignant hypertension. Lancet 2:803, 1979.

28. Segal JL: Hypertensive emergencies—practical approach to treatment. Postgrad Med 68:107, 1980.

29. Skinhøj E, Strangaard S: Pathogenesis of hypertensive encephalopathy. Lancet 2:461, 1973.

30. Strandgaard S, Olesen J, Skinhøj E, Lassen NA: Autoregulation of brain circulation in severe arterial hypertension. Br Med J 1:507, 1973.

31. Strandgaard S: Autoregulation of cerebral blood flow in hypertensive patients. The modifying influence of prolonged antihypertensive treatment on the tolerance to acute, drug-induced hypotension. Circulation 53:720, 1976.

32. Sundt TM Jr, Waltz AG: Cerebral ischemia and reactive hyperemia—Studies of cortical blood flow and microcirculation before, during and after temporary occlusion of middle cerebral artery of squirrel monkeys. Circ Res 28:426, 1971.

33. The treatment of malignant hypertension and hypertensive emergencies (editorial). JAMA 228:1673, 1974.

34. Vaamonde CA, David JD, Palmer RF: Hypertensive emergencies. Med Clin North Am 55:325, 1971.

35. Vidt DG: Managing the hypertensive emergency. Urban Health June, 15, 1979.

36. Vidt DG, Bravo EL, Fouad FM: Drug Therapy:Capropril. N Engl J Med 306:214, 1982.

37. Wilson DJ, Vidt DG: Control of severe hypertension with pulse doses of diazoxide. Clin Pharmacol Ther 23:135, 1978.

# Section III

# Controversies in Diagnosing Renal-Metabolic Disorders

# 7

# How Important Is Renal Biopsy in Managing Patients with Renal Disease?

# The Case for Its Aggressive Use

## David T. Lowenthal, M.D.
## Steven D. Saris, M.D.

## INTRODUCTION

Even though percutaneous renal biopsies have been performed in many centers for the past 30 years, controversy still exists over the safety and importance of this test.[11,31,42,45] In the 1950s, the question was: Is this procedure safe?[7] In the 1960s, the question was: Can we get any information from the biopsy? And, now the question is: Do we need the information? The answer to these questions is, emphatically, "Yes!" Clearly, not all patients with renal disease need a kidney biopsy since biopsies give us better information in certain disorders than others. The use of kidney biopsy as an agent for assessing renal disease can be of use with regard to the diagnosis, prognosis, and treatment of the individual patient.

In this chapter we will not discuss the role of renal biopsy in the early management (postoperative) of the transplant patient. Similarly, we will not argue the case of whether kidney biopsy is a valuable research tool since there can be no question that it is the "gold standard" for diagnosing and following the natural course and response to therapy of various renal diseases. We will consider, however, the general indications for biopsy (Table 7-1) and discuss the importance of biopsy in specific disease states such as systemic lupus erythematosus (SLE) and diabetes mellitus, as well as clinical situations such as proteinuria, hematuria, and renal insufficiency. The potential risks and complications associated with kidney biopsies are also considered.

## PREBIOPSY EVALUATION (See Table 7-2)

Prebiopsy evaluation is of prime importance. If the diagnosis can be established prior to biopsy and all other potentially treatable diseases are excluded, then the need for tissue can be avoided. Michael states that in his study of recurrent hematuria that biopsy may actually reduce the number of blood tests and radiologic studies required by the patient.[32] By establishing the diagnosis other studies can be avoided (even though the disease itself may be untreatable) and thereby save the patient time and expense.

An attempt was made to predict biopsy results using clinical criteria by Frey[15] et al. and by the International Study of Kidney Disease in Children.[38] Frey[15] suggests that membrano-proliferative glomerulonephritis may be differentiated from minimal change disease if one considers selectivity of proteinuria along with the presence of hematuria and hypocomplementemia. This is valuable information since minimal change disease in children is highly responsive to steroids. However, these findings are unfortunately nonspecific, overlapping with other causes of nephrotic syndrome such as focal sclerosis, epimembraneous glomerulonephritis,

**Table 7-1.** Indications for Percutaneous Renal Biopsy

Diagnosis
    Etiology
    Immunology
    Microbiology
Prognosis
    Histology and natural history
    Extent of structural damage
    Reversibility
    Recurrence in transplant
Treatment
    Specific therapy
    Response to therapy

and rapidly progressive glomerulonephritis. Therefore, these prebiopsy test results are really not very useful.

The most valuable prebiopsy evaluation is for hematuria. Extrarenal causes for blood loss and gross renal abnormalities must be excluded prior to biopsy of renal tissue by investigation of the coagulation system, arteriographically for intrarenal structural abnormalities and tumors, and cystoscopically for lower urinary tract causes of hematuria.

# DIAGNOSTIC INDICATIONS

## General Aspects

It is understandable that there are clinicians who honestly question the importance of making a definitive diagnosis in every patient. Without a diagnosis, however, we would resemble 19th-century physicians who had nothing better to offer patients than platitudes and a shoulder for lacrimation. Fairley[13] and Kincaid-Smith[24] made histopathological diagnoses in 266 cases out of 300 biopsy attempts. These results are similar to other previously reported large series. A more recent study by Paone and Meyer reported that of 89 adequate biopsy specimens, 77 afforded a diagnosis.[34] Therefore, it is evident that in spite of 30 years of experience and improvements, biopsy

is still not perfect but often it is the only way to make a correct diagnosis.

Parrish and Howe[35] reported that in 100 successful needle biopsies a diagnosis could not be made in only 9 percent. However, biopsy confirmed the clinical impression in 39 percent and most importantly, biopsy actually established the diagnosis in 52 percent of cases. A summary of Parrish and Howe's results is listed in Table 7-3. They found that the incorrect diagnosis was most often made in patients with hypertension, nephrosclerosis, and diabetes mellitus. They report that the prebiopsy diagnosis was correct anywhere from 20 to 100 percent of the time and, once the pathologic diagnosis was confirmed by biopsy, the clinician had a new diagnosis approximately 50 percent of the time. For example, of the 18 patients thought to have acute glomerulonephritis (AGN) prior to biopsy, only 16 were actually shown to have it. There were 20 patients in the study with biopsy proven AGN; 16 were correctly diagnosed (clinically), prior to biopsy and in 4 the clinical diagnosis had not been considered. Therefore, 89 percent of the patients were diagnosed correctly as having AGN clinically but 20 percent of AGN diagnosed histologically was missed clinically.

A more extreme example is diabetic glomerulosclerosis. This disorder was overdiagnosed, with only 20 percent of clinically suspected cases being confirmed on biopsy. Conversely, one-third of biopsy proven cases were unsuspected clinically. This report makes a very strong argument for doing renal biopsies.

Determining the etiology of a disease is the cornerstone for developing rational treatment. Renal biopsy, for example, may serve as the first indication of nephrotoxic renal failure, as caused by heavy metals, uric acid, and organic solvents. Similarly, acute interstitial nephritis caused by nonsteroidal antiinflamma-

**Table 7-2.** Clinical Renal Biopsy Report

Patient
    Age:               Surg Acession No.:    Kidney Biopsied:
    Hospital & No.      Date Obtained:        _____ Right _____Left
    Clinical Diagnosis    Doctor:
History of present illness:

Past history (occurrence and duration)
    Proteinuria:        Kidney Pain:      Arthritis:
    Hematuria:         Edema:           Rash:
    U.T. Infection:      Hypertension:     Toxemia:
                                Deafness:
Family History
    Diabetes:         Allergic History:    Deafness:
    Kidney Disease:    Hypertension:      Other:
Physical: General Condition
    BP:              Wt:              Ht:            T:
    Fundi:          Effusions:       Edema:        Rash:
    Arthritis:       Hepatomegaly:                 Splenomegaly:
    Palpable Kidneys:   Other Pertinent Findings:
Lab Data:
    Hgb:          FDP:           Albumin:      Phosphorus:
    Hct:          ASO Titer:      Globulin:      Glucose:
    WBC:        FANA:        Electrophoresis:  Na:
    Diff:         Rheum. Factor:   $\alpha 1\_\_\alpha 2\_\_\beta\_\_\gamma\_\_$  K:
      N__L__M__B__E__  Coomb's Test:    IgG__IgA__IgM__  Bicarb:
    Sed Rate:      BUN:          C'Profile:     Alk Phosphatase:
    Platelets:      Creat:         C3__C4__C3PA__  VDRL:
    Pro. Time:     Uric Acid:      C3NeF:       HBsAg:
    APTT:        Cholesterol     Calcium:      Cryoglobulin:
Urine:
    pH:           RBC's:                         Casts: Hyaline:
    Sp gr:        WBC's:                            Granular:
    Albumin      Epith Cells:                      RBC:
    Sugar:        OFB:                           WBC:
    Acetone:                                      Other:
Renal Function:
    Creat Clearance:   ml/min/1.73 m$^2$            IVP:

    24-hour Urine Protein:                    Kidney Size by X-Ray:
    24-hour Urine Volume:
    Protein Selectivity:
Cultures
    Urine:        Throat:         Blood:       Other:
Therapy
    Antibiotics:    Dialysis:                  Analgesics:
    Steroids:      Type:                   Transfusions:
    Diuretics:     Date:                   Mannitol:
                 Duration:                 Heavy metals:
                                    Cytotoxins:

    This clinical renal biopsy report is submitted with the renal biopsy specimen to facilitate accurate clinicopathologic correlation.
    (From Jenis EH, Lowenthal DT: Kidney Biopsy Interpretation. Philadelphia, F.A. Davis, 1976, p. 2.)

tory drugs[6] and such antibiotics as penicillin, methicillin, and ampicillin is diagnosed with assuredness only after biopsy. Indeed, biopsy confirmation of drug-induced acute interstitial nephritis ought to be obtained before permanently proscribing use of potentially life-saving drugs.

**Table 7-3.** Summary of Results

| | Diagnosed clinically | Correct | Correct (%) | Diagnosed Pathologically | Missed clinically | Missed clinically (%) |
|---|---|---|---|---|---|---|
| Normal | 3 | 3 | 100 | 10 | 7 | 67 |
| Acute glomerulonephritis | 18 | 16 | 89 | 20 | 4 | 20 |
| Chronic glomerulonephritis | 25 | 10 | 40 | 15 | 5 | 33 |
| Pyelonephritis | 10 | 6 | 60 | 10 | 4 | 40 |
| Nephrosclerosis | 6 | 4 | 50 | 24 | 20 | 90 |
| Malignant nephrosclerosis | 1 | 0 | 0 | 3 | 3 | 100 |
| Hemaglobinuric nephrosis | 2 | 2 | 100 | 4 | 2 | 50 |
| Diabetic glomerulosclerosis | 15 | 3 | 20 | 3 | 1 | 33 |

(From Parrish, A.E., Howe, J.S.: Kidney biopsy: A review of one hundred successful needle biopsies. Arch Intern Med 96:712, 1955. Copyright 1955, American Medical Association.)

The characteristic eosinophilic infiltration of the interstitium may be found.[25,30] Clinically, skin rash, eosinophilia, urinary eosiniphils, and a history of drug exposure may obviate the need for biopsy.

Occasionally a patient will appear to have some ill-defined systemic disease that cannot be diagnosed because laboratory results are nonspecific. Yet the kidney will be affected as gleaned from observing abnormal urine or blood chemistries. In this situation, the kidney biopsy may provide the first clue to the diagnosis of vasculitis, amyloidosis, or light chain disease which would otherwise be missed. Lynn et al. describe this in lupus as well.[28]

It is very important to determine the pathogenesis[8] of the disease even if the exact diagnosis is not established. With the development of plasmapheresis and immunosuppressive drugs, it is imperative to seek out immune complex deposits in the kidney biopsy.[27] Removal of circulating immune complexes or prevention of their formation may prove therapeutic. Regardless of whether the kidney is the specific antigenic stimulus for antibody formation or simply an "innocent bystander" (being damaged by immune complexes formed at extrarenal sites), histologic identification of these pathogenetic forces may influence therapy. The histopathologic diagnosis of membranous glomerulonephritis (MGN) may be primary or secondary to many systemic diseases, for example, connective-tissue disorders, diabetes mellitus and malignancy. Indeed, MGN and the nephrotic syndrome may be a harbinger of an occult lymphoma or carcinoma.[12]

Renal biopsy has been used in the past to confirm the diagnosis of pyelonephritis and cultures of the tissue have been used to identify the offending organism. Improved bacteriologic studies and development of more effective antibiotics have excluded pyelonephritis as an indication for biopsy today. In fact, infection is often listed as a relative contraindication to biopsy.

### Specific Disorders

**Proteinuria.** The clinician is frequently faced with a number of syndromes in which the need for kidney biopsy is considered (Table 7-4).

Proteinuria may be discovered on routine urinalysis even though the patient is asymptomatic. If 24-hour protein excretion is less than one gram or if protein excretion is posture dependent, then kidney biopsy is not necessary and the proteinuria should simply be followed at regular intervals. Protein excretion greater than one gram per day, however, is often associated with structural disease, and biopsy is recommended.

**Table 7-4.** Principal Indications for Renal Biopsy

| Clinical syndrome | Indications for biopsy |
|---|---|
| Asymptomatic proteinuria | Protein excretion more than 1 g/24 hours. |
| | Red blood cells in urine. |
| | Impaired renal function. |
| Asymptomatic hematuria | Intravenous pyelogram and cystoscopy do not show source. |
| | Proteinuria also present. |
| Unexplained azotemia | Persistant oliguria. |
| Nephrotic syndrome | Adults: unless cause is apparent from extrarenal manifestations; proteinuria usually is non-selective. |
| | Children: only if hematuria also present, or if proteinuria persists after trial of corticosteriod; proteinuria usually selective. |
| Acute renal failure | No obvious precipitating cause. |
| | Extrarenal obstruction excluded. |
| Chronic renal failure | Radiographically normal kidneys. |

Occult malignancy is now recognized as a not infrequent cause of MGN, making newly discovered proteinuria in the elderly a potentially ominous finding.[12] It follows that the biopsy diagnosis of MGN may lead to the discovery of a potentially curable form of cancer. Current evidence suggests that a brief, temporary period lasting 2 months of alternate day steroid therapy slows or prevents later deterioration of renal function in patients with idiopathic MGN.[9] Thus, in these two instances, histologic diagnosis strongly influences patient management and could profoundly improve prognosis. If proteinuria is associated with hematuria and/or impaired renal function, the prognosis is more ominous and biopsy is recommended.

When daily protein excretion is greater than 3.5 g, it is usually associated with other manifestations of the nephrotic syndrome. Nephrotic syndrome is a common problem in renal medicine and its differential diagnosis includes a long list of secondary systemic disorders afflicting the kidney as well as a variety of primary, intrinsic renal diseases. Diabetes and amyloidosis are common causes of this disorder. If these diagnoses can be confirmed by other means, biopsy may not be necessary. However, there are many other causes which can only be confirmed by biopsy. The major reason for examining renal tissue is that several causes of nephrotic syndrome are readily treatable.

Nephrotic syndrome in children is usually associated with selective proteinuria and is responsive to steroids. However, the diagnosis of minimal change disease is a pathologic diagnosis and is only made after observing normal or minimally altered glomeruli on routine stains and by seeing foot process fusion on electron microscopy. If proteinuria in a child persists after a trial of steroids or if hematuria is present, biopsy should be performed.

Adults with nephrotic syndrome usually have nonselective proteinuria and biopsy should be performed unless there is a clear-cut diagnosis apparent from extrarenal manifestations.

**Hematuria.**[32] Bleeding can originate from any portion of the urinary tract. Therefore, kidney biopsy should only be considered when intravenous pyelogram, culture, and cystoscopy are negative. If proteinuria is associated with hematuria, or if the red cells are in casts, then renal origin is much more likely and biopsy should be performed.

Paone found that none of his patients biopsied for hematuria alone had any change in therapy and half of the biopsies were nondiagnostic.[34] This does not agree with the work of Michael[32] who biopsed 33 patients with hematuria. Eighteen of these patients had glomerular deposits of IgA. This suggests that biopsy is a high-yield procedure once urine culture, X-ray and cystoscopy are shown to be negative. Early histologic diagnosis may prevent further expensive and potentially dangerous investigative procedures.

The significance and prognosis of IgA nephropathy associated with hematuria is uncertain at this time. Early reports suggesting IgA nephropathy was a benign condition have now been challenged.[20] Biopsy will help define the prevalence, natural history, and response to therapy of this disorder.

Marked increase in glomerular hematuria in patients with membranoproliferative glomerulonephritis or MGN could signal the onset of rapidly progressive glomerulonephritis. Biopsy will clarify whether this clinical diagnosis is accurate. If there is a change in histology, pulse steroid therapy or plasmapheresis may be of benefit.

**Renal Failure.** The precipitating cause(s) of acute renal failure is (are) often evident from the history and physical examination. On occasion, however, no precipitating event can be found or, conversely, several possible etiologic factors may be present but the importance of each may not be easily discerned. In this situation kidney biopsy will often be helpful. Azotemia with persistent oliguria has a very poor prognosis. Biopsy may confirm the cause (e.g., postinfectious, drug-induced) and thereby lead to effective therapy and a more knowledgeable definition of prognosis.

Biopsy will also be useful in the diagnosis of patients with chronic renal failure if the patient has normal-sized or enlarged kidneys. Biopsy of small shrunken kidneys is rarely diagnostic because end-stage kidneys are usually too

scarred for diagnostic considerations to be evaluated.

**Systemic Lupus Erythematosus**[36]. Probably the most controversial aspect of kidney biopsy concerns its importance in the diagnosis and management of lupus nephritis. Lynn et al. reported four cases of lupus presenting with manifestations of renal damage in the absence of systemic signs and symptoms.[28] Lupus nephritis would not have been diagnosed unless a biopsy had been performed. While there is little argument that this type of patient requires a tissue diagnosis, more controversy surrounds the management of the patient whose diagnosis has been made on clinical and chemical grounds? Should these patients have a biopsy regardless of whether they manifest signs of renal damage? Freis et al.[16] admit that the biopsy does yield important prognostic information but in their view it is only of marginal benefit and adds little to the clinical information. The problem with Freis' report is that only those patients already doing poorly were biopsied. Thus, by selecting patients with more obvious clinical deterioration, it is not surprising that the biopsy did not strikingly add to the patient's evaluation and management. One of the four studies reviewed by Freis actually did better in defining prognosis by biopsy than with the clinical data. Most importantly, Freis' report only addresses the question of biopsy as a prognostic indicator. The question of its role in diagnosis or treatment of histologic subtype is not dealt with.

Mahajan et al. studied renal biopsies in 90 consecutive patients with SLE.[29] All 90 patients had histologic changes consistent with lupus nephritis and 27 of these patients had no abnormalities of urine or of blood chemistries. Diffuse proliferative glomerulonephritis (DPGN) was found in more than 50 percent of the patients and it had the worst prognosis regardless of whether the patient had clinical manifestations or not. Twelve of the 27 patients without signs or symptoms of renal involvement had DPGN. Thus, 26 percent of all patients with DPGN did not manifest any urinary or serum abnormality at the time of study. DPGN in SLE is an indication for steroid therapy in many centers.

When intramembraneous deposits are seen by electron microscopy such aggressive therapies as plasmapheresis and immunosuppressive agents are often added. A patient with SLE manifesting proteinuria, cylindruria, hematuria with or without azotemia, could have focal DPGN or MGN. Since focal and membranous nephritis do not respond to steroid therapy, many, if not most, nephrologists and rheumatologists require a renal biopsy to rationally devise therapy.

Therefore, renal biopsy is an essential step in the evaluation of the patient with lupus because it will assist in the initial diagnosis, the evaluation of the extent of involvement and finally, it will help determine the best treatment for SLE.

**Diabetes Mellitus.** Renal biopsy has advanced our understanding of the pathogenesis and natural history of diabetic glomerulosclerosis, but most agree that the proteinuric diabetic without another apparent cause of renal disease need not be biopsied. The great frequency with which glomerulosclerosis complicates diabetes and our current lack of effective therapy, make biopsy an unnecessary invasive procedure in this setting. Parrish,[35] however, reports that renal biopsy substantiated the clinical diagnosis of diabetic glomerulosclerosis in only 20 percent of patients while 33 percent with histologically confirmed diabetic glomerulosclerosis were misdiagnosed clinically (Table 7-2). Whether clinicians would do

as badly in 1984 as in Parrish's 1955 study is a matter for speculation.

In summary, the course of diabetes mellitus and its complications follow a well-described pattern. In general, renal biopsy is not required to diagnose classic diabetic nephropathy. Development of proteinuria or renal failure early in the course of diabetes mellitus especially in the absence of retinopathy is, in our view, indication for renal biopsy, since diabetic nephropathy is less likely in this setting.[43]

**Nephrotic Syndrome**[47]: The International Study of Kidney Disease in Children,[38] a prospective epidemiological study, has suggested various criteria for the clinical diagnosis of the underlying glomerulopathology. This is especially valuable in those children whose nephrotic syndrome is associated with minimal change nephropathy .Furthermore, it has been shown that a biopsy can be valuable in anticipating the response prior to therapy when the clinical course has demonstrated a relapsing pattern wherein cyclophosphamide may be preferable to corticosteroids. Laboratory and clinical characteristics may help discriminate minimal change from other forms of glomerulonephropathies.[47] The absence of hypertension and the presence of hypercholesterolemia greater than 550 mg/dl may favor minimal change nephropathy. On the other hand, selectivity of proteinuria, the elevated plasma concentration of complement (C3), and the presence of hematuria were used to distinguish minimal change from mesangioproliferative glomerulonephritis. Corticosteroid therapy may slow the progression of renal dysfunction in membranous nephropathy, whereas its utility in focal sclerosis and mesangioproliferative glomerulonephritis is quite poor. However, the ultimate prognosis of these three diseases is similar and worsened but the presence of nephrotic syndrome rather than any particular characteristic on biopsy.

**Interstitial Nephritis:**[25,30] Tubulointerstitial nephropathy can occur as a prominent component of glomerular disease. Chronic progressive tubulointerstitial disease has often been mislabeled *chronic pyelonephritis* and often times is not attributable to an acute or chronic bacterial infection.[3] As in glomerular diseases some forms of tubulointerstitial nephropathy may have an immunological pathogenesis.[30] This has been demonstrated to be true in disorders due to hypersensitivity, for example, sulfonamides, penicillin, methicillin, drug-induced disorders. Immunologically mediated tubulointerstitial disease has been identified in transplant rejection, Sjögren's syndrome, and amyloidosis. On the other hand, chronic progressive disorders such as hereditary familial nephritis has a characteristic pathologic appearance and the diagnosis of Alport's syndrome can be made by renal biopsy.[20] Thus, there are various disorders involving the tubulointerstitial portion of the kidney which are primary abnormalities and confirmation of clinical impressions can be best achieved by renal biopsy.

# PROGNOSTIC INDICATIONS

Even though the diagnosis of multiple myeloma, SLE or diabetes mellitus may already be known, a kidney biopsy may still be indicated in order to determine the specific histology. The histologic information that has accrued from following the natural history of various diseases has indicated that certain histologic subtypes of a given disease carry a better prognosis than others. This be-

comes even more confusing since there is a possibility that histology can change over time and serial biopsies will be required in order to adequately manage the patients.

Fordham found that three histopathologists agreed well on the severity of the disease but they did not agree as well on the exact histologic diagnosis.[14] More importantly, however, the grading of disease severity correlated better with the clinical course than the prebiopsy blood chemistries would have suggested. They concluded, and we agree, that biopsy is a better predictor of future course than are blood chemistries.

By assessing the extent of structural damage, one can predict the reversibility of the disease process. Reversibility of disease was of prime significance in the early days of dialysis. The argument was that if the patient had reversible disease, dialysis was offered on a temporary basis. Irreversible disease, however, would necessitate chronic maintenance dialysis which was not readily available. Although this is no longer the case, it is still important to know the extent of renal damage to determine if chronic dialysis will become necessary. Armed with this information physicians can prepare patients both physically and emotionally.

Proteinuria, nephrotic syndrome, and azotemia during pregnancy may pose diagnostic and prognostic dilemmas.[24,26] Focal sclerosis[16,19] may adversely affect survival of renal allografts and various causes of interstitial nephritis[25] may confer a poor prognosis similar to glomerular disorders. These specific issues are addressed below.

## Pregnancy

Generally, physicians are reluctant to perform percutaneous renal biopsy during pregnancy due to early reports of an increased incidence of bleeding.[26] Therefore, our information concerning morphologic changes during pregnancy is somewhat limited. Nevertheless, Lindheimer and Katz[26] are quite specific in their recommendations for renal biopsy in women with renal complications of pregnancy. They suggested that biopsy is necessary when acute or chronic renal failure occurs in the first 34 weeks of gestation. Twenty percent of women who present with what appears to be preeclampsia actually have other renal lesions. Kincaid-Smith and Fairley[23] performed renal biopsy on 123 pregnant women with proteinuria. Thirty-seven percent had glomerulonephritis on biopsy. They found that arteriolar and immunologic changes did not adequately differentiate preeclampsia from glomerulonephritis. It there was even one glomerulus with hyalinization, sclerosis or fibrosis then glomerulonephritis was confirmed on biopsy and future prognosis was consistent with this diagnosis.

In their recommendations, Lindheimer and Katz[26] suggest steroid therapy for glomerular disease characterized by epithelial changes (other than preeclampsia) but no steroids if there is solely membranous changes. They also recommend discontinuance of pregnancy if there are arteriolar changes of preeclampsia at 28 to 32 weeks of gestation. Finally, they state that vascular changes indicate that future pregnancies are more hazardous.[24] Therefore, biopsy definitely can be useful in the diagnosis, prognosis, and treatment of the renal complications of pregnancy. When possible, every effort should be made to delay biopsy until after delivery, when complications of the procedure are reduced.

### Focal Sclerosis

Focal glomerulosclerosis[19,20] generally pursues a progressive downhill course to renal failure with persistent or recurrent episodes of proteinuria, hematuria, and the nephrotic syndrome. The actuarial five-year and ten-year survival rates are 60 to 70 percent and 10 to 50 percent, respectively. The disease is in general steroid resistant. Thus, it becomes important to distinguish the presence of this disorder from other causes of hematuria and nephrotic syndrome which may have very different prognoses.

### Transplantation

Renal transplantation is becoming an increasingly popular form of treatment for young patients with chronic renal failure. A question that is frequently raised is whether the primary renal disease will recur in the transplanted kidney. In diseases such as Goodpasture's syndrome, transplantation is not recommended as long as circulating antiglomerular basement membrane activity persists. A recent report suggests that if a transplant survives long enough, certain disorders will recur, for example, focal sclerosis, IgA nephropathy[1,17] and mesangial proliferative glomerulonephritis.[40] Therefore, kidney biopsy aids in the prognostic evaluation of patients being considered for renal transplantation.

Tubulointerstitial disorders[25] with a poor prognosis include analgesic abuse, radiation nephritis, disorders due to neoplasms, for example, leukemia, lymphoma, and multiple myeloma, and reflux nephropathy.[18] Renal biopsy can be of obvious help in identifying the presence and extent of renal involvement in these settings.

## THERAPEUTIC INDICATIONS

The common belief today is that biopsy, as well as any diagnostic study, should be performed only if it is going to affect patient management. We wholeheartedly agree, however, that treatment should be based on definite evidence and not mere statistical probability.

Kark and Muehrcke are convinced that each biopsy affects their patient's management.[21,22] Paone[34] reported that in 100 consecutive cases only 19 patients had a change in therapy as a direct result of the renal biopsy report. This does not mean that 81 percent of the biopsies are useless. It simply means that either the patient was already on the appropriate therapy or that therapy was not indicated. Also, it is important to point out that results of the kidney biopsy will affect the vigor with which one treats an individual patient.

Another reason to perform a kidney biopsy is to determine whether a given treatment is actually ameliorating the disease process. This is particularly true in disorders like SLE in which clinical parameters do not adequately reflect renal histologic changes.

The nephrologist's therapeutic armamentarium is just beginning to expand. Steroids have been the mainstay of therapy for vasculitis,[44] immune-complex glomerular and tubulointerstitial disorders yet there is a raging debate concerning their efficacy and indications. Much of this debate has been based on histologic diagnosis, without which a rational decision to use steroids is not possible. Cytotoxic agents such as azathioprine and cyclophosphamide are now being used more than ever in diseases such as Wegener's granulomatisis and biopsy is the best way to make the diagnosis and determine the need for these medications.

Fordham suggests that biopsy is a better predictor of prognosis and response to steroids in nephrotic syndrome than are clinical criteria.[14] Similarly, Seigel[39] reports that biopsy predicts the response to cyclophosphamide in relapsing minimal change disease more accurately than clinical findings.

Biopsy is also required in order to confirm the diagnosis of antiglomerular basement membrane disease which may respond to plasmapheresis. Nephrotoxins, for example, urate, calcium, paraproteins, can be demonstrated on kidney biopsy. Therefore, dialysis may be needed to clear the blood, or simply discontinuing present drug regimens will be necessary. And finally, as was mentioned above, the decision to transplant may be affected by the results of a kidney biopsy.

## COMPLICATIONS[2,10,41]

Once it has been decided that a renal biopsy is indicated, one must consider its potential risk. Biopsies were once felt to be too dangerous, with many early studies reporting serious complications. Bolton and Vaughan suggest that even though open biopsy is a major surgical procedure, it is actually safer than using the percutaneous route in their institution.[4] Clearly, open biopsy should be considered when contraindications to percutaneous biopsy exist.

Table 7-5 lists the commonly accepted contraindications to renal biopsy. An uncooperative patient will make localizing the kidney difficult and increases the risk of lacerating renal tissue. Under these conditions, open biopsy may be the wiser choice. Uncontrolled hypertension

**Table 7-5.** Contraindications to Renal Biopsy

Uncooperative patient (and inability to obtain
    consent)
Kidney not localized
Uncontrolled hypertension
Solitary kidney
Anasarca
Infection
Coagulopathy

**Table 7-6.** Complications of Renal Biopsy

| Lead Author | Year | #Pt | Adequate Tissue (%) | Morbidity (%) | Gross Hematuria (%) | Hematoma (%) | Trans-fused (%) | Surgery (%) | Death (%) | Other (%) |
|---|---|---|---|---|---|---|---|---|---|---|
| Altebarmakan[1] | 1981 | 632 | — | 8.5 | 5 | 1.5 | 1.0 | 0.2 | — | 1 Sepsis 1 Abscess |
| Bolton[2] | 1977 | 171 | 83 | 11 | 4.6 | 2.9 | 2.9 | 1 | — | |
| Diaz-Buxo[6] | 1975 | 1000 | 95 | 8.1 | 6.9 | 1.4 | — | 0.2 | 0.1 | 3 Oliguria 2 Obst. with clots |
| Welt[26] | 1968 | 8000 | 90 | — | 10-40 | 0.2 | — | 0.1 | 0.1 | 5 AV fistula |
| Muth[19] | 1965 | 500 | 95 | 4.6 | 3.8 | 0.4 | 0.4 | 0 | 0 | |
| Fairley[8] | 1962 | 300 | 88 | 4.3 | 1.3 | 0.7 | 0.3 | — | 0.3 | |
| Slotkin[24] | 1962 | 5000 | — | 0.7 | 2.5 | 0.5 | — | 0.3 | 0.1 | 1 Sepsis 1 Abscess |
| Brun[5] | 1958 | 510 | 40-67 | — | 7.9 | 0.2 | 2.2 | — | 0 | 2 Obst. with clots |
| Kark[14] | 1958 | 500 | 80 | 9.8 | 5.2 | 0.6 | 0.4 | 0 | 0 | 22 with pain 14 with colic 3 with increased hematuria |

apparently leads to greater bleeding problems, therefore, blood pressure should be controlled prior to the procedure. Since there is a finite risk of kidney loss during this procedure, one must take great care before attempting to biopsy a patient with only one kidney. Anasarca should be treated prior to biopsy since it makes the procedure technically more difficult. Infection should also be treated beforehand. Coagulopathy is an obvious contraindication to this procedure, however, Brezis[5] writes that he has successfully biopsied patients with prolonged thrombin time without complications.[5]

The most common complications of percutaneous kidney biopsy are listed in Table 7-6 along with their frequencies, as reported in some of the larger series. Microscopic hematuria has been reported in as many as 100 percent of cases.[22,33] However, gross hematuria is seen in only 4 to 8 percent of the patients and usually requires no specific treatment. The frequency of perirenal hematomas varies with the intensity with which it is searched for. With the advent of CT scans, the incidence has increased to 57 to 85 percent of percutaneously biopsied patients.[47] However, these are rarely symptomatic and rarely require therapy. Transfusion is required in 1 to 2 percent and the need for surgery is very infrequent. Nevertheless, there is a small but finite mortality associated with this procedure usually due to uncontrolled bleeding. If fluoroscopy is performed during biopsy, the risk of dye infusion is added to that of the biopsy. All things considered, this procedure is extremely safe when performed by an experienced clinician.

Note also the high percentage yield of adequate tissue in these studies (Table 7-6). In most series, adequate tissue was obtained in 80 to 95 percent. By adequate tissue we mean a specimen with 5 to 14 glomeruli which can be used in order to make a diagnosis.

## SUMMARY

Percutaneous kidney biopsy is a high-yield, low-risk procedure that gives the astute clinician a great deal of information that can be readily used in the diagnosis, prognosis, and treatment of his patients. The procedure is highly recommended in the patients with proteinuria, hematuria, renal insufficiency, or a secondary diagnosis in which the kidney is commonly but variably affected. While the clinician should avoid potential harm to his patients, he should also not withhold potential diagnostic tools which may prove beneficial.

## REFERENCES

1. Almkuist RD, Buckalew VM, Hirszel P, et al.: Recurrence of anti-glomerular basement membrane antibody mediated glomerulonephritis in an Isograft. Clin Immuno Immunopathol 18:54, 1981.
2. Alterbarmakien VK, Guthinger WP, Yakub YN, et al: Percutaneous kidney biopsies: Complications and their management. Urology 18:118, 1981.
3. Angell ME, Relman AS, Robbins SL: "Active" chronic pyelonephritis without evidence of bacterial infection. N Engl J Med 278:1301, 1968.
4. Bolton WK, Vaughan ED: A comparative study of open surgical and percutaneous renal biopsies. J Urol 117:696, 1977.
5. Brezis M: Prolonged thrombin time probably is no contraindication to kidney biopsy. N Engl J Med 304:462, 1981.
6. Brezin JH, Katz SM, Schwartz AB, et al: Reversible renal failure and nephrotic syndrome associated with non-steroidal anti-inflammatory drugs. N Engl J Med 301: 1271, 1979.
7. Brun C, Raaschou F: The results of five hundred percutaneous renal biopsies. Am J Med 24:676, 1958.

8. Cameron JS: The natural history of glomerulonephritis. In: Black D, Ed: Renal Disease. Blackwell Scientific Publications, Oxford, 1972, 295–329.

9. Collaborative study of adult nephrotic syndrome. A controlled study of short-term prednisone treatment in adults with membranous nephropathy. N Engl J Med 301:1301, 1979.

10. Diaz-Buxo JA, Danadio JV: Complications of percutaneous renal biopsy: an analysis of 1000 consecutive biopsies. Clin Nephrol 4:223, 1975.

11. Danovitch GM, Nissenson AR: The role of renal biopsy in determining therapy and prognosis in renal disease. Am J Nephrol 2:179, 1982.

12. Fagan J, Lewis EJ: Glomerulopathies of neoplasia. Kidney Int 11:297, 1977.

13. Fairley KF, Kincaid-Smith P: The clinical value of renal biopsy: experience in 300 cases. Med J Aust 49:897, 1962.

14. Fordham CC, Haseman J, Boerner R, et al: Renal biopsy in the nephrotic syndrome. Arch Intern Med 124:177, 1969.

15. Frey BM, Frey FJ, Zimmerman A, et al: Prediction of the histological type of glomerulonephritis: Multiple discriminant analysis of clinical and laboratory characteristics at time of diagnosis. Nephron 25:276, 1980.

16. Fries JF, Porta J, Liang MH: Marginal benefit of renal biopsy in systemic lupus erythematosus. Arch Intern Med 138:1386, 1978.

17. Hamburger J, Crosnier J, Noel LH: Recurrent glomerulonephritis after renal transplantation. Ann Rev Med 29:67, 1978.

18. Hutch JA, Miller ER, Hinman F Jr: Vesicoureteral reflux. Role in pyelonephritis. Am J Med 34:338, 1963.

19. Hyman LR, Burkholder PM: Focal sclerosing glomerulopathy with segmental hyalinosis. Lab Invest. 28:533, 1973.

20. Jenis E, Lowenthal DT: Kidney Biopsy Interpretation. FA Davis, Philadelphia, 1977.

21. Kark RM, Muehrcke RC, Pirani, CL, et al: The clinical value of renal biopsy. Ann Intern Med 43:807, 1955.

22. Kark RM, Muehrcke RC, Pollak VE, et al: An analysis of five hundred percutaneous renal biopsies. Arch Intern Med 101:439, 1958.

23. Kincaid-Smith P, Fairley KF: The differential diagnosis between preclamptic toxemia and glomerulonephritis in patients with proteinuria during pregnancy. In Lindheimer MD, Katz AI, Zuspan FP: Hypertension in Pregnancy. Wiley, New York, p 157, 1975.

24. Lindheimer MD, Katz AI, Zuspan FP: Hypertension in Pregnancy. Wiley, New York, p 157, 1975.

25. Kuhn K, Brod J: Interstitial nephropathies. Contributions to Nephrology no. 16, S. Karger, New York, 1979.

26. Lindheimer MD, Katz AI: Kidney function and disease in pregnancy. Lea & Febiger, Philadelphia, p 150, 1977.

27. Lockwood CM, Peters DK: Plasma exchange in glomerulonephritis and related vasculitides. Ann Rev Med 31:167, 1980.

28. Lynn RI, Siegel NJ, Hayslett JP: Lupus nephropathy as the initial manifestation of systemic lupus erythematosus. Yale J Biol Med 53:353, 1980.

29. Mahajan SK, Ordoney NG, Feitelson PJ, et al.: Lupus nephropathy without clinical renal involvement. Medicine 56:493, 1977.

30. McCluskey RT, Klassen J: Immunologically mediated glomerular, tubular and interstitial renal disease. N Engl J Med 288:564, 1973.

31. McGonigle R, Sharpstone P: Kidney biopsy. Br Med J 1:547, 1980.

32. Michael J, Jones NF, Davies DR, et al: Recurrent heamaturia: role of renal biopsy and investigative morbidity. Brit Med J 1:686, 1976.

33. Muth RG: The safety of percutaneous renal biopsy: An analysis of 500 consecutive cases. J Urol 94:1, 1965.

34. Paone DB, LeeRoy EM: The effect of biopsy on therapy in renal disease. Arch Intern Med 141:1039, 1981.

35. Parrish AE, Howe JS: Kidney biopsy: A review of one hundred successful needle biopsies. Arch Intern Med 96:712, 1955.

36. Pollak VE, Pirani CL, Schwartz FD: The natural history of the renal manifestations of systemic lupus erythematosus. J Lab Clin Med 63:537, 1964.

37. Rao KV, Crosson JT: Idiopathic membranous glomerulonephritis in diabetic patients. Report of three cases and a review of the literature. Arch Intern Med 140:624, 1980.

38. Report of the International Study of Kidney Diseases in Children: Nephrotic syndrome in children. Prediction of histopathology from clinical and laboratory characteristics at the time of diagnosis. Kidney Int 13:159, 1978.

39. Siegel NJ, Gaudo KM, Krassner LS, et al: Steroid dependent nephrotic syndrome in children: Histology and relapses after cyclophosphamide treatment. Kidney Int 19:454, 1981.

40. Solomon LR, Cairns SA, Lawler W: Reduction of post-transplant proteinuria due to recurrent mesangial proliferative (IgM) glomerulonephritis following plasma exchange. Clin Neph 16:44, 1981.

41. Slotkin EA, Madsen P.O.: Complications of renal biopsy: incidence in 5000 reported cases. J Urol 87:13, 1962.

42. Takacs FJ, Dowd JB, Zinman L: The liberal approach to renal biopsy. Lahey Clinic Found Bull 18:1, 1969.

43. Urizar RE, Schwarty A, Top F, et al: The nephrotic syndrome in children with diabetes mellitus of recent onset. N Engl J Med 281:173, 1969.

44. Verrier JJ, Cummins RH, Bacon PA, et al: Evidence for a therapeutic effect of plasmapheresis in patients with SLE. Q J Med, New 192:555, 1979.

45. Welt L: Renal biopsy. JAMA 205:220, 1968.

46. Wickre CG, Golper TA: Complications of percutaneous needle biopsy of the kidney. Am J Nephrol 2:173, 1982.

47. World MJ: Variables discriminating between cryptogenic glomerular lesions in adults in nephrotic syndrome. Q J Med 179:451, 1976.

# The Case Against Its Utility: Lupus Nephritis

Stanley P. Ballou, M.D.
Irving Kushner, M.D.

I would say that in the great majority of cases, the diagnosis reached by an experienced, competent physician from the history, his examination, and appropriate laboratory tests, will not be improved by renal biopsy in a manner that will affect significantly the management of the patient.[61]
Arnold R. Rich

## INTRODUCTION

Percutaneous renal biopsy has now been in use for just over three decades. The technical aspects of the procedure have been clearly defined and the procedure is now routinely employed by physicians at many institutions. The performance of renal biopsy is a standard component of training programs in nephrology. In view of the increasing use of this procedure over the past 30 years, it seems appropriate to critically examine the use of renal biopsy as a clinical tool. We will not address the investigational use of renal biopsy, an application which has undoubtedly brought about major advances in our understanding of renal disease, and about which there is little controversy. We will, however, reconsider the provocative statement by the late distinguished Professor of Pathology at Johns Hopkins University, cited above, which he delivered at a symposium assessing the first decade of use of percutaneous renal biopsy. That is, we will consider just how valuable the procedure of renal biopsy actually is in the diagnosis and management of individual patients with renal disease. Do histologic findings observed on renal biopsy provide information which influences clinical decisions regarding treatment and prognosis? Given our current state of knowledge, is this information not otherwise obtainable? In brief, is the patient better off for having undergone renal biopsy?

## HISTORICAL PERSPECTIVE

The potential application of renal biopsy as a clinical tool was recognized after the initial studies of Iverson and Brunn in 1951.[37] Over the ensuing decade, the technical aspects of the procedure were refined[53] and percutaneous biopsy was employed for evaluation of a great variety of renal diseases. An international symposium in 1961 summarized the experiences of a number of investigators who reported on the use of renal biopsy in many nephrologic disorders, and on its associated complications.[74] Since that time more sophisticated methods of evaluating renal tissue, for example, immunofluorescence and immunoenzymatic techniques, histochemistry, and electron microscopy, have been developed and employed with increasing frequency. The more widespread availability of percutaneous renal biopsy and the increased use of these sophisticated techniques for histologic evaluation has resulted in several distinct developments:

1. There have been great strides in the characterization and classification of renal histopathology, particularly of glomerular diseases. Thus J.S. Cameron, in referring to our understanding of the natural history of glomerulonephritis, has stated: "The greatest single advance has been the application and interpretation of renal biopsies."[13]

2. New disease entities have been defined, for example, IgA nephropathy, dense deposit disease, and crescentic glomerulonephritis, among others.

3. There has been a gradual delineation of the precise disease entities in which renal biopsy is thought to be of value in patient management, that is, in suggesting a diagnosis, influencing treatment or improving ability to prognosticate accurately. Table 7-7 lists a number of clinical nephrologic syndromes according to whether biopsy information is considered to be of value for patient management. The procedure appears to be of greatest potential value in the diffuse disease states such as the primary glomerulopathies. This might be anticipated from the knowledge that less than one ten thousandth of the total renal mass can be obtained by percutaneous needle biopsy.[27]

In the face of this wealth of information which has been accumulated over the past 30 years, we must wonder whether Dr. Rich has been left behind by the march of time. Is there still a rationale for a conservative approach to the clinical use of renal biopsy? We think there is. Renal biopsy is not without complications and is expensive. But perhaps most importantly, serious questions can be raised about how frequently patients are directly benefited by this procedure. Before addressing these questions, we will briefly consider the risk and expense of renal biopsy.

## COMPLICATIONS AND EXPENSE OF RENAL BIOPSY

Percutaneous renal biopsy is a relatively invasive procedure. Tissue, adequate for acceptable histopathologic interpretation, should contain at least 5 to 10 glomeruli[56] and can be obtained, under optimal circumstances, in 85 to 95 percent of patients. These figures are those from institutions reporting biopsies of large series of patients and therefore may represent the most favorable results. The approximate incidence of some of the more frequent complications has been compiled from several large series[10,12,15,18,20,39,41,44,51,57,70,] and surveys;[40,67]

**Table 7-7.** Clinical Use of Renal Biopsy

| |
|---|
| Of generally accepted value for |
|     Primary glomerulopathies |
|     Nephrotic syndrome of unknown etiology |
| Generally not indicated for |
|     Nephrolithiasis |
|     Cystic diseases |
|     Malignancy |
|     Infectious diseases |
|     Major vessel disease (hypertension, renal vein thrombosis) |
|     End-stage renal disease |
| Of uncertain value for |
|     Secondary glomerulopathies, e.g., lupus nephritis |
|     Distinguishing relative contribution of multiple disorders |

these are noted in Table 7-8. These figures are again probably optimal, being obtained largely from results published by centers where the procedure is performed frequently under standardized conditions.[11] The most common complication is bleeding. Microscopic hematuria occurs almost invariably, and perirenal or intrarenal hematomas have been documented by sophisticated procedures such as computed tomography[62] or ultrasonography[73] in 85 percent and 93 percent of patients, respectively. Gross hematuria, which occurs in about 5 to 10 percent of patients, is usually self-limited, but may persist for several days and necessitate transfusion in up to 2 percent of patients. While the incidence of more severe complications is relatively low, the performance of renal biopsy may lead directly to either nephrectomy or death in about 0.1 percent of patients[20,67] and the mortality has demonstrated no tendency to improve over the years.

Nor is the economic cost of renal biopsy trivial. The charge for the procedure itself is usually about $200 to $300, and for complete pathologic interpretation (including light, immunofluorescence and electron microscopy) $400 to $600. In addition, a minimum of one day of hospitalization is required, as well as associated laboratory tests such as blood counts, coagulation studies, and fluoroscopy. It is therefore obvious that the procedure may cost $1500 under optimal circumstances, making it certainly one of the more expensive nonoperative medical procedures.

Even if the complications and expense were negligible, the patient discomfort and morbidity associated with the procedure suggest that biopsy would probably not be performed if a diagnosis, prognosis, or therapeutic regimen could be reasonably established by less invasive means. For example, skin biopsy, a procedure clearly associated with negligible risk and expense, is neither necessary nor indicated in the diagnosis or management of impetigo, which is more appropriately diagnosed by bacteriologic culture.

In view of the known complications, economic expense and patient inconvenience associated with percutaneous renal biopsy, it is important to consider whether these costs are outweighed by the benefit it provides. Does the procedure provide information which is both of value in the management of individual patients and which is clearly superior to clinical information which can be obtained by other, simpler means? To address this question, we will examine the evolution of our perception of the clinical value of renal biopsy in systemic lupus erythematosus (SLE), as a well studied example.

## CLINICAL USEFULNESS OF RENAL BIOPSY IN MANAGEMENT OF LUPUS NEPHRITIS

The three ways that renal biopsy in lupus nephritis might affect patient management would be by confirming the diagnosis, by influencing therapy, or by improving our ability to prognosticate for individual patients. With our current state of knowledge and the availability of clinical and serological tests, biopsy is rarely indicated for the diagnosis of SLE in uncomplicated patients. Since therapeutic regimens in lupus nephritis are limited in number and nonspecific in effect, the major clinical value of biopsy in lupus nephritis has revolved about its capacity to provide valid prognostic information. We will consider the possible influence of biopsy findings on therapeutic decisions later; first, however, we will review the available data concerning the prognostic value of renal biopsy.

**Table 7-8.** Complications of Percutaneous Renal Biopsy*

| Complication | Approximate incidence (%) |
|---|---|
| Total | 8–10 |
| Gross hematuria | 5–10 |
| Perirenal hematoma | 1–2 |
| Transfusion requirement | 1–2 |
| Nephrectomy | 0–1 |
| Death | 0–1 |
| Others (Oliguria, obstruction, abscess, sepsis, infarction, A-V fistula, urine leak, puncture of other organ) | < 1 |

*Data compiled from series and surveys reporting greater than 100 cases (references 10,12,15,18,20,22,39,40,41,44,51,57,67,70).

Since the initial clinicopathologic studies of lupus nephritis by Muehrke and colleagues,[54,55] a number of investigators have sought to classify renal histology and correlate these findings with the clinical course of the disease.[19,60,64] The most common classification schema in current use is that initially suggested by Baldwin and colleagues[5] and subsequently modified by the World Health Organization.[49] Five major categories have been defined primarily by cellular proliferative and infiltrative changes within glomeruli as observed by light microscopy and include: (a) normal or minimal glomerular alteration; (b) mesangial proliferative glomerulonephritis; (c) focal proliferative glomerulonephritis; (d) diffuse proliferative glomerulonephritis; and (e) membranous glomerulonephritis. The demonstration by a number of investigators[1,4,43,66,68] of a correlation between the course of the renal disease and its histologic classification has led to the widespread belief that renal biopsy is indicated in most patients with lupus nephritis for prognostic purposes. Several authors[25,48] have demonstrated that such "severe" lesions as diffuse proliferative glomerulonephritis may be present in some patients without clinically apparent nephritis. This finding has suggested to some that biopsy may be routinely indicated in patients with lupus without regard to whether clinical evidence of renal involvement is present.[25]

In the past decade, however, a number of reports have raised distinct and disquieting concerns regarding the precise prognostic value of renal biopsy in individual situations. The possibility that some of these observations may apply to the interpretation of renal biopsy material in other renal diseases is real and therefore requires serious attention. Among these concerns are:

## Problems Associated with the Interpretation of Biopsy Histology

One problem in histology is *sampling error*, a potential difficulty associated with interpretation of any pathologic specimen obtained by needle biopsy. Early studies suggested that histologic findings observed on needle biopsy specimens were fairly representative of overall renal histology. However, a comparative study of pathology obtained by renal biopsy with that obtained at postmortem examination demonstrated an 84 percent correlation between the two in diffuse glomerular diseases, but only a 51 percent correlation in focal disorders.[42] Although it is widely assumed that histopathology in lupus nephritis is uniform and diffuse, there remains the distinct possibility that classification based upon only a small sample of tissue may not always be representative of the disease process. This difficulty is, of course, compounded if only a limited amount of glomerular tissue is obtained.

*Interobserver variation* is not an uncommon problem. While in many situations agreement among pathologists can be reached regarding broad classifications of histopathology, uncertainty remains regarding the possibility of inconsistent interpretation among different investigators. This problem has not been specifically addressed in lupus nephritis; disagreement among pathologists may occur in up to 35 percent of individual cases in other diseases.[26,33]

Difficulties may be posed by an *inability to classify histology into one of the defined categories.* The categories described above, like many histopathologic classifications, are obviously not always discretely definable; overlap between categories may occur in individual cases. The difference between focal proliferative and diffuse proliferative glomerulonephritis, for example, is not qualitative but one of degree. While 50 percent involvement has been used as the dividing line between focal and diffuse glomerular involvement,[50] this assessment on any given tissue specimen may be somewhat arbitrary. In addition, some biopsies may show both membranous and proliferative changes in glomeruli.

Precise classification therefore is clearly somewhat subjective. In some individuals renal histopathology may not fit well into one of the above categories. For example, patients with predominantly sclerotic glomerular changes, or predominantly interstitial disease, may be difficult to classify according to the above criteria, which focus primarily on cellular and capillary changes within glomeruli. It has therefore been said that precise classification may be unsatisfactory in up to 10 to 20 percent of biopsies.[50]

### The Problem of Transition between Classifications

It was initially assumed, based on serial biopsies and postmortem studies, that renal histopathology in individual lupus patients was relatively constant over time.[5,60] In more recent studies, however, a number of investigators have observed changes from one histopathologic category to another.[1,4,29,46,76] Changes from mesangial or focal proliferative to diffuse proliferative lesions are perhaps observed most frequently.[76] Transitions from proliferative categories to membranous nephritis also occur, perhaps as a result of therapy with corticosteroids[46] or immunosuppressive agents.[30] Frequent alterations in the underlying pathology lessen the value of a given biopsy. As Fries et al.[28] have suggested, a renal biopsy may represent only "a photograph of a motion picture."

### Uncertainty Regarding the Precise Prognostic Value of Standard Histologic Classifications

This is clearly the most serious indictment of the clinical use of renal biopsy in lupus nephritis, especially since, as noted previously, assessment of prognosis has generally been regarded as the major clinical benefit of renal biopsy in SLE. Lack of correlation of biopsy histology with both clinical findings and with eventual outcome has been observed. The relation between clinical tests of renal function and the severity of renal histologic abnormalities has been found imperfect by several investigators. Zweiman et al.[77] in an evaluation of 40 patients with SLE, found a lack of correlation between presence of clinical renal abnormalities and degree of renal pathologic change in 15. The outcome of these patients appeared to be more closely related to initial tests of renal function, regardless of the category of pathologic change. They therefore suggested that a clinician could not uniformly predict the likelihood of progressive renal disease in an individual lupus patient based on the microscopic findings from a renal biopsy at the time of initial evaluation.

More recent studies of clinicopathological correlations in lupus nephritis have reported the seemingly distressing finding that histologically "severe" lesions, such as diffuse proliferative glomerulonephritis, may occur in patients without any clinical evidence of renal disease.[25,48,75] For example, Mahajan et al.[48] reported renal biopsy findings for 90 lupus patients with and without clinical renal disease; 12 of the 27 patients with normal renal function and urinalysis were found to have diffuse proliferative glomerulonephritis on renal biopsy. One interpretation of this observation, based on the widely held view that this histologic finding has a poor prognosis, is that severe renal disease can exist in patients with SLE regardless of clinical renal abnormalities. Some would conclude that renal biopsy might truly be warranted in all patients with SLE in an attempt to detect such involvement. However, review of the subsequent course of these 12 patients indicates that their outcomes were more closely related to clinical parameters of renal dysfunction than to the initial histopathologic findings. Only 1 of the 12 patients subsequently developed renal failure and that patient did, in fact, manifest clinically evident renal abnormalities one year following the biopsy and 4 years prior to renal death. In contrast, 8 of 35 patients with diffuse proliferative glomerulonephritis and clinically evident renal disease eventually developed renal failure or renal death. A more appropriate interpretation of this study might therefore be that clinical features may be a useful guide to renal outcome and that the prognosis of diffuse proliferative glomerulonephritis is not uniformly bad. Other reports of patients with clinically occult diffuse proliferative glomerulonephritis have not provided follow-up information, so that the actual clinical significance of these observations cannot be established.[25]

Even more unsettling than the lack of correlation of histology with clinical findings is the lack of correlation recently noted between histologic classifications and eventual outcome. Hecht et al.[31] failed to observe a relation between long-term outcome and histopathologically "mild," "moderate," or "severe" disease by either light microscopy or election microscopy in 31 patients with lupus nephropathy. Cameron et al.,[14] using the widely recognized histologic classification described above, have found no correlation between histologic categories and eventual outcome in 71 patients with lupus nephritis. Finally, Magil et al.[47] observed that both survival and renal outcome were similar in 15 patients with focal proliferative glomerulonephritis and 15 patients with diffuse proliferative glomerulonephritis.

A different approach to assessing the prognostic value of renal biopsy has been taken by two groups that have addressed the question: Does renal biopsy provide information that is of greater prognostic value than that which can be obtained by clinical assessment alone? Fries et al.[28] compared the prognostic value of histologic classifications with that of clinical tests of renal function for three published series of patients[5,31,77] and 56 of their own patients. An accuracy coefficient[65] was employed which quantified the correlation between the observed clinical course and the predictive accuracy of either clinical or biopsy findings or both. They found that the predictive information afforded by histological classification did not add significantly at the margin to clinical information, and therefore suggested that histologic findings supply information which is essentially redundant to that obtained by clinical testing. These conclusions were reinforced by the findings of a recent survey which addressed the prognostic value of renal biopsy in very practical terms.[72] In this survey, involving 197 academic rheumatologists, the ability of physicians to accurately estimate clinical course and eventual outcomes for three representative patients with lupus nephritis on the basis of clinical information, was not improved by subsequently providing them with detailed renal histologic findings.

A final concern is whether the prognostic value of renal biopsy has suffered for want of emphasizing certain aspects of histopathology. Indeed, recent evidence suggests that certain histologic findings not previously included in traditional classifications may provide greater prognostic information concerning patient outcome. In brief, have we been looking for the right things in biopsy specimens? We would like to address this issue next.

# NEWER APPROACHES TO REEVALUATION OF RENAL BIOPSY INFORMATION IN SLE

One such approach has been the use of renal biopsy "scoring" to provide semiquantitative data concerning individual histopathologic findings.[52,58] Balow et al.[7] have devised a renal biopsy scoring system based on an "activity index" describing six lesions, and a "chronicity index" comprised of four discrete histologic lesions (Table 7-9). The individual abnormalities are scored from 0 to 3 + and summed to provide a total pathologic score. These authors suggested that this scoring system provided a clearer picture, with more specific details, than that conveyed by conventional histologic classifications. Their observations further suggested that evaluation of histologic features of chronicity could improve the prognostic value of renal biopsy when

compared with prognostications based upon conventional histologic classifications.[2]

A different approach to the evaluation of renal biopsies is that of multivariate analysis.[2a,6,71] Whiting-O'Keefe et al.[71] used a linear regression analysis which included a number of clinical variables to construct a linear model that predicted change in renal function one year after biopsy in 130 patients with lupus nephritis. When these investigators added individual renal histologic findings to the clinically determined regression model, they observed that the degree of glomerular sclerosis observed by light microscopy and quantity of subendothelial deposits assessed by electron microscopy both contributed significant predictive information to the clinical model. However, histologic classification according to the standard categories noted above did not contribute significantly to the regression model. They suggested that the greatest value of renal biopsy might be in the evaluation of degree of glomerular sclerosis and fibrosis. The strongest clinical predictors of outcome in their analysis were serum creatinine, a "laboratory activity" index consisting of serum com-

**Table 7-9.** Renal Biopsy Scoring System

| |
|---|
| Activity index |
|   Glomerular lesions |
|     Cellular proliferation |
|     Fibrinoid necrosis/nuclear karyorrhexis |
|     Hyaline thrombi/wire loops |
|     Cellular crescents |
|     Leukocyte infiltration |
|   Tubulointerstitial lesions |
|     Mononuclear-cell infiltration |
| Chronicity index |
|   Glomerular lesions |
|     Fibrous crescents/periglomerular fibrosis |
|     Sclerotic glomeruli |
|   Tubulointerstitial lesions |
|     Tubular atrophy |
|     Interstitial fibrosis |

(From Balow JE: In Decker JL, moderator: Systemic lupus erythematosus: Evolving concepts. Ann Intern Med 91:587, 1979.)

plement level and degree of hematuria, patient age and 24 hour urine protein excretion.

In a series of 25 patients, Ballou et al.[6] used a stepwise discriminant analysis to evaluate the relative prognostic value of various individual clinical and histologic findings in predicting the course of renal disease. At the time of renal biopsy, clinical findings of greatest prognostic value were serum creatinine and albumin concentrations, and patient age. These variables were among those identified as strong clinical predictors in the above linear model derived by Whiting-O'Keefe et al.,[71] except for serum albumin concentration, which can be shown to be inversely correlated with 24 hour urine protein excretion (Ballou, unpublished observations). Discriminant analysis of individual histologic findings revealed that glomerular sclerosis and mesangial cell proliferation provided the greatest predictive value concerning renal outcome. Classification on the basis of WHO criteria, however was not predictive of outcome. Although glomerular sclerosis was the histologic finding of greatest prognostic value, its addition to the clinical findings did not further improve outcome prediction.

Finally, Austin et al.[2a] used clinical and histologic data to generate multivariate survival models predictive of renal outcome for 102 lupus patients. The strongest clinical predictors were: age less than 24 years, male gender, and elevated serum creatinine level. Renal histology (categorized as activity and chronicity indexes) contributed significant prognostic information to the clinical predictors; however, only age and the histology chronicity index contributed significantly to a model, the predictions of which were similar to observed outcomes.

The results of these studies are basically in agreement, and suggest that certain clinical findings, such as serum creat-inine, and patient age, are of great prognostic value in the management of patients with lupus nephritis. Any improvement in prognostic ability to be gained from renal biopsy is more likely to be gained from assessment of histologic findings, related to chronicity, such as glomerular sclerosis, than by classification according to standard critieria.

It is of interest that glomerular sclerosis was among the histologic findings of greatest prognostic value in each of these studies. This finding has been noted to be associated with progressive renal disease and poor response to therapy by Morel-Maroger et al.[52] Baldwin and Gallo[3] have also emphasized the poor prognosis associated with this finding, and Zweiman et al.[77] observed that, among 11 patients with normal renal function at time of biopsy, the only patient to show subsequent deterioration was also the only patient with glomerular sclerosis. Finally, a recent study by Kant et al.[38] suggested that glomerular thrombosis as detected by the acid picro-Mallory stain described by Lendrum, may represent a precursor of glomerulosclerosis, and may therefore have distinct prognostic value in lupus and other glomerulonephritidies.

# GENERAL COMMENTS REGARDING PROGNOSTIC VALUE OF HISTOLOGY IN LUPUS NEPHRITIS

We have, until this point, considered only the prognostic value of renal histology as assessed by light microscopy. Both immunofluorescence and electron microscopy have been employed in clinicopathologic evaluations in lupus nephritis in recent years. Although some correlation has been observed between the amount and distribution of immune deposits as assessed by immunofluorescence and the clinical features and course of lupus nephritis,[32] the interpretation of the extent and location of these deposits is clearly somewhat subjective and difficult to quantitate by this technique.[50] Their prognostic value therefore remains uncertain. There is more evidence that large subendothelial electron dense deposits, as assessed by electron microscopy, may have distinct prognostic value in lupus nephritis.[9,19,21,24,31] However, some investigators have found little relation between this finding on an initial biopsy and eventual outcome,[23,43] and these changes may be observed, at least to some extent, in the majority of patients with SLE.[8,16] Furthermore, electron microscopy is not readily available in some institutions, is relatively expensive, and results may not become available for some time after performance of the biopsy.

In a consideration of the prognostic value of renal biopsy in lupus nephritis, we would be remiss not to consider an important possible explanation for the apparent reduced prognostic value noted in recent studies. This factor is related to the progressive improvement in prognosis of lupus nephritis over the years. It has become manifestly evident that the dismal prognosis previously associated with active lupus nephritis no longer holds true. In fact, the overwhelming majority of patients with lupus nephritis now do quite well, with reported five year survivals of 76 percent to 86 percent.[14,47,63,69] It is not clear whether the improved survival in recent years can be attributed to therapy, but whether it is or not is hardly the point. It is apparent that the prognostic distinctions between histologic subsets of renal SLE have been blunted by the overall improved outlook for such patients in recent years.

To summarize our current view of the prognostic value of renal biopsy in SLE: A number of phenomena, including (a) inconsistencies of interpretation; (b) transient nature of certain histologic findings; and (c) overall improvement in disease prognosis, have served to diminish the prognostic information traditionally associated with histologic classifications. It is now clear that certain clinical findings, particularly serum creatinine levels, have considerable prognostic value; histologic classifications apparently add little more prognostic information. Based on recent studies, it seems likely that any prognostic information to be obtained from renal biopsy is more likely to be derived from findings indicative of chronic irreversible changes such as glomerular sclerosis than by assessment of "active" lesions, which may be more conveniently indicated by serologic markers such as reduced concentrations of serum complement or elevated levels of anti-DNA antibodies.

## VALUE OF BIOPSY FOR DIAGNOSIS OR TREATMENT IN SLE

We have until now considered the renal biopsy in lupus primarily for its potential prognostic value. There seems little indication for biopsy for purely diagnostic purposes. Subtle changes within glomeruli may be found by electron microscopy or immunofluorescence in perhaps all patients with lupus, with or without nephritis;[8,16,34] their specificity remains unclear. In rare instances, however, biopsy may indicate the possible presence of another disease in addition to lupus.

Is biopsy in lupus patients a guide to therapy? The value of renal biopsy findings in influencing treatment in lupus nephritis remains unclear. We are aware of no study which has demonstrated that treatment decisions based on histologic classification alone have resulted in improved patient outcome. In most physicians' hands, treatment decisions over the course of time reflect serially assessed clinical symptoms and laboratory tests, and are also strongly influenced by the patient's response to the drugs employed, regardless of initial histologic findings. Thus, a patient whose proteinuria, sediment abnormalities and creatinine levels do not improve on initial therapy will usually receive more aggressive therapy, while patients whose abnormalities improve promptly will usually have their medications tapered and eventually discontinued. Nonetheless, the studies of Morel-Maroger et al.[52] do suggest that the finding of sclerotic lesions on biopsy indicates a lack of therapeutic responsiveness and implies that high dose corticosteroid therapy may be unwarranted.

## RENAL BIOPSY IN OTHER DISEASES

Can our concerns regarding the value of renal biopsy for clinical management of patients with lupus nephritis be generalized to the management of patients with other renal diseases? As stated above, the potential value of the procedure is clearly greatest for diffuse glomerular diseases. In such cases not only prognosis but also diagnosis becomes an important factor in the decision to biopsy. There has been less enthusiasm for initial renal biopsy in children with nephrotic syndrome, since a great majority of cases are related to minimal change disease, a steroid-responsive disorder.[17]

A multivariate analysis has been applied to diagnostic studies of nephrotic syndrome in children.[36] An equation obtained from this analysis yielded very good discrimination between patients with membranoproliferative glomerulonephritis and those with other forms of glomerular disease. It was suggested that this formula might permit the elimination of renal biopsy in those patients with

milder forms of glomerular disease who responded to initial steroid therapy.

The clinical value of renal biopsy for initial management of nephrotic syndrome has also been recently addressed in adults. A decision analysis was employed by Hlatky[33] and indicated that an initial trial of corticosteroid therapy without biopsy yields as many or more remissions, fewer complications and lower mortality than does either routine initial renal biopsy or routine biopsy limited to steroid-nonresponsive patients. It was therefore suggested that corticosteroid therapy, and response to this therapy, might obviate the need for biopsy as a guide to influence treatment decisions in adult nephrotic syndrome. Using a similar approach, Lau, et al. (43a) presented the illustrative case of a 53-year-old woman with idiopathic nephrotic syndrome. They employed sensitivity analyses to assess whether empiric initial therapy with corticosteroids might be a reasonable alternative to the conventional diagnostic strategy of performing a renal biopsy in such a situation. They concluded that the decision between the two strategies is essentially a toss-up. For this patient, with a life expectancy of more than 20 years, the difference in survival between strategies would be under three days. The approach to management is essentially the same as the approach to management of lupus nephritis described above; it is the response to therapy, rather than initial histologic findings, which dictate long-term management. Although the potential value of biopsy for establishing prognosis was not addressed in these studies it has been suggested that response to therapy may have substantial prognostic value.[35]

## CONCLUSION

The newer approaches to evaluation of renal histopathology described above, and the increasing availability of a number of new diagnostic techniques in nephrology, have encouraged a reevaluation of the precise clinical value of renal biopsy, not only in lupus nephritis but in other renal diseases as well. The conservative approach advocated here is not intended to interdict the performance of renal biopsy per se, but rather to caution against an unquestioning reliance on the clinical value of information obtained from it, and an inappropriate adherence to the view that biopsy is routinely important or necessary for the management of many patients. While renal biopsy is undoubtedly of diagnostic and probably prognostic value in some patients with diffuse primary glomerulopathies, the current ongoing enthusiasm for renal biopsy must be tempered with the realization that the major contribution of this procedure has been in the area of investigational medicine. The investigative potential of renal biopsy is far from exhausted. Further research employing electron microscopy, immunofluorescence, histochemistry, and other sophisticated modes of investigation, including statistical analyses, can be expected to provide even greater insight into the nature of renal disease in man. Perhaps we will arrive at the point when the information obtained from renal biopsy may be of unquestionable value in the management of most patients. At present, however, as far as overall benefit to the individual patient is concerned, Arnold Rich may still be right.

# REFERENCES

1. Appel GB, Silva FG, Pirani CL, et al: Renal involvement in systemic lupus erythematosus (SLE): A study of 56 patients emphasizing histologic classification. Medicine 57:371, 1978.
2. Austin HA, Joyce KM, Balow JE, et al: Prognostic features of renal histology in lupus nephritis (abstract). Arthritis Rheum 25 (suppl):S7, 1982.
2a. Austin HA, Muenz LR, Joyce KM, et al: Prognostic factors in lupus nephritis: Contribution of renal histologic data. Am J Med 75:382, 1983.
3. Baldwin DS, Gallo GR: Lupus nephritis. Clin Rheum Dis 1:639, 1975.
4. Baldwin DS, Gluck MC, Lowenstein J, et al: Lupus nephritis: Clinical course as related to morphologic forms and their transitions. Am J Med 62:12, 1977.
5. Baldwin DS, Lowenstein J, Rothfield NF, et al: The clinical course of the proliferative and membranous forms of lupus nephritis. Ann Intern Med 73:929, 1970.
6. Ballou S, Chung-Park M, Waggoner DM, et al: Prognostic value of clinical and renal biopsy findings in lupus nephritis. (abstract). Arthritis Rheum 23:651, 1980.
7. Balow JE: Clinicopathologic correlations in lupus nephritis. In Decker JL, moderator: Systemic lupus Erythematosus: Evolving concepts. Ann Intern Med 91:587, 1979.
8. Bardana EJ Jr, Bennett WM, Pirofsky B: Renal abnormalities in patients with systemic lupus erythematosus (SLE) with and without overt nephritis (abstract). Clin Res 22:589A, 1974.
9. Ben-Basset M, Rosenfeld J, Joshua H, et al: Lupus nephritis: Electron-dense and immunofluorescent deposits and their correlation with proteinuria and renal function. Am J Clin Pathol 72:186, 1979.
10. Bolton WK, Vaughn ED Jr: A comparative study of open surgical and percutaneous renal biopsies. J Urol 117:696, 1977.
11. Brewer DB: Renal Biopsy. 2nd Ed. The Williams & Wilkins Company, Baltimore, 1973.
12. Brun C, Raaschou F: The results of five hundred percutaneous renal biopsies. Arch Intern Med 102:716, 1958.
13. Cameron JS: The natural history of glomerulonephritis. p. 326. In Black, D., Ed.: Renal Disease, 3rd Ed., Blackwell Scientific Publications, Oxford, 1972.
14. Cameron JS, Turner DR, Ogg CS, et al: Systemic lupus with nephritis: A long-term study. QJ Med 148:1, 1979.
15. Carvajal HF, Travis LB, Srivastava RN, et al: Percutaneous renal biopsy in children.

An analysis of complications in 890 consecutive biopsies. Tex Rep Biol Med 29:253, 1971.

16. Cavallo T, Cameron WR, Lapenas D: Immunopathology of early and clinically silent lupus nephropathy. Am J Pathol 87:1, 1977.

17. Churg J, Habib R, White RHR: Pathology of the nephrotic syndrome in children. Lancet 1:1297, 1970.

18. Colodny AH, Reckler JM: A safe, simple and reliable method for percutaneous (closed) renal biopsies in children: Results in 100 consecutive patients. J Urol 113:222, 1975.

19. Comerford FR, Cohen AS: The nephropathy of systemic lupus erythematosus: An assessment by clinical, light and electron microscopic criteria. Medicine 46:425, 1967.

20. Diaz-Buxo JA, Donadio JV Jr: Complications of percutaneous renal biopsy: An analysis of 1,000 consecutive biopsies. Clin Nephrol 4:223, 1975.

21. Dillard MG, Tillman RL, Sampson CC: Lupus nephritis: Correlations between the clinical course and presence of electron-dense deposits. Lab Invest 32:261, 1975.

22. Dodge WF, Daeschner CW Jr, Brennan JC: Percutaneous renal biopsy in children. 1. General considerations. Pediatrics 30: 287, 1962.

23. Domoto DT, Kasgarian M, Hayslett JP, et al: The significance of electron dense deposits in mild lupus nephritis. Yale J Biol Med 53:317, 1980.

24. Dujovne I, Pollak VE, Pirani CL, Dillard MG: The distribution and character of glomerular deposits in systemic lupus erythematosus. Kidney Int 2:33, 1972.

25. Eiser AR, Katz SM, Swartz C: Clinically occult diffuse proliferative lupus nephritis: an age-related phenomenon. Arch Intern Med 139:1022, 1979.

26. Fordham CC, Haseman J, Boerner R, et al: Renal biopsy in the nephrotic syndrome. Arch Intern Med 124:177, 1969.

27. Freedman LR: Interstitial renal inflammation, including pyelonephritis and urinary tract infection. In Earley LE, Gottschalk CW, Eds: Strauss and Welt: Diseases of the Kidney, 3rd Ed, Little, Brown, Boston, 1979, p 835.

28. Fries JF, Porta J, Liang MH: Marginal benefit of renal biopsy in systemic lupus erythematosus. Arch Intern Med 138:1386, 1978.

29. Ginzler EM, Nicastri AD, Chen C-K, et al: Progression of mesangial and focal to diffuse lupus nephritis. N Engl J Med 291:693, 1974.

30. Hayslett JP, Kashgarian M, Cook CD, Spargo BH: The effect of azathioprine on lupus glomerulonephritis. Medicine 51:393, 1972.

31. Hecht B, Siegel N, Adler M, et al: Prognostic indices in lupus nephritis. Medicine 55:163, 1976.

32. Hill GS, Hinglais N, Tron F, Bach J-F: Systemic lupus erythematosus: Morphologic correlations with immunologic and clinical data at the time of biopsy. Am J Med 64:61, 1978.

33. Hlatky MA: Is renal biopsy necessary in adults with nephrotic syndrome? Lancet, 2:1264, 1982.

34. Holcraft RM, DuBois EL, Lundbert GD, et al: Renal damage in systemic lupus erythematosus with normal renal function. J Rheumatol 3:251, 1976.

35. Idelson BA, Smithline N, Smith GW, et al: Prognosis in steroid-treated idiopathic nephrotic syndrome in adults. Arch Intern Med 137:891, 1977.

36. International Study of Kidney Disease in Children: Nephrotic syndrome in children: Prediction of histopathology from clinical and laboratory characteristics at time of diagnosis. Kidney Int 13:159, 1978.

37. Iverson P, Brun C: Aspiration biopsy of the kidney. Am J Med 11:324, 1951.

38. Kant KS, Pollak VE, Weiss MA, et al: Glomerular thrombosis in systemic lupus erythematosus: Prevalence and significance. Medicine, 60:71, 1981.

39. Karafin L, Kendall AR, Fleisher DS: Urologic complications in percutaneous renal biopsy in children. J Urol 103:332, 1970.

40. Kark RM: Renal biopsy. JAMA, 205:220, 1968.

41. Kark RM, Muehrcke RC, Pollak VE, et al: An analysis of five hundred percutaneous renal biopsies. Arch Intern Med 101:439, 1958.

42. Kellow WF, Cotsonas NJ Jr, Chomet B, et

al: Evaluation of the adequacy of needle-biopsy specimens of the kidney: An autopsy study. Arch Intern Med 104:353, 1959.

43. Kimberly RP, Lockshin MD, Sherman RL, et al: "End-stage" lupus nephritis: Clinical course to and outcome on dialysis. Medicine, 60:277, 1981.

43a. Lau J, Levey AS, Kassirer JP, et al.: Idiopathic nephrotic syndrome in a 53-year-old woman: Is a kidney biopsy necessary? Medical Decision Making 2: 497, 1982.

44. Lee DA, Roger R, Agre KM, et al: Late complications of percutaneous renal biopsy. J Urol 97:793, 1967.

45. Lee P, Urowitz MB, Bookman AAM, et al: Systemic lupus erythematosus: A review of 110 cases with reference to nephritis, the nervous system, infections, aseptic necrosis and prognosis. QJ Med 46:1, 1977.

46. Lentz RD, Michael AF, Friend PS: Membranous transformation of lupus nephritis. Clin Immunol Immunopathol 19:131, 1981.

47. Magil AB, Ballon HS, Rae A: Focal proliferative lupus nephritis: A clinicopathologic study using the W.H.O. classification. Am J Med 72:620, 1982.

48. Mahajan SK, Ordonez NG, Feitelson PJ, et al: Lupus nephropathy without clinical renal involvement. Medicine 56:493, 1977.

49. McCluskey RT: Lupus nephritis. In Sommers SC, Ed: Kidney Pathology Decennial 1966–1975, Appleton-Century-Crofts, New York, 1975, p 435.

50. McCluskey RT: The value of renal biopsy in lupus nephritis. Arthritis Rheum 25:867, 1982.

51. McVicar M, Nicastri AD, Gauthier B: Improved renal biopsy technique in children. NY State J Med 74:830, 1974.

52. Morel-Maroger L, Mery J Ph, Droz D, et al: The course of lupus nephritis: contribution of serial renal biopsies. Adv Nephrol 6:79, 1976.

53. Muehrcke RC, Kark RM, Pirani CL: Technique of percutaneous renal biopsy in the prone position. J Urol 74:267, 1955.

54. Muehrcke RD, Kark RM, Pirani CL, Pollak VE: Lupus nephritis: A clinical and pathologic study based on renal biopsies. Medicine 36:1, 1957.

55. Muehrcke RC , Kark RM, Pirani CL, et al: Histological and clinical evolution of lupus nephritis. Ann Rheum Dis 14:371, 1955.

56. Muehrcke RD, Pirani CL: Renal biopsy: An adjunct in the study of kidney disease. p. 111. In Black D, Ed: Renal Disease, 3rd Ed, Blackwell Scientific Publications, Oxford, 1972.

57. Muth RG: The safety of percutaneous renal biopsy: an analysis of 500 consecutive cases. J Urol 94:1, 1965.

58. Pirani CL, Pollak VE, Schwartz FD: The reproductibility of semiquantitative analyses of renal histology. Nephron 1:230, 1964.

59. Pollak VE, Pirani CL, Kark RM: Effect of large doses of prednisone on the renal lesions and life span of patients with lupus glomerulonephritis. J Lab Clin Med 57:495, 1961.

60. Pollak VE, Pirani CL, Schwartz FD: The natural history of the renal manifestations of systemic lupus erythematosus. J Lab Clin Med 63:537, 1964.

61. Rich AR: Chairman's closing remarks. In Wolstenholme GEW, Cameron MP, Eds: Renal Biopsy: Clinical and Pathological Significance. Little, Brown, Boston, 1961, p 377.

62. Rosenbaum R, Hoffsten PE, Stanley RJ, et al: Use of computerized tomography to diagnose complications of percutaneous renal biopsy. Kidney Int 14:87, 1978.

63. Rothfield N: Clinical features of systemic lupus erythematosus. 1106. In Kelley WN, Harris ED Jr, Ruddy S, Sledge CB, Eds. Textbook of Rheumatology. WB Saunders, Philadelphia, 1981. p 1115.

64. Rothfield NF, McCluskey RT, Baldwin DS: Renal disease in systemic lupus erythematosus. N Engl J Med 269:537, 1963.

65. Shapiro AR: The evaluation of clinical predictions: A method and initial application. N Engl J Med 296:1509, 1977.

66. Sinniah R, Feng PH: Lupus nephritis: Correlation between light, electron microscopic and immunofluorescent findings and renal function. Clin Nephrol 6:340, 1976.

67. Slotkin EA, Madsen PO: Complications of renal biopsy: Incidence in 5000 reported cases. J Urol 87:13, 1962.

68. Striker GE, Kelly MR, Quadracci LJ,

Scribner BH: The course of lupus nephritis: A clinical pathological correlation of 50 patients. In Kincaid-Smith P, Mathew TH, Becker EL, Eds: Glomerulonephritis. Wiley, New York, 1973.

69. Wallace DJ, Podell TE, Weiner JM, et al: Lupus nephritis: Experience with 230 patients in a private practice from 1950 to 1980. Am J Med 72:209, 1982.

70. White RHR: Observations on percutaneous renal biopsy in children. Arch Dis Child 38:260, 1963.

71. Whiting-O'Keefe Q, Henke JE, Shearn MA, et al: The information content from renal biopsy in systemic lupus erythematosus: Stepwise linear regression analysis. Ann Intern Med 96:718, 1982.

72. Whiting-O'Keefe Q, Riccardi PJ, Henke JE, et al: Recognition of information in renal biopsies of patients with lupus nephritis. Ann Intern Med 96:723, 1982.

73. Winer RL, Handler SJ: Ultrasonic detection of complications following renal biopsy (abstract). Kidney Int 19:139, 1981.

74. Wolstenholme GEW, Cameron MP, Eds: Renal Biopsy: Clinical and Pathological Significance. Little, Brown, Boston, 1961.

75. Woolf A, Croker B, Osofsky SG, et al: Nephritis in children and young adults with systemic lupus erythematosus and normal urinary sediment. Pediatrics 64:678, 1979.

76. Zimmerman SW, Jenkins PG, Shelp WD, et al: Progression from minimal or focal to diffuse proliferative lupus nephritis. Lab Invest 32:665, 1975.

77. Zweiman B, Kornblum J, Cornog J, et al: The prognosis of lupus nephritis: role of clinical-pathologic correlations. Ann Intern Med 69:441, 1968.

# 8

# How Extensive Should the Work-Up Be for Hypercalciuric Patients with Nephrolithiasis?

# The Case for an Extensive Evaluation

## Charles Y.C. Pak, M.D.

Considerable progress has been made in urolithiasis research during the past decade. Much is now known regarding the physicochemical basis for crystallization of stone-forming salts in urine. Many physiologic or metabolic derangements which may predispose patients to stone formation have been identified. This information has permitted formulation of diagnostic criteria of different causes for nephrolithiasis based on physiologic derangements.

This progress has been particularly noteworthy in hypercalciuric nephrolithiasis. Thus, it has been suggested that hypercalciuria associated with nephrolithiasis may have different pathogenetic origins. Diagnostic protocols have been developed outlining an extensive evaluation aimed at differentiating the various forms of hypercalciuria. However, the wisdom of this approach has been questioned[39] because the existence of distinct forms of hypercalciuria remains unsettled and because it is not universally accepted that successful management of hypercalciuric nephrolithiasis requires an accurate definition of the underlying pathophysiology.

We have long espoused the view that an extensive evaluation is not only rational but may be crucial to ensure the satisfactory outcome of treatment. In defense of this view, we shall summarize the evidence that supports the following conclusions: (a) hypercalciuria has pathogenetic importance in stone formation; (b) various forms of hypercalciuric nephrolithiasis may be physiologically distinct; (c) reliable diagnostic protocols are available for identifying the different causes of hypercalciuria; (d) accurate diagnosis permits selective treatment based on the underlying pathophysiological derangement; and finally, (e) specific, selected treatment may be superior to more random therapies.

## DEFINITIONS AND RELATED CONCEPTS

Herein follows a brief review of certain of the terms and concepts used in this chapter to describe the physical chemistry of calcium nephrolithiasis.

### Saturation

Saturation is the state of solution in which maximal amounts of solute (e.g., stone-forming salts) have been dissolved. When saturated with regard to a given solute, rates of solution and precipitation are equal. When solid calcium phosphate is added to urine, the salt will continue to dissolve until the solution becomes saturated.

Supported by Grants USPHS PO1-AM20543 and MO1-RR00633.

287

## Activity Product

Activity Product refers to the product of the activities of each moiety of a stone-forming salt (e.g., calcium and oxalate). It is a measure of the state of saturation.

## Supersaturation

Supersaturation is the physical state in which more solute remains in solution than at saturation but without precipitation.

## Metastability

Metastability is the state of solution in which spontaneous precipitation of an ion pair does not occur during a defined period and under specific conditions. Metastability can be obtained despite supersaturation. Spontaneous precipitation will occur if the extent of supersaturation is raised sufficiently.

## Formation Product Ratio

The limit of metastability, or the minimum supersaturation required to elicit spontaneous precipitation of an ion pair from solution is called the *formation product ratio*. Below this limit, the solution remains metastable without spontaneous precipitation.

## FPR-APR Discriminant Score

The FPR-APR discriminant score is a quantitative measure of the propensity for spontaneous precipitation of calcium oxalate or brushite ($CaHPO_4 \cdot 2H_2O$) in urine. It is derived mathematically from the formation product ratio (FPR) and the activity product ratio (APR or state of saturation). The FPR or APR each contributes to spontaneous precipitation, since reduced limits of metastability or increased saturation would facilitate this process. The discriminant score assesses the effects of both FPR and APR. A positive value indicates increased likelihood of spontaneous precipitation, whereas a negative value reflects reduced likelihood.

## Permissible Increment

The permissible increment is a simple measure of spontaneous precipitation of calcium oxalate or brushite. The permissible increment in oxalate represents the amount of oxalate which needs to be added to urine to initiate spontaneous precipitation of calcium oxalate, whereas the permissible increment in calcium is the amount of added calcium required to cause spontaneous precipitation of brushite. The permissible increment in oxalate represents the amount of oxalate which needs to be added to urine to initiate spontaneous precipitation of calcium oxalate, whereas, the permissible increment in calcium is the amount of added calcium required to cause spontaneous precipitation of brushite.

## Calcium-Cyclic AMP Discriminant Score

The calcium-cyclic AMP discriminant score is a mathematical expression derived from the discriminant analysis of the relationship between fasting urinary calcium and cyclic AMP. A positive value indicates probable occurrence of renal hypercalciuria from parathyroid stimulation, whereas a negative value suggests normal response.

# PATHOGENETIC SIGNIFICANCE OF HYPERCALCIURIA

A valid case may be made for a strong cause and effect relationship between hypercalciuria and calcium stone formation.[36,38]

The physicochemical milieu of urine from patients with hypercalciuric nephrolithiasis may well potentiate the crystallization of stone-forming calcium salts. Their urine is characterized by supersaturation with calcium salts. Their urine is characterized by supersaturation with calcium phosphate (brushite) and calcium oxalate[26] and increased propensity for the spontaneous nucleation of these salts, as assessed by their FPR-APR discriminant score and permissible increment in calcium or oxalate (See definitions and related concepts).[33,21] That these characteristics are important determinants for stone formation is indicated by their degree of departure from normal, the positive correlation between the discriminant score of calcium oxalate and the severity of stone disease,[33] and by the close correlation between treatment-induced normalization of these parameters and clinical improvement (inhibition of stone formation).[23]

Hypercalciuria may be responsible for some or all of the enumerated physicochemical derangments. Urinary concentration of calcium has been shown to be directly correlated with urinary saturation and inversely correlated with the formation product ratio of brushite and calcium oxalate (see Definitions and Related Concepts).[38,26] Moreover, a significant relationship has been found between urinary calcium concentration and discriminant scores of permissible increments.[38] In our preliminary study, the exaggeration or induction of hypercalciuria was found to increase supersaturation[25] and reduce the limit of metastability (see Definitions and Related Concepts). The correction of hypercalciuria by appropriate treatment typically normalizes many of the aforementioned physicochemical disturbances.[33]

This conclusion, supporting an important role for hypercalciuria in stone formation, does not exclude or minimize the potential importance of other factors, such as relative hyperoxaluria, hyperuricosuria, and hypocitraturia. However, many patients with hypercalciuric nephrolithiasis present with hypercalciuria as the sole identifiable pathophysiological abnormality.[31] Despite reports to the contrary, urinary oxalate was not significantly increased in our patients with hypercalciuric nephrolithiasis,[15] probably because of self-imposed oxalate restriction. When the computer program of Finlayson was used for calculating activity products[14] (see Definitions and Related Concepts), a rise in calcium concentration was as equally effective as the increase in oxalate concentration in raising the saturation of calcium oxalate.[37]

# DISTINCT PHYSIOLOGIC BASIS FOR THE HYPERCALCIURIAS

It has been suggested that hypercalciuria associated with nephrolithiasis is heterogeneous and comprised of three major forms.[22] Hypercalciuria may be *resorptive*, *absorptive*, or *renal*, depending upon whether the principal derangement is excessive skeletal resorption and calcium mobilization, enhanced intestinal calcium absorption, or impaired renal tubular calcium reabsorption (i.e., the so-called renal leak).

**Resorptive hypercalciuria** associated with nephrolithiasis is almost always caused by primary hyperparathyroidism. Bone resorption is effected by enhanced osteoclast activity, stimulated by parathyroid hormone (PTH). Intestinal calcium absorption may also be increased secondary to PTH stimulation of the renal synthesis of 1,25-dihydroxyvitamin D (1,25 $(OH)_2D$).[17] Hypercalciuria often ensues, being largely caused by the hyperfiltration of calcium and perhaps by the suppressive effect of hypercalcemia

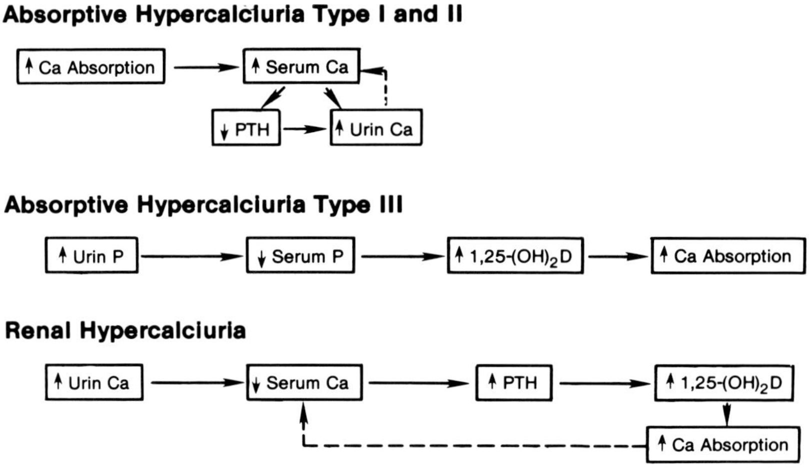

**Absorptive Hypercalciuria Type I and II**

**Absorptive Hypercalciuria Type III**

**Renal Hypercalciuria**

**Fig. 8-1.** Schemes for absorptive and renal hypercalciurias.

on renal tubular reabsorption of calcium. The latter may be a direct effect of hypercalcemic suppression of PTH secretion. Hypercalciuria is therefore primarily resorptive and secondarily, absorptive, as caused by PTH-induced vitamin D activation.

Absorptive and renal hypercalciuria constitute the two major variants of the condition termed idiopathic hypercalciuria[28] (Fig. 8-1). As the term implies, intestinal calcium absorption is presumed to be primarily increased in *absorptive hypercalciuria*. The resulting elevation in serum calcium concentration, though typically not into the hypercalcemic range, causes hypercalciuria by increasing the filtered load of calcium, and concurrently suppressing PTH secretion. Thus, this form of hypercalciuria is primarily absorptive and secondarily renal.

There are sufficient physiological and practical grounds for subdividing absorptive hypercalciuria into three subtypes.[36] Absorptive hypercalciuria, *Type I*, represents the classical form, whereby intestinal hyperabsorption and excessive renal excretion of calcium are encountered during ingestion of high as well as during low calcium diets.[31] In *Type II*, absorptive hypercalciuria, excessive calcium excre-

tion may be corrected by a low calcium diet, though continuously manifest on a high calcium intake.[15] In absorptive hypercalciuria, *Type III*, the presumed primary impairment in renal tubular reabsorption of phosphorus, stimulates renal synthesis of 1,25 $(OH)_2D$ which, in turn, increases calcium absorption.[3,41] There is some evidence to suggest that Type II may be a less severe form of the classical Type I. In this discussion, the term absorptive hypercalciuria shall refer to Types I and II but not Type III, unless otherwise stated.

The primary defect in *renal hypercalciuria* is impairment of tubular calcium absorption (renal leak). The resulting decline in serum calcium, albeit not into the hypocalcemic range, stimulates PTH secretion. Intestinal calcium absorption is usually secondarily increased by PTH stimulation of 1,25 $(OH)_2D$ synthesis,[46] allowing dietary calcium to contribute to the hypercalciuria. Thus, this form of hypercalciuria is primarily renal and secondarily, absorptive.

That the aforementioned hypercalciuric syndromes are separate and distinct entities, is supported by six lines of evidence.[28]

**Parathyroid Function.** Parathyroid hormone secretion should be normal or suppressed in absorptive hypercalciuria and stimulated in renal hypercalciuria consequent to serum calcium's tendency to increase and decrease, respectively.

In absorptive hypercalciuria, numerous studies have shown that serum immunoreactive PTH levels and urinary cyclic AMP excretion are normal.[7,22,24] Following an oral calcium load, urinary cyclic AMP is significantly lower in subjects with absorptive hypercalciuria than in nonhypercalciuric control subjects. The more profound reduction of cyclic AMP excretion probably reflected the greater suppression of PTH secretion in absorptive hypercalciurics, consequent to their greater fractional absorption of the dietary calcium load.[22]

In renal hypercalciuria, high serum PTH and urinary cyclic AMP excretion have been reported by several groups.[10,24,33] These biochemical changes may be corrected by either an oral calcium load or therapy with thiazide diuretics. Both treatments suppress PTH secretion by increasing serum calcium concentration, but since the latter acts by enhancing renal calcium reabsorption (i.e., diminishing the leak), the primary role of the renal calcium wastage is emphasized.

However, some normocalcemic patients may present with fasting hypercalciuria, indicative of a renal leak, but without evidence of parathyroid stimulation.[11,42,43] The relative prevalence of this subgroup among patients with hypercalciuric nephrolithiasis varies considerably from one laboratory to another. In our previous outpatient evaluation of 241 patients with nephrolithiasis,[31] 13 patients with "unclassified hypercalciuria" had the above features, as compared to 16 with renal hypercalciuria with secondary hyperparathyroidism (shown by high serum PTH and/or urinary cyclic AMP). We would suggest that the term *renal hypercalciuria* be reserved for calcium leak associated with secondary hyperparathy-

roidism. The possible causes for the fasting hypercalciuria without parathyroid stimulation will be discussed below.

**Evidence for Renal Calcium Leak.** The diagnosis of a renal calcium leak is predicated upon finding persistant hypercalciuria during fasting in normocalcemic subjects. As the duration of fasting is continued, calcium absorbed from the intestinal tract makes an ever-decreasing contribution to urinary calcium. In normocalcemic patients in whom the filtered load of calcium is not increased, a high fasting urinary calcium excretory rate indicates that a renal leak is present.[24] A high fasting urinary calcium has invariably been found in patients with renal hypercalciuria in whom the diagnosis was initially reached by independent methods. In contrast, urinary calcium excretion during fasting was usually within the normal range in patients with absorptive hypercalciuria. These results suggested that the renal tubular reabsorption of calcium may be impaired in renal hypercalciuria but not in absorptive hypercalciuria.[24]

It has been suggested that a renal leak of calcium may be caused by the excessive ingestion of sodium.[20] Indeed, when normal subjects take a high sodium diet the findings of renal hypercalciuria can be produced. These subjects manifest hypercalciuria, high serum 1,25 $(OH)_2D$ and enhanced intestinal absorption of calcium.[8] However, this contention is unlikely for the following reasons.

In our patients with renal hypercalciuria, fasting hypercalciuria was found while they were maintained or instructed to remain on the same sodium intake (100 mEq/day) as control subjects.[31] Twenty-four hour urinary sodium excretion was 141 ± 66 (S.D) mEq/day in subjects with renal hypercalciuria, values not significantly different from those of control subjects (106 ± 46 mEq/day).[31] Even though mean sodium excretion was 35 mEq/day greater in renal hypercalciurics, this small excess sodium intake does not substantially increase calcium excretion.[8] An exaggerated sodium load (250 mEq/day for 10 days) following a low sodium intake (9 mEq/day) caused a small but significant increase in fasting urinary calcium in normal subjects, however, fasting urinary calcium remained within normal limits.[9] Finally, no significant difference was found between fasting urinary calcium and fasting urinary sodium excretion among control subjects and patients with absorptive hypercalciuria.[8]

That renal hypercalciurics may have impaired proximal sodium and calcium reabsorption was further supported by the response of affected subjects to thiazide treatment. If sodium reabsorption at some site(s) proximal to the distal convoluted tubule was impaired, prevention of salt-wasting would, in part, require enhanced distal reabsorption, thereby recapturing the excess sodium reaching distal sites. The natriuretic response to thiazides, which inhibit sodium reabsorption in the distal convoluted tubule, therefore, should be exaggerated in subjects with concurrent proximal reabsorptive defects. In our preliminary study, an exaggerated natriuretic response to hydrochlorothiazide was encountered in subjects with renal hypercalciuria, but not in those with absorptive hypercalciuria or in subjects with fasting hypercalciuria with normal parathyroid function.

**Intestinal Calcium Absorption.** Intestinal absorption of calcium is invariably increased in absorptive hypercalciuria. Since calcium absorption and secretion occur simultaneously in the intestinal tract, net absorption can only be calculated by measuring the difference between calcium ingested and that appearing in the stool. Radioisotope studies measuring only the absorptive arm of the bidirectional process, overestimate net absorption.

That absorptive hypercalciuria is probably secondary to enhanced calcium absorption and not to diminished secretion is suggested by the fact that absorbed calcium typically exceeds urinary calcium.[22] The difference between absorbed calcium and urinary calcium (i.e., the calcium secreted by the intestine) has been shown to be somewhat lower in patients with absorptive hypercalciuria than in control subjects. This finding need not indicate the presence of a negative calcium balance, since it could reflect increased absorption of secreted calcium as well as dietary calcium. Although some patients with idiopathic hypercalciuria have been shown to be in negative calcium balance, they may not have suffered from absorptive hypercalciuria. Moreover, the results of calcium balance studies should be interpreted with caution because the balance techniques are relatively imprecise.

However, intestinal calcium absorption is increased in some but not all patients with renal hypercalciuria.[28] These results suggest that increased calcium absorption in renal hypercalciuria may not represent a primary derangement, but probably indicates a secondary event. The absorbed calcium is often less than the urinary calcium.

**Role of Vitamin D Metabolism.** In renal hypercalciuria, fractional intestinal calcium absorption was found to be directly correlated with the circulating concentration of 1,25 $(OH)_2D$.[28] Accordingly, the sequence of events leading to increased calcium absorption is likely to proceed as follows: The reduction of serum calcium concentration caused by the primary renal calcium leak, stimulates PTH secretion which, in turn, enhances renal synthesis of 1,25 $(OH)_2D$ and this hormone increases gastrointestinal (GI) calcium absorption. The validity of this hypothesis was shown by the restoration of normal serum 1,25 $(OH)_2D$ and intestinal calcium absorption following the correction of renal calcium leak with thiazide therapy.[46]

In absorptive hypercalciuria, a similar dependence on 1,25 $(OH)_2D$ cannot be invoked. Fractional calcium absorption, determined from the fecal recovery of orally administered radiocalcium, was not correlated with serum levels of 1,25 $(OH)_2D$.[17] In most patients, the fractional calcium absorption was inappropriately high for the level of serum 1,25 $(OH)_2D$.[17]

Studies of intestinal perfusion provided a further insight in the potential pathogenetic role of vitamin D in absorptive hypercalciuria.[6] Calcium absorption was found to be increased in jejunum but normal in ileum, whereas the jejunal absorption of magnesium, another divalent cation, was normal. The increased calcium absorption in jejunum was not attenuated by magnesium. This transport profile differs from the changes in calcium and magnesium absorption induced by vitamin D. Treatment of renal failure patients[40] and normal subjects[18] with 1,25 $(OH)_2D$ has been shown to augment calcium absorption in both jejunum and ileum and to enhance magnesium absorption. Moreover, the hyperabsorption of calcium in absorptive hypercalciuria may not be corrected by treatment with adrenocorticosteroids,[45] thiazide diuretics,[46] nor orthophosphate,[3] even though the latter reduces the serum concentration of 1,25 $(OH)_2D$.

However, serum 1,25 $(OH)_2D$ has been reported to be high in one-third to one-half of patients with absorptive hypercalciuria.[16,17,41] Although renal phosphate leak could explain this rise,[41] its presence has not been consistently demonstrated.[3] The cause for the high serum 1,25 $(OH)_2D$ remains largely unresolved.

**Different Responses to Treatment.** Absorptive hypercalciuria and renal hypercalciuria may be differentiated on the basis of these unique responses to certain forms of therapy.

In renal hypercalciuria, thiazide therapy "corrected" the renal calcium leak and restored to normal, parathyroid function, serum 1,25 $(OH)_2D$ concentration, and fractional GI calcium absorption.[46] In absorptive hypercalciuria, however, the serum concentration of 1,25 $(OH)_2D$ remained unchanged and the intestinal hyperabsorption of calcium persisted, despite reduction in urinary calcium.[46]

Sodium cellulose phosphate, a nonabsorbable resin with a high affinity for calcium, inhibits intestinal calcium absorption when given orally.[30] It caused a more prominent reduction in urinary calcium in absorptive hypercalciuria than in renal hypercalciuria.[28] Moreover, cellulose phosphate caused an exaggeration of secondary hyperparathyroidism (as indicated by urinary cyclic AMP excretion increasing from 7.98 ± 0.62 S.D. nmole/100 ml of glomerular filtrate to 10.58 ± 3.10 nmole/100 ml of glomerular filtrate) in renal hypercalciuria. In contrast, normal parathyroid function was maintained during treatment with sodium cellulose phosphate in absorptive hypercalciuria.[35]

**Sequelae of PTH Excess.** Although clinical bone disease is rare, quantitative measurement of bone density by photon absorptiometry has disclosed significantly reduced density in renal hypercalciurics (compared with age and sex-matched control groups).[19] The results indicated that secondary hyperparathyroidism had exerted deleterious effects on the skeleton. The lack of more substantial involvement was probably due to the compensatory intestinal hyperabsorption of calcium occurring from PTH-induced renal synthesis of 1,25 $(OH)_2D$.[46]

In contrast, bone density was not significantly different from that of controls in subjects with absorptive hypercalciuria.[19] This finding suggested that there is no prominent disturbance in bone metabolism or calcium balance in this form of hypercalciuria.

## DIFFICULTY WITH THE UNIFYING THEORY OF HYPERCALCIURIA

Disturbed proximal tubular transport of calcium and phosphate could explain many of the characteristic findings of idiopathic hypercalciuria. The variable extent to which secondary hyperparathyroidism occurred could be explained by the offsetting effects of primary calciuria and phosphaturia on PTH secretion. If hypercalciuria were the predominating defect, secondary hyperparathyroidism would blossom. On the other hand, prominence of phosphaturia could mask secondary hyperparathyroidism, by stimulating 1,25 $(OH)_2D$ synthesis and consequently augmenting intestinal absorption and skeletal mobilization of calcium, which would dampen PTH secretion.

The above scheme could account for the pathogenesis of renal hypercalciuria and of hypophosphatemic absorptive hypercalciuria (Type III), but not classic absorptive hypercalciuria (Type I). The unique features of absorptive hypercalciuria that justify its classification as a separate entity, include the following: (a) inappropriately low serum 1,25 $(OH)_2D$ for the level of intestinal calcium absorption;[17] (b) lack of significant skeletal involvement, as shown by normal fasting urinary calcium,[24] absorbed calcium exceeding urinary calcium,[22] and normal bone density;[19] (c) intact calcium conservation, indicated by the ability of sodium cellulose phosphate treatment to restore urinary calcium to normal without altering calcium balance;[30] (d) selective jejunal but not ileal hyperabsorption of calcium in the absence of altered magnesium absorption,[6,18,40] denoting a vitamin D-in-

dependent process; and (e) inability of orthophosphate therapy to correct the intestinal hyperabsorption of calcium, despite restoration of normal serum 1,25 $(OH)_2D$.[3]

Absorptive hypercalciuria may however, coexist with increased renal synthesis of $(OH)_2D$.[20,39] Such a picture could explain the presence of high serum 1,25 $(OH)_2D$ in some patients, and may contribute to the development of fasting hypercalciuria without parathyroid stimulation (to be described).

## DIAGNOSTIC SEPARATION OF THE HYPERCALCIURIAS

Reliable protocols are now available for the differentiation of the various forms of hypercalciuria[7,24,31] (Table 8-1). Our own ambulatory protocol requires three outpatient visits, and may be completed within one month.[27,38] This evaluation depends largely upon procedures that should be available in routine clinical laboratories. Certain specialized procedures may be obtained commercially. This work-up is cost-effective, since it can be conducted at a fraction of the cost incurred during hospitalization for renal colic.

### Diagnostic Criteria

Primary hyperparathyroidism may be recognized by the presence of hypercalcemia, hypophosphatemia, hypercalciuria, and increased or inappropriately high serum PTH and/or urinary cyclic AMP.[31] Hypercalcemic symptoms, peptic ulcer, or bone disease (osteitis, pathologic fractures, osteoporosis) may be present.

Absorptive hypercalciuria, Type I, is characterized by normal serum calcium, phosphorus, and normal fasting urinary

**Table 8-1.** Outline of Ambulatory Protocol for Differentiating the Hypercalciuric Syndromes

I. Procedures
  Visit 1: History and physical examination
       24-hour urine on random diet
  Visit 2: 24-hour urine on random diet
       Diet history and instruction
  Visit 3: 24-hour urine on restricted diet (400 mg Ca, 100 mEq Na/day)
       Fast and load

II. Laboratory Tests

| | BLOOD | | | | | URINE | | | | | | | |
| --- | --- | --- | --- | --- | --- | --- | --- | --- | --- | --- | --- | --- | --- |
| | CBC | SMA | PTH | Ca | UA | Cr | Na | pH | TV | Ox | cAMP | Citrate | Qual. Cystine |
| Visit 1 | X | X | X | X | X | X | X | X | X | | | | X |
| Visit 2 | | X | | X | X | X | X | X | X | | | | |
| Visit 3 | | X | | X | X | X | X | X | X | X | X | X | |
| Fast | | | | X | | X | | | | | X | | |
| Load | | | | X | | X | | | | | X | | |

Note. Cr: creatinine; Ox: oxalate; SMA: serum electrolytes, BUN, glucose; TV: total volume; UA: uric acid.

calcium excretion (< 0.11 mg/100 ml of glomerular filtrate),[24,31] that increases excessively following an oral calcium load (> 0.2 mg/mg creatinine).[24] Furthermore parathyroid function is normal or suppressed (serum PTH being below the upper limit of normal for a given assay, and the 24-hour urinary cyclic AMP, while ingesting a low calcium diet, is < 5.4 nmole/100 ml of glomerular filtrate).[22,31] Some patients may have a slightly increased fasting urinary calcium which probably reflects the incomplete clearance of absorbed calcium.[29]

More rigid dietary restriction of calcium and sodium, or fasting of longer duration, should restore fasting calcium excretion to normal while keeping parathyroid function within the normal range.

Absorptive hypercalciuria, Type II, is characterized by the same biochemical features as Type I, except for normocalciuria (< 200 mg/day) on a restricted calcium diet.[36] Apparently, intestinal calcium absorption during low calcium intake is normal, whereas that during high calcium intake increased. Indeed, if these patients are placed on a diet of 1000 mg calcium and 100 mEq sodium/day, urinary calcium exceeds 4 mg/kg/day or 250 mg/day. Urine volume is often < 1 liter/day, because some patients habitually take in less fluid.[31] Absorptive hypercalciuria associated with a low serum phosphorous concentration has been termed *hypophosphatemic absorptive hypercalciuria* or *absorptive hypercalciuria, Type III*.

Renal hypercalciuria is characterized by normocalcemia, high fasting urinary calcium excretion (> 0.11 mg/100 ml of glomerular filtrate) and increased circulating levels of PTH.[24] These results are indicative of a renal calcium leak with compensatory parathyroid stimulation. It should be noted that either the serum PTH or urinary cyclic AMP excretion must be elevated to diagnose renal hypercalciuria.[31] Bone density may be decreased in patients with renal hypercalciuria, and in some cases osteopenia may occur.[19]

## Fasting Hypercalciuria with Normal Parathyroid Function

Some patients with hypercalciuria manifest elements of both primary intestinal and renal defects.[11,36] Their urinary calcium excretion during fasting remains high, indicative of a primary renal calcium leak, but parathyroid function is normal or suppressed, suggesting increased calcium absorption. There are several possible explanations for this somewhat confusing picture.

The most likely cause for these observations is an incomplete clearance of absorbed calcium due to inadequate dietary preparation prior to the fasting urine collection.[29] We recommend that urine collections be obtained only after a minimum of 10 to 12 hours of fasting (except for distilled water), and after at least 1 week of adherence to a diet restricted in calcium (400 mg/day) and sodium (100 mEq/day).[27,31] Shorter periods of fasting and/or higher intakes of calcium may exaggerate fasting calciuria because the relatively large amount of calcium in the GI tract may continue to be absorbed in generous amounts. Moreover, calcium absorption may be high enough to compensate for the renal calcium leak and thereby prevent parathyroid stimulation. This problem may be resolved by the calculation of fasting urinary calcium-cyclic AMP discriminant score[29] (see Definitions and Related Concepts), prior preparation with sodium cellulose phosphate[31] or a fast of longer duration.

Other possible explanations for this "syndrome" include excessive skeletal mobilization of calcium, reduced responsiveness of parathyroid glands or renal adenyl cyclase to renal calcium leak, and an altered set point for PTH release. Enhanced renal synthesis of $1,25\ (OH)_2D$ may prove to be the cause for the increased skeletal mobilization of calcium in this syndrome.

# SELECTIVE TREATMENT OF HYPERCALCIURIAS

Elucidation of the physicochemical and physiologic basis for hypercalciuria and nephrolithiasis coupled with improved methods for diagnostic separation of hypercalciuric states, provides the basis for the "selective" treatment program.[34] In such a program, certain treatment is specifically chosen for each form of hypercalciuria based upon the chosen therapy's ability to correct the specific physicochemical and pathophysiologic disturbance underlying that disorder. This selective approach differs from more randomized treatment programs in which the same drug may be used in several forms of hypercalciuria even though its actions may be poorly defined.

On the basis of available data, we have chosen four selective treatment programs for hypercalciuric calcium nephrolithiasis.[34]

## Sodium Cellulose Phosphate for Absorptive Hypercalciuria Type I

Sodium cellulose phosphate (Mission Pharmacal Co., San Antonio, TX) a drug recently approved by the FDA, was considered to be selective for absorptive hypercalciuria Type I.[23,30,35] This nonabsorbable ion-exchange resin with a high binding affinity for calcium ions has been shown to correct the intestinal hyperabsorption of calcium (by binding calcium in the intestinal tract). It has been reported to restore to "normal" the physicochemical environment of urine, by reducing urinary saturation with brushite $(CaHPO_4 \cdot 2H_2O)$ and calcium oxalate, and by decreasing the propensity for the spontaneous nucleation of brushite and calcium oxalate. These conclusions are based upon measurements of the FPR-APR discriminant score (see Definitions and Related Concepts).[33] This treatment, however, may cause secondary hyperoxaluria and reduced magnesium excretion.[35] Thus, it has been our customary practice to moderately restrict dietary oxalate and to provide oral magnesium supplements (magnesium gluconate 1.0– 1.5 g twice/

day; not to be given with the cellulose phosphate).

The use of sodium cellulose phosphate should currently be restricted to those patients with absorptive hypercalciuria who present with normal fasting urinary calcium and normophosphatemia. The restoration of normal intestinal calcium absorption with sodium cellulose phosphate effectively lowers urinary calcium without significantly altering calcium balance, serum alkaline phosphatase, or bone density.[23,30,35]

In patients with fasting hypercalciuria or hypophosphatemia, there may be excessive skeletal mobilization of calcium. The use of sodium cellulose phosphate should be avoided unless such a skeletal involvement can be excluded.

## High Fluid Intake and/or Low Calcium Diet for Absorptive Hypercalciuria Type II

A low calcium intake (400 to 600 mg/day) in absorptive hypercalciuria Type II is ideally suited for these subjects, and indeed, normocalciuria is restored by this simple dietary restriction.[34] A high fluid intake (sufficient to achieve a minimum daily urine volume of two liters) is indicated since many of these patients have low 24-hour urinary volumes. An increased urine volume has been shown to reduce the urinary saturation of calcium oxalate, brushite, and monosodium urate and to inhibit spontaneous nucleation of calcium oxalate.[32]

## Orthophosphate for Absorptive Hypercalciuria Type III

Orthophosphate, the neutral salt of sodium and potassium phosphate, is the logical therapy for these subjects since phosphate inhibits synthesis of 1,25 $(OH)_2D$.[3] Moreover, it has been shown to reduce urinary saturation with calcium

oxalate and to inhibit spontaneous nucleation of brushite and calcium oxalate.[33] Oral therapy is initiated with 1.5 to 2.0 g daily of phosphorus, in three-to-four divided doses.

## Thiazide diuretics for Renal Hypercalciuria

Thiazide represents an ideal treatment program for renal hypercalciuria, since it corrects the renal leak of calcium, restore parathyroid function, serum 1,25 $(OH)_2D$ levels and calcium absorption to normal.[46] Thiazides have been shown to correct hypercalciuria, reduce urinary saturation, and enhance inhibitor activity against spontaneous nucleation of both calcium oxalate and brushite.[33] Hypocitraturia may develop, particularly when hypokalemia is present, and may oppose the beneficial response to therapy.[44] Thus, we routinely provide potassium supplementation even in the absence of symptomatic hypokalemia.

## Clinical Efficacy of Selective Treatments

The above selective treatment programs have been evaluated with a long-term prospective follow-up study.[34] The number of new stones formed was carefully assessed and compared with the number determined by history for the three years immediately preceding institution of selective therapy.

All four selective treatment programs effectively prevented new stone formation. Fifty-three to seventy-eight percent of patients remained in remission (did not form any more stones), and 77 to 100 percent of patients showed a reduced stone formation rate (Table 8-2). Each treatment produced a significant decline in the new stone formation rate. The actual number of stones formed during treatment was less than 39 percent of the number predicted to form from chance alone.

**Table 8-2.** Effect of Treatment on Clinical Course

| Condition | AH-I | AH-II | AH-III | RH |
|---|---|---|---|---|
| Treatment | SCP | Water & Diet | P | TZ |
| No. of patients | 18 | 24 | 8 | 13 |
| Pretreatment | | | | |
|     Total no. stones formed | 123 | 132 | 57 | 63 |
|     Duration, yr/pt | 3.00 | 3.00 | 3.00 | 3.00 |
|     Stone formation rate | | | | |
|       No./yr | $2.28 \pm 1.92$ | $1.83 \pm 3.29$ | $2.38 \pm 1.94$ | $1.61 \pm 1.90$ |
|       No./pt/yr | 2.28 | 1.83 | 2.38 | 1.62 |
| Treatment | | | | |
|     Total no. stones formed | 10 | 21 | 12 | 33 |
|     Duration, yr/pt | 2.37 | 2.32 | 4.13 | 4.16 |
|     Stone formation rate | | | | |
|       No./yr | $0.33 \pm 0.68$ | $0.52 \pm 1.09$ | $0.67 \pm 1.56\Gamma$ | $0.62 \pm 1.07$ |
|       No./pt/yr | 0.23 | 0.38 | 0.36 | 0.61 |
| Remission (%) | 77.8 | 70.8 | 62.5 | 53.8 |
| Reduced stone formation | | | | |
|     rate (%) | 100.0 | 91.7 | 100.0 | 76.9 |
| No. stones, observed/ | | | | |
|     predicted (%) | $10.3\Gamma$ | $28.3\Gamma$ | $28.2\Gamma$ | $38.5\Gamma$ |

Note. SCP, sodium cellulose phosphate; P, orthophosphate; TZ, thiazide; AH-I, absorptive hypercalciuria Type I; AH-II, absorptive hypercalciuria Type II; AH-III, hypophosphatemic absorptive hypercalciuria; RH, renal hypercalciuria. Values are presented as mean $\pm$ SD. For stone formation rate, the significant difference from pretreatment value produced by treatment is shown by (*) for $p<0.05$, $\Gamma$ for $p<0.001$. The significant difference between observed number of stones and predicted number, obtained by chi square, is shown by same symbols.

## Critique of the Prospective Clinical Trial

The favorable clinical response to selective treatment programs described above supports, but does not prove, the validity of the concept of a selective approach. Since randomized placebo control groups were not included and pretreatment history was obtained retrospectively without benefit of direct care, nonspecific influences associated with our close follow-up observation could have modified the clinical response to treatment. These nonspecific effects probably include change in dietary habits and fluid intake and improved patient compliance (from close follow-up). Positive "placebo effect" on the course of nephrolithiasis is well known.[13]

Although the need for assessing the placebo effect is clear, randomized trials with placebo controls pose formidable problems because of the difficulty in disguising test medications. Most patients can recognize sodium cellulose phosphate, thiazides or neutral phosphate.

Despite the lack of randomized control studies, several lines of evidence indicate that selective treatments had exerted a positive impact on the clinical course of stone disease. The clinical improvement (i.e., the reduced stone formation rate) produced by treatment was correlated well with objective measures of stone formation (i.e., reduced saturation of urinary calcium salts).[23,35] Our preliminary study suggests that the decline in urinary saturation of calcium salts occurring during treatment of absorptive hypercalciuria Type I with sodium cellulose phosphate resulted largely from the effect of treatment itself (reduction in urinary calcium) rather than from nonspecific influences (change in urine volume). When patients with absorptive hypercalciuria who had been on sodium cellulose phosphate were placed on alternative treatments, 57.1 per-

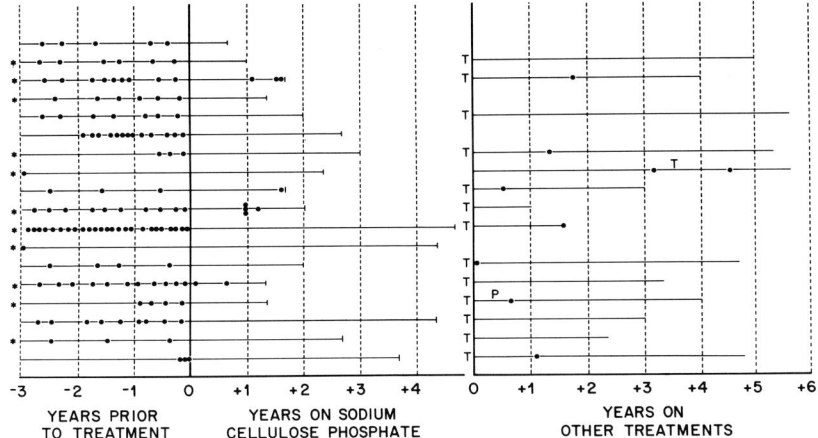

**Fig. 8-2.** Comparison of the effect of sodium cellulose phosphate with that of other treatments (T, thiazide or P, orthophosphate) on the new stone formation rate of absorptive hypercalciuria Type I. Each line represents studies in a single patient. Asterisk before each line represents studies in a single patient. Asterisk before each line indicates the presence of preexisting renal stone(s). Each point shows new stone formation.

cent developed new stones as compared with 22.2 percent during sodium cellulose phosphate treatment (Fig. 8-2).[38]

Finally, as previously discussed, a cogent argument may be made for a causal relationship between hypercalciuria and renal stone formation.[38] All four selective treatments effectively restore urinary calcium excretion to normal and correct many of the physicochemical disturbances occurring in the urine.

## Advantages of Selective Treatment Approach

The theoretical advantage of the selective approach is the as yet unproven assumption that treatments specifically chosen for their physicochemical and physiologic effects are less likely to cause side effects and more likely to overcome extrarenal manifestations of the disease process, than are more randomly chosen programs.

## Hazards of Therapy

Although concrete data are lacking, it is to be expected that certain randomized treatments working at cross-purposes to the underlying pathophysiologic defect, may be associated with significant hazards. Parathyroidectomy in patients with renal hypercalciuria may cause recurrence of renal leak of calcium and nephrolithiasis, because it does not correct the renal impairment.[2] Treatment of renal hypercalciuria with cellulose phosphate may cause negative calcium balance since the urinary excretion of calcium continues despite drug-induced reduction of GI absorption. Exaggerated secondary hyperparathyroidism and bone disease could easily develop in this setting. Orthophosphate therapy of normophosphatemic absorptive hypercalciuria may cause calcium retention, since high intestinal calcium absorption is maintained despite a reduction in urinary calcium.[3] Although the literature is discordant on this point, there are reports of parathyroid stimulation and soft-tissue calcification during the use of orthophosphate.[12]

Even though thiazides were considered to be "selective" for absorptive hypercalciuria Type I, it may not be an ideal therapy. Despite reduced calcium excretion, intestinal calcium absorption remained persistently elevated.[1] Preliminary study suggests that the "retained" calcium may accrete in bone.[37] Bone density, determined in the distal third of the radius by photon absorptiometry, increased significantly during thiazide treatment in absorptive hypercalciuria, with an annual increment of 1.34 percent. In contrast, bone density was not significantly altered in renal hypercalciuria where thiazides were shown to cause a decline in intestinal calcium absorption commensurate with a reduction in urinary calcium excretion. From a practical standpoint, the increment in bone density was small and was not associated with any apparent hazard. Nevertheless, this preliminary finding suggests that thiazides do not completely satisfy the criteria for selective therapy.

These potential complications of random treatments attest to the value of selective therapies.

### Extrarenal Manifestations

It is apparent that even if conservative treatments inhibit stone formation, specific treatments may be indicated for the prevention of nonrenal complications. Nephrolithiasis should be considered as a potential multisystem disease, in which stone formation is only one manifestation. In renal hypercalciuria, photon absorptiometry has demonstrated that reduced bone density may be a not uncommon complication.[19] Selective treatment with thiazide may avert this complication by restoring normal parathyroid function, as shown by stable bone density during a long-term follow-up.[37] Primary hyperparathyroidism is manifested clinically by peptic ulcer disease and bone disease, as well as by nephrolithiasis.[4] Parathyroidectomy typically averts all three manifestations. Though controversial, there is some evidence to suggest that bone may be adversely affected in patients with absorptive hypercalciuria Type III because of hypophosphatemia.[5] Orthophosphate therapy may retard this complication.

## REFERENCES

1. Barilla DE, Tolentino R, Kaplan RA, et al.: Selective effect of thiazide on the intestinal absorption of calcium in absorptive and renal hypercalciurias. Metabolism 27:125, 1978.
2. Barilla DE, Pak CYC: Pitfalls in parathyroid evaluation in patients with calcium urolithiasis. Urol Res 7:117, 1979
3. Barilla DE, Zerwekh JE, Pak CYC: A critical evaluation of the role of phosphate in the pathogenesis of absorptive hypercalciuria. Min Elec Metab 2:302, 1979.
4. Bone HG, Snyder WH, Pak CYC: Diagnosis of hyperparathyroidism. Ann Rev Med 28:111, 1977.
5. Bordier P, Ryckewart A, Gueris J, et al: On the pathogenesis of so-called idiopathic hypercalciuria. Am J Med 63:398, 1977.
6. Brannan PG, Morawski S, Pak CYC, et al: Selective jejunal hyperabsorption of calcium in absorptive hypercalciuria. Am J Med 66:425, 1979.
7. Broadus AE, Dominguez M, Bartter FC: Pathophysiologic studies in *idiopathic hypercalciuria.* J Clin Endocrinol Metab 47:751, 1977.
8. Breslau NA, McGuire JL, Zerwekh JE, et al: The role of dietary sodium on renal excretion and intestinal absorption of calcium and on vitamin D metabolism. J Clin Endocrinol Metab 55:369, 1982.
9. Breslau NA, Pak CYC: In preparation.
10. Coe FL, Canterbury JM, Firpo JJ, et al: Evidence for secondary hyperparathyroidism in idiopathic hypercalciuria. J Clin Invest 52:134, 1973.

11. Coe FL, Favus MJ, Crockett T, et al: Effects of low-calcium diet on urine calcium excretion, parathyroid function and serum 1,25(OH)$_2$D$_3$ levels in patients with idiopathic hypercalciuria and in normal subjects. Am J Med 72:25, 1982.

12. Dudley FJ, Blackburn CRB: Extraskeletal calcification complicating oral neutral-phosphate therapy. Lancet 2:628, 1970.

13. Ettinger B: Recurrent nephrolithiasis: Natural history and effect of phosphate therapy. A double-blind controlled study. Am J Med 61:200, 1976.

14. Finlayson B: Calcium stones: Some physical and clinical aspects. In David D, Ed: Calcium Metabolism in Renal Failure and Nephrolithiasis. New York, Wiley, 1979, p 337.

15. Galosy R, Clarke L, Ward DL, et al: Renal oxalate excretion in calcium urolithiasis. J Urol 123:320, 1980.

16. Gray RW, Wilz DR, Caldas AE, et al: The importance of phosphate in regulating plasma 1,25-(OH)$_2$-vitamin D levels in humans: Studies in healthy subjects, in calcium-stone formers and in patients with primary hyperparathyroidism. J Clin Endocrinol Metab 45:299, 1977.

17. Kaplan RA, Haussler MR, Deftos LJ, et al: the role of 1α, 25-dihydroxyvitamin D in the mediation of intestinal hyperabsorption of calcium in primary hyperparathyroidism and absorptive hypercalciuria. J Clin Invest 59:756, 1977.

18. Krejs GJ, Nicar MJ, Zerwekh JE, et al: Effect of 1,25-dihydroxyvitamin D$_3$ on calcium and magnesium absorption in the jejunum and ileum of healthy man. Am J Med, in press.

19. Lawoyin S, Sismilich S, Browne R, et al: Bone mineral content in patients with primary hyperparathyroidism, osteoporosis, and calcium urolithiasis. Metabolism 28:1250, 1979.

20. Muldowny FR, Freaney R, Moloney F: Importance of dietary sodium in the hypercalciuria syndrome. Kidney Int 22:292, 1982.

21. Nicar MJ, Hill K, Pak CYC: A simple technique for the assessment of the propensity for the crystallization of calcium oxalate and brushite in urine from the increment

in oxalate or calcium necessary to elicit precipitation. Metabolism 32:906, 1983.

22. Pak CYC, Ohata M, Lawrence EC, et al: The hypercalciurias: Causes, parathyroid functions and diagnostic criteria. J Clin Invest 54:387, 1974.

23. Pak CYC, Delea CS, Bartter FC: Successful treatment of recurrent nephrolithiasis (calcium stones) with cellulose phosphate. N Engl J Med 290:175, 1974.

24. Pak CYC, Kaplan RA, Bone H, et al: A simple test for the diagnosis of absorptive, resorptive and renal hypercalciurias. N Engl J Med 292:497, 1975.

25. Pak CYC: Idiopathic renal lithiasis: New developments in evaluation and treatment. In Fleisch H, Robertson WG, Smith LH, et al, Eds: Urolithiasis Research. New York, Plenum, 1976, p 213.

26. Pak CYC, Holt K: Nucleation and growth of brushite and calcium in urine of stone formers. Metabolism 25:665, 1976.

27. Pak CYC, Fetner C, Townsend J, et al: Evaluation of calcium urolithiasis in ambulatory patients. Comparison of results with those of inpatient evaluation. Am J Med 64:979, 1978.

28. Pak CYC: Physiological basis for absorptive and renal hypercalciurias. Am J Physiol 237:F415, 1979.

29. Pak CYC, Galosy RA: Fasting urinary calcium and cyclic AMP: A discriminant analysis for the identification of renal and absorptive hypercalciurias. J Clin Endocrinol Metab 48:260, 1979.

30. Pak CYC: Clinical pharmacology of sodium cellulose phosphate. J Clin Pharmacol 19:451, 1979.

31. Pak CYC, Britton F, Peterson R, et al: Ambulatory evaluation of nephrolithiasis: Classification, clinical presentation and diagnostic criteria. Am J Med 69:19, 1980.

32. Pak CYC, Sakhaee K, Crowther C, et al: Evidence justifying a high fluid intake in treatment of nephrolithiasis. Ann Intern Med 93:36, 1980.

33. Pak CYC, Galosy RA: Propensity for spontaneous nucleation of calcium oxalate. Quantitative assessment by urinary FPR-APR discriminant score. Am J Med 69:681, 1980.

34. Pak CYC, Peters P, Hurt G, et al: Is selec-

tive therapy of recurrent nephrolithiasis possible? Am J Med 71:615, 1981.

35. Pak CYC: A cautious use of sodium cellulose phosphate in the management of calcium nephrolithiasis. Invest Urol 19:187, 1981.

36. Pak CYC: Pathogenesis, consequences and treatment of the hypercalciuric states. Sem Nephrol 1:356, 1981.

37. Pak CYC, Nicar MJ, Northcutt C: The definition of the mechanism of hypercalciuria *is* necessary for the treatment of recurrent stone formers. In Ritz E, Massry SG, Eds: Pathophysiology of Renal Disease. Basel, Karger, 1982, p 136.

38. Pak CYC, Nicar MJ, Britton F: Clinical experience with sodium cellulose phosphate. World J Urol 1:180, 1983.

39. Peacock M: The mechanisms of hypercalciuria are unnecessary for treatment of recurrent renal calcium stone formers. In Ritz E, Massry SG, Eds: Pathophysiology of Renal Disease. Basel, Karger, 1982, p 152.

40. Schmulen C, Lerman M, Pak CYC, et al: Effect of 1,25-dihydroxyvitamin $D_3$ therapy on intestinal absorption of magnesium in patients with chronic renal disease. Am J Physiol 1:G349, 1980.

41. Shen FH, Baylink DJ, Nielsen RL, et al: Increased serum 1,25-dihydroxyvitamin D in idiopathic hypercalciuria. J Lab Clin Med 90:955, 1977.

42. Sutton RAL, Walker VR: Responses to hydrochlorothiazide and acetazolamide in patients with calcium stones. N Engl J Med 302:709, 1980.

43. Wasserstein AG, Agus ZS: Calcium balance during dietary calcium restriction in idiopathic hypercalciuria (Abstract). Min Elect Metab 6:271, 1981.

44. Yendt ER, Cohanim M: Prevention of calcium stones with thiazides. Kidney Int 13:397, 1978.

45. Zerwekh JE, Pak CYC, Kaplan RA, et al: Pathogenetic role of 1α,25-dihydroxyvitamin D in response to prednisolone therapy. J Clin Endocrinol Metab 51:381, 1980.

46. Zerwekh JE, Pak CYC: Selective effects of thiazide therapy on serum 1α,25-dihydroxyvitamin D and intestinal calcium absorption in renal and absorptive hypercalciurias. Metabolism 29:13, 1980.

# The Case for a Limited Evaluation

Alan G. Wasserstein, M.D.
Zalman S. Agus, M.D.

## INTRODUCTION

It is not uncommon in medicine that multiple therapeutic options are available to the physician, but definitive proof of the superiority of any one option is lacking. In these circumstances, it is tempting to believe that therapy may be tailored to specific subsets of the disease process in question. When these subsets may be defined in a logical and elegant manner, the appeal of "rational" therapy is almost irresistible. Thus, the initial enthusiasm for the diagnostic separation of "absorptive" and "renal" hypercalciuria is easy to understand.

With increasing experience, this enthusiasm has waned. The theoretical basis of the extensive evaluation of hypercalciuria has come into question, and the practical benefit of selective therapy has not been shown. We will argue against the extensive evaluation of hypercalciuria on theoretical and practical therapeutic grounds. On theoretical grounds, we have several objections to the classification of idiopathic hypercalciuria into renal and absorptive subgroups. (1) The definition of hypercalciuria is arbitrary and misleading. (2) The relation of hypercalciuria, in particular the 24-hour urine calcium excretion, to stone formation is uncertain. (3) Renal hypercalciuria, as defined by evidence of parathyroid hyperfunction, is extremely uncommon, but renal hypercal-

ciuria as defined by negative calcium balance or failure of calcium conservation on low intake may be typical of patients with idiopathic hypercalciuria. (4) Absorptive hypercalciuria (idiopathic hypercalciuria with normal or suppressed parathyroid function) is a misnomer insofar as increased bone resorption and/or renal tubular calcium leak are also present in the majority of patients and are not consequences of intestinal calcium hyperabsorption. On practical therapeutic grounds our objections to the classification of absorptive and renal hypercalciuria include the following. (1) The advantages of selective therapy of these subgroups have never been demonstrated in a controlled fashion. (2) Hypocalciuric therapy may be effective in normocalciuric as well as hypercalciuric stone formers. (3) Theoretical side effects of thiazide, such as calcium overload in absorptive hypercalciurics, have not had clinical significance in practice. (4) Alternative therapies whose use is suggested by the diagnostic categories, including sodium cellulose phosphate and dietary calcium restriction, have less empirical evidence of benefit and greater risk of side effects (negative calcium balance, hyperoxaluria) than does thiazide or phosphate therapy. The state of the evidence forces us to conclude that the "rational" approach to hypercalciuric nephrolithiasis has at present no rational basis.

# THEORETICAL CONSIDERATIONS

## Definition of Hypercalciuria

There is substantial overlap of urinary calcium excretion between stone-formers and normal controls.[36,49,52] In both groups, urinary calcium excretion is skewed to the right and Gaussian statistics cannot be applied. Hodgkinson and Pyrah[36] defined hypercalciuria as exceeding 300 mg/24 hours in men and 250 mg/24 hours in women; 10 percent of normal individuals had values exceeding these limits. These are not normal values in the usual sense, but an arbitrary definition. We have recently confirmed these values, virtually precisely, in a normal population which was age- and sex-matched with a group of recurrent stone-formers. Although daily urine calcium excretion was significantly higher in the stone-formers (260 versus 187 mg, p < 0.001), only 33 percent of stone-formers had values exceeding these arbitrary limits. Similarly, Morgan and Robertson[49] obtained a Gaussian distribution of urine calcium excretion by taking only an upper range of values; the median plus two standard deviations (SD) was 456 mg, and most stone-formers fell within this range. Since a majority of stone-formers have urine calcium excretion within the arbitrary normal range, and since a substantial "tail" in the normal population has hypercalciuria, it is evident that hypercalciuria cannot be regarded as a disease that in itself causes kidney stones. Most workers regard hypercalciuria as one urinary risk factor among several that predispose to renal calculi.[71,72] The relevant question then is not how high urinary calcium must be to cause stones, but whether there exists a threshold below which the risk of stone formation attributable to urine calcium excretion is negligi-

ble or zero. That is to say, a stone-former could have 24-hour urine calcium excretion of, say, 200 mg, close to the normal mean, and yet benefit from hypocalciuric therapy. For example, this level of urine calcium could impose minimal additional risk of stone formation in a normal individual, but in the presence of other risk factors, such as hyperoxaluria or absence of urinary inhibitors, pose a significant risk in the stone-former. There is little firm information on this point. Strauss et al.[79] have shown that treated stone-formers who relapsed had higher urine calcium excretion during treatment (216 mg/24 hours, 2.79 mg/kg BW) than did patients who did not relapse (186 mg/24 hours, 2.39 mg/kg BW). All these values are well within the conventional normal range. These data imply that "like blood pressure, calcium excretion is a graded risk factor throughout a wide range,"[79] and that the conventional upper limits of normal are not useful to guide therapy. However, these data do not address the question of initial therapy and do not indicate what values should constitute a threshold for therapy. Examination of the risk factor analysis of Robertson et al.[71] would suggest that the risk associated with hypercalciuria, though relatively low, rises steadily throughout the normal range of urine calcium excretion and rises sharply at values greater than two S.D. above the normal mean. However, in this study the statistical methods were suspect and the controls poorly defined. Pak et al.[62] have used a value of 200 mg/24 hours, which is in the general range suggested by the study of Strauss et al.[79] There is no evidence, however, that treatment of urine calcium excretion below 200 mg/24 hours would not also be efficacious. In this regard it is noteworthy that thiazides have been reported to ameliorate stone disease in normocalciuric patients;[15,87] however, such patients may have had urine calcium excretion in the high-normal range. Similarly, in vitro measurements of activity product ratio (APR) and formation product ratio (FPR) have shown a stone-forming propensity in the *majority* of patients with normocalciuric nephrolithiasis.[60] In this study, normocalciuria was defined as urine calcium excretion less than 200 mg/24 hours. Thus, there is some reason to believe that an arbitrary definition of hypercalciuria, especially if based on the upper limits of normal, could deprive some stone forming patients of potentially beneficial hypocalciuric therapy.

There are other important problems in the definition of hypercalciuria. There is a large intra-individual variation of urinary calcium, probably owing to the high intestinal calcium absorption in stoneformers. In normal individuals, urinary calcium represents 6 percent of dietary calcium, while in stone-formers urinary calcium represents 20 percent of dietary calcium.[52] Thus, during ambulatory evaluation, if dietary calcium varies by 200 mg on a putative diet (e.g., between 300 and 500 mg on a low calcium diet, between 800 and 1000 mg on normal calcium diet), the variation of urine calcium excretion will be 40 mg. Additional variation is introduced by incomplete urine collection, age,[12] seasonal factors (sunlight-induced vitamin D synthesis),[69] and salt intake.[50] In these circumstances, the allocation into alternative diagnostic categories according to an arbitrary demarcation of urine calcium excretion is potentially misleading. In this regard we have noted that a number of our patients have had sufficient spontaneous variation in urine calcium to alter an arbitrary diagnostic classification (unpublished observations).

## The Relationship of Hypercalciuria to Stone Formation

Let us assume, however, that hypercalciuria is clearly defined. The relationship of hypercalciuria to stone formation is not so straightforward as first appears. Certainly hypercalciuria is epidemiologically associated with nephrolithiasis,[12,36,49,52,71,72] although some workers believe that hypercalciuria is a less important risk factor for nephrolithiasis than are urine volume, oxalate, or uric acid. It is natural to suppose that hypercalciuria predisposes to renal stone formation by increasing urine saturation with respect to calcium-containing salts (calcium oxalate and brushite). Now, while it is true that urinary saturation with respect to calcium oxalate and brushite, expressed by the APR, is higher in stone-formers than in controls,[60,61,73] it is not so clear that hypercalciuria accounts for these differences. For example, the majority of control subjects also demonstrate supersaturation with calcium oxalate, and the overlap with stone-formers is substantial.[60,61] In addition, as noted above, patients with normocalciuric nephrolithiasis have increased APR for calcium oxalate and for brushite that are not different from those of hypercalciuric patients.[61] Pak and Galosy[60] have attempted to improve the discrimination between patients with nephrolithiasis and controls by combining APR and FPR for oxalate and brushite in a discriminant score. It should be noted that FPR reflects not urinary calcium but the presence of promoters or inhibitors of nucleation. Significantly, overlap between normocalciuric and hypercalciuric nephrolithiasis remains substantial, probably in consequence of increased *oxalate* excretion in both groups (see below), and the relative independence of FPR from urine calcium excretion. These data do not support the primacy of urine calcium excretion in determining stone forming propensity in nephrolithiasis. Indeed, if anything, they suggest that restriction of hypocalciuric therapy to hypercalciuric individuals may exclude some normocalciuric patients from a potentially beneficial therapeutic approach. It is also claimed that the decreased stone formation observed after hypocalciuric therapy supports the role of calcium excretion in formation of renal calculi.[60] This argument ignores the multiple potential benefits of these agents. For example, thiazide therapy reduces urine oxalate, and increases urinary volume, zinc, magnesium, and pyrophosphate.[87] Similarly, phosphate administration increases urinary pyrophosphate.[28]

It is obvious, however, that increments in urine calcium excretion must ultimately increase APR for calcium oxalate and brushite. Therefore, we must explain the relatively poor correlation of stone-forming propensity in vitro with urine calcium excretion. It is not difficult to imagine problems that would prohibit a simple relation between these measurements. For example, nucleation and crystal growth may begin in the collecting duct or on the wall of a papilla, and calcium concentrations in these local areas would be more important than the final urine concentration. Again, stone formation could occur during peak urine calcium excretion (probably postprandial), and the time average given by the total 24-hour calcium excretion may have only an indirect bearing on stone-forming propensity. Thus a patient could have normal 24-hour urine calcium excretion and yet have peak urine calcium concentrations that favor stone formation. The response of normocalciuric stone formers to hypocalciuric therapy may support hypotheses along these lines, although, again, these agents could have multiple beneficial effects beyond reduction of urine calcium. Finally, it is possible that the major contribution of hypercalciuria is not directly to enhance urinary saturation with respect to calcium-containing salts, but to serve as a marker for a more important determinant of stone formation, oxalate. This hypothesis has been advanced by Robertson and

Peacock.[70] These workers have suggested that urinary oxalate correlates better than urinary calcium with stone episode rate and with calcium oxalate crystalluria. Relatively small increases in urinary oxalate within the normal range may cause greater changes in urinary calcium oxalate saturation than do relatively large increments in urinary calcium to frank hypercalciuria. This paradox is explained by the presence of calcium in urine in substantial molar excess compared with oxalate. Thus, an increase in urine calcium brings about a reciprocal reduction in urine oxalate by complexation, and the calcium oxalate product is not markedly changed. An increase in urine oxalate does not have nearly so important an effect on the free urine calcium concentration, and therefore causes a relatively greater rise of the calcium oxalate product. In this scheme the major role of calcium metabolism in nephrolithiasis is in modulating oxalate excretion. The intestinal absorption of oxalate depends on the concentration of free oxalate in the intestinal lumen. Intestinal calcium hyperabsorption reduces intestinal luminal calcium and thereby promotes oxalate absorption. In support of these concepts, the majority of investigators have confirmed the presence of increased oxalate excretion in stone-formers[35,60,61,71,72,83] and its relation to increased intestinal calcium absorption.[35] Galosy et al.[30] failed to detect a difference in oxalate excretion between patients with nephrolithiasis and controls, but their patients were on oxalate-restricted diets. It is noteworthy that in studies from the same laboratory purporting to support the role of hypercalciuria in urinary saturation,[60,61] urinary oxalate was significantly greater than control in both hypercalciuric and normocalciuric nephrolithiasis. These considerations suggest that in the treatment of hypercalciuria, the manner of reduction of urine calcium may be as important as the degree of reduction. For example, reduction of intestinal calcium absorption might actually have a negative impact if accompanied by increments in urine oxalate. However, Pak et al. have challenged the concept that small increments in urine oxalate may have a greater effect on APR for calcium oxalate than do larger increments in urine calcium.[57]

## Inconsistencies in the "Renal" and "Absorptive" Categories of Hypercalciuria

Earlier studies suggested that patients with idiopathic hypercalciuria could be divided into two groups. Renal hypercalciuria was defined as a renal leak of calcium causing secondary hyperparathyroidism and secondary gastrointestinal hyperabsorption. In absorptive hypercalciuria, a primary increase in intestinal calcium absorption causes suppression of PTH and secondary increase in urine calcium excretion. As we will discuss below, this classification is no longer meaningful. Very few patients have elevated levels of PTH. The vast majority therefore would be classified as absorptive; yet in many of these patients recent studies have documented "fasting" calciuria and/or negative calcium balance, indices which are not compatible with a primary increase in intestinal absorption.

**"Renal" Hypercalciuria.** One of the purposes of the extensive evaluation of hypercalciuria is the recognition of renal leak, for which therapy with thiazides is logical. This type of hypercalciuria is characterized by primary renal leak of calcium, secondary hyperparathyroidism, and secondary intestinal calcium hyperabsorption, presumably due to stimulation of $1,25 (OH)_2D$ synthesis. An early report[16] found that 40 percent of patients with idiopathic hypercalciuria have elevated serum immunoreactive parathyroid hormone (iPTH) and therefore suggested that primary renal calcium leak was a major form of idiopathic hypercalciuria. However, this very high incidence probably reflected problems with the PTH radioimmunoassay. In subsequent reports, elevated iPTH or urinary cyclic adenosine monophosphate (UcAMP) have been uncommon findings. Sutton and Walker,[80] Strauss et al.,[79] and Lau et al.[39] did not find any cases of hyperparathyroidism in series of 32, 27, and 100 patients, respectively. Burckhardt and Jaeger[13] found one such case in a series of 150 patients. Pak et al.[59] have recently reported that the frequency of renal hypercalciuria, characterized by increased serum iPTH or UcAMP, is 8 percent in patients with nephrolithiasis. These discrepancies must reflect differences in the PTH immunoassay or in the interpretation of UcAMP values. A proportion of such cases may be due to subtle primary hyperparathyroidism. In a recent report, Broadus et al.[11] described ten such patients, in whom only 20 percent of repeated calcium determinations were elevated. In three patients, serum calcium was consistently normal. Unfortunately, ionized calcium was not measured. The majority of patients presented with renal calculi and resembled what has been described as renal hypercalciuria, except that the elevated UcAMP was not normally suppressed by oral calcium load. However, given the variability of autonomy of hyperplastic or adenomatous parathyroid glands, this criterion may not be adequate to distinguish subtle primary hyperparathyroidism from renal hypercalciuria. The persistence of hypercalciuria after successful parathyroid surgery favors (but does not prove) the diagnosis of renal hypercalciuria with secondary parathyroid stimulation,[8] but others[66] were unable to confirm the importance of this phenomenon. Interestingly, there is a higher proportion of females with "renal" than with "absorptive" hypercalciuria, consistent with the possibility that some renal hypercalciuria represents or is at least in the spectrum of subtle primary hyperparathyroidism.[55]

Renal hypercalciuria has also been defined by elevation of the fasting calcium/creatinine ratio (Ca/Cr), but this criterion has had only secondary value. In some patients, elevated fasting Ca/Cr has coexisted with normal parathyroid indices but has been rationalized as a consequence of delayed gastrointestinal (GI) absorption. Hypercalciuria in these cases was classified as absorptive. Difficulties in this interpretation will be considered below.

The infrequency of secondary hyperparathyroidism in idiopathic hypercalciuria leads us to doubt the importance of *primary* renal leak of calcium in any but rare cases. Nevertheless, renal tubular defects may be present in most patients with idiopathic hypercalciuria. At least three laboratories have established the presence of such renal tubular defects. Lau et al.[39] have found impaired proximal tubular fluid absorption in both "fasting" and "diet-dependent" hypercalciuria, but not in normocalciuric nephrolithiasis. Phosphate administration normalized urine calcium excretion, but did not correct fasting hypophosphatemia or the proximal tubular defect. These observations show that the defect was not a consequence of hypercalciuria or of previous stone passage; in addition, phosphate depletion was unlikely to have caused the defect but may not have been corrected by phosphate administration. Sutton and Walker[80] found that urinary excretion of sodium, calcium and magnesium was enhanced to a greater degree after hydrochlorothiazide in idiopathic hypercalciuria than in control, and to a lesser degree after acetazolamide. They therefore deduced the presence of a proximal tubular defect. In agreement with Lau et al.,[39] they found apparent tubular defects in both "fasting" and "diet-dependent" hy-

percalciuria but not in normocalciuric nephrolithiasis. A recent preliminary report[53] found both proximal and distal tubular defects, including impairment of PAH secretion, glucose absorption, and urine acidification and concentrating ability; in contrast to other reports, both hypercalciuric and normocalciuric stoneformers demonstrated these defects. It is important to note in these investigations that the study populations did not have evidence of hyperparathyroidism and therefore would qualify as "absorptive" hypercalciuria, whether fasting or diet-dependent; nevertheless, renal tubular defects were observed. The precise mechanism whereby renal tubular defects contribute to idiopathic hypercalciuria is uncertain. A direct effect to cause renal calcium leak is one possibility; alternatively, renal phosphate wasting could lead to idiopathic hypercalciuria through a variety of pathways (see below).

**Absorptive Hypercalciuria.** In so-called absorptive hypercalciuria, primary intestinal hyperabsorption of calcium is thought to cause increased urinary calcium excretion, presumably by increasing the filtered load of calcium as well as by inducing relative hypoparathyroidism. The prediction of suppressed parathyroid function has been fulfilled by several groups,[18,74] but other observations cast doubt on the hypothesis of isolated, primary intestinal calcium hyperabsorption. Thus, positive or zero calcium balance would be expected. But in the era before parathyroid function could be assessed, negative calcium balance was noted in the majority of patients with idiopathic hypercalciuria;[17] most of these patients presumably had "absorptive" hypercalciuria (normal or suppressed parathyroid function). More recently, fasting hypercalciuria has been frequently observed in the absence of secondary hyperparathyroidism.[18,39,80] For example, patients with so-called absorptive hypercalciuria have higher mean fasting Ca/Cr ratios than do controls, though within the normal range; and some of these patients have fasting Ca/Cr ratios that are clearly out of the normal range.[55,62,80] It has been argued that this fasting calciuria represents delayed intestinal hyperabsorption, and can be abolished by the administration of sodium cellulose phosphate.[55] However, it should be noted that even after sodium cellulose phosphate, 24-hour urine calcium excretion remains higher in "absorptive" hypercalciuria than in controls (106 mg vs 62 mg).[62] Furthermore, during dietary calcium restriction for 7 to 9 days, we[85] and Coe et al.[18] have noted that urine calcium excretion exceeds dietary intake in the majority of patients with idiopathic hypercalciuria with normal or low serum iPTH or UcAMP. The proportion of patients with such negative calcium balance represents a minimum estimate, as more radical calcium restriction might have exposed the defect in a larger number. The maintenance of low calcium intake for one week seems to us long enough to exclude the presence of delayed intestinal hyperabsorption. Thus, we believe that the classification of absorptive and renal hypercalciuria is flawed: A substantial proportion of patients (if not all) with "absorptive" hypercalciuria have apparent renal leak of calcium. Conversely, renal leak of calcium, as defined by negative calcium balance or fasting calciuria, may be demonstrated in a majority of patients with idiopathic hypercalciuria despite normal parathyroid function.[18,85]

One additional qualification must be added: The finding of fasting hypercalciuria or negative calcium balance in idiopathic hypercalciuria does not necessarily imply the presence of a renal calcium leak. Increased bone resorption (presumably via a PTH-independent mechanism) could produce similar findings. Although one would hope to detect an elevated serum calcium or filtered load of calcium in this circumstance, enhanced bone resorption could enhance renal calcium excretion without a *detectable* change in serum calcium. The recent work of Lemann and his colleagues is instructive in this regard.[1,45] These workers gave calcitriol to normal volunteers and produced serum levels of 1,25 dihydroxy vitamin D (1,25 $(OH)_2D$) comparable to those in idiopathic hypercalciuria. Although fasting serum calcium was not significantly changed, urine calcium excretion was markedly enhanced and indeed negative calcium balance ensued on a low calcium intake. The latter effect was presumed to be due to the effect of 1,25$(OH)_2D$ to enhance bone resorption, though an additional effect on renal calcium handling could not be excluded. Since circulating 1,25$(OH)_2D$ is elevated in idiopathic hypercalciuria, it is reasonable to suppose that a similar state of resorptive hypercalciuria exists in this condition. Indeed, some years ago Liberman et al.[44] showed by calcium kinetic studies that idiopathic hypercalciuria is generally characterized by increased bone turnover as well as intestinal calcium hyperabsorption. However, evidence of increased bone resorption in idiopathic hypercalciuria has been equivocal. Whether bone mass is reduced in "absorptive" hypercalciuria is controversial.[41,74] In addition, direct histologic evidence of bone resorption has usually been lacking,[46] though in one study increased bone resorption was demonstrated histologically in a hypophosphatemic subgroup of idiopathic hypercalciuria.[8] It is possible that bone turnover is enhanced in "absorptive" (normoparathyroid) idiopathic hypercalciuria, but not to a degree that usually produces histological evidence of bone resorption. In any case, enhanced bone resorption would not account for tubular defects other than calciuria[39,53,80] that have been observed in idiopatic hypercalciuria.

Whether fasting calciuria with normal parathyroid function represents renal leak or bone resorption, it cannot be attributed to primary intestinal calcium hyperabsorption. Yet this is the category to which most patients with idiopathic hypercalciuria are now assigned. We prefer to regard apparent "renal leak" of calcium (as well as other tubular defects) as a feature of idiopathic hypercalciuria, not the property of a particular subset.

**Alternative Models of Idiopathic Hypercalciuria: The Role of 1,25(OH)$_2$D and Phosphate Depletion.** The hypothesis that intestinal calcium hyperabsorption is the primary abnormality in idiopathic hypercalciuria is also at variance with two major (though sometimes disputed) features of normoparathyroid idiopathic hypercalciuria: increased[32,37,38,74] or normal[18] serum 1,25(OH)$_2$D and decreased $T_M PO_4/GFR$,[10,18,37,39,74] with or without hypophosphatemia. To the contrary, suppression of parathyroid function would be expected to reduce serum 1,25(OH)$_2$D and enhance $T_M PO_4/GFR$. The possibility therefore arises that stimulation of 1,25(OH)$_2$D production and/or renal phosphate wasting are primary events and intestinal calcium hyperabsorption a secondary consequence.

Any model of the pathogenesis of idiopathic hypercalciuria must include these features: increased circulating 1,25(OH)$_2$D, reduced serum phosphate and $T_M PO_4/GFR$, renal tubular defects, and fasting calciuria with normal or suppressed parathyroid function. We believe that these observations fall naturally into a coherent and unitary synthesis.

**Role of Elevated Serum 1,25(OH)$_2$D.** Since 1,25(OH)$_2$D is the major modulator of intestinal calcium absorption in normal man, it is natural to assume that elevated serum 1,25(OH)$_2$D mediates enhanced intestinal calcium absorption in idiopathic hypercalciuria. However, this supposition has been challenged, the countervailing

view being that the enhanced intestinal calcium absorption of idiopathic hypercalciuria (absorptive hypercalciuria, normoparathyroid idiopathic hypercalciuria) is independent of vitamin D or, at least, falls into one of two subsets according to vitamin D dependence or independence. For example, it has been argued that while intestinal calcium hyperabsorption is universal in absorptive hypercalciuria, frankly elevated serum 1,25(OH)$_2$D was present in only one-third of such patients.[32,38] Furthermore, even when increased, serum 1,25(OH)$_2$D levels were insufficient to account for the observed magnitude of intestinal calcium absorption in some of the patients.[5] However, both we (unpublished observations) and others[37] have found frankly increased circulating 1,25(OH)$_2$D levels in the large majority (80 percent) of patients with absorptive (normoparathyroid) hypercalciuria. Furthermore, current technology does not distinguish free from total 1,25(OH)$_2$D, while only the free moiety may be biologically active. Thus, correlations of serum level with biological effect can only be approximate at the present time. Another argument against the importance of circulating 1,25(OH)$_2$D in idiopathic hypercalciuria has been the demonstration that administration of prednisolone did not reduce intestinal calcium absorption in idiopathic hypercalciuria, but did so in another vitamin D-dependent hyperabsorptive state, sarcoidosis.[89] However, glucocorticoids act in sarcoidosis by reducing 1,25(OH)$_2$D synthesis, an effect which they do not have in idiopathic hypercalciuria or in normal controls. Steroids did not reduce serum 1,25(OH)$_2$D or intestinal calcium absorption in normal controls,[89] but one would not thereby infer that 1,25(OH)$_2$D has no role in intestinal calcium absorption in normal man. A third argument adduced to support the concept of primary intestinal calcium hyperabsorption in idiopathic hypercalciuria is the localization in the intestine of the site of calcium hyperabsorption. Brannan et al.[9] found that intestinal calcium hyperabsorption in idiopathic hypercalciuria was restricted to the jejunum, whereas in patients with chronic renal failure treated with calcitriol there was also calcium hyperabsorption in the ileum. However, this study also contains some data (unidirectional fluxes) favoring an effect in the ileum, and more importantly, was not adequately controlled. Perhaps the best argument in favor of vitamin D-independent intestinal calcium hyperabsorption in idiopathic hypercalciuria is that phosphate administration reduced serum $1,25(OH)_2D$ but, in agreement with several prior studies,[51,65] did not reduce intestinal calcium absorption.[5] It should be noted, however, that phosphate administration has also failed to inhibit intestinal calcium absorption in normal man;[27] these studies preceded the ability to measure $1,25(OH)_2D$.

On balance, the evidence against the role of elevated serum $1,25(OH)_2D$ in intestinal calcium hyperabsorption in idiopathic hypercalciuria is thin and unpersuasive. We favor the view that $1,25(OH)_2D$ does indeed mediate calcium hyperabsorption. A vitamin D-independent subset of absorptive hypercalciuria remains possible but unlikely, as frankly reduced serum $1,25(OH)_2D$ should have been observed in such a group. Mediation of intestinal calcium hyperabsorption by $1,25(OH)_2D$ avoids the necessity of postulating two unrelated abnormalities in normoparathyroid hypercalciuria. In addition, the elevation of serum $1,25(OH)_2D$ helps to explain other features of idiopathic hypercalciuria, including increased bone turnover,[44] negative calcium balance during dietary calcium restriction,[1,18,45,85] and associated hyperoxaluria due to enhanced intestinal calcium absorption.[1] Thus, the abnormality of $1,25(OH)_2D$ metabolism accounts for both intestinal cal-

cium hyperabsorption (on normal calcium intake) and fasting calciuria or negative calcium balance (on restricted calcium intake). However, certain features of idiopathic hypercalciuria cannot be attributed to elevations of circulating $1,25(OH)_2D$, such as multiple renal tubular transport defects. For example, the administration of calcitriol to normal volunteers did not reproduce phosphate wasting or hypophosphatemia.[1]

**Renal Phosphate Wasting.** Hypophosphatemia was included in Albright's early description of the syndrome of idiopathic hypercalciuria.[2] Numerous investigators have confirmed the findings of reduced serum phosphate and/or $T_MPO_4/GFR$.[10,18,39,52,74] Indeed, in studies where a significant difference between stone-formers and controls was not obtained,[5] it is likely that a type II error, due to insufficient sample size, was present. Negative phosphate balance on a normal diet[24] and impaired phosphate conservation during dietary phosphate deprivation[43] have also been demonstrated. Lau et al.[39] showed that this renal phosphate wasting was independent of PTH. Serum iPTH was normally suppressed by calcium infusion, but $T_MPO_4/GFR$, though increased from baseline, remained persistently reduced compared to normal controls. On the other hand, a preliminary report[37] has suggested that phosphate wasting in idiopathic hypercalciuria could be due to hypersensitivity to the action of PTH (see below), but the evidence is more indirect.

The features of experimental phosphate depletion in humans and animals bear a striking resemblance to idiopathic hypercalciuria. Intestinal calcium absorption is enhanced, both because of phosphate depletion per se and increased $1,25(OH)_2D$ production;[6,29,81] serum iPTH is suppressed;[22] proximal and distal renal tubular defects are induced;[31] and bone turnover is enhanced.[20] Striking hypercalciuria ensues, the consequence of absorptive, bone resorptive, and renal mechanisms. It is tempting to speculate that renal phosphate wasting in idiopathic hypercalciuria could produce phosphate depletion and thereby reproduce the known features of the syndrome. For example, fasting serum phosphate has been inversely correlated with urinary calcium excretion,[74] with calciuric response to an oral calcium load,[10] and with circulating $1,25(OH)_2D$.[32,74] Moreover, phosphate administration ameliorates some features of idiopathic hypercalciuria. For example, phosphate administration has a significant hypocalciuric effect in idiopathic hypercalciuria,[26,51,82] but relatively little hypocalciuric effect in normocalciuric normal volunteers[27] or in normocalciuric stone-formers.[26,51,82] Phosphate administration also reduces serum $1,25(OH)_2D$ levels in idiopathic hypercalciuria.[5] In patients with idiopathic hypercalciuria with reduced $T_MPO_4/GFR$, histologic bone lesions similar to those of phosphate depleted animals were demonstrated and were ameliorated by phosphate administration.[8] These observations are consistent with repletion of a preexisting phosphate deficit, but could also reflect a pharmacologic effect of phosphate administration.

On the other hand, phosphate administration has not corrected impaired proximal renal tubular fluid absorption[39] nor, as noted above, intestinal calcium hyperabsorption.[5,51] Furthermore, others have failed to correlate fasting serum phosphate or $T_MPO_4/GFR$ with serum $1,25(OH)_2D$, intestinal calcium absorption, or fasting urine calcium.[5] Finally, frank reduction of serum phosphate and/or $T_MPO_4/GFR$ have been variable findings in idiopathic hypercalciuria.[8,10,40] Some workers[8] have classified their patients as to those with normal or with reduced values, while others[10] have noted reduced serum phosphate and $T_MPO_4/GFR$ but, because these were inconsistent

findings, questioned their pathogenetic significance. Barilla et al.[5] doubted the presence of significant phosphate depletion because serum phosphate and $T_MPO_4/GFR$, initially low-normal, rose significantly on a constant and relatively low phosphate intake. These results do suggest that low $T_MPO_4/GFR$ in idiopathic hypercalciuria can adapt appropriately to changes in dietary phosphate: fasting serum phosphate and $T_MPO_4/GFR$ normally react in what seems a paradoxical fashion to phosphate availability, rising during mild phosphate deprivation, and this normal response was observed in idiopathic hypercalciuria. However, the set-point for renal phosphate transport does appear to be abnormally low in idiopathic hypercalciuria on a random (outpatient, high-phosphate) diet, and the rise in serum phosphate and $T_MPO_4/GFR$ during phosphate restriction does not rule out underlying phosphate depletion.

**Synthesis.** The variable occurrence of increased circulatory $1,25(OH)_2D$ or of hypophosphatemia has led to the proliferation of subgroups of idiopathic hypercalciuria with normal or suppressed parathyroid function ("absorptive" hypercalciuria). When circulating $1,25(OH)_2D$ and serum phosphate are in the normal range, "absorptive" hypercalciuria is attributed to primary intestinal hyperabsorption, but additional subgroups may be distinguished on the basis of either elevated $1,25(OH)_2D$ or of frank hypophosphatemia. In our view, the delineation of these subgroups depends on a misinterpretation of the significance of normal ranges. For example, we have noted that mean serum phosphate and $T_MPO_4/GFR$, though within the normal range, were significantly reduced in idiopathic hypercalciuria compared to normocalciuric stone-formers.[39] This observation is comparable to those of Bordier et al.[8] and Broadus et al.[10] Rather than divide our patients into those with normal or reduced

$T_MPO_4/GFR$, however, we believe they share a common pathogenesis. Since even small reductions in $T_MPO_4/GFR$ within the normal range could lead to phosphate depletion, phosphate wasting could be of general significance in idiopathic hypercalciuria even though frankly low serum phosphate or $T_MPO_4/GFR$ are not universal. In support of this possibility, it is remarkable that small doses of antacids can produce significant hypercalciuria in the absence of detectable negative phosphate balance.[78] Although loss of phosphate in the urine may not be strictly comparable to failure of intestinal phosphate absorption, even relatively mild phosphate wasting could conceivably account for hypercalciuria in stone-formers.

Similarly, the fact that circulating 1,25 $(OH)_2D$ is not elevated in *all* patients with idiopathic hypercalciuria signifies only that elevations of 1,25$(OH)_2D$ within the normal range may also produce hypercalciuria. In this regard it is noteworthy that in our experience mean circulating 1,25 $(OH)_2D$ in normocalciuric stone-formers is in the upper part of the normal range (unpublished observations). In addition, as noted above, several other observations militate against the existence of a 1,25$(OH)_2D$-independent subgroup of idiopathic hypercalciuria: frankly reduced or even low-normal values of 1,25 $(OH)_2D$ have not been observed, and total circulating 1,25$(OH)_2D$ may not reflect the biologically active, free moiety.

Thus, we find no convincing evidence of primary intestinal calicum hyperabsorption independent of 1,25$(OH)_2D$ or phosphate depletion. Nor do we believe that it is profitable to distinguish 1,25$(OH)_2D$-mediated hypercalciuria from a hypophosphatemic subgroup. Rather, it is attractive to unite the observations of reduced $T_MPO_4/GFR$ and increased serum 1,25$(OH)_2D$ in a single hypothesis. We speculate that the primary abnormality in idiopathic hypercalciuria is a proximal tubular defect in phosphate transport, not unlike that in Fanconi syndrome and hypophosphatemic rickets. However, in contrast to those disorders, and for reasons not yet explained, 1,25 $(OH)_2D$ synthesis in the proximal tubule is usually enhanced by the consequent intracellular phosphate depletion. This hypothesis is consistent with the putative effect of intracellular phosphate depletion on the renal 25-hydroxy-D-1$\alpha$ hydroxylase.[6,29,81] Systemic (as opposed to renal proximal tubular) phosphate depletion may or may not be present and contribute in a variable degree to the observed abnormalities. Indeed, the consequences of both 1,25 $(OH)_2D$ excess and of phosphate depletion are quite similar and often indistinguishable. In some patients, phosphate depletion per se may be the predominant cause of hypercalciuria, and 1,25$(OH)_2D$ production may remain within the normal range because of 1,25$(OH)_2D$-independent effects of phosphate depletion to enhance intestinal calcium absorption and bone resorption and suppress PTH secretion. However, it is also possible that patients with normal total serum 1,25 $(OH)_2D$ actually have elevated levels of the free hormone. Taken together with the difficulty of measuring intracellular phosphate, or of correcting phosphate depletion in the presence of ongoing renal phosphate wasting, it is difficult to disentangle the contributions of 1,25$(OH)_2D$ excess and phosphate depletion per se at present. However, we suspect that the proximal phosphate transport defect contributes to the syndrome mainly by enhancing 1,25$(OH)_2D$ synthesis. This hypothesis is economical in that proximal tubular phosphate depletion could account for a defect in fluid absorption.[31,39,80] However, it is also possible that enhanced 1,25$(OH)_2D$ synthesis, impaired fluid absorption, and phosphate wasting are all independent manifestations of a primary, intrinsic proximal tubular defect. Insogna et al.[37] have suggested a third possibility. Noting that 1,25 $(OH)_2D$ levels and nephrogenous cyclic AMP were strikingly sensitive to variations of dietary calcium intake, they suggested that idiopathic hypercalciuria may be due to hypersensitivity to the effect of PTH. Because of the results of calcium infusion (above),[39] we doubt this mechanism but further work is necessary.

These models, as well as the empirical observations which we have summarized, imply that the classification of idiopathic hypercalciuria into absorptive and renal subsets is a hopeless enterprise. An absorptive component will be detected as a consequence of increased serum 1,25 $(OH)_2D$ or possibly phosphate depletion. An apparent "renal calcium leak" can also be detected in a majority of patients with normal parathyroid function, as a consequence of enhanced bone resorption (due to increased circulating $1,25(OH)_2D$ or to phosphate depletion) or of impairment of renal tubular calcium transport (due to an intrinsic tubular defect, phosphate depletion, or PTH suppression). It is vain to single out one of the multiple consequences of $1,25(OH)_2D$ excess or phosphate depletion as the dominant mechanism in a subset of patients. It is also misleading to assign primacy to any one mechanism (absorptive, renal, or resorptive), since these defects can be exposed under different circumstances and are not responsible for one another. Thus, the predominant cause of hypercalciuria on a high calcium intake may be intestinal hyperabsorption, but on a low calcium intake a renal leak or bone resorption become apparent. The "renal leak" of calcium does not account for gut absorption as a secondary consequence and it would be inaccurate to classify idiopathic hypercalciuria as either absorptive or renal. We suggest that this diagnostic distinction be abandoned.

# THERAPEUTIC CONSIDERATIONS

## Clinical Trials

Diagnostic classification of idiopathic hypercalciuria is intended to guide selective therapy. In a recent comprehensive description of selective therapy of hypercalciuria,[63] thiazides were recommended for renal hypercalciuria, sodium cellulose phosphate for relatively marked absorptive hypercalciuria (type I), dietary calcium restriction for relatively mild absorptive hypercalciuria (type II), allopurinol for contributory hyperuricosuria, and nonspecific therapy (high fluid intake and/or low calcium diet) for normocalciuric nephrolithiasis. As we have tried to argue, the theoretical grounds for these recommendations are dubious; as we shall now try to show, the empirical results of therapeutic trials are, if anything, still less convincing.

At the outset it must be stated flatly that there are few, if any, adequate trials of prophylactic therapy in nephrolithiasis. There is a widespread clinical impression that thiazide diuretics are effective in hypercalciuric nephrolithiasis and perhaps in normocalciuric nephrolithiasis as well.[15,48,87] In a recent preliminary report,[14] nine studies of thiazides were analyzed. Neither the seven studies which found a beneficial effect nor the two (randomized controlled) studies which found no effect had a study design adequate to justify their conclusions. Most of the studies have had no true control group. In view of the marked placebo effect in stone prophylaxis, upwards of 50 percent,[26,76] this is a glaring omission. Stone frequency falls after therapeutic intervention, but this apparent benefit may be due to cointerventions (such as enhanced fluid intake) or to spontaneous cycling of disease activity. Ettinger[26] has suggested that a minimum follow-up of three years is necessary to avoid the latter effect, and in many one-group studies the *mean* duration of follow-up is less than three years.[15,63]

The major recent report on selective therapy by Pak et al.[63] suffers from these same defects: (1) potentially effective cointerventions; (2) inadequate duration of follow-up; and (3) absence of suitable controls. In all groups, patients were advised to increase fluid intake, restrict oxalate intake, and avoid high salt intake and vitamin C supplements. The mean duration of follow-up in various groups ranged from 1.70 to 3.37 years. In all groups marked and significant reductions of stone formation rate occurred and were attributed to the specific therapy employed. There is no justification for this conclusion. The data are entirely consistent with placebo effect or with the beneficial effect of increased fluid intake or oxalate restriction. Indeed the one departure in the study from the program of selective therapy gives an opposite conclusion to that reached by the authors: Because of a short supply of sodium cellulose phosphate, some patients with the more severe form of absorptive hypercalciuria (type I) were treated with thiazides, and these patients had a substantial reduction in stone frequency that does not appear to be significantly different from the response to cellulose phosphate. Aside from this one group, there is no comparison of alternative therapy in comparable patients. This study design, proceeding from the laudable motive of giving each patient the best individualized therapy according to the investigators' initial conceptions, cannot be taken as supporting the benefit of selective therapy. The study was intended to apply certain ideas, not to test them, and cannot add or detract from its initial rationale.

An alternative method of testing selective therapy is to compare the effects of alternative agents on *in vitro* measures of stone forming propensity. Of course, this is a second-best approach, the relation of *in vitro* tests to stone formation *in vivo* being indirect and uncertain. Pak and Galosy[60] correlated APR-FPR discriminant scores with stone forming severity and found favorable decrements in this index with "appropriate" therapy. Once again, however, they did not compare alternative therapy within a diagnostic subgroup. Also, the number of patients tested was small.

## Specific Agents

**Thiazide Diuretics.** Since there is no convincing empirical evidence of the clinical superiority of selective therapy for idiopathic hypercalciuria, we must fall back on the theoretical arguments on which specific recommendations have been made. Thiazide diuretics reduce urine calcium excretion both by inducing volume contraction and thereby enhancing proximal tubular calcium reabsorption as well as by directly enhancing distal tubular calcium reabsorption.[19] Thiazides reduce urine calcium excretion comparably in absorptive and in renal hypercalciuria.[4] Nevertheless, it has been suggested that thiazide therapy be restricted to patients with renal hypercalciuria (hypercalciuria with normocalcemia and hyperparathyroidism). Thus, thiazide therapy in renal hypercalciuria has been reported to reduce UcAMP, serum $1,25 (OH)_2D$, and intestinal calcium absorption.[4,88] These effects were not observed in absorptive hypercalciuria (idiopathic hypercalciuria with normal or suppressed parathyroid function). The basis for the effects of thiazides in renal hypercalciuria was presumed to be suppression of parathyroid hormone production by retained calcium.

In view of the marked sensitivity of nephrogenous cAMP and 1,25 (OH)$_2$D to dietary calcium in absorptive hypercalciuria in the study of Insogna et al.,[37] it is difficult to see why thiazides did not have a comparable effect in absorptive hypercalciuria. If 1,25 (OH)$_2$D is not reduced, it is also odd that hypercalcemia has not been more frequently reported during thiazide administration in absorptive hypercalciuria. Further studies of the effects of thiazides on 1,25 (OH)$_2$D metabolism are necessary. Be that as it may, it has been feared that thiazide administration could produce progressive positive calcium balance in absorptive hypercalciuria due to continued intestinal calcium hyperabsorption and reduced urine calcium excretion. In support of this possibility, Pak et al.[57] have recently reported that bone density increased at a low but significant rate during thiazide therapy in absorptive hypercalciuria, while no change was observed in renal hypercalciuria. Although no adverse clinical consequences of calcium overload have been reported during thiazide therapy in absorptive hypercalciuria, the use of thiazides in this setting has been questioned. On the other hand, patients with idiopathic hypercalciuria may have negative calcium balance to begin with,[17] a tendency which could be ameliorated by thiazides.

We would tend to agree with the assessment that thiazide therapy does not correct the underlying abnormalities in idiopathic hypercalciuria with normal or suppressed parathyroid function. Thus, circulating 1,25(OH)$_2$D levels are probably not reduced by thiazides,[42,88] though this observation requires confirmation; and phosphate depletion may be exacerbated to the extent that thiazides at least initially enhance phosphate excretion.[87] However, the recommendation to restrict thiazide therapy to renal hypercalciuria puts the proponents of selective therapy in the odd position of denying to the vast majority of patients with calcium nephrolithiasis the agent which has been most widely used and achieved the greatest popularity. Nor is the evidence for this recommendation very firm. For example, Yendt[87] has reported reduced intestinal calcium absorption in the majority of idiopathic hypercalciuria after 12 to 24 months of therapy. Although specific diagnostic categories were not assigned, it is likely that the majority of these patients did in fact have absorptive hypercalciuria (normal or suppressed parathyroid function). Ehrig et al.[25] reported the failure of thiazide to reduce intestinal calcium absorption in approximately half of their patients with idiopathic hypercalciuria, but most of their studies were not carried out long enough to see the effect described by Yendt.[87] Taken together with a preexisting tendency to negative calcium balance and with the absence of significant clinical consequences of calcium overload, these data suggest that the fear of positive calcium balance has been overstated. Moreover, when we consider the effectiveness of thiazides in reducing urine calcium excretion in absorptive hypercalciuria, as well as the multiple other potential benefits of thiazide therapy (reduced oxalate excretion,[87] enhanced pyrophosphate excretion,[17] and enhanced urine volume[9]), it does not seem reasonable to restrict the use of these agents to one very infrequent form of idiopathic hypercalciuria. Indeed, as indicated above, there are theoretical as well as empirical grounds for offering the drug to the normocalciuric as well as hypercalciuric patient.

**Orthophosphate (Neutral or Alkaline).** Phosphate administration reduces urine calcium excretion in hypercalciuric stone-formers,[26,34,51,82] but has little hypocalciuric effect in normal individuals or in normocalciuric stone-formers.[26,27,51,82] The mechanism of hypocalciuria may be increased renal tubular calcium reabsorption, either a direct effect of phosphate as shown by micropuncture in parathyroidectomized animals[86] or a consequence of parathyroid stimulation; decreased bone resorption;[67] or decreased intestinal calcium absorption. The effect of phosphate administration on intestinal calcium absorption is unclear. Ettinger[26] found a greater decrement of urine calcium excretion in stone formers with increased as compared with normal intestinal calcium absorption. This difference was attributed to complexation of phosphate with intestinal calcium to produce insoluble complexes. Heyburn et al.[34] recently reported that phosphate administration reduced radiocalcium absorption in recurrent stone-formers. However, in other studies calcium absorption was not reduced by phosphate administration, either in normal individuals,[27] in idiopathic hypercalciuria,[51] or in absorptive hypercalciuria.[5] Similarly, urine oxalate excretion has been unchanged[77] or enhanced,[34] consistent with the absence or presence, respectively, of an effect on intestinal calcium absorption. Therefore, currently available data are contradictory as to whether orthophosphate, like thiazides, causes decreased urine calcium excretion, unchanged intestinal calcium absorption and positive calcium balance;[5,27,51] or like cellulose phosphate, causes decreased intestinal calcium absorption and hyperoxaluria.[34]

Like thiazides, phosphate may also act by means other than its hypocalciuric effect. Phosphate administration increases urinary pyrophosphate,[28,34] an inhibitor of calcium phosphate nucleation. To the extent that brushite serves as a nidus for calcium oxalate stone formation, this effect may be beneficial in the prevention of calcium oxalate as well as calcium phosphate urolithiasis.[54] Such an effect could account for the clinical impression that phosphate is beneficial in normocalciuric as well as in hypercalciuric nephrolithiasis, although a significant hypocalciuric effect is observed only in hypercalciuric patients.[82]

Also as with thiazides, clinical experience has been generally favorable, though not without dissenting opinions. Thomas[82] reviewed several studies as well as his own experience and concluded that orthophosphate provided effective therapy in idiopathic nephrolithiasis, regardless of the presence of hypercalciuria. Heyburn et al.[34] reported that neutral phosphate administration reduced stone episode rate; urine oxalate was slightly but significantly elevated, but marked reduction of urine calcium and increase of urine pyrophosphate were thought to account for overall benefit. However, Ettinger[26] failed to demonstrate a beneficial effect of phosphate as compared with placebo in a double-blind controlled study. It should be noted that this study used acid phosphate, which was subsequently shown by Lau et al. to have less hypocalciuric effect than neutral phosphate.[40]

The use of orthophosphate has several practical and theoretical disadvantages. The agent causes diarrhea, particularly in doses exceeding 2 g daily. The high sodium content of neutral phosphate may counteract its hypocalciuric tendency. One complication which is commonly cited but which probably should be discounted is extraskeletal calcification. Review of the one paper to show this effect[23] shows that only four patients were reported, that truly massive doses of orthophosphate (15 g daily) were employed, that the major site of calcification was conjunctival, and that though one patient developed renal calcification, there was no change in renal function in any. Thus the danger of extraskeletal calcification has been much exaggerated. A more serious objection is the possibility of causing or exacerbating hyperparathyroidism, particularly in patients with baseline parathyroid stimulation (renal hypercalciuria). In normal subjects, acute phosphate administration lowered serum ionized calcium and elevated serum iPTH.[68] As is well known, chronic phosphate retention has been implicated as a major cause of secondary hyperparathyroidism in chronic renal failure.[75] The evidence in patients with nephrolithiasis is uncertain. Thus chronic phosphate administration has been reported to elevate serum iPTH or urine cyclic AMP[5,8] or to have no effect on serum iPTH.[5,8,77] Since chronic phosphate administration has been associated with reduced[5,77] or unchanged[8,39] fasting serum phosphate, it is conceivable that PTH-independent adaptation to increased dietary phosphate[84] could abort parathyroid stimulation in patients with normal renal function. Furthermore, there is no evidence to suggest that phosphate-induced parathyroid stimulation is clinically significant. For example, phosphate administration does not increase urinary hydroxyproline.[82] Significantly, phosphate administration to patients with idiopathic hypercalciuria with frankly reduced serum phosphate or $T_MPO_4/GFR$ was associated with *decreased* bone resorption by histological examination, even though serum iPTH was increased. This observation could conceivably reflect a direct effect of phosphate on bone[67] or a reduction of circulating 1,25(OH)$_2$D.[5] In summary, there is little evidence to suggest that phosphate administration causes either negative calcium balance or secondary hyperparathyroidism in the large majority of patients with idiopathic hypercalciuria. Even in patients with preexisting hyperparathyroidism (renal hypercalciuria), a deleterious effect of phosphate administration has not been shown. It may be prudent to withhold phosphate therapy in this latter group of patients but, as noted above, the frequency of baseline hyperparathyroidism in idiopathic hypercalciuria is extremely low.

**Sodium Cellulose Phosphate.** This agent binds calcium in the intestinal lumen, thereby reducing intestinal calcium absorption and calcium excretion.[3,7,21,51,56,58,65] In a small number of balance studies, fecal calcium excretion was increased and urine calcium excretion

reduced to a similar degree, calcium balance therefore remaining unchanged. Reduced calcium absorption stimulates parathyroid function and urinary excretion of cyclic AMP.[55] Urinary oxalate excretion is enhanced in consequence of increased intestinal oxalate absorption.[33] Intestinal magnesium absorption is reduced and both oxalate restriction and magnesium supplements have been recommended during therapy with this agent.

The efficacy of cellulose phosphate is disputed. A favorable therapeutic result has been reported by Pak and his colleagues,[56,58,63] but the duration of follow-up was for the most part less than 3 years, there was no control group, and urine oxalate excretion rose significantly. By contrast, Bachman et al. reported 47 percent stone recurrence at 2 years despite a 40 percent reduction of urine calcium excretion. However, these authors did not restrict dietary oxalate or provide magnesium supplements.

There are considerable theoretical drawbacks to the use of cellulose phosphate. Perhaps most important is the secondary hyperoxaluria, which may not be fully corrected by dietary oxalate restriction. As noted above, oxalate may have a more important role than calcium in the formation of calcium oxalate stones in urine.[70] In addition, despite the evidence of unchanged calcium balance in a small number of patients,[21,51,65] negative calcium balance remains a serious risk. It must be remembered that patients with idiopathic hypercalciuria and normal or suppressed parathyroid function failed to conserve urinary calcium when placed on a severe dietary calcium restriction.[18,85] Indeed, in light of these results, it is difficult to understand why patients on cellulose phosphate have not manifested negative calcium balance. There is a small but significant increment in urine phosphate with cellulose phosphate therapy, probably because of some hydrolysis of this agent in the intestinal lumen;[56] however, this quantity of urine phosphate does not seem enough to account for the effective calcium conservation that has been observed. Decreased bone density has not been observed with cellulose phosphate,[56] but the duration of follow-up was less than 3 years. Because of the fear of negative calcium balance and exacerbation of hyperparathyroidism, this agent has been recommended only for patients with so-called absorptive hypercalciuria (type I).[63] However, in view of the evidence that even patients carrying this diagnostic designation may fail to conserve calcium on low calcium diet, we would be hesitant to recommend the drug to any patient with idiopathic hypercalciuria.

**Nonspecific Therapy: Dietary Calcium Restriction and Increased Fluid Intake.** Reduction of dietary calcium intake is advisable in patients who have hypercalciuria due to excessive calcium ingestion. However, a reduction of dietary calcium intake below the usual range has not been shown to be of benefit and has drawbacks similar to those of cellulose phosphate. First, oxalate excretion is enhanced; and a small increment in oxalate excretion may in fact worsen stone forming propensity even if urine calcium excretion is reduced.[47] Second, the evidence that most stone-formers are in negative calcium balance[17] and that during low calcium diet urine calcium excretion exceeds dietary calcium intake[18,85] suggests that negative calcium balance may be a consequence of dietary calcium restriction. Hence, while dietary calcium surfeit should be avoided, it is difficult at present to recommend calcium restriction.

Increased fluid intake has been shown to reduce the stone-forming propensity of urine *in vitro*,[64] but has not been tested in a controlled clinical trial. The marked placebo effect in urolithiasis is striking, however, and one wonders to what degree increased fluid intake contributes to this phenomenon. In one study,[15] increased fluid intake failed where thiazide diuretics succeeded in reducing stone formation in normocalciuric nephrolithiasis. However, urine volume was not increased in the former group. One must wonder about the enthusiasm and precision with which physicians prescribe increased fluid intake: they may be reluctant to conclude a sophisticated evaluation with advice so mundane as to seem a folk remedy. Nevertheless, the prescription of increased fluid intake does require some care. Alcohol- or sugar-containing beverages should be avoided because of the calciuric effect of these substances; in hardwater areas, distilled water may be necessary. A timed schedule of water intake including bedtime and 3:00 or 4:00 A.M. doses is optimal for the well-motivated patient. Repeated determinations of urine volume to ensure compliance are necessary. However, the aversion to fluids of some stone-formers is well known, decreased fluid intake being one of the major risk factors for stone formation,[72] and this therapeutic regime may well meet with failure due to poor patient compliance.

## Approach to Idiopathic Hypercalciuria

These considerations suggest the following approach. In the recurrent stone former, serum calcium, phosphate, uric acid and creatinine, urinalysis and stone analysis (if available) should be obtained. An abdominal film should be compared with previous films for evidence of metabolic activity (appearance of new stones or growth of existing stones). The presence of metabolic activity will guide further evaluation and therapy, as described below. In a 24-hour urine on a random diet, calcium, creatinine, sodium, uric acid, oxalate, urine volume, and perhaps citrate should be assessed. Urine acidifying ability should be assessed, at least by fasting urine pH, as should qualitative urine cystine. Creatinine is needed to assess completeness of urine collection, sodium because of its influence on urine calcium excretion, and uric acid, oxalate, urine volume, and possibly citrate because they are independent risk factors for stone formation. As indicated above, the definition of hypercalciuria is not clear. By the usual criterion of normal, mean plus 2 S.D., most stone-formers do not have hypercalciuria; on the other hand, the lower limit at which the marginal benefit of hypocalciuric therapy would exceed the risk and inconvenience of such therapy may not be much above the normal mean. In the absence of clear information, we recommend an upper limit of urine calcium excretion of 200 mg or 2.5 mg/kg BW daily.

Specific therapy should probably be restricted to patients with metabolic activity. The contrary view is that hypercalciuria or other metabolic abnormality merits therapy even in the absence of demonstrable stone growth. At present, this is a matter of physician preference. If therapy is thought to be indicated, either for metabolic activity or for hypercalciuria, we initiate a program of increased fluid intake; moderate salt restriction; avoidance of dietary oxalate; discontinuation of antacids or large vitamin A, D, or C supplements if present; and an agent such as a thiazide or neutral phosphate, particularly if urine calcium excretion exceeds 200 mg daily. This regimen should be implemented in the large majority of patients in whom treatment is indicated. However, the presence of other abnormalities such as cystinuria, hyperuricosuria, or renal tubular acidosis may require additional measures. It should be noted that the decision to use a thiazide or neutral phosphate does not require the demonstration of hypercalciuria. This is reasonable on theoretical grounds, since reduction of urinary

calcium excretion even within the normal range may reduce stone-forming propensity, and since both agents could potentially act through mechanisms other than reduction of urine calcium. Use of these agents regardless of urine calcium excretion is also reasonable on practical grounds, since normocalciuric stone-formers have been reported to respond to either agent.[15,82,87] On the other hand, nonspecific therapy (high fluid intake and dietary oxalate restriction) has been effective in uncontrolled studies of normocalciuric stone-formers, and some physicians may choose to withhold thiazide or phosphate in stone-formers whose daily calcium excretion is less than 200 mg.

Except in special cases, there is little to choose between thiazides and neutral phosphate. The presence of allergy to sulfa drugs contraindicates the use of thiazides. The presence of urinary infection with urease-producing organisms, or struvite stones, contraindicates the use of phosphate. Likewise, phosphate should be avoided in patients with renal failure or hyperphosphatemia. A point in favor of thiazides is that there is no danger of exacerbation of hyperparathyroidism in the unusual case where baseline parathyroid function is elevated. Indeed, regardless of whether hyperparathyroidism represents normocalcemic primary hyperparathyroidism or renal hypercalciuria, thiazides should be effective in reducing stone formation. If hypercalcemia supervenes, parathyroid exploration may be necessary. By contrast, phosphate therapy in these patients could exacerbate hyperparathyroidism. On the other hand, there is no evidence (only a theoretical fear) that phosphate therapy causes negative calcium balance or clinically significant exacerbation of hyperparathyroidism even in this setting. Some physicians may wish to determine serum iPTH or UcAMP before initiating phosphate therapy; in our experience, the incidence of hyperparathyroidism in idiopathic hypercalciuria is so low that this precaution may not be necessary. Another approach is simply to use thiazide as the first-line drug in all cases, reserving phosphate for those cases (less than 10 percent)[87] where thiazide diuretics are not tolerated. On the other hand, a case can be made for phosphate as the first-line drug: thiazides are known to increase serum lipids and glucose concentration and the effect of this agent on the development of atherosclerotic disease is unknown. Similarly, the use of phosphate avoids the possibility of allergic reactions such as may be seen with thiazides.

We do not recommend sodium cellulose phosphate or low calcium diet. Our reservations are in part theoretical: Just as thiazides are feared to cause positive calcium balance in so-called absorptive hypercalciuria (though no clinical consequences have been observed), so cellulose phosphate is feared to cause negative calcium balance, although this has not been demonstrated in the few patients who have been studied. Nevertheless, we are swayed by the potential of cellulose phosphate or calcium restriction to increase urine oxalate, an effect which may more than outweigh the benefit of reduced urine calcium excretion.

It may be inquired why an initial determination of urinary calcium, sodium, or volume is necessary if therapy with thiazide or phosphate will be initiated even in normocalciuric individuals. One reason for such an evaluation is that a baseline is useful to judge the response to therapy. Although we cannot be certain that reduction of urine calcium excretion accounts for the reduced rate of stone formation, the observation that urine calcium excretion is higher in relapsing stone formers suggests (but does not prove) that this may be the case. Thus, an inadequate hypocalciuric response to therapy may require additional intervention. Of course,

the definition of an adequate hypocalciuric response is somewhat arbitrary. Based on the results of Strauss et al.[79] a daily urine calcium excretion of 200 mg or 2.5 mg/kgBW on thiazide therapy may be an appropriate goal. Whether such a goal is also appropriate or necessary during phosphate therapy is unknown. Failure to achieve an adequate hypocalciuric response to thiazide often reflects failure of sodium restriction. In occasional cases thiazide administration fails to reduce urine calcium excretion sufficiently despite salt restriction. In these cases the addition of another agent may be useful. Amiloride is a potassium-sparing diuretic which has a hypocalciuric effect independent of thiazide. This drug is a logical addition to thiazide therapy and the combination of hydrochlorothiazide 50 mg and amiloride 5 mg has been found useful in an uncontrolled study.[48]

Thus, therapeutic considerations provide no justification for classification of idiopathic hypercalciuria into absorptive and renal subgroups. This classification aims to restrict hypocalciuric therapy to those with proven hypercalciuria; but urine calcium excretion may be a graded risk factor throughout the normal range and available agents may have multiple beneficial effects apart from reduction of urine calcium excretion. The attempt to restrict thiazide therapy to that small group of patients with "renal" hypercalciuria, when the drug is probably effective in the vast majority of patients with idiopathic nephrolithiasis, also seems inappropriate. Likewise, the attempt to find a group of patients in whom cellulose phosphate is safe seems misguided: Such a subgroup (pure "absorptive" hypercalciuria) may not exist, the agent has serious theoretical drawbacks, and most importantly, experience with this agent is too limited to recommend it over thiazide or phosphate therapy. We prefer a straightforward and unitary therapeutic approach, consistent with our unitary view of idiopathic hypercalciuria. Although theoretically phosphate has the appeal of treating idiopathic hypercalciuria at a more fundamental level, we find little to choose between thiazide and phosphate. In most patients either agent will be of benefit and we cannot endorse any sophisticated attempt to determine which patient should receive which drug. Current approaches to achieve this goal have not been shown to be necessary in the practical management of idiopathic nephrolithiasis, though they may be valuable as research tools.

# ACKNOWLEDGMENTS

The writing of this chapter and research reported was supported in part by an NIH Research Grant HL00340 and an NIH Training Grant AM05634.

# REFERENCES

1. Adams ND, Gray RW, Lemann J Jr, et al: Effects of calcitriol administration on calcium metabolism in healthy men. Kidney Int 21:90, 1982.
2. Albright FP, Henneman P, Benedict P, et al: Idiopathic hypercalciuria. Proc R Soc Med 46: 1077, 1953.
3. Bachman U, Danielson VG, Johansson G: Treatment of recurrent calcium stone formation with cellulose phosphate. J Urol 123: 9, 1980.
4. Barilla DE, Tolentino R, Kaplan RA, et al: Selective effect of thiazide on the intestinal absorption of calcium in absorptive and renal hypercalciurias. Metabolism 27: 125, 1978.
5. Barilla DE, Zerwekh JE, Pak CYC: A critical evaluation of the role of phosphate in the pathogenesis of absorptive hypercalciuria. Min Electrolyte Metab 2: 302, 1979.
6. Baxter LA, DeLuca HF: Stimulation of 25-hydroxy vitamin $D_3$-1 hydroxylase by phosphate depletion. J Biol Chem 251: 3158, 1976.
7. Blacklock NJ, MacLeod MA: The effect of cellulose phosphate on intestinal absorption and urinary excretion of calcium. Some experience in its use in the treatment of calcium stone formation. Br J Urol 46: 385, 1974.
8. Bordier P, Ryckewart A, Gueris J, et al: On the pathogenesis of so-called idiopathic hypercalciuria. Am J Med 63: 398, 1977.
9. Brannan PG, Morawski S, Pak CYC, et al: Selective jejunal hyperabsorption of calcium in absorptive hypercalciuria. Am J Med 66: 425, 1979.
10. Broadus AE, Dominguez M, Bartter FC: Pathophysiological studies in idiopathic hypercalciuria: use of an oral calcium tolerance test to characterize distinctive hypercalciuric subgroups. J Clin Endocrinol Metab 47: 751, 1978.
11. Broadus AE, Horst RL, Littledike ET, et al: Primary hyperparathyroidism with intermittent hypercalcemia: Serial observations and simple diagnosis by means of an oral calcium tolerance test. Clin Endocrinol 12: 225, 1980.
12. Bulusu L, Hodgkinson A, Nordin BEC, et al: Urinary excretion of calcium and creatinine in relation to age and body weight in normal subjects and patients with renal calculi. Clin Sci 38: 601, 1970.
13. Burckhardt P, Jaeger P: Secondary hyperparathyroidism in idiopathic renal hypercalciuria: Fact or theory? J Clin Endocrinol Metab 53: 550, 1981.
14. Churchill DN: Effectiveness of thiazides in preventing recurrent calcium urolithiasis: The quality of the evidence. Am Soc Nephrol Abstr 15: 26A, 1982.
15. Coe FL: Treated and untreated recurrent calcium nephrolithiasis in patients with idiopathic hypercalciuria, hyperuricosuria, or no metabolic disorder. Ann Intern Med 87: 404, 1977.
16. Coe FL, Canterbury JM, Firpo JJ, et al: Evidence for secondary hyperparathyroidism in idiopathic hypercalciuria. J Clin Invest 52: 134, 1973.
17. Coe FL, Favus MJ: Disorders of stone formation. In Brenner, BM, Rector FC, Eds.: The Kidney. Saunders, Philadelphia, 1981, p 1971.
18. Coe FL, Favus MJ, Crockett T, et al: Effects

of low-calcium diet on urine calcium excretion, parathyroid function and serum 1,25 $(OH)_2D_3$ levels in patients with idiopathic hypercalciuria and in normal subjects. Am J Med 72: 25, 1982.

19. Costanzo LS, Windhager EE: Calcium and sodium transport by the distal convoluted tubule of the rat. Am J Physiol 235: F492, 1977.

20. Cuisinier-Gleizes P, Thomasset M, Sainteny-Debove F, et al: Phosphorus deficiency, parathyroid hormone and bone resorption in the growing rat. Calcif Tissue Res 20: 235, 1976.

21. Dent CE, Harper CM, Parfitt AM: The effect of cellulose phosphate on calcium metabolism in patients with hypercalciuria. Clin Sci 27: 417, 1964.

22. Dominguez JH, Gray RW, Lemann J Jr: Dietary phosphate deprivation in women and men. Effects on mineral and acid-balances, parathyroid hormone, and the metabolism of 25-OH vitamin D. J Clin Endocrinol Metab 47: 751, 1976.

23. Dudley FJ, Blackburn CRB: Extraskeletal calcification complicating oral neutral phosphate therapy. Lancet 2: 628, 1970.

24. Edwards NA, Hodgkinson A: Studies of renal function in patients with idiopathic hypercalciuria. Clin Sci 29: 327, 1965.

25. Ehrig U, Harrison JE, Wilson DR: The effect of long-term thiazide therapy on intestinal calcium absorption in patients with recurrent renal calculi. Metabolism 23: 139, 1974.

26. Ettinger B: Recurrent nephrolithiasis: natural history and effect of phosphate therapy. A double-blind controlled study. Am J Med 61: 200, 1976.

27. Farquharson RF, Salter WT, Aub JC: Studies of calcium and phosphorus metabolism. XIII The effect of ingestion of phosphate on the excretion of calcium. J Clin Invest 10: 251, 1931.

28. Fleisch H, Bisaz S, Care AD: The effects of orthophosphate on urinary pyrophosphate excretion and the prevention of urolithiasis. Lancet 1: 1065, 1964.

29. Friedlander EJ, Henry HL, Norman AW: Studies on the mode of action of calciferol: effects of dietary calcium and phosphorus on the relationship between the 25-hydroxy vitamin $D_3$-1α-hydroxylase and production of chick intestinal calcium binding protein. J Biol Chem 252: 8677, 1977.

30. Galosy R, Clarke L, Ward DL, et al: Renal oxalate excretion in calcium urolithiasis. J Urol 123: 320, 1980.

31. Goldfarb S, Westby GR, Goldberg M, et al: Renal tubular effects of chronic phosphate depletion. J Clin Invest 59: 770, 1977.

32. Gray RW, Wilz DR, Caldas AE, et al: The importance of phosphate in regulating plasma 1,25 $(OH)_2$ vitamin D levels in humans: Studies in healthy subjects, in calcium stone-formers, and in patients with primary hyperparathyroidism. J Clin Endocrinol Metab 45: 299, 1977.

33. Hayashi Y, Kaplan RA, Pak CYC: Effect of sodium cellulose phosphate on crystallization of calcium oxalate in urine. Metabolism 24: 1273, 1975.

34. Heyburn PJ, Robertson WG, Peacock M: Phosphate treatment of recurrent calcium stone disease. Nephron 32: 314, 1982.

35. Hodgkinson A: Evidence of increased oxalate absorption in patients with calcium-containing renal stones. Clin Sci Mol Med 54: 291, 1978.

36. Hodgkinson A, Pyrah LN: The urinary excretion of calcium and inorganic phosphate in 344 patients with calcium stone of renal origin. Br J Surg 46: 10, 1958.

37. Insogna K, Lang R, Kliger A, et al: Evidence for hypersensitivity of 1,25 $(OH)_2D$ production in absorptive hypercalciuria. Clin Res 30: 525A, 1982.

38. Kaplan RA, Haussler MR, Deftos LJ et al: The role of 1,25-dihydroxyvitamin D in the mediation of intestinal hyperabsorption of calcium in primary hyperparathyroidism and absorptive hypercalciuria. J Clin Invest 59: 756, 1977.

39. Lau YK, Wasserstein A, Westby GR, et al: Proximal tubular defects in idiopathic hypercalciuria: Resistance to phosphate administration. Min Electrolyte Metab 7: 237, 1982.

40. Lau YK, Wolf C, Nussbaum P, et al: Differing effects of acid versus neutral phosphate therapy of hypercalciuria. Kidney Int 16: 736, 1979.

41. Lawoyin S, Sismilich S, Browne R, et al: Bone mineral content in patients with pri-

mary hyperparathyroidism, osteoporosis, and calcium urolithiasis. Metabolism 28: 1250, 1979.

42. Lemann J Jr, Gray RW, Adams ND: Lack of effect of hydrochlorothiazide on plasma 1,25 $(OH)_2$ vitamin D concentrations in patients with nephrolithiasis. Abstract, IV Int Congr Nephrol, p.E-2, 1979.

43. Lemann J Jr, Gray RW, Wilz DR: Evidence for a renal $PO_4$ leak in patients with calcium nephrolithiasis. p. 34, Proc. 3rd Int. Workshop on Phosphate and Other Minerals, Madrid, 1977.

44. Liberman UA, Sperling O, Atsmon A, et al: Metabolic and kinetic studies in idiopathic hypercalciuria. J Clin Invest 47: 2580, 1968.

45. Maierhoffer WJ, Gray RW, Cheung HS, et al: Elevated serum 1,25-$(OH)_2$-vitamin D concentrations in healthy men stimulate bone resorption. Clin Res 30: 527A, 1982.

46. Malluche HM, Tschoepe W, Ritz E, et al: Abnormal bone histology in idiopathic hypercalciuria. J Clin Endocrinol Metabolism 50: 654, 1980.

47. Marshall RW, Cochran M, Hodgkinson A: Relationship between calcium and oxalic acid intake in the diet and their excretion in the urine of normal and renal stone-forming subjects. Clin Sci 43: 91, 1972.

48. Maschio L, Tessitore N, D'Angelo A, et al: Prevention of calcium nephrolithiasis with low-dose thiazide, amiloride and allopurinol. Am J Med 71: 623, 1981.

49. Morgan B, Robertson WG: The urinary excretion of calcium. Clin Orth Rel Res 101: 254, 1974.

50. Muldowney FP, Freaney R, Moloney MF: Importance of dietary sodium in the hypercalciuria syndrome. Kidney Int 22: 292, 1982.

51. Nassim JR, Higgins BA: Control of idiopathic hypercalciuria. Br Med J 1: 675, 1965.

52. Nordin BEC: Hypercalciuria. Clin Sci Mol Med 52: 1, 1977.

53. Pabico RC, McKenna BA: Proximal and distal nephron functions are abnormal in patients with idiopathic nephrolithiasis .Am Soc Nephrol Abstr 15: 38A, 1982.

54. Pak CYC: Hydrochlorothiazide therapy in nephrolithiasis. Effect on the urinary activity product and formation product of brushite. Clin Pharmacol Ther 14: 209, 1972.

55. Pak CYC: Physiological basis for absorptive and renal hypercalciurias. Am J Physiol 237: F415, 1979.

56. Pak CYC: Clinical pharmacology of sodium cellulose phosphate. J Clin Pharmacol 19: 451, 1979.

57. Pak CYC: A critical evaluation of treatment of calcium stones. In Massry SG, Ritz E, John H, Eds: Phosphate and Minerals in Health and Disease. Plenum, New York, 1980, p 451.

58. Pak CYC, Delea CS, Bartter FC: Successful treatment of recurrent nephrolithiasis (calcium stones) with cellulose phosphate. N Engl J Med 290: 175, 1975.

59. Pak CYC, Fetner C, Townsend J, et al: Evaluation of calcium urolithiasis in ambulatory patients. Comparison of results with those of inpatient evaluation. Am J Med 64: 979, 1978.

60. Pak CYC, Galosy RA: Propensity for spontaneous nucleation of calcium oxalate. Quantitative assessment by urinary FPR-APR discriminant score. Am J Med 69: 681, 1980.

61. Pak CYC, Holt K: Nucleation and growth of brushite and calcium in urine of stone-formers. Metabolism 25: 665, 1976.

62. Pak CYC, Ohata M, Lawrence EC, et al: The hypercalciurias: causes, parathyroid functions and diagnostic criteria. J Clin Invest 54: 387, 1974.

63. Pak CYC, Peters P, Hurt G, et al: Is selective therapy of recurrent nephrolithiasis possible? Am J Med 71: 615, 1982.

64. Pak CYC, Sakhaee K, Crowther C, et al: Evidence justifying a high fluid intake in the treatment of nephrolithiasis. Ann Intern Med 93: 36, 1980.

65. Parfitt AM, Higgins BA, Nassim JR, et al: Metabolic studies in patients with hypercalciuria. Clin Sci 27: 463, 1964.

66. Parks J, Coe F, Favus M: Hyperparathyroidism in nephrolithiasis. Arch Intern Med. 140: 1479, 1980.

67. Raisz LG, Neimann I: Effect of phosphate, calcium and magnesium on bone resorption and hormonal responses in tissue culture. Endocrinology 85: 446, 1969.

68. Reiss E, Canterbury JM, Bercovitz MA, et al: The role of phosphate in the excretion of parathyroid hormone in man. J Clin Invest 49: 2146, 1970.
69. Robertson WG, Gallagher JC, Marshall DH: Seasonal variations in urinary excretion of calcium. Br Med J 4: 436, 1974.
70. Robertson WG, Peacock M: The cause of idiopathic calcium stone disease: hypercalciuria or hyperoxaluria. Nephron 26: 105, 1980.
71. Robertson WG, Peacock M, Heyburn PJ, et al: Risk factors in calcium stone disease of the urinary tract. Br J Urol 50: 449, 1978.
72. Robertson WG, Peacock M, Heyburn PJ, et al: Epidemiological risk factors in calcium stone disease. Scand J Urol Nephrol Suppl 53: 15, 1980.
73. Robertson WG, Peacock M, Marshall RW, et al: Saturation-inhibition index as a measure of the risk of calcium oxalate stone formation in the urinary tract. N Engl J Med 294: 249, 1974.
74. Shen FH, Baylink DJ, Nielsen RL, et al: Increased serum 1,25-dihydroxyvitamin D in idiopathic hypercalciuria. J Lab Clin Med 90: 955, 1977.
75. Slatopolsky E, Rutherford WE, Hruska K, et al: How important is phosphate in the pathogenesis of renal osteodystrophy? Arch Intern Med 138: 848, 1978.
76. Smith MJV: Placebo versus allopurinol for renal calculi. J Urol 117: 690, 1977.
77. Smith LH, Thomas WC, Jr, Arnaud CD: Orthophosphate therapy in calcium renal lithiasis. In Urinary Calculi, International Symposium on Renal Research. Basel, Karger, 1973, p 188.
78. Spencer H, Kramer L, Norris C, et al: Effect of small doses of aluminum containing antacids on calcium and phosphorus metabolism. Am J Clin Nutr 36: 32, 1982.
79. Strauss AL, Coe FL, Deutsch L, et al: Factors that predict relapse of calcium nephrolithiasis during treatment. A prospective study. Am J Med 72: 17, 1982.
80. Sutton RAL, Walker VR: Responses to hydrochlorothiazide and acetazolamide in patients with calcium stones. N Engl J Med 302: 709, 1980.
81. Swaminathan R, Sommerville BA, Care AD: Metabolism *in vitro* of 25-hydroxycholecalciferol in chicks fed on phosphorus deficient diets. Clin Sci 54: 197, 1978.
82. Thomas WC: Use of phosphate in patients with calcareous renal calculi. Kidney Int 13: 390, 1978.
83. Tiselius HL: Oxalate and renal stone formation. Scand J Urol Nephrol Suppl 53: 135, 1980.
84. Trohler U, Bonjour JP, Fleisch H: Inorganic phosphate homeostasis. Renal adaptation to the dietary intake in intact and thyroparathyroidectomized rats. J Clin Invest 57: 264, 1976.
85. Wasserstein AG, Agus ZS: Calcium balance during dietary calcium restriction in idiopathic hypercalciuria. Mineral Electrolyte Metab 6: 271, 1981.
86. Wong NL, Quamme GA, O'Callaghan TJ, et al: Renal tubular transport and phosphate depletion: a micropuncture study. Can J Phys Pharmacol 58: 1063, 1980.
87. Yendt ER, Cohanim M: Prevention of calcium stones with thiazides. Kidney Int 13: 397, 1978.
88. Zerwekh JE, Pak CYC: Selective effects of thiazide therapy on serum 1,25-dihydroxy vitamin D and intestinal calcium absorption in renal and absorptive hypercalciurias. Metabolism 29: 13, 1980.
89. Zerwekh JE, Pak CYC, Kaplan RA, et al: Pathogenetic role of 1,25-dihydroxy vitamin D in sarcoidosis and absorptive hypercalciuria: different response to prednisolone therapy. J Clin Endocrinol Metab 51: 381, 1980.

# Section IV

## Controversies in Treating Renal-Electrolyte Disorders

# 9

# Mild Hypokalemia in Nonedematous, Nondigitalized Patients

# The Case for a More Conservative Approach to Prophylaxis and Therapy

David H. Lawson, M.D.

Cardiac failure accounts for some 5 percent of admissions to medical wards, being more prevalent in the elderly and in those with preexisting hypertension. The standard approach to treatment of acute cardiac failure is the use of loop diuretics such as furosemide. Indeed, furosemide is one of the most commonly prescribed drugs in hospital medical wards—a review of data from the Boston Collaborative Drug Surveillance Program (BCDSP) shows that 22 percent of medical inpatients studied by one of the participating centers in that program had received furosemide during hospitalization.[17] Likewise, hypertension is one of the most common conditions receiving long-term treatment with drugs in the Western world. Foremost amongst the drugs in common use to treat hypertension are the thiazide diuretics.

Presumably, because of widespread awareness that hypokalemia may result from therapy with furosemide or thiazides, routine potassium chloride supplementation is virtually the norm in diuretic recipients both in and out of hospital. In the series cited above in which 22 percent of medical admissions received furosemide, 28 percent of all medical patients received potassium chloride. This enthusiastic (some might say overenthusiastic!) use of potassium supplements has been taught to a generation of medical students. Writing a potassium chloride prescription for a diuretic recipient now seems to be a reflex reaction for many physicians.

## PHYSIOLOGIC AND PATHOPHYSIOLOGIC ASPECTS (FIG. 9-1)

Let us more carefully examine the evidence and assumptions upon which this virtually automatic use of potassium supplements is based. Current physiological evidence from animal experiments suggests that potassium filtered at the glomerulus is completely reabsorbed in the proximal tubule. Potassium appearing in the final urine derives from that which is secreted by distal tubular epithelium. In animals receiving diuretics such as furosemide or thiazides, there is an increase in the amount of potassium secreted distally.[21] Depending upon intake and absorption of dietary potassium, this increased output could lead to potassium depletion were it to continue for significant periods of time. Moreover, diuretic-induced hydrogen ion secretion causes a metabolic alkalosis which further exacerbates tubular potassium elimination. Thus, in animals receiving diuretic therapy for short spells there is usually a net negative balance of potassium due to its increased urinary elimination.

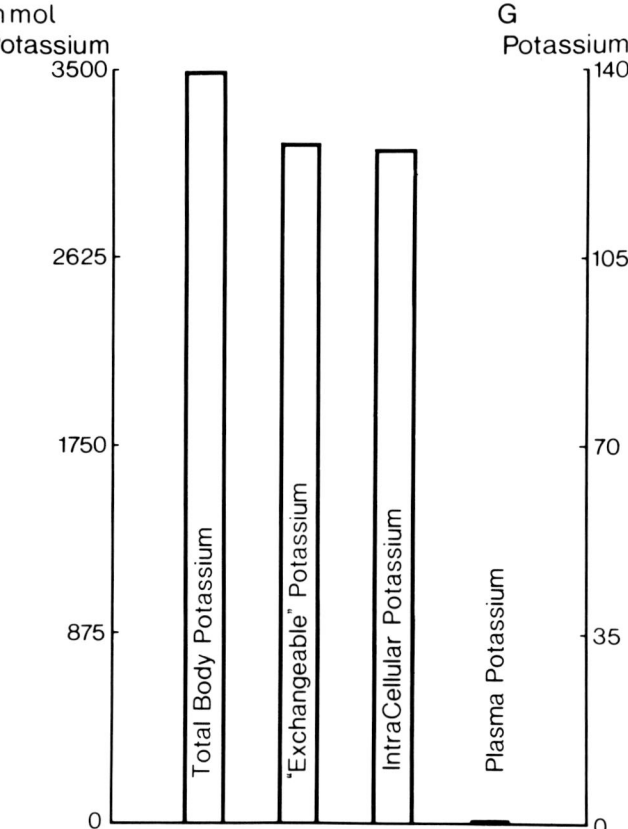

**Fig. 9-1.** Distribution of body potassium content in average 70 kg man (derived from Bowman WC, Rand MJ: Textbook of Physiology and Pharmacology. 2nd Ed. Blackwell Scientific Publications, London 1980.)

So far, the need for potassium chloride supplementation for diuretic recipients is internally consistent and makes good physiological sense. Problems arise however when we try to translate the results of these short-term animal experiments to the human situation.

One of the two major difficulties in evaluating the human data is arriving at accurate and reproducible estimates of a given patient's potassium status. The other significant problem relates to the issue of whether an observed potassium deficit is indeed attributable to the diuretic or rather to the underlying condition for which the drugs were prescribed.

Three main measures of potassium status are available. Measurements of serum potassium concentration are accurate and reproducible but only an infinitesi-

mally small portion of total body potassium is present in the serum or plasma[2,34] and the resulting values do not accurately reflect whole body content (Fig. 9-1). Estimation of intracellular potassium concentration in red and white blood cells is reproducible and in some investigations has correlated well with other more sophisticated estimates of whole body potassium status.[7,28] However, more work must be done in this area before these assays gain widespread popularity. "Exchangeable potassium" measurements using isotope dilution techniques ($^{42}$K) are mainly research tools and cannot be used to assess serial changes in body potassium status over short time periods. Moreover, the results with $^{42}$K have a wider range of variability than does the measurement of whole body potassium using the naturally occurring isotope of potassium ($^{40}K$). This latter technique requires sophisticated equipment which is not readily available. For these reasons most reported studies of potassium metabolism in diuretic recipients have relied heavily on serial measurements of serum potassium concentration and the terms *hypokalemia* and *potassium deficit* have erroneously become virtually synonymous to most physicians.

## HYPOKALEMIA AFTER LONG-TERM DIURETIC USE

Based on their literature review, Morgan and Davidson observed that the mean fall in serum potassium concentration after furosemide therapy was 0.3 mmol/L and after thiazides, 0.6 mmol/L.[22] Moreover, there was little correlation between dose or duration of treatment and changes in serum potassium levels. In the papers, prescribed doses of potassium were relatively ineffective in correcting the hypokalemia. Nevertheless, concentrations of serum potassium below 3.0 mmol/L were unusual in patients receiving diuretics for hypertension or heart failure. They therefore suggested that the description "hypokalemia" should be confined to those patients with serum potassium concentrations below 3.0 mmol/L rather than the more customary level of 3.5 mmol/L. These observations, made to a large extent on data from European publications, are compatible with information available from North America. Thus, for example, Greenblatt and his colleagues analyzing data from the Boston Collaborative Drug Surveillance Program reported that hypokalemia was noted in 3.6 percent of 2367 consecutive furosemide recipients.[8] Of particular interest was their observation that supplementary potassium chloride or coadministration of potassium-sparing diuretics did not completely prevent the hypokalemia but appeared merely to marginally reduce its frequency and more importantly, to delay its onset. These workers confirmed the absence of a clear dose-response relationship between furosemide treatment and hypokalemia.

In 1978 the Danish workers Krakauer and Lauritzen reviewed the effects of diuretic therapy in a group of 489 outpatients over the age of 65 years.[13] They reported that one-third of these individuals were taking diuretic treatment regularly and of those, two-thirds also had received a prescription for potassium supplements.[13] The mean serum potassium concentration of the diuretic recipients averaged 0.1 to 0.3 mmol/L below those of the nonrecipients, the greatest disparity occurring in female subjects. Serum potassium concentrations below 3.5 mmol/L were noted in 15 percent of subjects (2 percent in men and 13 percent in women). A total of seven of the 489 patients had serum potassium concentrations below 3.0 mmol/L (1.4 percent), all being diuretic recipients. Finally and most importantly, there were no differences in the serum potassium concentrations in these subjects when analyzed according to whether or not they received prescriptions for potassium supplements. This study highlights several interesting observations. Hypokalemia, independent of diuretic therapy, was most common in women, and women also showed the greater fall in mean potassium concentration after diuretic use. Finally, potassium supplementation was uniformly ineffective in preventing diuretic-induced hypokalemia. Whether this failure was due to noncompliance with therapy or the inherent inefficacy of the supplements could not be shown by this study. And indeed regardless of its cause the answer to the question "If I prescribe potassium supplements for my diuretic recipients, does this keep their serum potassium concentrations normal?" was answered.

One attempt to answer this question was mounted by Schwartz and Swartz in 1974 when they reported on the use of potassium chloride elixir in treating thiazide-induced hypokalemia.[33] The main difficulty with this study was that they regarded all potassium concentrations below 3.8 mmol/L as indicating "hypokalemia," a level substantially higher than now would be regarded as requiring treatment.

Sandor et al. made serial measurements of plasma and whole body potassium in 158 hypertensive outpatients over a period of 2 years, while they received diuretics.[31] Although these patients showed no fall in whole body potassium content, they manifested wide and unpredictable fluctuations in plasma potassium concentration that were independent of diet or use of supplementary potassium. There was a tendency for the lowest plasma potassium concentrations to be observed within the first 3 months of treatment, thereafter the values appeared to rise somewhat before stabilization.

In a large study of hypokalemia in a general hospital, my colleagues and I reported that of 58,167 patients who had at least one electrolyte sample analyzed, only 73 patients (0.1 percent) had a plasma potassium concentration below 2.0 mmol/L and in only 10 patients (0.01 percent) was this degree of hypokalemia attributable to a diuretic.[19] In each of these patients, the history was complex and the patient gravely ill. No otherwise stable patient had this degree of severe hypokalemia solely caused by diuretic treatment. Further analysis of this data showed that a discharge diagnosis of cardiac disease, both hypertensive and cardiac failure, was no more common than expected among patients with plasma potassium concentrations of 2.0 to 2.4

mmol/L or 2.5 to 2.9 mmol/L. Thus, in hospitalized subjects there was no evidence to suggest that plasma potassium concentrations below 3.0 mmol/L occurred with a greater than expected frequency in those with cardiac failure.

## CAUSES OF HYPOKALEMIA AFTER DIURETIC USE

Accepting that a small degree of hypokalemia occurs following diuretic therapy, is this due directly to the diuretics or could it be due to the underlying cardiac disease or indeed to the effects of hospitalization per se? Unfortunately, answers to these questions are difficult to obtain. Morgan and his colleagues reviewed the literature relating to potassium depletion in heart failure and attempted to assess its relation to long-term diuretic therapy.[23] They reported that although many studies demonstrate that patients with heart failure have 20 to 30 percent less exchangeable body potassium than healthy, sex-matched control subjects, the total body potassium was within 5 percent of predicted values once their weight is taken into account (i.e., within experimental error). Whereas previously it had been assumed that the "reduction" in exchangeable potassium was due to diuretic treatment, other possibilities exist. Morgan and his colleagues argued that the difference was largely due to failure to match patients and controls in terms of age and body habitus. When this was done much of the observed deficit disappeared and most of the outstanding differences could be accounted for by a reduction in potassium content due to muscle wasting consequent to chronic heart failure. The rate at which the injected isotope equilibrates with exchangeable potassium pools may differ in patients receiving diuretics, thereby spuriously lowering the calculated body content. Thus, none of the 29 studies reviewed by Morgan and his colleagues provided convincing evidence that severe cellular potassium depletion was common in those patients with heart failure receiving long-term diuretic treatment.

In 1976 my group reported a long-term study of 21 patients with cardiac failure receiving diuretics to maintain them edema free.[16] Serial samples of plasma, blood cell, and total body potassium were made over a period of one year and the results compared with a series of 10 control subjects. Initially, all diuretic recipients received potassium supplements, but these were soon withdrawn in 17 of the 21. In none of the patients receiving diuretics alone was there a statistically significant alteration in any of the parameters of potassium handling assessed. Of the four subjects who continued with potassium supplements, one had persistent heart failure and persistent hypokalemia which proved unresponsive to potassium supplements together with potassium-sparing diuretics. This patient had profound cardiac failure and it is likely that the hypokalemia was due more to this factor than to diuretic therapy per se. The possibility that a paradoxical stimulation of potassium excretion was effected by aldosterone antagonists must also be considered.[29]

Davidson and his colleagues studied plasma and total body potassium in 151 patients with heart disease, half of whom were taking diuretics with potassium supplements.[3] They reported that after allowance was made for age and body size, the diuretic group showed a total body potassium which was 3 to 5 percent (100 to 150 mmol/L) lower than the nondiuretic group. Thirteen of the 83 diuretic recipients had plasma potassium concentrations below 3.5 mmol/L. There was no relationship between the dose of potas-

sium supplements prescribed and total body potassium measurements.

To these studies must now be added the recent observation that hospital inpatients who develop hypokalemia may do so spontaneously.[24] Review of 70 unselected patients in a Leeds hospital with plasma potassium concentrations below 2.8 mmol/L showed that normokalemia was commonly achieved even in the absence of supplementary potassium. It was concluded that the hypokalemia arose as a result of transient shifts of potassium into cells under a variety of stimuli associated with the acute admissions. Although none of these patients had taken diuretics it is likely that had they been doing so, the hypokalemia would have been attributed to the diuretic.

From these reports we can conclude that

1. Short-term diuretic treatment in animals results in increased urinary potassium elimination.

2. A similar situation pertains to humans.

3. A reduction in serum potassium concentration averaging 0.3 to 0.6 mmol/L is not infrequent in diuretic recipients, the fall being greater with the longer-acting thiazide diuretics than with loop diuretics such as furosemide.

4. This fall in serum potassium concentration is not dependent on dose or duration of diuretic treatment.

5. There is no good correlation between any fall in serum potassium concentration and change in whole body potassium status.

6. The fall in serum potassium concentration may result in "hypokalemia" depending upon the initial serum potassium concentration and the definition of 'hypokalemia' adopted.

7. Serum potassium concentrations below 3.0 mmol/L are extremely uncommon in patients receiving diuretic treat-

ment for hypertension or cardiac failure unless coincidental severe salt restriction is undertaken.

8. It is not possible to predict which individual patients are going to develop hypokalemia at the outset of diuretic therapy.

9. Chronic cardiac failure per se will lead to muscle wasting with loss of intracellular potassium resulting in lower than expected values for exchangeable and —to a lesser extent—total body potassium. These alterations are not the result of diuretic therapy but are directly attributable to the cardiac failure per se.

# RISKS OF HYPOKALEMIA

What are the risks of mild hypokalemia to the patients? Although a wide variety of symptoms such as general malaise, lethargy, loss of concentration, and weakness have been ascribed to hypokalemia, there is no good evidence that an average fall in serum potassium concentration of the order of 0.6 mmol/L is associated with general symptoms. Thus although profound hypokalemia, especially were it to develop insidiously and be associated with renal disease,[30] may well cause symptoms in the patient; the mild drop in serum potassium concentration found in patients with cardiac failure has never been shown to do so. Recently, however, concern has surfaced that even a mild and otherwise asymptomatic decrease in serum potassium concentration may be associated with a reduced threshold for cardiac dysrhythmias which could prove fatal after an acute myocardial infarction.[5,11] These observations remain largely uncontrolled and controversial. In particular, the temporal relationships between the onset of the hypokalemia and the serious ventricular ectopic activity has not been demonstrated convincingly.[10]

The published data have not excluded other more likely causes of the dysrhythmias, or factors which may independently produce hypokalemia and arrhythmias such as excess catecholamine secretion. The one situation where there is good evidence to link hypokalemia with clinically serious ventricular dysrhythmias is in patients receiving digoxin or other digitalis-containing preparations.[6,20] Thus, in patients with cardiac failure who are receiving digoxin or other cardiac glycosides, while also taking diuretic drugs, every effort should be taken to ensure that serum potassium concentrations remain stable. This ideal is difficult to achieve, however. It is therefore reassuring to see the substantial number of studies published recently which indicate that in the majority of patients with heart failure —those who remain in sinus rhythm —regular long-term use of cardiac glycosides is of little value[4] and can be discontinued.[12]

In view of the major interest in this topic of arrhythmias in relation to hypokalemia it is perhaps surprising that so little animal work has been done to attempt to elucidate several of the unknown facets of the problem. For example, does hypokalemia per se induce ventricular dysrhythmias in the intact heart, in the heart which has sustained a recent infarction, or in neither situation? Is there a dose-response relationship between hypokalemia and dysrhythmias or is hypokalemia merely a marker for some more subtle biochemical derangement such as hypomagnesemia or hypocalcemia? Does hypokalemia itself cause dysrhythmias independently of intracellular potassium status or is the key issue the concentration of potassium in the cells of the conducting system? I await with interest the results from such animal studies. It is certainly surprising that none of the major pharmaceutical firms which have such an interest in this area—exemplified as it is

**Table 9-1.** Approximate Amounts of Potassium and Chloride in Foodstuffs

| Food | $K^+$ content mmol/100 g | $K^+$ per average serving (mmol) | Cl per average serving (mmol)[a] |
|---|---|---|---|
| Sardines | 14 | 14 | — |
| Beef | 11 | 11 | — |
| Peanut butter | 17 | 7 | — |
| Chocolate | 11 | 4 | 1 |
| Brazil nuts | 17 | 7 | 1 |
| Potatoes | 25 | 50 | 8 |
| Parsley | 22 | 5 | 1 |
| Onions | 35 | 6 | — |
| Mushrooms | 13 | 9 | 0.5 |
| Leeks | 20 | 14 | 1 |
| Carrots | 25 | 25 | 3 |
| Brussels sprouts | 42 | 45 | 4 |
| Broccoli | 10 | 10 | 2 |
| Beetroot | 7 | 4 | 1 |
| Oranges | 3 | 3 | — |
| Peaches | 27 | 20 | 0.2 |
| Bananas | 15 | 15 | 6 |
| Apricots | 30 | 30 | — |

Daily potassium requirements 800 to 1300 mg (20 to 33 mmol).
[a]Assuming no salt added in cooking.

by the large amount of advertising I receive about potassium salts and "potassium-sparing" diuretics—have sponsored such important research.

# SOURCES OF POTASSIUM

## Diet (Table 9-1)

Patients acquire most of their potassium in their diets. A daily intake of 0.8 to 1.3 g (20–33 mmols) potassium is required to maintain health. Normal Western diets contain between two and three times this amount. Foods rich in potassium include apricots, bananas, peaches, beans, brussels sprouts, carrots, onions, potatoes, spinach, tomatoes, and bread. Thus, for example, 100 g of brussels sprouts contains an average of 42 mmol of potassium. This is equivalent to 6 Slow-K tablets (Ciba-Geigy). However, it must not be assumed that all dietary potassium is available, since much is complexed with such salts as citrate which limit its absorption.

## Potassium Supplements (Table 9-2)

Potassium is a difficult substance to prescribe for patients. The organic salts such as the acetate, citrate or gluconate are quite impalatable and therefore unsuitable for routine use. Moreover, since a potassium deficit is usually accompanied by loss of chloride, it is difficult to correct that deficit unless chloride is also prescribed. Use of salts other than the chloride may pardoxically stimulate tubular potassium secretion thereby exacerbating negative potassium balance.[32] For this reason potassium chloride is the preferred salt for prophylaxis against or treatment of hypokalemia. Unfortunately this salt is also unpalatable. For a time an enteric-coated formulation of the chloride salt enjoyed considerable vogue, but this preparation was poorly absorbed and caused intestinal ulceration and hemorrhage resulting in its withdrawal from the market in the mid-1960s. Recently three preparations for oral potassium supplementation have become widely accepted. First, and most popular of all, is the use of a slow-

**Table 9-2.** Potassium Supplements and Potassium-Sparing Diuretics

| Medication | Daily dose (range) | Cost per dose* (dollars) | Comments |
|---|---|---|---|
| **Potassium-Sparing Diuretics** | | | |
| Triamterene | 50 to 300 mg | 0.14/100 mg | Risk of hyperkalemia is high in patients with renal failure and diabetes. |
| Spironolactone | 50 to 300 mg | 0.40/ 50 mg | |
| Amiloride | 5 to  20 mg | 0.25/5 mg | Slower onset and greater frequency of side effects make spironolactone less desirable. |
| **Potassium Supplements** | | | |
| Liquids | | | |
| KCl Elixir | 30 to 90 ml 20 mmol/15ml) | 0.65/15 ml | Poor palatability and GI upset common |
| Kaon Elixir | 30 to 90 ml (20 mmol/15ml) | 0.35/15 ml | More palatable than KCl but gluconate anion is converted to $HCO_3$ which is excreted with $K^+$. Thus, KCl is a more effective supplement. |
| Tablets/Capsules | | | |
| Slow-K (KCl in wax matrix | 3 to 12 tabs (8 mmol/tab) | 0.43/tab | More palatable than liquid KCl. May cause GI erosions. |
| Micro-K Extentabs (microencapsulated KCl). | 3 to 12 tabs (8 mmol/tab) | 0.11/tab | Well tolerated. May be less likely to cause GI erosions than Slow-K. |
| K-Lyte ($K^+$ $HCO_3$ and | 1 to 3 tabs (25 mmol/tab) | 0.50/tab | $K^+$ not well retained due to diuresis of accompanying anions. |
| Klorves (KCl powder) | 1 to 3 packets of powder (20 mmol per packet) | 0.55/packet | Effervescent mixture |

*Price based on Temple Hospital formulary (1983).

release preparation in which the potassium chloride is dispersed in a wax matrix (Slow-K, Ciba-Geigy). Second, is the use of fixed dose combinations of diuretics and potassium chloride in a wax matrix. It is claimed that this preparation improves compliance while imposing a lesser dose requirement for potassium supplementation. Third, is the effervescent tablet which may be useful for the elderly but is inconvenient for individuals who are out and about performing their daily chores away from home. Finding a source of water to dissolve the tablet may be inconvenient or embarassing for the active subject.

These therapies are not without their problems. For example, there is remarkably little in the literature to demonstrate that the potassium present in these wax matrix preparations is freely available for absorption. Ben Ishay and Engelman[1] studied 10 patients, comparing the "bioavailability" of similar doses of a slow release potassium chloride preparation suspended in a wax matrix (Slow-K, Ciba-Geigy) with that of a 10 percent solution. Comparable increments in urine and plasma potassium were obtained suggesting that the bioavailability of the slow release compound was similar to that of the oral solution. Unfortunately, there are very few confirmatory reports in the literature.

It has been widely held that wax-imbedded potassium chloride preparations caused minimal, if any, intestinal toxicity. This notion was directly tested by McMahon et al.[26] with a double-blind study comparing the endoscopic changes in the upper gastrointestinal tract caused by a wax matrix preparation with those caused by a microencapsulated formulation of potassium chloride. They found a large number of such gastric mucosal lesions as hyperemia, edema, erosions and small ulcers in patients receiving the widely used wax-matrix preparation. Although the significance of such lesions can be questioned, the fact remains that they are present and could produce major symptoms, especially if recipients have any delay in gastrointestinal emptying. Ulceration of the esophagus is known to accompany ingestion of such preparations by subjects with retarded esophageal emptying.[25]

Recognizing that potassium supplements have their inherent problems, we next turn to the potassium-sparing diuretics in hopes of safely effecting potassium retention during therapy with other potassium-wasting diuretics. Theoretically, this seems a good option but, as I shall demonstrate, this therapy is associated with much greater risk and expense than simple potassium chloride replacement. It can safely be concluded that we have as yet no suitable, nontoxic method of acquiring additional potassium salts other than by the time-honored manner: the diet. A summary of available potassium supplements and sparing diuretics is outlined in Table 9-2.

# HYPERKALEMIA

In 1974, I reviewed the records of 16,000 consecutive medical inpatients studied by the BCDSP.[15] Of these, 31 percent (4921 patients) had received potassium chloride during their hospital stay. Potassium was given prophylactically in 87 percent of recipients. Hyperkalemia (plasma potassium > 5.5 mmol/L) was reported in 74 of 1910 patients (3.9 percent) who received only oral potassium chloride and 71 of 819 (8.7 percent) who received both oral and parenteral potassium (the later being prescribed during the course of intravenous fluid therapy). Overall, 3.6 percent of recipients of potassium developed significant hyperkalemia during their admission. The mean level of hyperkalemia was 6.0 mmol/L (SEM ±

0.1 mmol/L). In 15 percent of the total, the hyperkalemia was of such severity as to be life-threatening or to have been partially responsible for the patient's death. This study caused significant interest since hyperkalemia had previously been regarded as a rare event and not one regularly associated with potassium therapy. The hyperkalemia was noted more often in the elderly, and in those with renal impairment but was independent of sex or primary reason for hospitalization. The only difficulty with interpreting this information was that it was of necessity derived from patients with a large variety of underlying diseases. Likewise, Greenblatt and Koch-Weser,[9] analyzing similar patients noted that hyperkalemia occurred in 8.6 percent of 788 spironolactone recipients. The hyperkalemia was more common in patients with renal impairment and indeed was noted in 42 percent of patients with renal impairment who were receiving both spironolactone and potassium chloride. These studies emphasize that hyperkalemia, previously thought to occur mainly when bolus injections of potassium salts[14] were given, may also occur after relatively small doses of oral potassium salts.

The Boston program now has sufficient information to examine the risks of hyperkalemia and hypokalemia in patients hospitalized as a result of congestive cardiac failure per se.[19] Over the study period, 4.5 percent of 3879 patients hospitalized with cardiac failure developed hypokalemia and 3.7 percent developed hyperkalemia. Thus, in 3879 patients with congestive heart failure being treated in University teaching hospitals, drug-attributed hypo- and hyperkalemia occurred with approximately equal frequency. Of particular interest and possible clinical relevance, was the observation that drug-attributed hypokalemia was more common in females and independent of renal function whereas hyper-

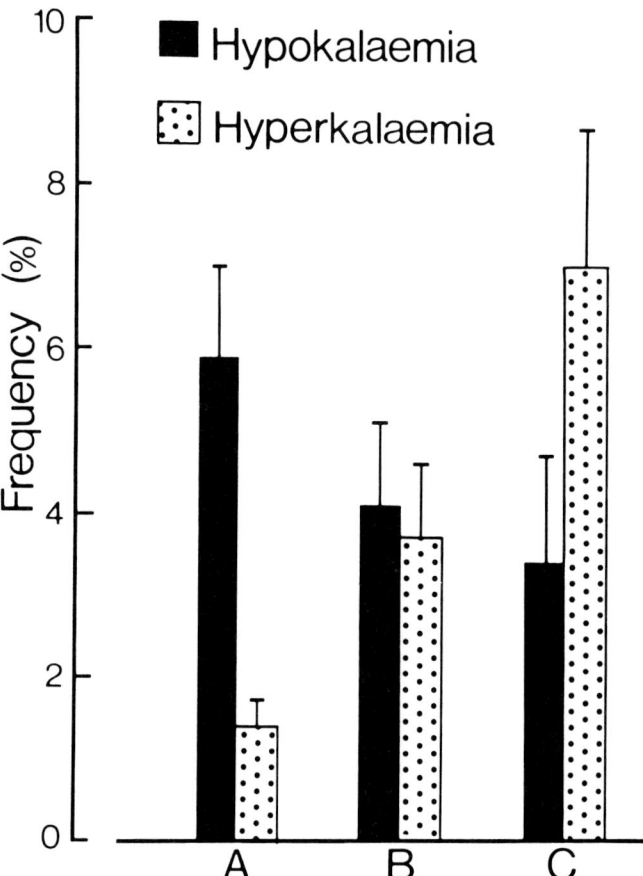

**Fig. 9-2.** Drug-attributed alterations in potassium handling in cardiac failure (A) Potassium losing diuretics without KCl. (B) Potassium losing diuretics with KCl. (C) Potassium-sparing diuretics with potassium losing diuretics.

kalemia was somewhat more frequent in males and was impressively related to renal function. Life-threatening degrees of hypokalemia and hyperkalemia occurred with approximately equal frequencies, that is, two per 1000 patients treated.

This report, from probably the largest series of patients with cardiac failure reviewed in one study, emphasizes the fact that such patients are at risk from developing both hypokalemia and hyperkalemia. The hypokalemia was most common in patients receiving loop diuretics without potassium supplements and the hyperkalemia in those receiving potassium-sparing diuretics (Table 9-3 and Fig. 9-2). Actually a major contributing cause of the hyperkalemia was the routine prescription of potassium supplements in the early phases of therapy for cardiac failure, prior to establishing a significant diuresis and prior to assessing the patient's potassium and renal status. In my view, potassium supplements should not be prescribed to patients receiving diuretics for heart failure until a diuresis has been established and their renal-electrolyte status defined.

It must be appreciated that this study examined only inpatients.[19] The author is unaware of any comparable series of observations on outpatients and indeed such a study would be a formidable undertaking. Many technical problems limit accurate assessment of serum potassium concentration in outpatients. Any delay in assaying serum samples and/or any major alteration in the ambient temperature of

**Table 9-3.** Drug Attributed Alterations in Potassium Handling in
Heart Failure

| Hypokalemia 175    (4.5%) | | Hyperkalemia 144    (3.7%) |
|---|---|---|
| 78/1318—5.9% | Potassium losing diuretics without KCl | 18/1269—1.4% |
| 69/1699—4.1% | Potassium losing diuretics with KCl | 65/1741—3.7% |
| 28/ 826—3.3% | Potassium sparing diuretics ± potassium losing diuretics | 61/ 869—7.0% |

Derived from Lawson DH, O'Connor PC, Jick H: Drug-attributed alterations in potassium handling in congestive cardiac failure. Eur J Clin Pharmacol 23:21, 1982.

the blood sample may result in potassium leakage from the red blood cells, thereby masking hypokalemia or resulting in artifactual hyperkalemia.

Recently my group has reported the results of a prospective survey of hyperkalemia occurring in a teaching hospital over a period of one year.[27] We found 406 patients with significant, nonartifactual, hyperkalemia amongst 29,063 consecutive patients (1.4 percent). As anticipated, hyperkalemia was primarily related to impaired renal function. A total of 44 percent of patients had impaired renal elimination of potassium as the primary etiological factor in their hyperkalemia. Nevertheless, drug treatment played almost as significant a part in the etiology of the hyperkalemia as did renal impairment. Indeed 37 percent of patients had their hyperkalemia attributed in large part to potassium supplements either oral potassium chloride (21 percent), intravenous potassium chloride (8 percent) or aldosterone antagonists (8 percent).

From these reports we can conclude that

1. The minimal fall in serum potassium concentrations often seen in diuretic recipients does not cause any symptoms recognized by the patient.

2. Reports that this small fall in serum concentrations may cause serious ventricular dysrhythmias under certain conditions are uncontrolled and may well arise as a result of unrecognized associated disorders. More detailed studies are required before these reports can be accepted.

3. Further studies of the role of altered serum and intracellular potassium concentration on cardiac rhythm are urgently required in animals.

4. Digitalis-induced cardiac arrhythmias can be precipitated by relatively small alterations in serum potassium concentrations.

5. Supplementary potassium is best given in the diet. If oral potassium salts are required, a wax-matrix base in which potassium chloride is suspended is probably best although early reports suggest that a microencapsulated formulation may reduce gastrointestinal irritation even further.[26]

6. Attempts to prevent the modest hypokalemia complicating use of furosemide or ethacrynic acid by adding aldosterone antagonists or replacing loop diuretics with triamterene or amiloride, are inadvisable in view of the greater costs and the risk of hyperkalemia.

7. Hyperkalemia occurs most frequently when inpatients with heart failure are given potassium supplements or potassium-sparing diuretics before a diuresis is established and/or before knowledge of serum potassium and renal status is available.

8. Life-threatening hypokalemia and hyperkalemia occur with approximately equal frequency in hospitalized patients treated for cardiac failure.

9. Hyperkalemia is strongly correlated with impaired renal function.

10. Over one-third of hospitalized patients with significant hyperkalemia developed this abnormality secondary to the inappropriate use of potassium supplements or potassium sparing diuretics.

## COSTS OF POTASSIUM SUPPLEMENTS AND POTASSIUM-SPARING DIURETICS

Purely on economic grounds alone, the widespread prophylactic use of potassium and potassium-sparing diuretics must be called into question. Harrington et al.[10] cited data from IMS America in 1982 indicating that approximately 7.5 million prescriptions for potassium supplements and 19 million prescriptions for potassium-sparing diuretics were written annually. The single indication for these prescriptions was "essential benign hypertension" and this represented a yearly cost of over 250 million dollars. These data do not include diuretics, diuretic combinations, and potassium supplements for other indications such as heart failure and they refer only to the United States. Worldwide, the cost of these drugs exceeds one billion dollars annually. Better use could be found for such a vast sum.

## TREATMENT OF ASYMPTOMATIC HYPOKALEMIA

As has been indicated in many of the studies cited above, the risk of hypokalemia developing in long-term diuretic recipients is low. The magnitude of the risk depends upon the criteria accepted for the term "hypokalemia." It is my contention that this should be a plasma potassium concentration of 3.0 mmol/L or less and not the more usually quoted levels of 3.5 or 3.8 mmol/L.

If a long-term diuretic recipient is found on routine testing to have a plasma potassium concentration of 2.9 mmol/L, I advise that this be repeated within a short time. If it remains unchanged and there are no obvious causes such as persistent vomiting or diarrhea, or recent alterations in dietary habits, a search should be made to determine whether the patient has evidence of secondary hyperaldosteronism or any other cause of hypokalemia. Treatment by potassium supplementation is justified until the patient's serum potassium concentration returns to the normal range. Thereafter this supplement can be withdrawn and the patient kept under close surveillance. Such a situation does not arise frequently in clinical practice.

Where a long-term diuretic recipient has been found to have a plasma concentration between 3.1 and 3.5 mmol/L in the absence of other causes, I normally advise that no active treatment is necessary and the patient merely be watched unless also taking long-term digoxin therapy. In those specific circumstances, supplementary potassium is justified on a regular prophylactic basis.

## CONCLUSIONS

In any cost-benefit analysis this massive cost in dollar terms can only be justified if it is shown that patient's symptoms are relieved following potassium supplementation and/or they are at lesser risk than their nonsupplemented counterparts. It is my view that the evidence purported to justify this widespread "habit" is not yet available and is unlikely to become so. I would therefore propose that the routine prophylactic use of potassium supplements in outpatients receiving diuretics for the treatment of hypertension or for maintenance of an edema-free state in compensated heart failure, should be severely restricted. Such drugs are indicated primarily for diuretic recipients who are also

1. suffering from a major degree of hepatic disease accompanied by ascites and hypoalbuminemia
2. receiving concurrent therapy with cardiac glycosides
3. unable to consume a normal balanced diet for periods exceeding one week
4. suffering from diarrhea of measurable severity or duration.

When a patient is hospitalized with acute heart failure and receives urgent diuretic therapy, potassium supplements should not be administered until the serum potassium, urea and creatinine concentrations are available and a satisfactory diuresis is established.

When a nonedematous, nondigitalized patient receiving diuretics is found to have mild hypokalemia, short-term use of oral potassium salts such as a wax-matrix potassium chloride prescription (Slow-K, Ciba-Geigy) is clearly justified. However, detailed assessment of the patient is necessary to discover why the hypokalemia occurred. Thus, in such patients it is important to ensure that they are taking an adequate diet, are free from gastrointestinal disease, do not abuse laxatives and have no major underlying organic pathology such as Conn's syndrome.

Having satisfied oneself on these points, potassium supplements can be withdrawn once the serum potassium concentration returns to normal. The patient should then be kept under detailed observation for a few months to ensure that the hypokalemia does not recur. Routine potassium supplements should not be used as a substitute for careful assessment of this type of patient.

# REFERENCES

1. Ben Ishay D, Engelman K: Bioavailability of potassium from a slow release tablet. Clin Pharm Therap 14:250, 1973.
2. Bowman WC, Rand MJ: Textbook of Physiology and Pharmacology. 2nd Edition. Blackwell Scientific Publications, London, 1980.
3. Davidson C, Burkinshaw L, McLachlan MSF, et al: Effect of long-term diuretic treatment on body potassium in heart disease. Lancet 2: 1044, 1976.
4. Dobbs SM, Kenyon WI, Dobbs RJ: Maintenance digoxin after an episode of heart failure: Placebo controlled trial in outpatients. Br Med J 1: 749, 1977.
5. Duke M: Thiazide-induced hypokalemia. Association with acute myocardial infarction and ventricular fibrillation. JAMA, 239:43, 1978.
6. Fisch C, Greenspan K, Kurebel SB, et al: Effect of digitalis on conditions of the heart. Proc Card Dis 6: 343, 1964.
7. Flear CTG, Florence I, Williams JA: Water, sodium potassium and chloride content of skeletal muscle in fit and ill subjects. J Clin Pathol 21: 555, 1968.
8. Greenblatt DJ, Duhme D, Allen MD, et al: Clinical toxicity of furosemide in hospitalized patients. Am Heart J 94: 6, 1977.
9. Greenblatt DJ, Koch-Weser J: Adverse reactions to spironolactone, JAMA 225: 40, 1973.
10. Harrington JT, Isner JM, Kassirer JP: Our national obsession with potassium. Am J Med 73: 155, 1982.
11. Holland OB, Nixon JV, Kuhnert L: Diuretic-induced ventricular ectopic activity. Am J Med 70: 762, 1981.
12. Johnston GD, McDevitt DG: Is maintenance digoxin necessary in patients with sinus rhythm? Lancet, 1: 567, 1979.
13. Krakauer R, Lauritzen M: Diuretic therapy and hypokalaemia in geriatric out-patients. Dan Med Bull 25: 126, 1978.
14. Lankton JW, Siler JN, Neigh JL: Hyper-

kalemia after administration of potassium for non-rigid parenteral fluid conditions. Anaesthesiology, 39: 660, 1973.

15. Lawson DH: Adverse reactions to potassium chloride. Q J Med 43: 433, 1974.

16. Lawson DH, Boddy K, Gray JMB, et al: Potassium supplements in patients receiving long-term diuretics for oedema. Q J Med 45: 469, 1976.

17. Lawson DH, Jick H: Drug surveillance for adverse drug effects: A study of medical inpatients. J Clin Pharm 3: 203, 1978.

18. Lawson DH, Henry DA, Lowe JM, et al: Severe hypokalemia in hospitalized patients. Arch Intern Med 139: 978, 1979.

19. Lawson DH, O'Connor PC, Jick H: Drug-attributed alterations in potassium handling in congestive cardiac failure. Eur J Clin Pharmacol 23: 21, 1982.

20. Lown B, Weller JM, Wyatt N, et al: Effects of alterations of body potassium on digitalis toxicity. J Clin Invest 31: 648, 1952.

21. Morgan T, Berliner RW: A study of continuous microperfusion of water and electrolyte movements in the loop of Henle and distal tubule of the rat. Nephron, 6: 388, 1969.

22. Morgan DB, Davidson C: Hypokalemia and diuretics: An analysis of publications. Br Med J 1: 905, 1980.

23. Morgan DB, Burkinshaw L, Davidson C: Potassium depletion in heart failure and its relation to long-term treatment with diuretics: A review of the literature. Postgrad Med J 54: 72, 1978.

24. Morgan DB, Young RM: Acute transient hypokalaemia: New interpretation of a common event. Lancet 2: 1044, 1982.

25. McCall AJ: Slow-K ulceration of oesophagus with aneurysmal left atrium. Br Med J 3: 230, 1975.

26. McMahon FG, Ryan JR, Akdamar K, et al: Upper gastrointestinal lesions after potassium chloride supplements: A controlled clinical trial. Lancet, 2: 1059, 1982.

27. Paice B, Gray JMB, McBride D, et al: Hyperkalaemia in hospitalised patients. Br Med J, in press.

28. Patrick J, Jones NF, Bradford B, et al: Leucocyte potassium in uremia: comparisons with erythrocyte potassium and total exchangeable potassium. Clin Sci 43: 669, 1972.

29. Ramsey LE, Harrison IR, Shelton JR, et al: Paradoxical potassium excretion in response to aldosterone antagonists. Eur J Clin Pharmacol 11: 101, 1977.

30. Relman AS, Schwartz WB: The nephropathy of potassium depletion. J Clin Invest 34:954, 1955.

31. Sandor FF, Pickens PT, Crallan J: Variations of plasma potassium concentrations during long-term treatment of hypertension with diuretics without potassium supplements. Br Med J 284: 709, 1982.

32. Schwartz WB, van Ypersele de Striou CE, Kassirer JP: Role of anions in metabolic alkalosis and potassium deficiency. N Engl J Med J, 286: 1189, 1983.

33. Schwartz AB, Swartz CD: Dosage of potassium chloride elixir to correct thiazide-induced hypokalemia. JAMA 230: 702, 1974.

34. Widdowson EM, McCance RA, Spray CM: The chemical composition of the body. Clin Sci 10: 113, 1951.

# The Case for Routinely Normalizing Serum Potassium

## O. Bryan Holland, M.D.

In the last few years several studies have challenged the previous prevailing opinion[32,36,47] that diuretic-induced hypokalemia is innocuous when it occurs in asymptomatic, nondigitalized patients. Diuretic-induced hypokalemia is a common clinical problem, occurring in 30 to 50 percent of patients treated with diuretics.[32] Unfortunately, in spite of the widespread clinical relevance of diuretic-induced hypokalemia, previous therapeutic recommendations were based on "clinical impressions" and retrospective studies[18,80] correlating ventricular arrhythmias observed on routine electrocardiograms with serum potassium determinations done at about the same time. However, a review of present evidence leads to the clear conclusion that potassium depletion with diuretic therapy may lead to a number of problems which require normalization of the serum potassium concentration to minimize their expression.

## EFFECTS OF HYPOKALEMIA

The suggestion that hypokalemia is innocuous is curious. Potassium is the major intracellular cation, and a rich experience indicates that it has important roles in maintaining cellular integrity as well as in influencing a variety of cellular processes, including neuromuscular excitability, energy provision, carbohydrate and protein metabolism, and acid-base status.

Potassium depletion may change neuromuscular excitability in several ways. As resting membrane potential moves toward the depolarization threshold, excitability for depolarization increases. Initially, extracellular potassium depletion is more prominent than intracellular depletion, which increases the ratio of intracellular to extracellular potassium and increases resting transmembrane potential.[6,33] However, the activity of ATPase, a family of membrane enzymes for transport of various ions and other substances across cell membranes may decrease with potassium depletion,[37,38] which decreases transmembrane potential. Potassium depletion diminishes the activity of choline acetylase and thus the synthesis of acetylcholine, the neurotransmitter for cholinergic neuromuscular depolarization.[61] The net effect of these changes may lead to variable results, though the usual effect is a depression of neuromuscular function. Potassium depletion interferes with the transfer of high energy phosphate essential for ATP provision[8,51] or for phosphorylation of creatine[7] to provide energy for muscle contraction. This transfer of high energy phosphate is important in carbohydrate metabolism. Potassium is also involved in carbohydrate metabolism through its effects on acetylkinase, which catalyzes the fusion of acetate and coenzyme A for citrate production from oxalacetate in the tricarboxylic acid cycle[59] and by its importance in glycogen synthesis[10,29,31,39,52,78] and in facilitating insulin release.[16,40,41,70] Acid-base status is altered by potassium depletion in that alkalosis ensues secondary to increased activity of renal glutaminase, which increases ammonia production and hydrogen ion excretion,[45] and from an increase in tubular hydrogen versus potassium exchange for sodium.[52,69,81] Experimental potassium depletion leads to decreased protein synthesis and growth retardation.[12,78] In addition to these more generalized effects, potassium depletion produces characteristic effects upon the heart, neuromuscular system, kidney, gastrointestinal tract, and pancreatic islets.

## Cardiac Effects

Potassium depletion initially leads to an increase in resting membrane potential,[33] which should protect against ventricular ectopic activity (VEA) by increasing the change required to reach the depolarization threshold. Furthermore, potassium depletion increases the usual slight myocardial cellular asymmetry in depolarization and repolarization. This change is reflected in an increase in the relative refractory period. The net effect of these changes is that the chance of occurrence of reentry mechanisms is increased.

Cardiac pathological findings are relatively similar with experimental potassium depletion in the rat[55] and in humans with potassium depletion from chronic gastrointestinal losses or other etiologies.[48,57,64] The pathologic findings include an early period of cellular swelling with loss of striations, glycogen accumulation, and nuclear fading to eventual disappearance. Beginning with the loss of striations, cells consisting mainly of tissue macrophages along with

sarcolemma nuclei and occasional polymorphonuclear leukocytes collect around the affected fibers. MacPherson[55] has emphasized that there is little if any destruction of the connective tissue framework, though it may undergo considerable collapse, and there is preservation of the blood supply. Thus, it appears that there is considerable ability for myocardial regeneration, in contrast to myocardial infarction lesions, in that scar formation is minimal to completely absent. These lesions occur in a patchy distribution throughout the ventricles, though the largest are subendocardial, especially in the papillary muscles and trabeculae. Atrial lesions also occur but they are usually smaller. The severity and number of these experimental cardiac lesions are intensified by exercise[26] and by sodium loading.[13]

A 25 percent reduction in myocardial potassium content produces mitochondrial vacuolization and dissolution of cristae accompanied by ballooning of spaces adjacent to sarcolemmal membranes and dilatation of sarcoplasmic vesicles. Furthermore, mitochondrial and micrososomal ATPase is reduced by about 25 percent.[37] These changes may play a significant role in the depression of myocardial contractility[1,35,38,49] and tendency to develop pulmonary edema with exercise[49] which has been noted with experimental potassium depletion. An additional functional impairment which has been noted is decreased vascular reactivity.[28,30] All of these factors may lead to a slight blood pressure fall with potassium depletion,[28,65] though excess potassium administration has also been noted to lower the blood pressure slightly.[74] However, in the latter case, simultaneous sodium depletion cannot be ruled out as the cause for the blood pressure fall.

The clinical assessment of the severity of these cardiovascular changes secondary to potassium depletion has been difficult. Electrocardiographic changes characteristic of hypokalemia have been noted to occur in only about 50 percent of patients with significant total body potassium depletion.[71] In the past it was felt that ventricular arrhythmias were not particularly common in nondigitalized, hypokalemic patients. This opinion was based on some retrospective studies[18,80] in which a routine electrocardiogram was correlated with potassium determinations done at approximately the same time. However, more recent studies using more accurate techniques such as 24 hour ambulatory ECG monitoring and ECG monitoring during exercise testing have documented that ventricular arrhythmias occur in a significant number of patients with diuretic-induced hypokalemia, even in patients without symptoms and physical findings suggestive of cardiovascular disease.

One of these studies[42] involved patients with mild to moderate hypertension and a history of diuretic-induced hypokalemia. The patients were taken off previous diuretic therapy and potassium repleted for a period of 2 to 3 weeks during an initial one month placebo phase. At the end of this placebo phase, baseline ambulatory ECG monitoring was normal. Exercise testing with simultaneous ECG monitoring documented that the patients did not appear to have underlying coronary artery disease or exercise-induced ventricular ectopic activity (VEA). The patients were then treated with hydrochlorothiazide (HCTZ, 100 mg/day) for a period of 4 weeks to induce hypokalemia, and at the end of this time the ambulatory ECG monitoring, plasma potassium determinations, and exercise testing were repeated. Seven of 21 HCTZ-treated patients had developed VEA at this time, and four of the seven were noted to have complex VEA (ventricular tachycardia, ventricular couplets,

multifocal premature ventricular beats), arrhythmias which have been associated with sudden death (Fig. 9-3). Exercise testing during the phase of hypokalemia was less sensitive in identifying VEA since only 2 of the 7 patients had ventricular arrhythmias during exercise testing. The patients were then potassium repleted with spironolactone, and the effect of potassium repletion was assessed by periodic additional 24 hour ambulatory ECG monitoring. Complex VEA was abolished by potassium repletion, and there was a statistically significant decrease in the frequency of VEA with potassium repletion in 6 of these 7 patients (Fig. 9-3). Interestingly, the one exception was a case who was noted to have persistent unifocal ventricular premature beats (VPBs) varying from 31 to 220 unifocal VPBs per hour during four ambulatory ECG monitorings done over a period of 13 weeks during the phase of potassium repletion. The addition of propranolol for an additional 6 week period still did not cause the ambulatory ECG monitoring to return to the pattern characteristic of the baseline phase. It thus appeared that this patient had undergone some kind of cardiac change as a result of HCTZ-induced hypokalemia that resulted in the production of VEA which persisted for an exceedingly long period of time, even after potassium repletion. One is tempted to speculate that this change might have been explained by the focal cardiac lesions which have been observed with potassium depletion.[48,55,57,64] This study has been criticized[36] by the suggestion that spontaneous variation in the ambulatory ECG monitoring might explain the study results since more than one ambulatory ECG monitoring was not done in the baseline phase to document the baseline pattern in great detail. However, unifocal VPBs occurred with an average frequency of 14.7 beats/hour/24 hour ECG monitoring while the patients were

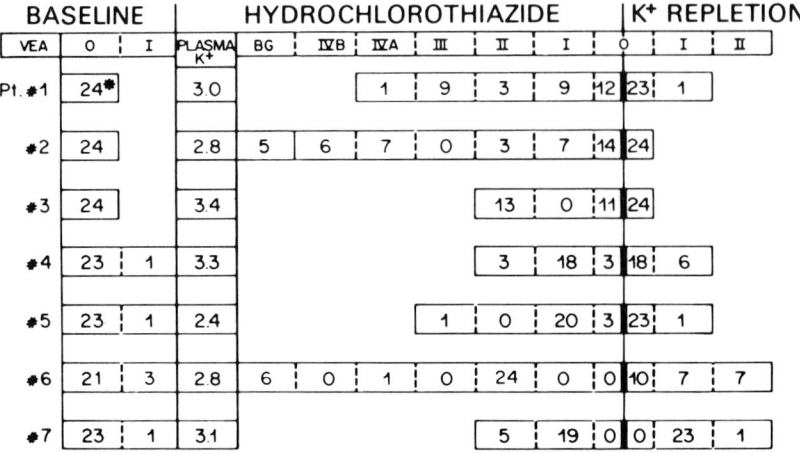

| | BASELINE | | | HYDROCHLOROTHIAZIDE | | | | | | | K+ REPLETION | |
|---|---|---|---|---|---|---|---|---|---|---|---|---|
| VEA | O | I | PLASMA K+ | BG | IVB | IVA | III | II | I | O | I | II |
| Pt. #1 | 24* | | 3.0 | | | 1 | 9 | 3 | 9 | 12 | 23 | 1 |
| #2 | 24 | | 2.8 | 5 | 6 | 7 | O | 3 | 7 | 14 | 24 | |
| #3 | 24 | | 3.4 | | | | 13 | O | 11 | 24 | | |
| #4 | 23 | 1 | 3.3 | | | | 3 | 18 | 3 | 18 | 6 | |
| #5 | 23 | 1 | 2.4 | | | 1 | O | 20 | 3 | 23 | 1 | |
| #6 | 21 | 3 | 2.8 | 6 | O | 1 | O | 24 | O | O | 10 | 7 | 7 |
| #7 | 23 | 1 | 3.1 | | | | 5 | 19 | O | O | 23 | 1 |

VEA GRADE I = ≤30 Unifocal VPB / hr.    II = >30 Unifocal VPB / hr. or >1 VPB /min.
III = Multifocal    IVA = Couplets    IVB = Ventricular Tachycardia    BG = Bigeminy
* Hr./ 24 hr. OF VEA OF THAT GRADE

**Fig. 9-3.** Development of ventricular ectopic activity (VEA) in 7 of 21 patients with uncomplicated essential hypertension and normal baseline 24-hour ambulatory monitoring (AM) treated with hydrochlorothiazide (50 mg twice a day) and the subsequent therapeutic response to potassium repletion with spironolactone. The level of plasma potassium noted at the time of ambulatory monitoring during hydrochlorothiazide treatment is indicated. The grades of ventricular ectopic activity attained and the numbers of hours of that grade during 24-hour ambulatory monitoring is depicted. (With permission, from: Holland OB, Nixon JB, Kuhnert L: Am J Med 70:762, 1981.)

hypokalemic vs an average at 0.5 unifocal VPB's/hour/24 hour ECG monitoring while the patients were normokalemic, a statistically significant difference. Thus, the study results did not appear to be explained by spontaneous variation.

The occurrence of VEA during hypokalemia has been assessed with static and dynamic exercise testing in an additional study.[43] Thirty-eight patients were administered HCTZ at dosages from 50 to 200 mg daily to attempt to achieve blood pressure normalization. These patients had no historical, laboratory, or physical abnormalities suggesting cardiac disease. Static and dynamic exercise testing was done before the initiation of HCTZ and then repeated when the patients were receiving either 50 or 100 mg HCTZ daily. Before HCTZ therapy there

was no significant change in the frequency of unifocal VPBs during the exercise testing. However, during HCTZ therapy there was a significant increase in unifocal VPBs with both static and dynamic exercise testing which correlated with the fall in serum potassium from HCTZ (Fig. 9-4). Multifocal VPBs were observed in 4 patients. Thus, this study also demonstrated that patients with diuretic-induced hypokalemia have VEA of a type which has been associated with sudden death.

Preliminary results[84] of a large Medical Research Council trial of treatment of hypertension also suggest that the incidence of VEA is increased by thiazide therapy and that hypokalemia might play an important role in the genesis of this VEA. In 164 patients studied during

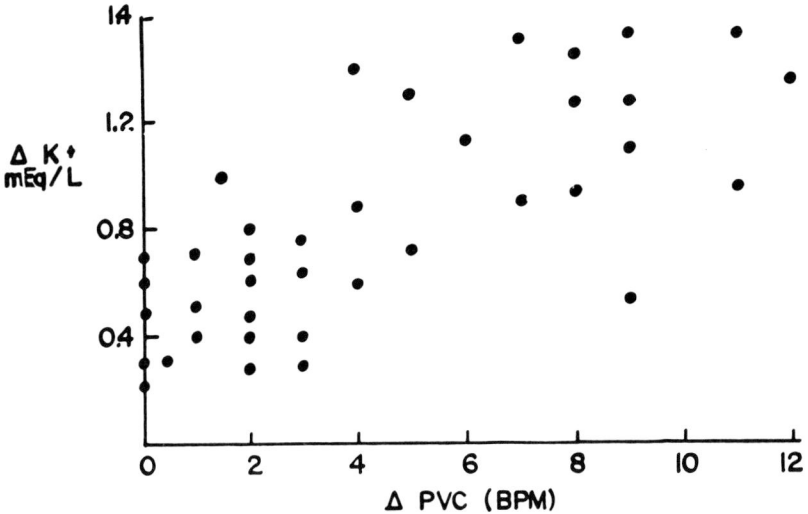

**Fig. 9-4.** Correlation between change in serum potassium and frequency of ventricular premature contractions in 38 mild to moderate hypertensive patients. (From: Hollifield JW, Slaton PE. Thiazide diuretics, hypokalemia, and cardiac arrhythmias. Acta Med Scand Suppl 647: 67, 1981.)

chronic thiazide therapy, the prevalence of VPBs was greater in thiazide-treated than in placebo-treated patients. In addition, "special" VPBs (multifocal, couplets, R on T, bigeminy) were even more common in a selected group of 20 hypokalemic patients treated with thiazide in comparison to the group treated with placebo. An enhanced incidence of ventricular arrhythmias has also been noted with diuretic-induced hypokalemia in another study.[14] In this latter study, older patients and those with evidence of underlying cardiovascular disease were noted to be at risk. In contrast, an increased incidence of ventricular arrhythmias was not noted with diuretic-induced hypokalemia in one study.[63] However, documentation of a normal 24 hour baseling ambulatory ECG was not done in this study. Spontaneous variation in ambulatory ECG monitoring increases greatly when abnormalities are present.[11] Thus, spontaneous variation in the ambulatory ECG monitoring would have tended to obscure the effects of diuretic treatment in this latter study. In addi-

tion, since potassium chloride instead of a potassium-sparing diuretic was used for potassium repletion, simultaneous magnesium depletion may have prevented myocardial potassium repletion. Thus, several studies now indicate that ventricular arrhythmias may occur as complications of chronic diuretic-induced hypokalemia. Though it is true that a large prospective study has not documented that diuretic-induced VEA leads to an enhanced incidence of sudden death, there is no reason to think that diuretic-induced VEA is innocuous. In fact, in Lown's study of patients with sudden death, 24 percent had hypokalemia associated with chronic diuretic therapy for hypertension.[54] Thus, hypokalemia should be treated to avoid ventricular arrhythmias.

Another line of evidence which strongly suggests that the serum potassium should be maintained within the normal range concerns the incidence of malignant ventricular arrhythmias in patients who present with acute myocardial infarction. Patients, such as those with essential hypertension, who are receiving chronic diuretic therapy represent a population much more likely to sustain an acute myocardial infarction at some point in their life. There are now a number of well documented studies[21,44,62,66,76] which indicate that hypokalemic patients with a myocardial infarction have a marked increase in the chance of developing malignant ventricular arrhythmias in comparison to normokalemic patients. In one such study[76] the records of 151 patients entering a coronary care unit were reviewed retrospectively, and it was found that 67 percent of patients with a serum potassium of less than 3.1 mEq/L had ventricular tachycardia or ventricular fibrillation compared to 40 percent of patients with a serum potassium between 3.1 to 3.5 mEq/L and 20 percent of normokalemic patients. In another similar study of 918 pateints,[62] a similar relationship of hypokalemia to malignant ventricular arrhythmias was demonstrated, with an overall incidence of malignant ventricular arrhythmias in 29 percent of hypokalemic patients versus 17 percent of normokalemic patients (Fig. 9-5). These types of studies have been criticized[36] in that in some studies the presence of hypokalemia was not documented before the onset of malignant ventricular arrhythmias, and the arrhythmias were not documented to subside immediately with potassium administration. However, this latter large study was a prospective study with serum potassium determined at the time of admission. It is unrealistic to think that ventricular fibrillation or tachycardia would be managed with potassium chloride alone in the setting of acute myocardial infarction to explore the influence of hypokalemia.

The level of potassium depletion sufficient to provoke VEA remains controversial. Life-threatening[17] as well as more benign[42] VEA has been noted with borderline hypokalemia, and a correlation between the magnitude of change in the serum potassium and the incidence of exercise-provoked VPBs has been found.[43] Studies in digitalis-treated patients indicate that alkalosis, reflecting intracellular potassium depletion, is an additional factor exclusive of the serum potassium concentration that should be considered.[9] Thus, even mild potassium depletion may be arrhythmogenic. Therefore these numerous studies provide additional evidence that patients receiving chronic diuretic therapy should have their serum potassium maintained in the normal range.

## Neuromuscular Function

Muscle weakness is a well-recognized symptom of moderate to severe potassium deficiency. Adverse consequences of mild potassium depletion are less appreciated. Potential problems with milder potassium deficiency include the danger of rhabdomyolysis with exercise as well as the likelihood that maximal exercise capacity would be impaired. A major factor increasing muscle blood flow in exercising muscles is augmentation of cellular potassium release.[50] Potassium deficient muscle might thus be expected to allow a lesser increase in blood flow and lead to diminished exercise capacity with relative ischemia, facilitating rhabdomyolysis.[50] Thus, maintenance of normokalemia will minimize this problem.

## Renal Effects

Interestingly, a number of renal structural and functional effects have been demonstrated with potassium depletion even when total kidney potassium determinations remain normal or only slightly reduced.[69,81] Thus, the mechanism of renal injury must involve certain vital subcellular functions in a

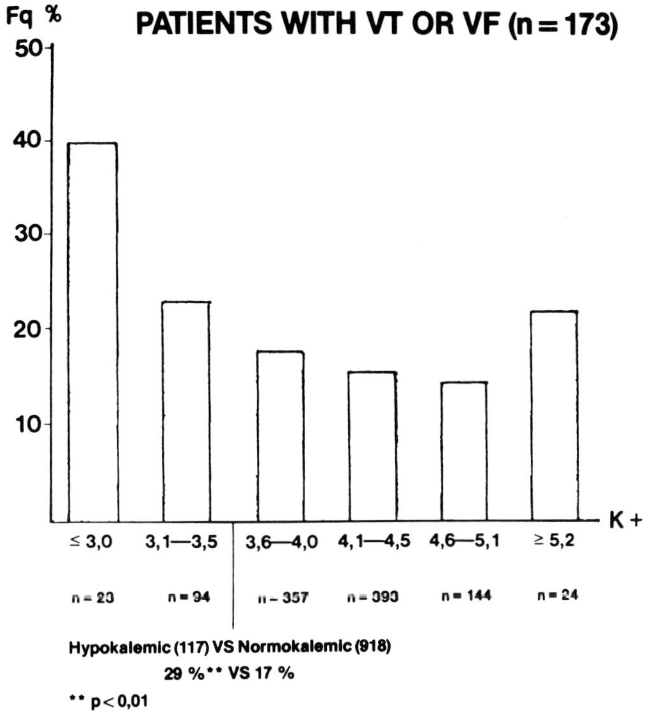

Fq %   **PATIENTS WITH VT OR VF (n = 173)**

**Fig. 9-5.** Incidence of ventricular tachycardia or ventricular fibrillation during hospital stay in relation to admission serum potassium values. (With permission, from: Nordrehaug JE Malignant arrhythmias in relation to serum potassium values in patients with an acute myocardiac infarction. Acta Med Scand Suppl 647: 101, 1981.)

manner different from skeletal muscle or other tissues that characteristically exhibit more prominent total potassium depletion, or there may be heterogeneity in the tendency of the different types of cells within the kidney to become potassium depleted. The kidneys of rats with experimental potassium depletion are typically enlarged and exhibit vacuolar changes in the collecting ducts and proximal convulated tubules.[69,81] These lesions include an intracellular accumulation of large granules, presumably altered mitochondria, which frequently cause luminal obstruction, dilatation of more proximal ducts and ultimate cell rupture followed by regenerative hyperplasia and occasional calcification. Similar lesions have been observed in the kidneys of potassium-depleted humans, though changes in the proximal tubules are much more prominent.[69,81] Since there is some suggestion that there is an enhanced incidence of pyelonephritis with kaliopenic nephropathy,[86] these lat-

ter findings may have been secondary to superimposed pyelonephritis or continued susceptibility to renal infections. With potassium repletion the renal lesions are largely reversible in most patients.[68]

In addition to these structural changes, various functional changes occur with potassium depletion.[45,52,69,81] A variety of renal enzymatic changes have been reported, although the level of potassium depletion which initiates these changes is not presently established. Levels of alkaline phosphatase, acid phosphatase, glutaminase, and carbonic anhydrase are increased. Tubular secretion of paraaminohippurate (PAH) is impaired. The urinary concentrating mechanism is impaired; bicarbonate excretion is impaired, and ammonium excretion is enhanced, presumably reflecting the increased activity of renal glutaminase.[45] With potassium repletion, renal function appears to return essentially to normal unless there has been superimposed pyelonephritis. Thus, a variety of renal structural and functional abnormalities have been noted with hypokalemia. Though the level of hypokalemia necessary to induce these abnormalities and to enhance the susceptibility to pyelonephritis is not fully defined, it would appear judicious to maintain the serum potassium in the normal range to minimize the chance of any of these problems.

### Gastrointestinal Effects

Potassium depletion appears to cause little structural damage to the gastrointestinal tract, though several functional defects have been identified, the most prominent of which is a decrease in intestinal motility. The mechanism of this motility disturbance is poorly explained at the present time, though it is possible that it results from diminished acetylcholine synthesis.[61] In addition, potassium depletion diminishes gastric acid secretion and is reflected by a decrease in potassium concentration of gastric fluids.[15]

### Effects on Carbohydrate Metabolism

Potassium depletion has a diabetogenic effect.[16,29,31,34,40,41,67,70,72,77,78] Potassium is deposited in the liver with glycogen, and there are conflicting studies suggesting that potassium depletion either decreases[10,31] or increases[29,31,78] glycogenesis. However, the relevance of these observations with more severe potassium depletion to the in vivo effects of milder potassium depletion is not clear at the present time. Nonetheless, there is good evidence that even slight hypokalemia can be diabetogenic in some patients, primarily through diminishing insulin release.[16,40,41,70,77,78] These chronic modest rises in blood sugar may provide a cardiovascular risk by enhancing atherosclerosis. Several recent large studies[56,58] have demonstrated that treatment of pa-

tients with exceedingly mild hypertension with diuretic agents may not improve cardiovascular mortality but may actually lead to an enhanced risk. These recent studies have reawakened interest in adverse cardiovascular effects of chronic diuretic therapy. As discussed above, some of the excess in cardiovascular mortality can be explained by an increased incidence of sudden death due to ventricular arrhythmias. However, all of the increased cardiovascular mortality is not secondary to sudden death, and so other factors that would enhance the risk of myocardial infarction should be sought. Chronic thiazide diuretic therapy has been associated with modest rises in serum cholesterol and triglyceride concentrations.[3] In addition, worsening of glucose tolerance in these patients[60] may be reflected by a significant increase in glycosylated hemoglobin concentration.[3] Potassium depletion alone appears to be highly important in the genesis of this glucose intolerance, and some investigators[40] feel that it provides the total explanation. The importance of potassium depletion in diminishing beta cell sensitivity for insulin release in humans has been elucidated further recently with the hyperglycemic clamp technique.[40] Normal subjects administered 100 mg hydrochlorothiazide daily had diminished insulin release when hypokalemic, but no change in insulin release when simultaneous potassium supplements were provided.[40] Though potassium depletion may not be the only factor causing the diabetogenic effect of diuretics, maintenance of normal serum potassium concentration during chronic diuretic therapy will minimize this important diabetogenic factor.

## SUMMARY

Potassium depletion produces widespread structural changes and/or dysfunction in a number of organ systems. Unfortunately, the levels of in vivo potassium depletion required to lead to these changes remain uncertain in several instances. Some of these changes have been demonstrated only with in vitro experiments in which marked potassium deficiency has been produced. However, it is a mistake to dismiss all of these changes as being unlikely to occur in the intact animal in the face of more modest potassium depletion. For example, significant changes in insulin release have been noted with only modest hypokalemia.[16,40,67,77] Furthermore, there is considerable heterogeneity in the tendency of various organs to become potassium depleted, and there are clear examples of significant dysfunction occurring in the face of only slight changes in total organ potassium content. For example, abnormalities in kidney structure and function have been identified in the hypokalemic dog in the presence of essentially normal total organ potassium stores.[69,81] Similarly, myocardium is relatively resistent to potassium depletion in comparison to skeletal muscle,[49,81] but ventricular arrhythmias have been noted with mild hypokalemia (plasma potassium of 3.0 to 3.5 mEq/L)[9,17,42,43] even in patients without apparent underlying cardiac disease. Patients with abnormal hearts would be expected to have even greater problems with developing VEA while hypokalemic.[11] Most diuretic-treated patients would have the potential for occult cardiac disease. The expense and potential risk of periodic careful studies to evaluate cardiac status does not seem warranted to identify a subgroup that might be less susceptible to VEA. Furthermore, the difficulty in determining clinically the level of potassium depletion is further compounded by the fact that the plasma or serum potassium determination is the only tool that is widely available. Though the plasma potassium determination is the more preferable of the two since it is not subject to a variable rise in potassium concentration during clot retraction, serum potassium determinations are performed more commonly at present because of greater ease with autoanalyzer determinations. Though there is a correlation between the intensity of total body potassium depletion and serum potassium, the variation is sufficient so that some individuals might have significant organ depletion in the face of only slight hypokalemia.[71] The previous clinical impression that hypokalemia was innocuous appears to have been based significantly on previous studies showing that total body potassium depletion was modest with chronic diuretic therapy[32,36,47,85] and that, in general, patients appeared to suffer no dramatic ill effects. However, a number of lines of evidence have now suggested convincingly that chronic, subclinical potassium depletion may produce adverse effects ranging from a slow diabetogenic acceleration of atherosclerosis to eventual, dramatic clinical manifestations due to ventricular arrhythmias. Thus, the chronic effects of potassium depletion may be difficult to appreciate clinically so that a reliable decision can be made about the need for potassium repletion. The only practical approach appears to be to maintain the serum potassium concentration in the normal range. Even in the face of this, there may be problems with potassium depletion in certain cell populations or their subcellular organelles. However, unless some manifestation such as worsening of glucose tolerance is noted, there is no way clinically to quantitate these lesser degrees of potassium depletion.

## RELATIONSHIP OF POTASSIUM DEFICIENCY TO MAGNESIUM DEFICIENCY

Dyckner and Wester[22-24] have reported extensive studies of the correlation of serum potassium, serum magnesium, muscle potassium, and muscle magnesium in diuretic-treated patients with congestive heart failure, essential hypertension and other causes of secondary aldosteronism. Their studies, as well as older studies[20,46,73,75,79] indicate that diuretics can lead to simultaneous depletion of both potassium and magnesium in serum and/or skeketal muscle. The incidence of magnesium depletion in patients with uncomplicated essential hypertension treated chronically with modest dosages of thiazide diuretics is presently unknown. Furthermore, the correlation between skeletal muscle magnesium and myocardial magnesium remains poorly defined in humans. A fall in serum magnesium concentration does not appear to occur as early in the course of diuretic therapy as does hypokalemia. Nonetheless, significant muscle magnesium depletion can occur in the face of normal serum magnesium concentration. There is a relatively good correlation between skeletal muscle potassium and magnesium content[2,22,82,83] though there is controversy about whether potassium[2] or magnesium[82,83] leads to the deficiency of the other cation. One postulate[82,83] is that magnesium deficiency decreases sodium-potassium ATPase, which diminishes intracellular potassium content. In any case intracellular potassium depletion may not correct with potassium supplementation until magnesium repletion is provided.[2,22,23,24,82,83] Magnesium depletion has also been associated with ventricular arrhythmias, perhaps secondary to the simultaneous depletion of intracellular potassium.[5,23,24,25,53] As a consequence, pure potassium repletion may have little effect upon ventricular arrhythmias associated with simultaneous muscle potassium and magnesium depletion, whereas initial magnesium repletion allows the repletion of muscle potassium and the resolution of ventricular arrhythmias.[5,23,24,25,46,53]

Thus, some patients may benefit from simultaneous potassium and magnesium repletion.

# TREATMENT RECOMMENDATIONS

A number of more recent studies suggest that the previous clinical impression that hypokalemia is innocuous in nondigitalized patients is erroneous. The serum potassium concentration should be checked in diuretic-treated patients within 1 to 2 weeks after initiation of diuretic therapy, and hypokalemic patients should be treated to restore normokalemia. Serum potassium concentration and total body potassium depletion usually remain relatively constant after the first month of diuretic therapy.[85] Thus, once normokalemia is restored, only occasional monitoring of serum potassium is necessary. In the majority of patients, the addition of a potassium-sparing diuretic provides some advantages over the addition of potassium chloride supplements for the following reasons:

1. The diuretic-treated patient has secondary aldosteronism and thus a highly efficient mechanism for excreting potassium supplements. A potassium-sparing diuretic is more likely to allow normokalemia to be restored in spite of this secondary aldosteronism.[4]

2. Patient compliance is better with potassium-sparing diuretics than with potassium supplements.

3. Certain patients may have simultaneous potassium and magnesium deficiencies. The potassium-sparing diuretics also conserve magnesium.[19] This may provide more effective control of complications of potassium depletion by allowing better intracellular potassium repletion.

However, some patients develop side effects with potassium-sparing diuretics, and these agents may be more likely to cause hyperkalemia in patients with diminished renal function. Thus, potassium chloride supplements may be more satisfactory in some patients. All diuretic-treated patients do not become hypokalemic, so some form of potassium repletion should not be prescribed routinely since hyperkalemia can also lead to lethal ventricular arrhythmias. However, the chance of developing complications from hyperkalemia when potassium-sparing diuretics or potassium supplements are given only to hypokalemic patients is very small. Nonetheless, serum potassium must be monitored to document that normokalemia has been achieved.

In summary, potassium depletion can lead to a number of adverse clinical effects. Since some of these occur with minimal potassium depletion, normokalemia should be restored in all diuretic-treated patients to minimize the chance of these complications.

# REFERENCES

1. Abbrecht PH: Cardiovascular effects of chronic potassium deficiency in the dog. Am J Physiol 223:555, 1972.
2. Alfrey AC, Miller NL, Butkus D: Evaluation of body magnesium stores. J Lab Clin Med 84:153, 1974.
3. Ames RP, Hill P: Improvement of glucose tolerance and lowering of glycohemoglobin and serum lipid concentrations after discontinuation of antihypertensive drug therapy. Circulation 65: 899, 1982.
4. Antcliff AC, Hamilton M, Beevers DG, et al: The use of amiloride hydrochloride in the correction of hypokalaemic alkalosis induced by diuretics. Postgrad Med J 47: 644, 1971.
5. Bigg RPC, Chia R: Magnesium deficiency: Role in arrhythmias complicating acute myocardial infarction? Med J Aust 1: 346, 1981.
6. Bilbrey GL, Herbin L, Carter NW, et al: Skeletal muscle resting membrane potential in potassium deficiency. J Clin Invest 52: 3011, 1973.
7. Boyer PD, Lardy HA, Phillips PH: The role of potassium in muscle phosphorylations. J Biol Chem 146: 673, 1942.
8. Boyer PD, Lardy HA, Phillips PH: Further studies on the role of potassium and other ions in the phosphorylation of the adenylic system. J Biol Chem 149: 529, 1943.
9. Brater DC, Morrelli HF: Digoxin toxicity in patients with normokalemic potassium deficiency. Clin Pharmacol Ther 22: 21, 1976.
10. Buchanan JM, Hastings AB, Nesbett FB: The effect of the ionic environment on the synthesis of glycogen from glucose in rat liver slices. J Biol Chem 180: 435, 1949.
11. Calvert A, Lown B, Gorlin R: Ventricular premature beats and anatomically defined coronary heart disease. Am J Cardiol 39: 627, 1977.
12. Cannon PR, Frazier LE, Hughes RH: Influence of potassium on tissue protein synthesis. Metabolism 1: 49, 1952.
13. Cannon PR, Frazier LE, Hughes RH: Sodium as a toxic ion in potassium deficiency. Metabolism 2: 297, 1953.
14. Caralis P, Perez-Stable E, Materson B: Ventricular ectopy and diuretic-induced hypokalemia in hypertensive patients. Clin Res 29: 832A, 1981.
15. Carone FA, Cooke RE: Effect of potassium deficiency on gastric secretion in the rat. Am J Physiol 172: 684, 1953.
16. Conn JW: Hypertension, the potassium ion and impaired carbohydrate tolerance. N Engl J Med 273: 1135, 1967.
17. Curry P, Stubbs W, Fitchett D, et al: Ventricular arrhythmias and hypokalaemia. Lancet, 2:231, 1976.
18. Davidson S, Surawicz B: Ectopic beats and atrioventricular conduction disturbances. Arch Intern Med 120: 280, 1967.
19. DeVane J, Ryan MP: The effects of amiloride and triamterene on urinary magnesium excretion in conscious saline-loaded rats. Br J Pharmacol 72: 285, 1981.
20. Duarte CG: Effects of ethacrynic acid and

furosemide on urinary calcium, phosphate and magnesium. Metabolism 17: 867, 1968.

21. Duke M: Thiazide-induced hypokalemia: Association with acute myocardial infarction and ventricular fibrillation. JAMA 239: 43, 1978.

22. Dyckner T, Wester PO: The relation between extra and intracellular electrolytes in patients with hypokalemia and/or diuretic treatment. Acta Med Scand 204: 269, 1978.

23. Dyckner T, Wester PO: Ventricular extrasystoles and intracellular electrolytes in hypokalemic patients before and after correction of the hypokalemia. Acta Med Scand 204: 375, 1978.

24. Dyckner T, Wester PO: Ventricular extrasystoles and intracellular electrolytes before and after potassium and magnesium infusions in patients on diuretic treatment. Am Heart J 97: 12, 1979.

25. Dyckner T, Wester PO: Magnesium deficiency contributing to ventricular tachycardia. Acta Med Scand 212: 89, 1982.

26. Follis RH Jr: Effect of exercise on rats fed a diet deficient in potassium. Proc Soc Exper Biol Med 51: 71, 1942.

27. Fourman P, McCance RA, Parker RA: Chronic renal disease in rats following a temporary deficiency of potassium. Br J Exp Pathol 37: 40, 1955.

28. Friedman M, Freed SC, Rosenman RH: Effect of potassium administration on (1) peripheral vascular reactivity and (2) blood pressure of the potassium-deficient rat. Circulation 5: 415, 1952.

29. Fuhrman FA: Glycogen, glucose tolerance and tissue metabolism in potassium-deficient rats. Am J Physiol 167: 314, 1951.

30. Fukuchi S, Hanata M, Takahashi H, et al: The relationship between vascular reacitvity and extracellular potassium. Tohuku J Exp Med 85: 181, 1965.

31. Gardner LI, Talbot NB, Cook CD, et al: The effect of potassium deficiency on carbohydrate metabolism. J Lab Clin Med 35: 592, 1950.

32. Gifford RW: A guide to the practical use of diuretics. JAMA 235: 1890, 1976.

33. Glaser GH, Stark L: Excitability in experimental myopathy. Neurology 8: 708, 1958.

34. Goldner MG, Zarowitz H, Akgun S: Hyperglycemia and glycosuria due to thiazide derivatives administered in diabetes mellitus. N Engl J Med 262: 403, 1960.

35. Gunning JF, Harrison CE Jr, Coleman HN III: The effects of chronic potassium deficiency on myocardial contractility and oxygen consumption. J Mol Cell Cardiol 4: 139, 1972.

36. Harrington JT, Isner JM, Kassirer JP: Our national obsession with potassium. Am J Med 73: 155, 1982.

37. Harrison CE Jr, Novak LP, Connelly DC, et al: Adenosinetriphosphatase activity of cellular organelles in experimental potassium depletion cardiomyopathy. J Lab Clin Med 75: 185, 1970.

38. Harrison CE Jr, Cooper G, IV, Zujko KJ, et al: Myocardial and mitochondrial function in potassium depletion cardiomyopathy. J Mol Cell Cardiol 4: 633, 1972.

39. Hastings AB, Buchanan JM: The role of intracellular cations on liver glycogen formation in vitro. Proc Nat Acad Sci 28: 478, 1942.

40. Helderman JH, Elahi D, Andersen DK, et al: Prevention of the glucose intolerance of thiazide diuretics by maintenance of body potassium. Diabetes 32: 106, 1983.

41. Hiatt N, Davidson MB, Chapman LW, et al: Epinephrine enhancement of potassium-stimulated immunoreactive insulin secretion. Diabetes 27: 550, 1977.

42. Holland OB, Nixon JV, Kuhnert L: Diuretic-induced ventricular ectopic activity. Am J Med 70: 762, 1981.

43. Hollifield JW, Slaton PE: Thiazide diuretics, hypokalemia and cardiac arrhythmias. Acta Med Scand Suppl 647: 67, 1981.

44. Hulting J: In-hospital ventricular fibrillation and its relation to serum potassium. Acta Med Scand Suppl 647: 109, 1981.

45. Iacobellis M, Muntwyler E, Griffin GE: Kidney glutaminase and carbonic anhydrase activity and tissue electrolyte composition in potassium-deficient dogs. Am J Physiol 183: 395, 1955.

46. Iseri LT, Freed J, Bures AR: Magnesium deficiency and cardiac disorders. Am J Med 58: 837, 1975.

47. Kassirer JP, Harrington JT: Diuretics and potassium metabolism: A reassessment of the need, effectiveness and safety of potassium therapy. Kidney Int 11: 505, 1977.

48. Keye JD Jr: Death in potassium deficiency: Report of a case including morphologic findings. Circulation 5: 766, 1952.

49. Knochel JP, Foley FD Jr; & Lipscomb K: High resting cardiac output with exercise-induced pulmonary edema in the conscious, potassium-deficient dog. Mineral Electrolyte Metab 1: 336, 1978.

50. Knochel JP, Schlein EM: On the mechanism of rhabdomyolysis in potassium depletion. J Clin Invest 51: 1750, 1972.

51. Lardy HA, Ziegler JA: The enzymatic synthesis of phosphopyruvate from pyruvate. J Biol Chem 159: 343, 1945.

52. Leaf A, Santos RF: Physiologic mechanisms in potassium deficiency. N Eng J Med 264: 335, 1961.

53. Levine SR, Crowley TJ, Hai HA: Hypomagnesemia and ventricular tachycardia. Chest 81: 244, 1982.

54. Lown B, Calvert AF, Armington R, et al: V. Monitoring for serious arrhythmias: Monitoring for serious arrhythmias and high risk of sudden death. Circulation [Suppl III] 51 & 52: 189, 1975.

55. MacPherson CR: Myocardial necrosis in the potassium-depleted rat: A reassessment. Br J Exp Pathol 37: 279, 1956.

56. The Management Committee: The Australian therapeutic trial in mild hypertension. Lancet 1: 1261, 1980.

57. McAllen PM: Myocardial changes occurring in potassium deficiency. Br Heart J 17: 5, 1955.

58. Multiple Risk Factor Intervention Trial Research Group: Multiple risk factor intervention trial: Risk factor changes and mortality results. JAMA 248: 1465, 1982.

59. Muntz JA: Effect of ions on the activity of enzymes derived from cardiac tissue. Ann NY Acad Sci 72: 415, 1959.

60. Murphy MB, Lewis PJ, Kohner E, et al: Glucose intolerance in hypertensive patients treated with diuretics; a fourteen-year follow-up. Lancet 2: 1293, 1982.

61. Nachmansohn D, John HM: Studies on choline acetylase: Effects of amino acids on the dialyzed enzyme. Inhibition by α-Keto acids. J Biol Chem 158: 157, 1945.

62. Nordrehaug JE: Malignant arrhythmias in relation to serum potassium values in patients with an acute myocardial infarction. Acta Med Scand Suppl 647: 101, 1981.

63. Papademetriou V, Khatri I, Freis ED: Cardiac arrhythmias in diuretic induced hypokalemia (abstr). Am J Cardiol 49:924, 1982.

64. Perkins JG, Petersen AB, Riley JA: Renal and cardiac lesions in potassium deficiency due to chronic diarrhea. Am J Med 8: 115, 1950.

65. Perera GA: Depressor effects of potassium-deficient diets in hypertensive man. J Clin Invest 32: 633, 1953.

66. Rao SK: The arrhythmic danger of hypokalemia. Med Res Opin Suppl 1 7: 83, 1981.

67. Rapoport MI, Hurd HF: Thiazide-induced glucose intolerance treated with potassium. Arch Intern Med 113: 405, 1964.

68. Relman AS, Schwartz WB: The nephropathy of potassium depletion. N Engl J Med 255: 195, 1956.

69. Relman AS, Schwartz WB: The kidney in potassium depletion. Am J Med 24: 764, 1958.

70. Saglid U, Andersen V, Andreasen PB: Glucose tolerance and insulin responsiveness in experimental potassium depletion. Acta Med Scand 169: 243, 1961.

71. Schwartz WB, Levine HD, Relman AS: The electrocardiogram in potassium depletion. Am J Med 16: 394, 1954.

72. Shapiro AP, Benedek TG, Small JL: Effect of thiazides on carbohydrate metabolism in patients with hypertension. N Eng J Med 265: 1028, 1961.

73. Sheehan J, White, A: Diuretic-associated hypomagnesaemia. Br Med J 285: 1157, 1982.

74. Skrabal F, Auböck J, Hörtnagl H: Low sodium/high potassium diet for prevention of hypertension: Probable mechanisms of action. Lancet 2: 895, 1981.

75. Smith WO, Kyriakopoulos AA, Hammarsten JF: Magnesium depletion induced by various diuretics. Oklahoma State Med Assoc J 55: 248, 1962.

76. Solomon RJ, Cole AG: Importance of potassium in patients with acute myocardial infarction. Acta Med Scand Suppl 647: 87, 1981.

77. Spergel G, Bleicher SJ, Goldberg M, et al: The effect of potassium on the impaired

glucose tolerance in chronic uremia. Metabolism 16: 581, 1967.

78. Spergel G, Schmidt P, Stern A, et al: Effects of hypokalemia on carbohydrate and lipid metabolism in the rat. Diabetes 16: 312, 1967.

79. Sullivan JM, Dluhy RG, Wacker WEC, et al: Interrelationships among thiazide diuretics and calcium, magnesium, sodium, and potassium balance in normal and hypertensive man. J Clin Pharmacol 18: 530, 1978.

80. Weaver WF, Burchell HB: Serum potassium and the electrocardiogram in hypokalemia. Circulation 21: 505, 1960.

81. Welt LG, Hollander W Jr, Blythe WB: The consequences of potassium depletion. J Chronic Dis 11: 213, 1960.

82. Whang R, Welt, LG: Observations in ex-perimental magnesium depletion. J Clin Invest 42: 305, 1963.

83. Whang R, Morosi HJ, Rodgers D, et al: The influence of sustained magnesium deficiency on muscle potassium repletion. J Lab Clin Med 70: 895, 1967.

84. Whelton PK, Brennan P, Miall WE, et al: Thiazide induced arrhythmias. Clin Res 30: 341A, 1982.

85. Wilkinson PR, Issler H, Hesp R, et al: Total body and serum potassium during prolonged thiazide therapy for essential hypertension. Lancet 1:759, 1975.

86. Woods JW, Welt LG, Hollander W Jr, et al: Susceptibility to experimental pyelonephritis during and after potassium depletion. J Clin Invest 38: 1056, 1959.

# 10

# Alkali Therapy of the Organic Acidoses: A Critical Assessment of the Data and the Case for Judicious Use of Sodium Bicarbonate

Robert G. Narins, M.D.
Edward R. Jones, M.D.
Leslie P. Dornfeld, M.D.

## INTRODUCTORY PRINCIPLES AND STATEMENT OF THE ARGUMENT

When metabolic acids are added to body fluids at rates which exceed their removal, fixed acids accumulate causing predictable changes in serum electrolytes and acid-base parameters.[33] Except for the most severe degrees of acidosis, each mEq/L increment in the serum acid anion concentration, reduces the serum bicarbonate concentration by a like amount.[38]

The rate and efficiency with which lost bicarbonate is replenished is vitally dependent upon the character of accumulated acid anion and upon the presence of normally functioning kidneys (Table 10-1). Any combination of the following three processes may be utilized to reestablish body bicarbonate stores.

### Metabolic Conversion of Organic Anions to Bicarbonate

The following equations illustrate the steps involved in the oxidative metabolism of sodium lactate to bicarbonate.

(1) $H_3C-COH_2-COO^-Na^+ + 3O_2 \rightarrow 3CO_2 + 2H_2O + NaOH$
(2) $CO_2 + H_2O \leftrightarrow H_2CO_3$
(3) $H_2CO_3 + NaOH \rightarrow NaHCO_3 + H_2O$

---

Sum: Sodium Lactate $+ 3O_2 \rightarrow 2CO_2 + 2H_2O + NaHCO_3$

Lactate serves as the prototype for such commonly encountered organic acid anions as β-hydroxybutyrate, acetoacetate and citrate, which under normal conditions, are all very rapidly metabolized to bicarbonate. Indeed, infusion of 50 to 100 mEq/hr of sodium lactate is so briskly consumed that serum levels rise by less than 0.5 mEq/L.[47] Administration of insulin to diabetics in ketoacidosis or normalization of tissue perfusion in lactic acidosis allows for rapid oxidation of accumulated organic acid anions and metabolic resynthesis of titrated bicarbonate. Thus, to the extent that all organic anions produced during acidosis are retained and then metabolized, all titrated bicarbonate ought to be rapidly restored. Urinary loss of organic anions, that is, ketonuria or lactaturia, deprives the subject of "potential alkali," and thereby limits the host's capacity to metabolically replace all lost bicarbonate.

This metabolic process, of course, is not available in the inorganic acidoses. The hydrochloric acidosis complicating such disorders as diarrhea, adrenal insufficiency, and interstitial nephritis replaces bicarbonate with the nonmetabolizable chloride anion. Normalization of bicarbonate stores in this setting is vitally dependent upon renal synthesis and exogenous administration.

## Renal Resynthesis

The ability of renal tubular epithelia to generate $H_2CO_3$ by hydrating neutral $CO_2$ and then to separate and transport in opposite directions the acid's ionic moieties ($H^+$ and $HCO_3^-$) forms the basis for the renal regulation of serum bicarbonate concentration (Fig. 10-1). Protons derived from $H_2CO_3$ are secreted into the distal tubular lumen in exchange for filtered sodium which, in turn, enters peritubular capillaries along with $HCO_3^-$ anions derived from cellular $H_2CO_3$.

Thus, the epithelial process of luminal $H^+$, $Na^+$ exchange at once acidifies the glomerular filtrate while the contraluminal egress of $NaHCO_3$ alkalinizes blood. If the source of luminal sodium derives from filtered acid salts (e.g., sodium acetoacetate, the organic acid salt formed when acetoacetic acid titrates sodium bicarbonate, or sodium chloride, the inorganic acid salt formed when the base neutralizes hydrochloric acid) the sodium reabsorption and simultaneous $H^+$ secretion reforms the acid in the tubular lumen. Cellular bicarbonate is returned with reabsorbed sodium to the systemic circulation via the renal venous effluent. This reformed luminal acid is titrated or "absorbed" by renal $NH_3$ buffer and excreted as $NH_4$ acetoacetate or $NH_4Cl$. In this manner, each millimole of acid excreted is matched by a millimole of bicarbonate returned to the systemic circulation. In the organic acidoses, renal alkali synthesis summates with that bicarbonate generated metabolically, but in the inorganic acidoses, the only endogenous source of alkali derives from the kidneys. It should be noted that the kidneys take hours to days to replenish depleted bicarbonate stores making this process decidedly slower than metabolic alkali synthesis.

## Exogenous Alkali

The direct infusion or ingestion of $NaHCO_3$ will, of course, restore serum bicarbonate concentrations to normal. Such organic acid salts as sodium lactate, citrate, or acetate are alkalinizing only by consequence of their oxidative conversion to bicarbonate. The pK's of the acids from which these salts are derived are so low as to render the salts intrinsically ineffective as buffers at physiologic pH's.

As depicted in Table 10-1, the character of the acidosis dictates the means and rate by which hypobicarbonatemia may

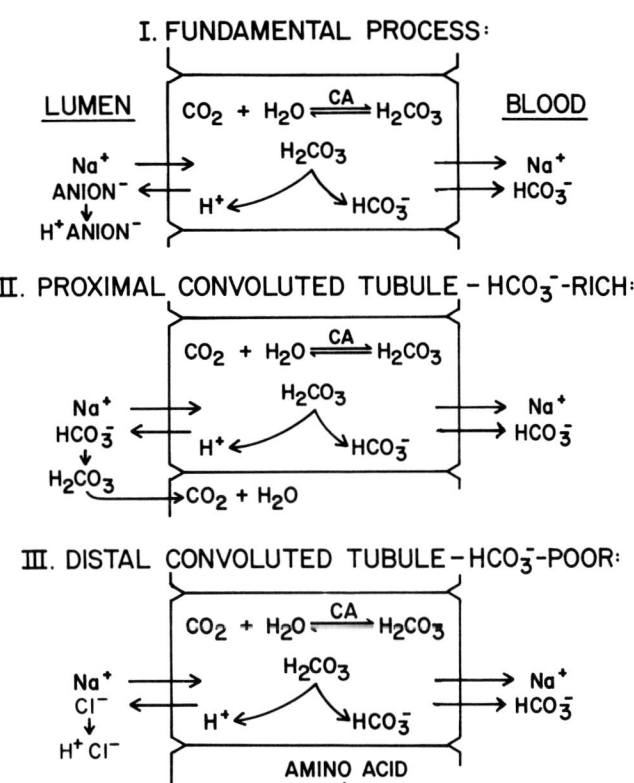

**Fig. 10-1.** Renal bicarbonate reabsorption and synthesis: Top panel: Fundamental process involved in both reabsorption and synthesis entails hydration of $CO_2$ with subsequent formation of $H^+$ and $HCO_3^-$ from the $H_2CO_3$. Luminal $Na^+/H^+$ exchange and peritubular transfer of $NaHCO_3$ completes the process. Middle Panel: $H^+$ secreted into $HCO_3^-$ rich proximal lumen allows for the depicted reabsorption of filtered $NaHCO_3$. Bottom panel: Secretion of $H^+$ into $HCO_3^-$ poor distal tubular lumen allows for acid excretion along with titrated $NH_3$ buffer and net addition of $HCO_3^-$ to blood. Abbreviation: CA: Carbonic anhydrase.

be normalized. Organic acidoses may utilize all three restorative options, whereas inorganic acidoses are restricted to renal synthesis and exogenous alkali for replenishing bicarbonate losses. When inorganic acidosis complicates acute or chronic renal failure, serum bicarbonate concentration will remain frozen at low levels unless exogenous alkali is administered. The need for alkali therapy in severe inorganic acidosis, especially when complicated by varying degrees of renal failure, is now generally accepted. Debate continues to rage, however, over the advisability of such therapy for the organic acidoses. There are those who argue that once the precipitating defect is nullified, that is, when insulin is administered to a diabetic in ketoacidosis or hypoxia or hypotension is corrected in certain forms of lactic acidosis, the metabolic and renal regeneration of bicarbonate will normalize serum

levels without need for exogenous alkali. Indeed, they go on to say that alkali therapy brings with it a number of untoward effects that invests the treatment with more lethality than is manifested by the disease for which it is being given.

Advocates of alkali therapy, however, dismiss discussions of untoward effects as unproven funereal maunderings which ring trivial in comparison to the life-threatening hemodynamic and metabolic effects of severe acidosis. The remainder of this chapter presents a critical review of the pros and cons (Table 10-2) of alkali therapy of organic acidosis using ketoacidosis and lactic acidosis as prototypical forms. In our view, the available data, on balance, favor the judicious use of alkali in severe organic metabolic acidosis. The arguments marshalled against bicarbonate therapy, we believe, are generally based on misconceptions, distortions

**Table 10-1.** Means of Replenishing Depleted Bicarbonate Stores in the Metabolic Acidoses

| Forms of Metabolic Acidosis | Metabolic $Ket^- \to HCO_3^-$ Rate: Rapid (mins– hrs.) | Renal $HCO_3^- \to$ Blood $H^+ \to$ Urine Rate: Slow (hrs– days) | Exogenous Infuse, Ingest $NaHCO_3$ Rate: Variable |
|---|---|---|---|
| Organic Acidoses $H^+Ket^- + Na^+HCO_3^- \to$ $Na^+Ket^- + CO_2 + H_2O$ | + | + | + |
| Inorganic acidoses $H^+Cl^- + Na^+HCO_3^- \to$ $Na^+Cl^- + CO_2 + H_2O$ | 0 | + | + |
| Inorganic acidoses plus renal failure | 0 | 0 | + |

of experimental studies, and flimsy bridges of faith constructed to prematurely apply experimental observations to the care of desperately ill patients.

# ARGUMENTS AGAINST THE USE OF BICARBONATE

## Salt and Water Overload

It has been argued that parenteral administration of sodium bicarbonate puts patients at risk of extracellular fluid (ECF) overload. This point is, of course, invalid in diabetic ketoacidosis (DKA) where ongoing glycosuria and ketonuria cause net losses of sodium and potassium to approximate 8 and 6 mEq/kg, respectively, and losses of body water to approach 75 to 100 ml/kg.[11,15,30] Replenishing a portion of lost sodium with bicarbonate can hardly be viewed as "salt and water overload."

It is true, however, that very large quantities of sodium bicarbonate may be needed to treat some patients with lactic acidosis and in this setting the risk of pathologically expanding the ECF space is real. Combining the use of potent diuretics with administered alkali usually is effective in preventing excessive retention of salt. Parenteral sodium bicarbonate may be infused at rates equal to diuretic-induced sodium chloride losses. In this manner, body sodium content remains constant while infused bicarbonate re-

**Table 10-2.** The Pros and Cons for Alkali Therapy of Organic Acidosis

| Cons | Pros |
|---|---|
| Sodium bicarbonate causes salt and water overload | When chloride replaces organic anions, $NaHCO_3$ therapy becomes more important. |
| Overshoot alkalosis develops in the reparative stage of acidosis | |
| Alkali therapy worsens hypokalemia | Alkali therapy reverses the harmful cardiovascular effects of acidosis |
| Hypercapnia is caused by administered bicarbonate | |
| CSF acidosis is precipitated by parenteral alkali | Sensitivity of blood pH to small absolute changes in $PCO_2$ and $HCO_3$ puts severely acidotic patients in great jeopardy |
| Tissue hypoxia indirectly results from administered alkali | |
| Alkali therapy paradoxically stimulates endogenous organic acid production. | |

places excreted chloride. Peritoneal or hemodialysis may be required for patients in whom renal failure precludes use of diuretics.

## Overshoot Alkalosis

In the reparative phase of metabolic acidosis it is very common for blood pH to more rapidly normalize than $HCO_3$ concentration or $PCO_2$. During therapy, the stimulation of respiration, initially provoked by metabolic acidosis, persists for hours despite a rising plasma bicarbonate concentration (Table 10-3). This disproportionate elevation of bicarbonate causes the $PCO_2/HCO_3$ ratio to decrease, thereby reducing the hydrogen ion concentration.[41,53] The injudicious administration of large amounts of $NaHCO_3$ can exaggerate this phenomenon.

During the repair of organic acidosis, serum bicarbonate concentration increases as accumulated acid anions are oxidized. Serum bicarbonate concentration therefore, will be determined by the summation of metabolically generated alkali and that given parenterally. Resulting hyperbicarbonatemia and persisting hypocapnia may combine to produce severe alkalemia. Use of 100 to 250 mEq of $NaHCO_3$ rarely provokes significant overshoot alkalosis.

## Hypokalemia

Derangements of internal and external potassium balance complicate organic acidoses and their therapy. The ECF contraction caused by the glycosuric-osmotic diuresis in DKA activates the renin-angiotensin-aldosterone cascade, which in turn provokes a striking kaliuresis. Continued polyuria, independent of mineralocorticoid secretion, will also stimulate renal potassium losses.[54] Indeed, it has been estimated that patients with DKA suffer a 5 to 10 mEq/kg body weight deficit of potassium.[11,15,30]

Hyperkalemia is more likely to complicate an inorganic rather than an organic acidosis, whereas hypokalemia complicates the reparative phase of each form of metabolic acidosis. Intracellular buffers absorb a major portion of an imposed acid load. In inorganic acidosis the transmembrane potential difference is reduced by consequence of the positive charge brought into cells by entering protons. Restriction of inorganic anions (e.g., $Cl^-$) to the extracellular space, by consequence of their relative impermeance to cell membranes, enhances extracellular negativity. This disruption of the normal transmembrane charge favors the passive egress of potassium from the cell into the ECF. Since organic anions (lactate, ketones) are more permeable to cells, the transcellular electrical gradient is not altered and maldistribution of potassium is not enhanced. Thus, for a given degree of acidemia, infusions of HCl are more likely to cause hyperkalemia than are infusions of lactic or ketoacids.[39]

With therapy of metabolic acidosis, alkalinization of the ECF enhances the intracellular movement of potassium. This redistribution is, of course, enhanced by insulin treatment in DKA.

While it is true that exogenous alkali in conjunction with reparative endogenous bicarbonate generation enhances the tendency to hypokalemia, use of judicious amounts of $NaHCO_3$ exerts little effect on serum potassium concentration (Table 10-4). When an average of 200 mEq of $NaHCO_3$ was given over a 24 hr period to 11 patients with severe DKA, external and internal potassium balance did not differ from that of 7 patients given saline without alkali.[48] Use of 400 mEq of $NaHCO_3$ during the first day's therapy, clearly enhanced the intracellular transfer of potassium, necessitating infusion of more KCl to maintain normokalemia.[48]

There is no substitute for carefully monitoring serum electrolyte and acid-

**Table 10-3.** Components of Overshoot Alkalosis

| Study Parameters | | Normal | Diabetic Ketoacidosis | | |
|---|---|---|---|---|---|
| | | | Initial | NaHCO$_3$ Therapy | Metabolic Oxid. of Ketones |
| Na | (mEq/L) | 140 | 140 | 145 | 145 |
| Cl | (mEq/L) | 105 | 105 | 100 | 105 |
| HCO$_3$ | (mEq/L) | 25 | 5 | 15 | 30 |
| Anion Gap (mEq/L) | | 10 | 30 | 30 | 10 |
| PCO$_2$ (mm Hg) | | 40 | 16 | 27 | 34 |
| pH | | 7.40 | 7.11 | 7.37 | 7.57 |

base parameters during therapy of any severe acidosis. Physicians knowledgeable of the pathophysiologic forces affecting potassium balance in the organic acidoses, should be able to sustain normokalemia despite insulin therapy and a rising serum bicarbonate concentration. Potassium infusions can easily be adjusted to keep pace with ongoing urinary losses and with intracellular shifts. With reasonable vigilance, there is no persuasive evidence to show that addition of 150 to 250 mEq of NaHCO$_3$ prevents maintainance of normokalemia in the organic acidoses.

## Bicarbonate-Induced Hypercapnia

It has been argued, with some justification, that bicarbonate therapy of metabolic acidosis in patients with advanced acute or chronic lung disease, may worsen preexisting hypercapnia. The CO$_2$ produced when infused bicarbonate combines with hydrogen ions, is cleared by normal lungs, but may be retained in the presence of pulmonary disease. Patients with stable, steady state hypercapnia excrete their normal minute-to-minute CO$_2$ production but to accomplish this, they require an elevated PCO$_2$. In terms of the nephrologist, their pulmonary "clearance" of CO$_2$ is diminished. Just as the addition of extra urea to the blood of patients with stable, steady-state renal failure transiently increases the BUN, so should the addition of CO$_2$ (derived from administered bicarbonate) only transiently increase arterial PCO$_2$, in steady state pulmonary disease.

The rapidity with which HCO$_3$-derived CO$_2$ is excreted has not been well

**Table 10-4.** Effect of Administered NaHCO$_3$ on Potassium Balance during the First 24 Hours of Therapy of DKA

| Group | Mean Administered Dose | | | Potassium | | |
|---|---|---|---|---|---|---|
| | Insulin (units) | Sodium (mEq) | Bicarbonate (mEq) | Infused[b] (mEq) | Excreted (mEq) | Retained (mEq) |
| Saline[a] (7) | 234 | 856 | 0 | 238 | 135 | 103 |
| Alkali | | | | | | |
| Low Dose (11) | 287 | 826 | 200 | 225 | 136 | 89 |
| High Dose (7) | 288 | 731 | 400 | 343 | 153 | 190 |

(From Soler NG, Dixon K, Bennett MA, et al: Potassium balance during treatment of diabetic ketoacidosis:with special reference to the use of bicarbonate. Lancet 2:665, 1972.)
[a]Number of patients indicated by parentheses.
[b]Amount required to maintain normal serum K$^+$.

studied, but the results of two experiments are informative. Bishop et al. rapidly administered 1 mEq/kg of $NaHCO_3$ to intubated dogs being ventilated at fixed minute volumes.[12] Within 15 seconds of receiving the bolus of alkali, arterial $PCO_2$ rose to $49 \pm 10$ mm Hg from control values of $27 \pm 7$ mm Hg, but within 10 minutes had fallen to $37 \pm 6$ mm Hg.[8] Adrogué et al. infused over 10 minutes, 5 mmol/kg of $NaHCO_3$ to dogs made chronically hypercapnic by exposure to high $PCO_2$ atmospheres in an environmental chamber.[2] No detectable change in arterial $PCO_2$ ($70 \pm 2.8$ mm Hg) was noted by 30 minutes after infusion. A number of additional studies have evaluated the effects of large loads of $NaHCO_3$ on $PCO_2$ in infants with respiratory distress syndromes.[17,24,49] Hubel et al. found that $PCO_2$ was not significantly increased despite parenteral administration of 5 to 8 mEq/kg/24 hrs of $NaHCO_3$ to infants with this disorder.[24] Other authors using similar loads of alkali reported mild (10 to 15 percent) to severe (20 to 30 percent) increments in $PCO_2$.[17,49] These data are difficult to interpret since it was not made clear that the patients had steady-state hypercapnia and the administration of alkali at once generated $CO_2$ but also raised systemic pH, which in turn may have decreased ventilation.

Thus, in that small population of patients with mixed metabolic and respiratory acidosis, bicarbonate therapy is likely to transiently elevate $PCO_2$ without changing arterial pH. Since $CO_2$ is more penetrable of cells than is bicarbonate, this short-lived increment in $PCO_2$ may also cause a short-lived fall in intracellular pH. Therapy of mixed acid-base disorders is predicated upon simultaneously ministering to each of the primary disorders.[33] The presence of hypercapnia in the face of hypobicarbonatemia is often associated with profound acidemia and is an indication for supporting respiration, that is, re-

moving the cause of hypoventilation or initiating mechanical ventilation. Thus, the practice of good medicine dictates that in this mixed acid-base disorder, therapy be applied simultaneously to the pulmonary and to the metabolic disorders. Improved gas exchange ought to prevent bicarbonate-induced hypercapnia.

## Cerebrospinal Fluid Acidosis

It has long been known that systemic and CSF pHs change concordantly during development and treatment of respiratory acid-base disorders.[43] Discordant changes, however, are noted during the inception of acute metabolic acidosis and when alkali therapy is given in treatment of chronic metabolic acidosis.[43] These observations are best understood in light of two facts: (1) $CO_2$ easily penetrates the blood-brain barrier, allowing systemic hypercapnia and hypocapnia to almost instantaneously change the CSF $PCO_2$. Thus, systemic and CSF pH's rapidly fall in respiratory acidosis and rapidly rise in respiratory alkalosis; (2) bicarbonate crosses the blood-brain barrier with difficulty, indeed it takes hours to days for systemic-CSF equilibration to occur. Thus, the earliest phase of acute metabolic acidosis is associated with systemic hypobicarbonatemia but an unchanged CSF bicarbonate concentration. Systemic acidification stimulates ventilation by triggering those chemoreceptors in direct contact with blood and those communicating with the interstitial fluid of the brain.[16] The systemic hypocapnia resulting from stimulated respiration quickly lowers CSF $PCO_2$ thereby lowering the $PCO_2/HCO_3$ ratio, causing alkalinization of the CSF. Thus, acute metabolic acidosis simultaneously acidifies blood, and interstitial fluid (brain and peripheral) while paradoxically alkalinizing CSF.[19] In time, CSF bicarbonate concentration falls and pH either normalizes or acidifies.[18]

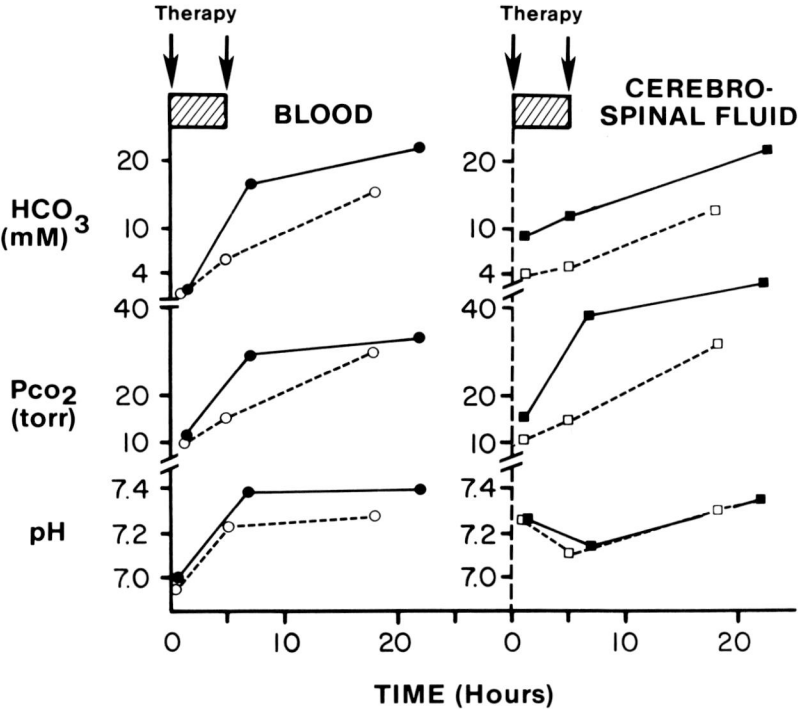

**Fig. 10-2.** Effect of systemic alkali therapy on CSF acidity in DKA. Arterial blood and CSF were simultaneously sampled at the indicated times. Therapy: Patient 1 (°⋯°) received 180 mmol NaHCO₃ and 300 units of regular insulin and Patient 2 (°—°) received 123 mmols of NaHCO₃ and 300 units ot regular insulin. (Reprinted, by permission of the New England Journal of Medicine, from Posner JB, Plum F: Spinal fluid pH and neurologic symptoms in systemic acidosis. N Engl J Med 277:605, 1967.)

During the reparative phase of metabolic acidosis, blood and interstitial bicarbonate concentrations rise more briskly than that in the CSF. The diminution of alveolar ventilation consequent to the rising plasma bicarbonate concentration, allows blood and CSF $PCO_2$ to increase equivalently. Thus, in this early stage of repair, blood and interstitial pH are increasing while the greater increment in $PCO_2$ than in bicarbonate, lowers CSF pH. This paradoxical acidification is neutralized in time as increasing amounts of bicarbonate enter the CSF.

In 1967, Posner and Plum described—among other patients—two diabetics in severe ketoacidosis who received 123 and 180 mEq of NaHCO₃ over ap-

proximately 4 hours (Figure 10-2). Interpreted in the light of our current understanding of blood-CSF acid-base relationships, it is not surprising that acute bicarbonate therapy worsened CSF acidosis while alkalinizing blood. Because both patients exhibited transient neurological deterioration when their CSF pH fell, the authors expressed concern regarding rapid administration of sodium bicarbonate.[44]

The importance of this observation has been distorted by some authors.[23] Evidence indicates that equivalent degrees of CSF acidification occur whether serum bicarbonate is rapidly increased with exogenous alkali or more slowly increased by endogenous metabolism and renal function (Table 10-5).[5,36] Indeed, in these cited studies, despite decreases in CSF pH to values as low as those seen in Posner and Plum's two diabetics, all 15 patients manifested improved CNS function. While paradoxical acidification of the CSF may somehow affect cerebration, it should be remembered that brain interstitial fluid pH during $NaHCO_3$ therapy, is more reflective of blood pH than that of spinal fluid.[16] It is our impression that many physicians have used Posner and Plum's two diabetics who transiently became mildly stuporous as evidence for the malignant effects of alkali therapy. Of the many and profound metabolic changes that accompany DKA, it seems inappropriate to blame CSF acidification for a mild change in cerebration. One would be hard-pressed to find two other patients so superficially studied but who have so profoundly influenced therapy of a life-threatening disease. The following quote from Doctors Posner and Plum indicates that unlike many others, they have no illusions regarding the magnitude of their observation:

> The correction of metabolic acidosis, although raising the serum pH, can paradoxically lower the extracellular pH of the brain. During this period, transient neurologic depression may appear, but this is neither profound nor dangerous and does not outweigh the requirement for prompt correction of serum acidosis.[42]

## Alkali-Induced Tissue Hypoxia

Synthesis of several observations has led to the speculative conclusion that acute alkali therapy of chronic metabolic acidosis could theoretically cause tissue hypoxia.[6] The findings upon which this theory is based include the following: (1) Changes in red blood cell (RBC) pH directly and *rapidly* alter hemoglobin's affin-

**Table 10-5.** CSF pH and Conciousness during Therapy of DKA with and without $NaHCO_3$

| | Effects of Alkali Therapy (n=9)[a] | | | Therapy without Alkali (n=6)[b] | | |
|---|---|---|---|---|---|---|
| | Admission values[c] | | 4 hrs after $NaHCO_3$ (225–400 mEq)[c] | Admission values[c] | | 4 to 9 hrs later (no $NaHCO_3$)[c] |
| Arterial Blood | | | | | | |
| $HCO_3$ (mM)[d] | 5.6 | | 16.0 | 5 | | 12 |
| | 1 | | 2 | 1 | | 2 |
| $PCO_2$ (mm Hg) | 12 | | 21 | 14 | | 23 |
| | 1 | | 1 | 1 | | 3 |
| pH | 7.06 | | 7.41 | 7.09 | | 7.29 |
| | 0.03 | | 0.04 | 0.04 | | 0.03 |
| Spinal fluid | | | | | | |
| $HCO_3$ (mM)[d] | 10 | | 10 | 12 | | 15 |
| | 1 | | 1 | 2 | | 2 |
| $PCO_2$ (mm Hg) | 24 | | 35 | 23 | | 32 |
| | 2 | | 3 | 2 | | 4 |
| pH | 7.27 | Δ pH | 7.15 | 7.35 | Δ pH | 7.27 |
| | 0.01 | $-0.12 \pm 0.05$[e] | 0.03 | 0.03 | $-0.08 \pm 0.02$[e] | 0.05 |
| Level of Conciousness | | Improved | | | | Improved |

[a]Data from Assal J, Aoki TT, Manzano FM, et al: Metabolic effects of sodium bicarbonate in management of diabetic Ketoacidosis Diabetes 23: 405, 1974.

[b]Ohman JL Jr, Marliss EB, Aoki TT, et al: The cerebrospinal fluid in diabetic ketoacidosis. N Engl J Med 284: 283, 1971.

[c]Mean ± SEM indicated.

[d]$HCO_3$ expressed per liter of water (serum value |x|1.07 = value in terms of blood water). Mean ± SEM indicated.

[e]Difference between admission and subsequent pH values. Mean ± SEM.

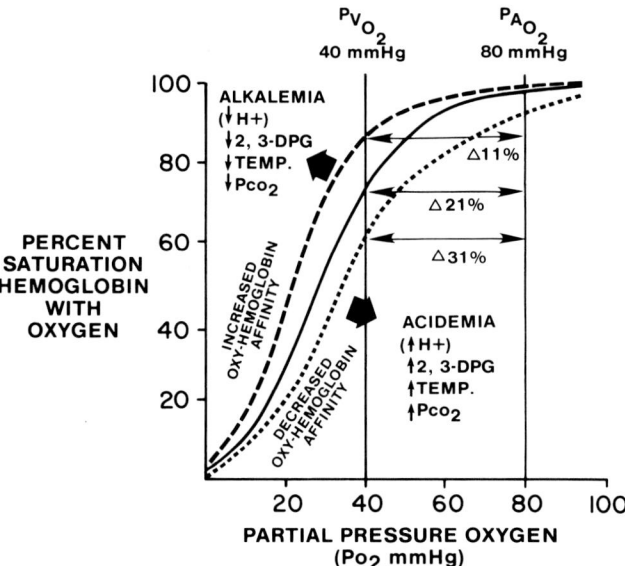

**Fig. 10-3.** Oxy-hemoglobin dissociation curve: The effect of various modifiers of oxy-hemoglobin dissociation on the sigmoid curve relating $PO_2$ to hemoglobin saturation with $O_2$. Modifiers noted in the left upper portion shift the curve to the left (- - -) while those noted on the right shift curve to the right. Passing from an arterial $O_2$ tension of 80 mm Hg ($PaO_2$) to a venous $O_2$ tension of 40 mm Hg ($PvO_2$) normally allows for a 21 percent ($\Delta$21%) desaturation of hemoglobin, whereas acidemia and alkalemia increase and decrease desaturation by 10 percent respectively. See text for details. Abbreviation: 2,3-DPG: 2,3-Diphosphoglyceric acid.

ity for oxygen. This Bohr effect allows for acid pH to diminish and alkaline pH to increase oxyhemoglobin binding (Fig. 10-3).[9] (2) Changes in RBC pH *slowly* alter glycolytic rates; such that acidosis inhibits and alkalosis enhances glycolysis.[27] Since the enzyme which is most sensitive to acid-base changes is phosphofructokinase, and since this regulatable step precedes the formation of 2,3-diphosphoglyceric acid (2,3-DPG) (Fig. 10-4), acidosis eventually decreases and alkalosis eventually increases RBC levels of this phosphorylated intermediate.[27] (3) The effect of 2,3-DPG on hemoglobin affinity for oxygen is similar to that of protons, that is, increased RBC levels (like acid pH) diminish hemoglobin avidity for oxygen while decreased RBC levels (like alkaline pH) enhance hemoglobin avidity for oxygen[13] (Figs. 10-3, 10-4).

Changes in hydrogen ion concentration cause slight alterations in the configuration of the hemoglobin molecule which limits oxygen's accessibility to its binding sites.[50] A decrease in blood pH of 0.1 to 0.2 units allows for an additional 10 percent of bound oxygen to be liberated, whereas a similar increase in pH reduces

oxygen delivery by a like amount (Fig. 10-3). This Bohr effect is rapidly switched on and off, that is, it occurs within minutes of the acid-base perturbation and is sustained in chronic acidosis or alkalosis. Thus, if all else were equal, tissue oxygenation would be enhanced by acute metabolic acidosis and depressed by acute metabolic alkalosis. When the acid-base derangement is sustained beyond 12 to 24 hours, induced changes in RBC glycolysis and 2,3-DPG levels eradicate the pH effects on oxygen binding to hemoglobin. With chronicity of metabolic acidosis, rates of RBC glycolysis are reduced causing 2,3-DPG levels to decrease which, in turn, enhances oxy-hemoglobin association.[16] The presence of these two offsetting chemical changes, that is, acid RBC pH and low RBC levels of 2,3-DPG, cancel each other's effect. Thus, the enhanced tissue oxygenation seen with acute metabolic acidosis is neutralized by the metabolic events attending chronic acidosis.[16]

The argument logically follows that since $NaHCO_3$ therapy can rapidly return RBC pH toward normal—thereby rapidly erasing the Bohr effect—but only slowly

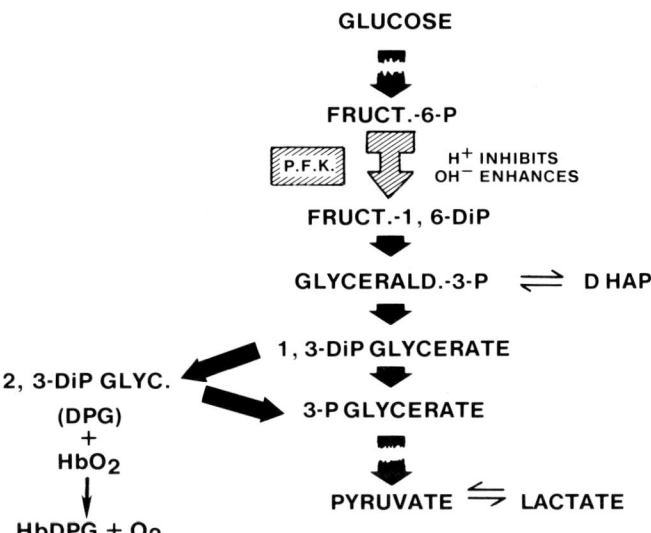

**Fig. 10-4.** Erythrocyte Glycolysis: Simplified diagram of the metabolic conversion of glucose to pyruvate and lactate. See text for details. Abbreviations: DHAP: dihydroxyacetone phosphate; 1,3-Dip glycerate: 1,3-diphosphoglycerate; Fruct-1,6DiP: fructose-1,6-diphosphate; Fruc-6-P: fructose-6-phosphate; glycerald-3-P: glyceraldehyde-3-phosphate; HbO$_2$: oxyhemoglobin; HbDPG: reduced hemoglobin, bound to DPG; PFK: phosphofructokinase; 3-P-glycerate: 3-phosphoglycerate.

replenish depleted RBC stores of 2,3-DPG, hemoglobin affinity for oxygen will be acutely increased. During this transient period when pH improvement precedes 2,3-DPG replenishment, tissue oxygenation may be impaired.[6]

Study of this chemical interplay between RBC protons and phosphorylated intermediates is of great interest and most certainly has sparked our understanding of oxygen transport and delivery. One must, however, be extremely wary of applying these principles to the treatment of DKA before appropriate studies have demonstrated their validity. For reasons outlined below, we believe that premature and excessive importance has been attributed to the potential for alkali therapy of organic acidosis to induce tissue "asphyxia."

The sustained hyperventilation and increased PaO$_2$ associated with DKA (see above) and the enhanced cardiac output consequent to the restoration of ECF volume and pH (see below) should increase tissue oxygen delivery regardless of modest increments in hemoglobin's affinity for oxygen. Importantly, Munk et al. have shown that hemoglobin binding of oxygen during the repair of ketoacidosis is modestly enhanced regardless of whether or not NaHCO$_3$ is administered.[29]

Another fact, yet to be acknowledged by proponents of the alkali-tissue hypoxia theory, is that glycosylated hemoglobin (Hb$_{A1c}$) unlike normal hemoglobin, is barely influenced by changes in RBC 2,3-DPG levels.[10] Bunn and Briehl have shown that the oxygen affinity of Hb$_{A1c}$ is one-fifth as responsive to changes 2,3-DPG levels as normal hemoglobin A.[10] Since 15 to 20 percent of hemoglobin is glycosylated in hyperglycemic diabetics, the alkali-tissue hypoxia theory seems less applicable to the care of DKA.[22]

We recently tested whether acute alkali therapy of chronic acidosis impairs tissue oxygenation.[7] Rats were made chronically acidotic by adding ammonium chloride to their ad lib drinking water for one week. Half the rats were gavage-fed an isotonic solution of NaHCO$_3$ in amounts predetermined to normalize serum bicarbonate concentration and pH and then strenuously exercised for 5 minutes. The other group of chronically acidotic rats received equal volumes of NaCl prior to treadmill exercise. One would predict that exercise-induced lactic acidosis would be worsened by acute alkali therapy were it to induce tissue hypoxia. Indeed, both groups performed equally well and postexercise blood lactate levels were virtually identical.[7] These data suggest that acute correction of chronic acidosis does not significantly compromise tissue oxygenation.

Thus, although theoretical arguments can be developed suggesting that alkali therapy may impair tissue oxygen delivery, evidence supporting its clinical significance is flimsy at best. For reasons outlined above, we disagree with those who argue for limited use of alkali in severe ketosis for fear of inducing tissue hypoxia.

### Alkali Stimulation of Endogenous Organic Acid Production

The question of whether a negative feedback relationship exists between acid-base parameters in the ECF and endogenous organic acid synthesis was recently addressed by Hood et al.[25] Fasting obese subjects were given 2 mmol/kg of either NaCl, NaHCO$_3$, or NH$_4$Cl over one week to determine whether alkali therapy stimulated and acid therapy inhibited fasting ketone acid production. Predictably, alkali and acid therapy caused slight degrees of hyperbicarbonatemia and hypobicarbonatemia, respectively. Daily net ketoacid production was strikingly increased in those ingesting alkali and decreased in subjects receiving acid, suggesting that a servo-mechanism indeed exists between net acid-synthesis and some function of acid-base balance (Fig. 10-5). The mechanism whereby the ketogenesis "recognizes" the acid or alkaline load has yet to be defined. Alkali loading could enhance net ketone synthesis by stimulating free fatty acid mobilization and its hepatic conversion to ketoacids and/or inhibiting the extrahepatic catabolism of the acid anions.

The interpretation of this interesting observation is problematic. Those interpreting it broadly could argue that NaHCO$_3$ is contraindicated in treating ketoacidosis since its use in fasting ketosis stimulates production of the offending acid. In our view this would be a most inappropriate application of these findings. Therapy of severe DKA includes use of *insulin* along with appropriate amounts of bicarbonate. Insulin suppresses free fatty acid mobilization and conversion to ketones in the liver while simultaneously enhancing extrahepatic ketone oxidation.[12] These advantageous effects of insulin more than outweigh any mild disadvantageous ketogenic effects that alkali therapy may have.

Along similar lines, Fields et al. and Fraley et al. have recently demonstrated that parenteral administration of even massive amounts of alkali does not easily increase serum bicarbonate concentration in patients with cancer-associated chronic lactic acidosis.[20,21] Both studies demonstrate a direct stoichiometric relationship between the alkali infused and the acid produced, presumably by the tumor.[20,21] Although the mechanism whereby NaHCO$_3$ therapy stimulated lactic acid synthesis was not clearly demonstrated, a small rise in blood pH may have stimulated tumor glycolysis (see above).

While the ability of exogenous alkali to ameliorate the hypobicarbonatemia of many forms of lactic acidosis is well documented,[14] there is good reason not to give massive doses of NaHCO$_3$. Assuming that the increased net lactic acid production stimulated by alkali therapy reflects increased tumor biosynthesis, then, as Field et al. point out, lactate must be coming from amino acid and glucose precursors.[20] To the extent that patients with cancer-associated chronic lactic acidosis are already malnourished, stimulation by bicarbonate of the tumor's parasitic consumption of important substrates, could prove disastrous. We would agree that

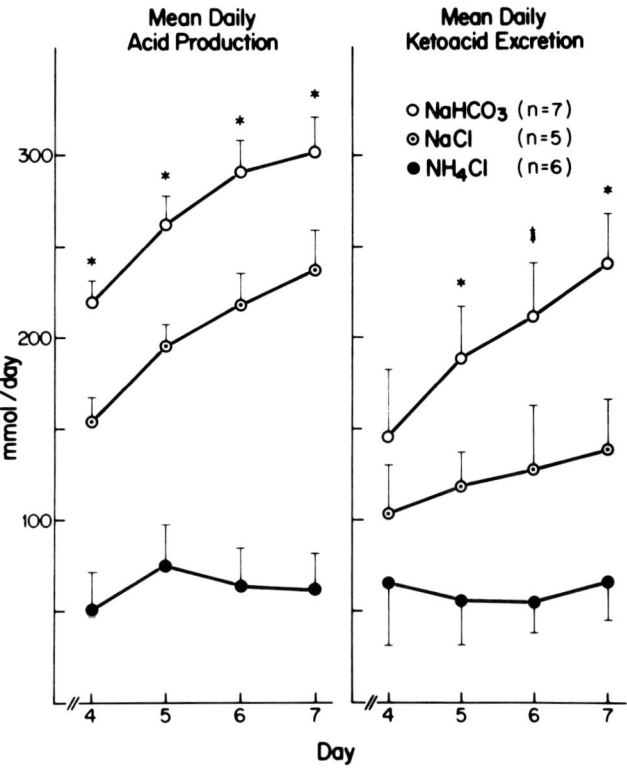

**Fig. 10-5.** Effect of acidosis and alkalosis on total daily acid production and ketoacid excretion during fasting. Subjects fasted for seven days. Alkali, salt, and acid given as 2 mmols kg daily. *p<0.001; ‡, p<0.005. (From: Hood VL, Danforth E Jr., Horton, ES, & Tannen RL: Impact of hydrogen ion on fasting ketogenesis: Feedback regulation of acid production. Am J Physiol 242:F238, 1982).

the dose of bicarbonate chosen ought to be the smallest amount that effects the highest achievable serum bicarbonate concentration. This dose can only be defined by trial.

Experimental lactic acidosis induced by intravenous phenformin (phenethylbiguanide) following surgical pancreatectomy, is not improved by NaHCO$_3$ therapy.[4] Indeed, liver and RBC pH, portal vein blood flow and cardiac output are worsened by NaHCO$_3$ as compared to therapy with equimolar amounts of NaCl.[4] The meaning of this observation is not entirely clear to us. Intravenous phenformin is a myocardial toxin and it may well be that alkali therapy enhances the drug's accessibility to myocardial cells or somehow sensitizes the heart to the drug's noxious action.[3,32] Indeed, phenformin is a weak base and if bicarbonate therapy alkalinized the urine, drug clearance may be impaired exposing the heart

to a greater dose. In any case, this experimental disorder may have little to do with lactic acidosis as it occurs in humans.

Dichloroacetate (DCA) enhances the oxidation of lactate and in a true sense, serves the patient suffering lactic acidosis in a manner analogous to insulin's role in DKA. Results from a recent study showing that dogs with experimentally induced lactic acidosis fared far better with DCA therapy alone, than with NaHCO$_3$ therapy alone, should come as no surprise.[40] Would anyone doubt that diabetics suffering severe ketoacidosis are more likely to survive when treated with insulin than with NaHCO$_3$? No one advocating the use of alkali in organic acidosis *ever* suggested that it be used as a *substitute* for insulin, or DCA. Most certainly, advocates of alkali therapy suggest it be used as an adjunct to those treatments aimed at reversing the increased synthesis of organic acids. For this reason, studies comparing therapy with alkali alone and DCA alone [40] have little bearing on the issues under discussion.

# ARGUMENTS FOR THE USE OF BICARBONATE

## Mixed Hyperchloremic High Anion Gap Acidoses

The argument that therapy of organic acidoses with exogenous alkali is unnecessary since metabolic oxidation of retained organic acid anions generates needed bicarbonate, has been softened by recent studies of DKA.[1] Adrogué et al. demonstrated that prior to therapy, 52 percent of patients with DKA had a hyperchloremic (i.e., nonanion gap) component to their metabolic acidosis.[1] After 4 and 8 hours of standard therapy, the percentage increased to 82 percent and 91 percent, respectively.[1] Continued urinary loss of ketone salts, with retention of administered NaCl, at once squanders potential alkali (i.e., ketone anions), reduces the anion gap as measurable chloride anions replace usually unmeasured ketone anions, but serum bicarbonate concentration remains unchanged and low. The host's capacity to replenish depleted alkali stores by metabolic processes diminishes in parallel with the emergence of this hyperchloremic phase. By progressively shifting dependence for bicarbonate synthesis from metabolic to renal mechanisms, patients lose their capacity to rapidly normalize depleted stores of alkali. It has indeed been demonstrated that without exogenous alkali therapy, serum bicarbonate concentration rises more slowly in those diabetics with hyperchloremic acidosis than those with simple high anion gap acidoses.[1] The rate of recovery is apt to be even slower in elderly diabetics and in those with obvious chronic renal damage, that is, in groups with compromised renal acid excretion and bicarbonate generation. These observations ought to soften the hearts of even the most impassioned assailants of bicarbonate therapy.

## Cardiovascular Effects of Acidosis

Among the most menacing effects of metabolic acidosis are its disruptive hemodynamic actions. A recent critical review concluded that severe metabolic acidosis impairs myocardial contraction, reduces cardiac output, and, by simultaneously causing arteriolar dilatation, results in dangerous degrees of hypotension.[34] Additional pernicious effects of acidosis include bradycardia and sensitization to various malignant ventricular arrhythmias and venoconstriction.[34] The latter effect causes redistribution of venous blood from a peripheral to a central location, thereby increasing the workload of a failing myocardium.

The cellular entry of calcium ions and the binding of calcium to the sarcolemma plays a key role in myocardial and arteriolar contraction.[28,52] The uptake of calcium cations via specific membrane channels is stimulated by catecholamines and competitively inhibited by hydrogen ions.[35,52] Protons also interfere with calcium binding to the sarcolemma.[28] This interplay among acid, catecholamines, and calcium may well underlie the myocardial depressant effect of metabolic acidosis and the vasodilatation and hypotension that complicate the organic acidoses.

It has been repeatedly observed that contraction of the isolated heart as well as in vitro contraction of animal and human myocardial strips are impaired by even small decrements of the medium pH.[26,37] In vivo studies, however, indicate that little change in cardiac function occurs until arterial pH decreases to less than 7.20.[34] Adrenal medullary release of epinephrine is stimulated by acidosis and the positive inotropic effect of catecholamines appears to offset the direct negative effects of acid on the heart.[31] As blood pH falls below 7.20 the direct negative inotropic effect of acidosis is unmasked.[34] It can be argued that a critical concentration of protons is required to competitively impair cate-chole-stimulated calcium uptake. It is not clear whether preexisting myocardial damage—as might be seen in long-standing diabetes mellitus—sensitizes the heart to acidosis. It is clear, however, that pretreatment with β-adrenergic blocking agents does sensitize to systemic acidosis. Indeed, myocardial contraction and cardiac output are impaired by lesser decrees of acidemia.[45,51]

Like myocardial contraction, arteriolar contraction is also disturbed when blood pH falls below 7.20.[51] It follows that the hypotension seen at low blood pH is associated with well-perfused limbs, giving the appearance of "warm-shock." Acidification increases the tone of peripheral veins, an effect that is independent of the presence of catecholamines.[46] Thus, peripheral venoconstriction forces more

blood centrally, thereby increasing the myocardial workload.

As blood pH is reduced to below 7.20 the combination of increased central blood volume and decreased myocardial contraction, predisposes patients with metabolic acidosis to congestive heart failure. The pH of 7.20 therefore, is a reasonable therapeutic endpoint. Bicarbonate ought to be given in amounts that raise pH to this value. The elderly and patients receiving β-adrenergic blocking drugs appear to be more sensitive to acidosis and may well require a more normal pH to normalize myocardial function.[34]

### Severe Metabolic Acidosis Sensitizes pH to Small Additional Changes in Bicarbonate Concentration or PCO₂

The constraints of the enforced relationship between blood hydrogen ion concentration, PCO₂ and bicarbonate concentration, render arterial acidity exquisitely sensitive to even mild additional changes in alkali or PCO₂ reserves. The Henderson equation:

$$(H^+) = \frac{24\ PCO_2}{(HCO_3^-)}$$

demands that the *ratio* of PCO₂ to HCO₃⁻ concentration define blood pH. In severe metabolic acidosis the bicarbonate concentration is primarily reduced to very low values while the PCO₂ is secondarily decreased to low pressures. It follows that otherwise small absolute decrements in bicarbonate concentration or increments in PCO₂, can markedly alter the *ratio* of PCO₂ to HCO₃⁻ and thereby effect major and life-threatening changes in blood (H⁺). Table 10-6 illustrates this point. The superimposition of what, under normal circumstances, would be a trivial degree of lactic acidosis, causes precipitous reduction of blood pH. Although the 2.5 mM accumulation of lac-

tate reduces blood bicarbonate concentration only by a mere 2.5 mM, since the (H⁺) is defined by the *ratio* of PCO₂ to HCO₃⁻, and since the denominator is halved, the ratio must double. Thus, this otherwise minor reduction in bicarbonate concentration doubles the (H⁺) defining a fall in blood pH from 7.11 to 6.81. The dehydrated diabetic in ketoacidosis with a serum bicarbonate concentration of 5 mM and a PCO₂ of 16 mm Hg is at risk of precipitously lowering blood pH should a 2 to 3 mM accumulation of acid take place. The consumption of blood bicarbonate occurs much faster than does pulmonary compensation, allowing the full brunt of the hypobicarbonatemia to

**Table 10-6.** Sensitivity of pH to Small Additional Changes in Bicarbonate or PCO$_2$ in Severe Metabolic Acidosis. H$^+$ = 24 PCO$_2$/HCO$_3$$^-$

| Acid-base Parameters | Normal | Simple Severe DKA | Mild Lactic Acidosis Plus Simple Severe DKA | Mild PCO$_2$ Retention plus Simple Severe DKA | Therapy with Modest Amounts of NaHCO$_3$ |
|---|---|---|---|---|---|
| HCO$_3$ (mM) | 24.0 | 5.0 | 2.5 | 5.0 | 8.0 |
| PCO$_2$ (mm Hg) | 40 | 16 | 16 | 32 | 16 |
| H$^+$ (nM) | 40 | 77 | 154 | 154 | 48 |
| pH | 7.40 | 7.11 | 6.81 | 6.81 | 7.32 |

cause pH to fall. Since cellular and bone buffers absorb increasing quantities of generated protons, it takes a substantial load of organic acid to effect this 2.5 mM fall in bicarbonate.[34] Nonetheless, the severely acidotic dehydrated diabetic with compromised myocardial function must be at added risk of generating a lactic acidosis.

Small absolute increments in PCO$_2$ also dramatically increase the ratio of PCO$_2$ to HCO$_3$ and thereby define a precipitous fall in pH. The increase in arterial PCO$_2$ from 16 mm Hg to 32 mm Hg doubles the PCO$_2$/HCO$_3$ ratio and severely acidifies blood (Table 10-6).

The last column in Table 10-6 indicates how alterations in the PCO$_2$/HCO$_3$ ratio may be used advantageously. Addition of 150 to 300 mmol of NaHCO$_3$ to insulin, potassium and saline therapy of DKA can raise an adult's serum bicarbonate concentration by 3 mM and (Table 10-6) raise blood pH into a much safer zone. In our view, addition of this modest amount of alkali to the therapeutic regimen adds little risk but brings with it an added measure of safety that may prove life-saving for some patients.

We fully recognize that the majority of ketoacidotics do well with simple use of saline, insulin, and potassium. The number of patients with an absolute need for exogenous alkali is uncertain, and, given the enormous difficulties with such studies, is not likely to be defined.

We believe the risks of severe meta-bolic acidosis far outweigh the theoretical risks of alkali therapy and therefore continue to recommend judicious use of sodium bicarbonate in treating the organic acidosis.

# REFERENCES

1. Adrogué HJ, Wilson H, Boyd AE, et al: Plasma acid-base patterns in diabetic ketoacidosis. N Engl J Med 307:1603, 1982.
2. Adrogué HJ, Brensilver J, Cohen JJ et al: Influence of steady-state alterations in acid-base equilibrium on the fate of administered bicarbonate in the dog. J Clin Invest 71:867, 1983.
3. Arieff AI, Park R, Leach WJ, et al: Pathophysiology of experimental lactic acidosis in dogs. Am J Physiol F135, 1980.
4. Arieff AI, Leach W, Park R, et al: Systemic effects of NaHCO$_3$ in experimental lactic acidosis in dogs. Am J Physiol 242:F586, 1982.
5. Assal J, Aoki TT, Manzano FM, et al: Metabolic effects of sodium bicarbonate in management of diabetic ketoacidosis. Diabetes 23:405, 1974.
6. Bellingham AJ, Detter JC, Lenfant C: Regulatory mechanisms of hemoglobin oxygen affinity in acidosis and alkalosis. J Clin Invest 50:700, 1971.
7. Benjamin J, Kopyt N, Jones ER, et al: Tissue O$_2$ delivery is stable despite rapid correction of chronic metabolic acidosis. Abstracts, Am Soc Nephrol 136A, 1982.
8. Bishop RL, Weisfeldt, ML: Sodium bicarbonate administration during cardiac arrest. Effect on arterial pH, PCO$_2$ and osmolality. JAMA 235:506, 1976.

9. Bohr C, Hasselbalch K, Krogh A: Ueber emen in biologischen beziehung wichtigen einfluss, den die kohlen saverespannune des blutes anf dessen samer-stoffbinding ubt. Skand Arch Physiol 16:402, 1904.

10. Bunn HF, Briehl RW, Larrabee P, et al: The interaction of 2,3-diphosphoglycerate with various human hemoglobins. J Clin Invest 49:1088, 1970.

11. Butler AM, Talbot NB, Barnett CH, et al: Metabolic studies in diabetic coma. Trans Assoc Am Physicians 60:102, 1947.

12. Cahill GF Jr: Ketosis. Kidney Int 20:416, 1981.

13. Chanutin A, Curnish RR: Effect of organic and inorganic phosphates on the oxygen equilibrium of human erythrocytes. Arch Biochem Biophys 121:96, 1967.

14. Cohen RD, Woods HF: Clinical and biochemical aspects of lactic acidosis. Chap. 8. Blackwell Scientific Publications, Oxford, England, 1976.

15. Danowski TS, Peters JH, Rathbun JC, et al: Studies in diabetic acidosis and coma with particular emphasis on the retention of administered potassium. J Clin Invest 28:1, 1949.

16. Dempsey JA, Forster HV: Mediation of ventilatory adaptations. Physiol Rev 62:262, 1982.

17. Evans RS, Oliver RE, Appleyard WJ, et al: Effects of intragastric and intravenous sodium bicarbonate on rate of recovery from post-asphyxial acidosis in the neonate. Arch Dis Child 45:321, 1970.

18. Fencl V, Vale JR, Broch JA: Respiration and cerebral blood flow in metabolic acidosis and alkalosis in humans. J Appl Physiol 27:67, 1969.

19. Fencl V: Distribution of $H^+$ and $HCO_3^-$ in cerebral fluids. In Siesjo BK, Sorensen SC, Eds: Homeostasis of the Brain. Copenhagen, Munksgaard, 1971, pp 175–179.

20. Fields ALA, Wolman SL, Halperin ML: Chronic lactic acidosis in a patient with cancer: Therapy and metabolic consequences. Cancer 47:2026, 1981.

21. Fraley DS, Adler S, Bruns FJ, et al: Stimulation of lactate production by administration of bicarbonate in a patient with a solid neoplasm and lactic acidosis. N Engl J Med 303:1100, 1980.

22. Gabbay KH, Hasty K, Breslow JL: Glycosylated hemoglobins and long-term blood gluose control in diabetes mellitus. J Clin Endocrinol Metab 44:859, 1977.

23. Goldberger E: Metabolic acidosis syndromes. In Goldberger E, Ed: A Primer of Water, Electrolyte and Acid-Base Syndromes. Philadelphia, Lea and Febiger, 1980, p. 25.

24. Hobel CJ, Oh W, Hyvarinen MA, et al: Early versus late treatment of neonatal acidosis in low-birth-weight infants: Relation to respiratory distress syndrome. J. Pediatrics 81:1178, 1972.

25. Hood VL, Danforth E Jr, Horton ES, et al: Impact of hydrogen ion on fasting ketogenesis: feedback regulation of acid production. Am J Physiol 11:F238, 1982.

26. Johannson M, Nilsson E: Acid-base changes and excitation-contraction coupling in rabbit myocardium. I. Effect on isometric tension development at different contraction frequencies. Acta Physiol Scand 93:295, 1975.

27. Minakami S, Yoshikawa H: Studies on erythrocyte glycolysis. III. The effects of active cation transport, pH and inorganic phosphate concentration on erythrocyte glycolysis. J Biochem 59:145, 1966.

28. Mitchell JH, Wildenthal K, Johnson RL Jr: The effects of acid-base disturbances on cardiovascular and pulmonary function. Kidney Int 1:375, 1972.

29. Munk P, Freedman MH, Levison H, et al: Effect of bicarbonate on oxygen transport in juvenile diabetic ketoacidosis. J Pediatrics, 84:510, 1974.

30. Nabarro JDN, Spencer AG, Stowers JM: Metabolic studies in severe ketosis. Q J Med 21:225, 1952.

31. Nahas GG, Zaguy D, Milhaud A, et al: Acidemia and catecholamine output of the isolated canine adrenal gland. Am J Physiol 213:1186, 1967.

32. Narins RG, Szidon JP, Relman AS: Unpublished observations.

33. Narins RG, Emmett M: Simple and mixed acid-base disorders: A practical approach. Medicine 59:161, 1980.

34. Narins RG, Bastl CP, Rudnick MR, et al:

Acid-base metabolism. In Gonick HC, Ed: Current Nephrology. Vol 5. New York, Wiley, 1982, p 79.

35. Nayler WG, Ferrari R, Poole-Wilson PA, et al: A protective effect of a mild acidosis on hypoxic heart muscle. J Mol Cell Cardiol 11:1053, 1979.

36. Ohman JL Jr, Marliss EB, Aoki TT, et al: The cerebrospinal fluid in diabetic ketoacidosis. N Engl J Med 284:283, 1971.

37. Opie LH, Kadas T, Geevers W: Effect of pH on the function and glucose metabolism of the heart. Lancet 2:551, 1963.

38. Osnes J, Hermansen L: Acid-balance after maximal exercise of short duration. J Appl Physiol 32:59, 1972.

39. Oster JR, Perez GD, Vaamonde CA: Relationship between blood pH and potassium and phosphorus during acute metabolic acidosis. Am J Physiol F235:345, 1978.

40. Park R, Arieff AI, Leach W, et al: Treatment of lactic acidosis with dichloroacetate in dogs. J Clin Invest 70:853, 1982

41. Pierce NF, Fedson DS, Brigham KL, et al: The ventilatory response to acute base deficit in humans. Time course during development and correction of metabolic acidosis. Ann Intern Med 72:633, 1970.

42. Plum F, Posner JB: Diagnosis of Stupor and Coma. Philadelphia, FA Davis, 1975, p 204.

43. Posner JB, Swanson AG, Plum F: Acid-base balance in cerebrospinal fluid. Arch Neurol 12:479, 1965.

44. Posner JB, Plum F: Spinal-fluid pH and neurologic symptoms in systemic acidosis. N Engl J Med 277:605, 1967.

45. Rocamora JM, Downing SE: Preservation of ventricular function by adrenergic influences during metabolic acidosis in the cat. Circulation Res 24:373, 1969.

46. Sharpey-Schaffer EP, Semple SJG, Halls RW, et al: Venous constriction after exercise; its relation to acid-base changes in venous blood. Clin Sci 29:397, 1965.

47. Soffer LJ, Dantes DA, Sobotka H: Utilization of intravenously injected D-lactate as a test of hepatic function. Arch Intern Med 62:918, 1938.

48. Soler NG, Dixon K, Bennett MA, et al: Potassium balance during treatment of diabetic ketoacidosis: with special reference to the use of bicarbonate. Lancet 2:665, 1972.

49. Stoneman MER, Owens RM: Effects of intragastric sodium bicarbonate in infants with respiratory distress. Arch Dis Child 43:155, 1968.

50. Valeri CR: Hemoglobin. In Brobeck JR, Ed: Best and Taylor's Physiological Basis of Medical Practice. Baltimore, Williams and Wilkins, 1979, pp 4–43.

51. Wildenthal K, Mierzwiak DS, Myers RW, et al: Effects of acute lactic acidosis on left ventricular performance. Am J Physiol 214:1352, 1968.

52. Williamson JR, Safer B, Rich T, et al: Effects of acidosis on myocardial contractility and metabolism. Acta Med Scand Suppl 587:95, 1975.

53. Winters RW, Lowder JA, Ordway NK: Observations on carbon dioxide tension during recovery from metabolic acidosis. J Clin Invest 37:640, 1958.

54. Wright FS: Sites and mechanisms of potassium transport along the renal tubule. Kidney Int 11:415, 1977.

# 11

# Treatment of Hyponatremia

# The Case for a More Conservative Approach

## Michael D. Norenberg, M.D.

Hyponatremia is one of the most common electrolyte disorders encountered in a general hospital.[4] It may occur acutely following the rapid intake of hypotonic fluids (bladder irrigations, intravenous fluid therapy, beer drinkers, hemo- or peritoneal dialysis and psychogenic polydipsia) and in acute SIADH. Alternatively it may develop chronically, often in patients who have other serious medical conditions and who frequently are on diuretics. Patients with hyponatremia may present with mild nonspecific symptoms such as anorexia, nausea, vomiting, weakness, muscular cramps and twitching, myoclonus and asterixis.[4,24] Confusion and delirium may predominate often mimicking a psychotic state.[63] Occasionally it may present as a life-threatening condition with stupor, coma, and seizures.[4,24] The development of symptoms is dependent on the level of serum sodium and more importantly on the rate at which the hyponatremic level is achieved.[8,24] Patients acutely hyponatremic may show severe symptoms even with levels of 120 to 125 mEq/L whereas in cases of more slowly developing hyponatremia, patients may reach levels as low as 110 and still be relatively asymptomatic.

Animal studies have shown a 50 percent mortality following severe acute hyponatremia.[3] The situation in humans is less clear. Fatal cases have been described by Helwig et al.,[29] Lipsmeyer and Acker-man,[37] Raskind,[48] and Arieff et al.[3] While some of these fatalities were indeed clearly the result of hyponatremia, many of these patients had received therapy, some of it aggressive, and consequently it is difficult to say whether the poor outcome of those patients was truly due to the hyponatremia itself or to its correction. Thus, while there is no argument that severe, symptomatic hyponatremia, especially when acute, needs prompt attention, it is the manner in which these patients should be corrected that is controversial.

Our concern with the issue of correction of hyponatremia came about from an analysis of patients with central pontine myelinolysis (CPM), a potentially serious neurological disorder.[46] Our study disclosed that CPM in every instance was associated with a rapid rise in serum sodium usually from hyponatremic levels and frequently following aggressive correction of hyponatremia. This observation was then subsequently supported by experimental studies showing that hyponatremic rats wherein the serum sodium was raised rapidly developed lesions similar to CPM in man.[32,33]

In this chapter we will: (1) provide evidence that CPM is due to a rapid rise in serum sodium; (2) review and analyze the available literature dealing with correction of hyponatremia; and (3) suggest therapeutic recommendations whereby severe, symptomatic hyponatremia may be successfully treated while hopefully at the same time avoiding the development of CPM.

# CENTRAL PONTINE MYELINOLYSIS

CPM was initially described by Adams and coworkers in 1959.[1] The lesion consists of a symmetrical zone of demyelination in the pontine base. The periphery of the pons is always spared and frequently there is sparing of the corticospinal tracts (Fig. 11-1). Histologically there is evidence of myelin breakdown, loss of oligodendrocytes, endothelial nuclear swelling, infiltration by macrophages, slight reactive astrocytosis with the eventual conversion into a glial scar. There is no inflammation. Neuronal cell bodies and axons are usually intact although in severe cases there may be considerable loss of neurons leading to cavitation. Involvement of other parts of the nervous system has frequently been described, a feature recently emphasized by Wright and coworkers.[64] These extrapontine lesions are typically found in the thalamus, striatum and the gray-white junctions of the cerebellum and cerebrum. Extrapontine involvement is usually limited to severe cases.

The clinical expression of this disorder ranges from asymptomatic (i.e., a small incidental lesion found at autopsy) all the way to a devastating disorder resulting in a "locked-in syndrome." The condition is often ushered in by changes in mental state, particularly confusion and agitation. This then may be followed by flaccid or spastic quadriparesis, hyperreflexia, and extensor plantar responses. There is often evidence of bulbar involvement with facial and tongue weakness, dysphagia, and dysarthria. The diagnosis of CPM may be suspected by the constellation of signs and symptoms and its presence may be detected by means of CT scanning particularly when coronal views are examined.[56]

While the condition is not necessarily fatal a high mortality is associated with it, probably due to other serious medical illnesses that these patients often have. Some improvement in their neurologic state often occurs and occasional rather dramatic improvements have been noted (personal observation). There is no known treatment of CPM, although a brief report indicates the potential usefulness of corticosteroids.[50]

## Etiological Considerations

The etiology of CPM has been an enigma. It was early recognized that it never occurred in isolation but instead appeared to complicate another preexisting serious medical condition.[26,44] Additionally, almost all cases developed in a hospital setting, that is, practically no patients were ever admitted to the hospital with clinical signs and symptoms of CPM.[44]

A number of etiologic factors have been suggested over the years including malnutrition, alcoholism, liver disease, vascular insufficiency, and a number of toxins.[1,17,26,34,44,52,53,57] However, none of these proposed factors has been consistently identified in all of the reported cases.

Electrolyte abnormalities also have been frequently mentioned although no clear consistent pattern has been recognized.[9,11,15,23,40,42,47,51] In 1977 we emphasized the association with hyponatremia.[12] In our study of 16 CPM patients, all of them had hyponatremia during their last hospitalization. However, an analysis of the time course of hyponatremia and CPM was not made. Messert and coworkers[41] in 1979 also made cogent arguments in favor of a crucial role for hyponatremia in the development of CPM.

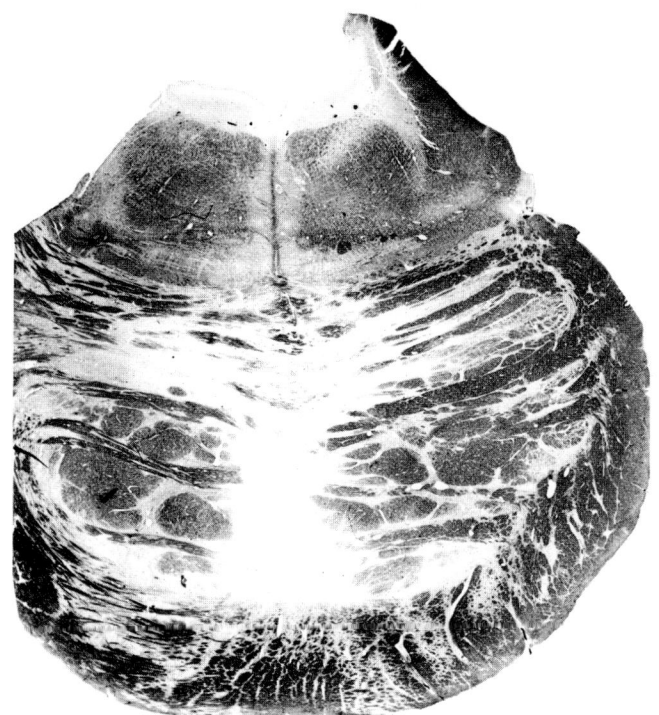

**Fig. 11-1.** Myelin-stained section of human pons showing symmetrical zone of myelin loss in pontine base.

There were, however, some problems in accepting that hyponatremia alone was the cause of CPM:

1. Shortly after we had published our report on the association of hyponatremia with CPM we identified a number of patients who died with severe hyponatremia (105 to 115 mEq/L) but did not show any significant pathological changes (except perhaps for slight edema) and specifically disclosed no evidence of CPM.

2. While hyponatremia was found in all our cases, in 9 of the 16 patients it was rather mild (127 to 130 mEq/L). That degree of hyponatremia is exceedingly common and yet CPM is rare.

3. In the review of the literature that we performed there were many cases wherein normonatremia was observed and in three patients, hypernatremia was described instead.

4. If hyponatremia alone was responsible for CPM, one might predict that some of the patients would have been hospitalized with clinical evidence of CPM. That has rarely, if ever, been described and instead the patients develop CPM while in the hospital.

5. The pathology of hyponatremia in both man and experimental animals is often unremarkable. Relatively minor changes are observed and the only consistent observation has been the presence of cerebral edema which often is only slight.[3,19,20,29,31,38,49,60] Focal neuropathological alterations have not been described. In unpublished studies carried out with Dr. Roger E. Riepe, we specifically looked for the possible development of CPM in experimental animals which had been made hyponatremic. Despite using many protocols (varying the severity and duration of hyponatremia) we were singularly unsuccessful in producing any demyelinative lesions. (Subtle astroglial changes resembling Alzheimer type II changes were the only abnormalities found.)

6. Hyponatremia has been present for a long time and yet CPM appears to have been nonexistent prior to the 1950s.[2]

## Analysis of CPM Patients and Experimental Studies

The above issues raise serious questions about hyponatremia being the sole causal factor in CPM. Yet, we still believed that in some fashion hyponatremia was indeed playing some role in its development. We then carried out a retrospective study comparing hyponatremic patients who subsequently developed CPM with hyponatremic patients who did not develop CPM.[46] We reviewed the neuropathology protocols over the previous 7 years and were able to identify 12 patients who had sufficient clinical and electrolyte information for evaluation. All patients had been hyponatremic for a week or more. Analysis of the sodium data from these 12 patients revealed that in every instance, a rapid and sustained rise in serum sodium had occurred 3 to 10 days prior to the development of symptoms

consistent with CPM (and subsequently verified at autopsy). In all 12 cases, a rise of at least 20 mEq/L was achieved within 3 days and in some of these patients, considerably greater increases within a shorter period of time were observed. In addition, and perhaps a crucial observation, was the fact that in 11 of the 12 patients some degree of hypernatremia had developed (147 to 160 mEq/L). A particularly illustrative case strongly indicating to us that it was not hyponatremia but the rise in serum sodium that was critical was that of a patient who had been hyponatremic for at least 2 weeks but was neurologically intact and without any evidence of CPM. It was only after the period of sodium rise that CPM developed (Fig. 11-2).

It should be emphasized that in every instance CPM occurred while the patient was in the hospital and none of the patients were ever admitted with clinical symptoms suggesting CPM. Moreover, the rise in sodium was not always due to aggressive correction of hyponatremia, although that certainly was the case in some patients. In at least 5 of the patients

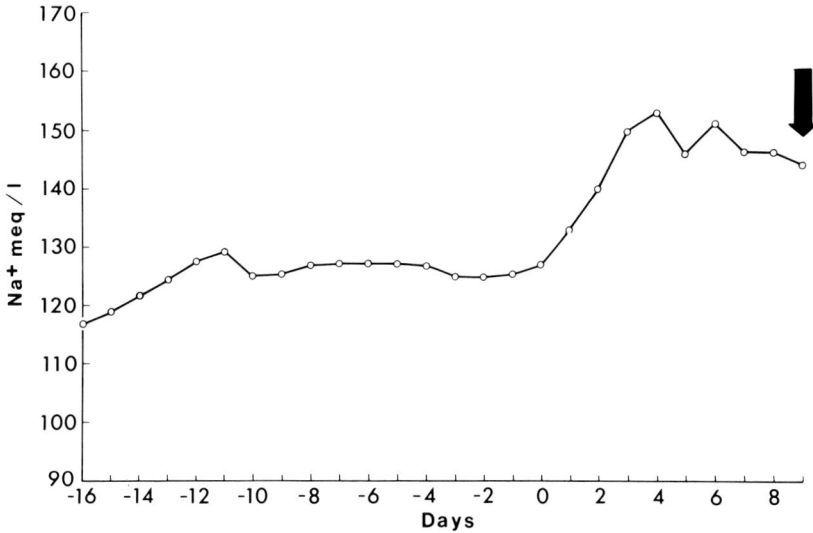

**Fig. 11-2.** Patient with hyponatremia of at least 16 days duration who developed clinical evidence of CPM 5 days after the peak in serum sodium elevation. Day 0 indicates the onset of the abrupt rise in sodium.

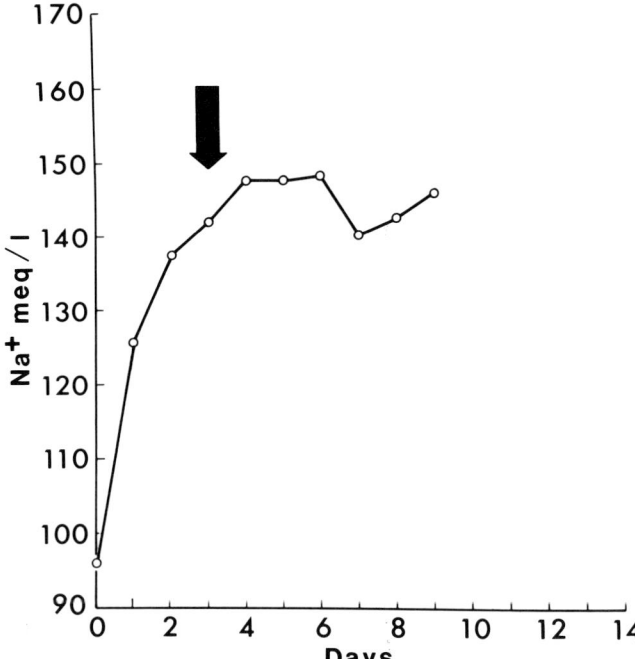

**Fig. 11-3.** Severly hyponatremic patient who developed CPM on the third day after aggressive correction (50 mEq/L rise). Autopsy disclosed a large CPM lesion.

the rise in sodium seemed to be related to the administration of lactulose as part of the therapy for hepatic encephalopathy. Lactulose has been shown to cause hypernatremia resulting from hypotonic water losses.[59] In general, there was a rough correlation between the magnitude and speed with which the final sodium level was achieved and how soon the disorder presented clinically and the severity of the disease (Figs. 11-3,11-4).

By contrast, in a group of hyponatremic patients who did not develop CPM (otherwise similar with respect to level and chronicity of hyponatremia, underlying medical conditions, age, and sex) there was little to no rise in serum sodium (Fig. 11-5). Two patients differed slightly from the rest of the group. One patient showed a rapid rise in sodium of about 25 mEq/L over a 2-day period but 1 day after reaching 150 mEq/L, the sodium value fell again into the hyponatremic range. It thus appeared that a sustained rise in serum sodium may be essential for CPM to develop. Another patient showed a substantial rise in serum sodium (22 mEq/L) but this rise was achieved slowly (over 7 days) suggesting a prompt rise as a prerequisite for CPM.

A review of the literature disclosed that in every case with sufficient electrolyte data (17 patients), a similar sequence of events occurred, namely, the patients were admitted with hyponatremia or developed hyponatremia in the hospital (except 1 patient), were rapidly corrected and then subsequently developed CPM.

It thus appeared to us that the principal distinguishing feature between these two patient populations was the rate and magnitude of sodium rise and the length of time that the sodium levels remained elevated. Additionally, in almost all patients the sodium rose into the hypernatremic range. This study also gave further support to the view that hyponatremia alone is not the sole factor in the development of CPM. Illustrative was the large number of hyponatremic patients in whom lesions of CPM were not found. Additionally, we found that several of our

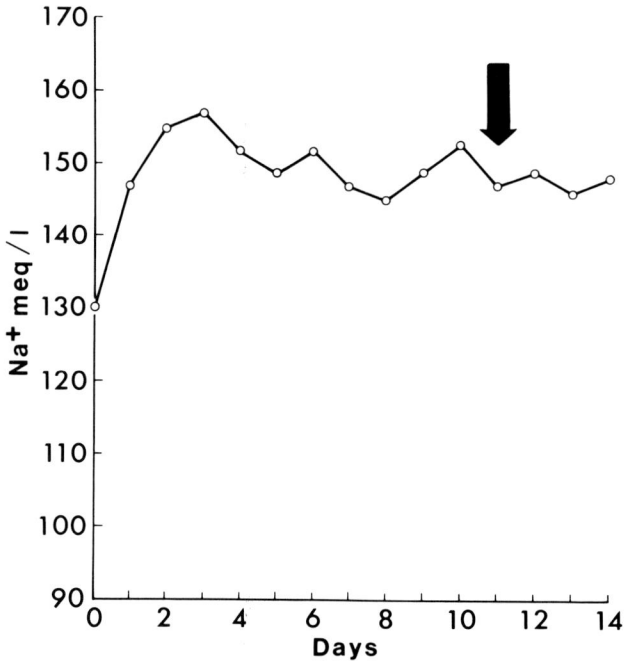

**Fig. 11-4.** Mildly hyponatremic patient whose serum sodium rose 28 mEq/L probably due to lactulose therapy, but clinical evidence of CPM presented only 8 days after the maximum rise in sodium. Autopsy showed a moderately sized CPM lesion.

patients had only borderline hyponatremia (130 mEq/L). Finally, there is the case of the chronically hyponatremic patient who only developed CPM following the sodium rise.

More recently, I have had the opportunity to identify a case of pathologically verified CPM who had been well-studied clinically and who was not at any time hyponatremic. His serum sodium had risen from an admission value of 139 mEq/L to 171 on the tenth hospital day (presumably on the basis of lactulose therapy). The patient died on the 20th hospital day. At autopsy a recent, small (clinically insignificant) CPM lesion was found. It thus would appear that hyponatremia while almost always clinically present, may not be an absolute prerequisite.

To experimentally test the view that it was the rapid rise in serum sodium (rather than hyponatremia) which was responsible for the production of CPM, we studied rats which were made hyponatremic for 3 days by the administration of pitressin and water and which were sub-

sequently quickly corrected with hypertonic saline. The majority of these animals developed symmetrical demyelinative lesions similar to CPM in man[32,33] (Fig. 11-6). Electron microscopic studies showed that oligodendrocytes were the cellular elements most vulnerable to these experimental procedures.[43] Rats kept hyponatremic for a comparable period of time as well as rats allowed to slowly correct themselves failed to develop any demyelinative lesions. Studies by Laureno using a similar protocol in dogs also showed the presence of demyelinative lesions in brain.[36]

It is unknown how these electrolyte alterations bring about demyelinative lesions. We have postulated that a rapid rise in serum sodium may cause an osmotic injury to endothelium.[44] This endothelial injury may release a myelinolytic factor. Preliminary studies in our laboratory have indeed shown an increased amount of endothelial-associated plasminogen activator.[45] Plasmin (its formation catalyzed by plasminogen activator) is ca-

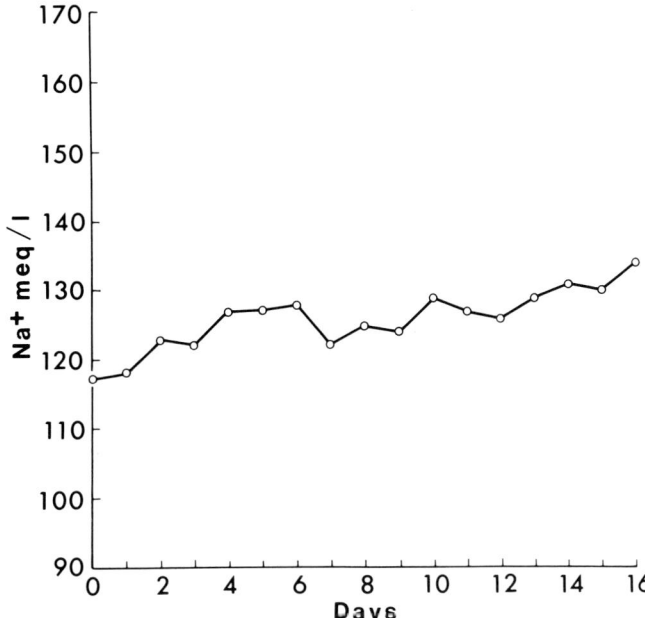

**Fig. 11-5.** Hyponatremic patient showing a gradual rise in sodium. Death was due to renal failure and pancreatitis. Autopsy showed no evidence of CPM.

pable of hydrolyzing myelin basic protein.[13]

It seems apparent that the weight of evidence is strongly in favor of the view that it is the rapid rise in serum sodium from hyponatremic levels which is responsible for CPM. The serum sodium in CPM is usually characterized by: (1) a preceding period of hyponatremia present for days or weeks prior to the rise, (2) a rise of at least 20 mEq/L achieved within 3 days, (3) such rise in the sodium level once achieved remains at approximately the same level (i.e., there is no subsequent significant drop in the serum sodium), and (4) at least in our patients, the final sodium level is usually in the hypernatremic range.

### Analysis of Successfully Treated Hyponatremic Patients

We now have to reconcile the above conclusions with a number of reports demonstrating that many patients seem to do well clinically following the rapid correction of hyponatremia. Perhaps an anal-

ysis of these cases and comparison with ours might provide a clue to the proper parameters of sodium elevation involved in the development of CPM.

The data of these successfully corrected patients are presented in the Table 11-1. Many of these patients indeed showed marked increases in serum sodium that were achieved within a very short period of time. It might thus be argued that it was this rapid treatment (within 36 hours) that resulted in a good outcome. However, while some of our CPM patients achieved the sodium rise more slowly (over 3 days), 3 of our patients had rises of 25 mEq/L or greater in less than 24 hours indicating that rapid treatment alone did not differentiate our CPM patients from these successfully corrected patients. Two items, however, did distinguish these two patient populations. (1) The sodium value after correction in most of the successfully treated patients remained in the hyponatremic range (mean = 132.6 mEq/L) with only 2 patients having been overcorrected. By contrast, 11 of our 12 CPM patients devel-

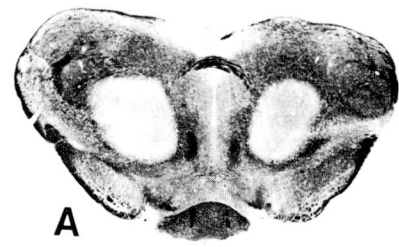

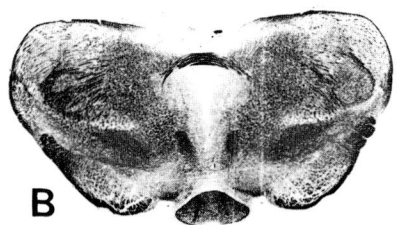

**Fig. 11-6.** (A) Myelin-stained cross section of the brainstem-hypothalamic junction of a rapidly corrected hyponatremic rat showing symmetrical zones of myelin loss. (B) Normal control. (From Kleinschmidt-DeMasters BK, Norenberg, MD: Rapid correction of hyponatremia causes demyelination: Relation to central pontine myelimolyses. Science 211:1068–1070, 1981. Copyright 1981 by the American Association for the Advancement of Science.

oped some degree of hypernatremia following the rise in sodium. (2) Perhaps even more important is that in almost all patients included in the Table, the time period of hyponatremia lasted only for several hours to a few days at most, whereas in all of our CPM patients hyponatremia had been present for a considerably longer period of time (one week or more). It is noteworthy that the only patient in this successfully treated group who probably had chronic hyponatremia, had a sodium rise of only 18 mEq/L.

Consistent with the view that chronicity of hyponatremia followed by a rapid correction predisposes to neurological deficits are the reports by Arieff and Witte[5] and Ashraf et al.[6] Fourteen patients were described who had hyponatremia for at least 5 days prior to their rapid (within 36 hours) correction. Final sodium values were not stated other than their being greater than 130 mEq/L. All 14 either died or were left with significant neurological deficits.

It was the contention of the above-mentioned authors that it was the prolonged period of hyponatremia alone that was responsible for their patients' unfavorable outcome. As has already been argued we believe that it was instead the rapid correction given to these chronically hyponatremic patients which may have resulted in their neurological deficits. It is of interest that some of their patients (as well as some of ours) often showed marked improvement in their mental status following the administration of hypertonic saline only to come down several days later with a totally different set of neurologic symptoms often focal in nature. This would suggest that perhaps something other than hyponatremia was responsible for these new clinical findings. It is possible that some of their patients may have developed CPM. The availability of CT scans or detailed postmortem findings might have aided in the interpretation of these cases.

In contrast to the uniformly poor out-

**Table 11-1.** Hyponatremic Patients Successfully Treated with Rapid Correction[a]

| Reference | Patient | Type of Hyponatremia[b] | Rise of Sodium (mEq/L) | Sodium Value at Correction (mEq/L) | Time of Correction (Hours) |
|---|---|---|---|---|---|
| Wynn and Rob[65] | 1 | Acute[b] | 33 | 143 | 24 |
| Wynn and Rob[65] | 2 | Acute | 19 | 136 | 20 |
| Wynn and Rob[65] | 3 | Acute | 20 | 142 | 8 |
| Wynn and Rob[65] | 4 | Acute | 15 | 133 | 3 |
| Wynn and Rob[65] | 5 | Acute | 13 | 120 | 24 |
| Swanson and Iseri[55] | 1 | Acute | 30 | 131 | 6 |
| Swanson and Iseri[55] | 2 | Acute | 13 | 140 | 10 |
| Carter[14] | | Acute | 20 | 137 | 24 |
| Langgard and Smith[35] | 1 | Acute | 45 | 150 | 36 |
| Langgard and Smith[35] | 2 | Acute | 35 | 147 | 8 |
| Hobson and English[30] | | Acute | 21 | 130 | 12 |
| Walters et al.[58] | | Acute | 31 | 130 | <24 |
| Summer and Smythe[54] | 1 | Acute | 27 | 124 | " |
| Summer and Smythe[54] | 2 | ? | 28 | 127 | " |
| Beresford[10] | 1 | Acute | 15 | 130 | 24 |
| Devereaux and McCormick[18] | | Acute | <21 | 121 | 20 |
| Hantman et al.[28] | 1 | Acute | 13 | 134 | 7 |
| Hantman et al.[28] | 2 | Acute | 8 | 130 | 5 |
| Hantman et al.[28] | 3 | Acute | 11 | 132 | 6 |
| Hantman et al.[28] | 4 | Acute | 12 | 129 | 10 |
| Hantman et al.[28] | 5 | Probably acute | 13 | 130 | 8 |
| Ashraf et al.[6] | 4 | Probably acute | >21 | >130 | <36 |
| Ashraf et al.[6] | 5 | Probably acute | >14 | 130 | " |
| Decaux et al.[16] | 1 | ? | 11 | 130 | 24 |
| Decaux et al.[16] | 2 | ? | 15 | 137 | " |
| Decaux et al.[16] | 3 | ? | 20 | 133 | " |
| Decaux et al.[16] | 4 | ? | 16 | 139 | " |
| Decaux et al.[16] | 5 | Probably acute | 16 | 132 | " |
| Decaux et al.[16] | 6 | ? | 27 | 136 | " |
| Decaux et al.[16] | 7 | Probably acute | 15 | 135 | " |
| Weizman et al.[62] | | Probably acute | 37 | 141 | " |
| Ayus et al.[7] | 1 | Acute | 42 | 130 | 15 |
| Ayus et al.[7] | 2 | Acute | 32 | 128 | 12 |
| Ayus et al.[7] | 3 | Acute | 40 | 135 | 24 |
| Ayus et al.[7] | 4 | Acute | 25 | 123 | 5 |
| Ayus et al.[7] | 5 | Acute | 21 | 124 | 13 |
| Ayus et al.[7] | 6 | ? | 22 | 131 | 12 |
| Ayus et al.[7] | 7 | Probably chronic | 18 | 127 | 12 |

[a]Rapid correction = within 36 hours.
[b]Acute = less than 2–3 days; chronic = 1 week or more.

come of rapidly corrected chronically hyponatremic patients are the results from the same laboratory on 51 chronically hyponatremic patients all but 5 of whom received conservative therapy.[3] Four patients died of problems unrelated to electrolyte disturbances. The remainder did well. Five patients did receive hypertonic saline and did well. Unfortunately, the rate and magnitude of correction of these patients were not provided in their report.

At present there is no adequate explanation why chronic hyponatremic patient appear to respond poorly to a sudden osmotic stress. As we have speculated elsewhere,[32,44] the preceding period of hyponatremia may have caused CNS injury, perhaps to astrocytes,[61] which in some fashion prevented the brain from making appropriate adaptive responses (e.g., the generation of idiogenic osmoles) that could have minimized the effects of a severe osmotic challenge.

In sum, several factors acting together appear to predispose hyponatremic patients to the subsequent development of CPM: duration of preceding hyponatremia, magnitude and rate of sodium rise and final sodium value. Since one of our CPM patients and one described in the literature[27] had final sodium values of 135 mEq/L or less, the role of overcorrection is unclear. Moreover, since only two of the successfully treated cases of acute hyponatremia was overcorrected, we do not as yet know what role excessive correction may have on acutely hyponatremic patients.

## THERAPEUTIC RECOMMENDATIONS

Based on the foregoing discussion a number of therapeutic recommendations may be made. To begin with, asymptomatic hyponatremia requires little treatment (water restriction only) or no treatment at all.[25] Symptomatic hyponatremia needs to be treated. The method suggested by Ayus and coworkers[7] and Arieff and Schmidt[4] appears safe, particularly when dealing with acute hyponatremia. Yet, this therapy needs to be carefully and meticulously monitored to avoid the possibility of over-correction that might result in hypernatremia. It might be better yet to treat these patients just fast enough to improve the patient's neurological status (often with as little as a rise of only 10 to 15 mEq/L and at times even less). Once there has been a stabilization in the patient's neurological state, there is no further need for aggressive therapy and correction may be allowed to proceed at a slow pace by means of water restriction. In addition, the possible complication of congestive heart failure following a high load of salt needs to be kept in mind especially in individuals having a history of heart disease. Lastly, although this is more of a theoretical than a real problem, there is the potential development of intracerebral hemorrhages following the administration of hypertonic saline. Hemorrhages have indeed been reported with hypernatremia[21,22,39] but not thus far with rapid correction of hyponatremia.

With regard to the management of patients with chronic hyponatremia a considerably greater degree of caution needs to be exercised and a conservative approach would appear to be prudent. Moveover, these patients appear to tolerate hyponatremia reasonably well. Our studies have indicated that these chronically hyponatremic patients run a great risk in developing CPM following rapid rises in sodium. It is possible that CPM may develop in these patients even though the final sodium levels are in the normo- or hyponatremic range. Guidelines on how fast and how high the sodium may safely be raised are simply not available at present. These patients have to be treated but the aim should only be improvement of their neurologic status rather than attainment of some preconceived serum sodium level.

## SUMMARY AND CONCLUSIONS

Analysis of patients with CPM has shown a strong association with a rapid rise in serum sodium concentration, frequently the result of aggressive correction of hyponatremia. CPM developed in those patients who had been chronically hyponatremic prior to the rise in sodium concentration and in many instances the rise entered the hypernatremic range. These findings have been supported by experimental studies in rats and dogs. It appears that a rapid elevation of sodium into the 120 to 130 mEq/L range may be safely accomplished in the acutely hyponatremic patients. The grave risk in aggressive correction, however, is that these patients may inadvertently become hypernatremic if not carefully monitored and thereby potentially develop CPM. Guidelines for patients with chronic hyponatremia still need to be defined. It is argued that rapid correction in these patients may be particularly hazardous. Correction should thus be carried out with extreme caution and guided by the patient's clinical state rather than by the serum sodium value.

# REFERENCES

1. Adams RD, Victor M, Mancall EL: Central pontine myelinolysis: A hitherto undescribed disease occurring in alcoholic and malnourished patients. Arch Neurol Psychiat 81:154, 1959.
2. Aleu FP, Terry RD: Central pontine myelinolysis. A report of two cases. Arch Pathol 76:140, 1963.
3. Arieff AI, Llach F, Massry SG: Neurological manifestations and morbidity of hyponatremia: Correlation with brain water and electrolytes. Medicine 55:121, 1976.
4. Arieff AI, Schmidt RW: Fluid and electrolyte disorders and the central nervous system. In Maxwell MH, Kleeman CR, Eds: Clinical Disorders of Fluid and Electrolyte Metabolism. New York, McGraw-Hill, 1980 p 1409.
5. Arieff AI, Witte JM: Death or permanent neurologic disability despite correction of protracted hyponatremia. Kidney Int 16:955, 1979.
6. Ashraf N, Locksley R, Arieff AI: Thiazide-induced hyponatremia associated with death or neurologic damage in outpatients. Am J Med 70:1163, 1981.
7. Ayus JC, Olivero JJ, Frommer JP: Rapid correction of severe hyponatremia with intravenous hypertonic saline solution. Am J Med 72:43, 1982.
8. Baskin JL, Keith HM, Scribner BH: Water metabolism in water intoxication: review of basic concepts. Am J Dis Child 83:618, 1952.
9. Behar A, Bental E, Aviram A: Central pontine myelinolysis: A case report. Acta Neuropathol 3:343, 1964.
10. Beresford HR: Polydipsia, hydrochlorothiazide, and water intoxication. JAMA 214:879, 1970.
11. Berry K, Olszewski J: Central pontine myelinolysis. A case report. Neurology 13:531, 1963.
12. Burcar PJ, Norenberg MD, Yarnell PR: Hyponatremia and central pontine myelinolysis. Neurology 27:223, 1977.
13. Cammer W, Bloom BR, Norton WT, Gordon S: Degradation of basic protein in myelin by neutral proteases secreted by stimulated macrophages: a possible mechanism of inflammatory demyelination. Proc Natl Acad Sci 75:1554, 1978.
14. Carter TJ: Water intoxication. Br Med J 2:367, 1959.
15. Conger JD, McIntyre JA, Jacoby WJ: Central pontine myelinolysis associated with inappropriate antidiuretic hormone secretion. Am J Med 47:813, 1969.
16. Decaux G, Unger J, Brimioulle S, et al: Hyponatremia in the syndrome of inappropriate secretion of antidiuretic hormone. JAMA, 247:471, 1982.
17. DeReuck J, VanderEecken, H, Thiery E, et al: Central pontine myelinolysis and its arterial blood supply. Acta Neurol Psychiat Belg 75:193, 1975.
18. Devereaux, MW, McCormick RA: Psychogenic water intoxication. Am J Psychiat 129:628, 1972.
19. Dila CF, Pappius HM: Cerebral water and electrolytes: The experimental model of inappropriate secretion of antidiuretic hormone. Arch Neurol 26:85, 1972.
20. Dodge PR, Crawford JD, Probst JH: Studies in experimental water intoxication. Arch Neurol 3:513, 1960.
21. Finberg L: Pathogenesis of lesions in the nervous system in hypernatremic states. I. Clinical observations of infants. Pediatrics 23:40, 1959.
22. Finberg L, Luttrell CN, Redd H: Pathogenesis of lesions in the nervous system in hypernatremic states. II. Experimental studies of gross anatomic changes and alteration of chemical composition of the tissues. Pediatrics 23:46, 1959.
23. Finlayson MH, Snider S, Oliva LA, et al:

23. Cerebral and pontine myelinolysis: Two cases with fluid and electrolyte imbalance and hypotension. J Neurol Sci 18:399, 1973.

24. Fishman RA: Neurological manifestations of hyponatremia. In Vinken PJ, Bruyn GW, Eds: Handbook of Clinical Neurology. Vol. 28 (Part 2). Amsterdam, North-Holland, 1976, p 495.

25. Flear CTG, Gill GV: Hyponatremia: Mechanisms and management. Lancet 2:26, 1981.

26. Goebel HH, Herman-Ben Zur P: Central pontine myelinolysis, p 285. In Vinken PJ, Bruyn GW, Eds: Handbook of Clinical Neurology. Vol. 28. Amsterdam, North-Holland, 1976.

27. Gross SG, Bell RD: Central pontine myelinolysis and rapid correction of hyponatremia. Texas Med 78:59, 1982.

28. Hantman D, Rossier B, Zohlman R, et al: Rapid correction of hyponatremia in the syndrome of inappropriate secretion of antidiuretic hormone. Ann Intern Med 78:870, 1973.

29. Helwig FC, Schutz CB, Curry DE: Water intoxication: Report of a fatal human case with clinical, pathological and experimental studies. JAMA, 104:1569, 1935.

30. Hobson JA, English JT: Self-induced water intoxication: case study of a chronically schizophrenic patient with physiological evidence of water retention due to inappropriate release of antidiuretic hormone. Ann Intern Med 58:324, 1963

31. Holliday MA, Kalayci MN, Harrah J: Factors that limit brain volume changes in response to acute and sustained hyper- and hyponatremia. J Clin Invest 47:1916, 1968.

32. Kleinschmidt-DeMasters BK, Norenberg MD: Rapid correction of hyponatremia causes demyelination: Relation to central pontine myelinolysis. Science, 211:1068, 1981.

33. Kleinschmidt-DeMasters BK, Norenberg MD: Neuropathologic observations in electrolyte-induced myelinolysis in the rat. J Neuropathol Exp Neurol 41:67, 1982.

34. Landers JW, Chason JL, Samuel VN: Central pontine myelinolysis: A pathogenetic hypothesis. Neurology 15:968, 1965.

35. Langgård H, Smith WO: Self-induced water intoxication without predisposing illness. Report of two cases. N Engl J Med 266:378, 1962.

36. Laureno R: Experimental pontine and extra-pontine myelinolysis. Trans Am Neurol Assoc 105:354, 1980.

37. Lipsmeyer E, Ackerman GL: Irreversible brain damage after water intoxication. JAMA 196:286, 1966.

38. Luse SA, Harris B: Brain ultrastructure in hydration and dehydration. Arch Neurol 4:139, 1961.

39. Luttrell CN, Finberg L: Hemorrhagic encephalopathy induced by hypernatremia: Clinical, laboratory and pathological observations. Arch Neurol Psychiat 81:424, 1959.

40. McCormick WF, Danneel CM: Central pontine myelinolysis. Arch Intern Med 119:444, 1967.

41. Messert B, Orrison WW, Hawkins MJ, et al: Central pontine myelinolysis: Considerations on etiology, diagnosis and treatment. Neurology 29:147, 1979.

42. Monseu G, Flament-Durand J: Pathogenesis of central pontine myelinolysis: a clinical and pathological description of three cases. Pathol Eur 6:75, 1971.

43. Norenberg MD: Ultrastructural observations in electrolyte-induced myelinolysis. J Neuropathol Exp Neurol 50:319, 1981.

44. Norenberg MD: An osmotic endothelial injury hypothesis. A pathogenetic mechanism in central pontine myelinolysis. Arch Pathol 40:66, 1983.

45. Norenberg MD, Bell PK: Plasminogen activator and steroids in electrolyte-induced myelinolysis. Proceedings 9th Int Cong Neuropathol 76, 1982.

46. Norenberg MD, Leslie KO, Robertson AS: Association between rise in serum sodium and central pontine myelinolysis. Ann Neurol 11:128, 1982.

47. Paguirigan A, Lefken EB: Central pontine myelinolysis. Neurology 19:1007, 1969.

48. Raskind M: Psychosis, polydipsia, and water intoxication: Report of a fatal case. Arch Gen Psychiat 30:112, 1974.

49. Rymer MM, Fishman RA: Protective adaptation of brain to water intoxication. Arch Neurol 28:49, 1973.

50. Schneck SA, Burks JS, Yarnell PR: Ante-

mortem diagnosis of central pontine mye-linolysis. Neurology 28:389, 1978.

51. Sherins RJ, Verity MA: Central pontine myelinolysis associated with acute haem-orrhagic pancreatitis. J Neurol Neurosurg Psychiat 31:583, 1968.

52. Shurtliff LF, Ajax ET, Englert E Jr, et al: Central pontine myelinolysis and cirrhosis of the liver: A report of four cases. Am J Clin Pathol 46:239, 1966.

53. Sima A, Bradvik B: Central pontine mye-linolysis: A case report. Acta Pathol Micro-biol Scand A 84:73, 1976.

54. Summer GL, Smythe McC: Inappropriate antidiuretic hormone secretion. J So Caro-lina Med Assoc 62:455, 1966.

55. Swanson AG, Iseri OA: Acute encephalop-athy due to water intoxication. N Engl J Med 258:831, 1958.

56. Thompson DS, Hutton, JT Sears JC, et al: Coronal computerized tomography in the antemortem diagnosis of central and extra-pontine myelinolysis. Arch Neurol 38:243, 1981.

57. Tomlinson BE, Pierides AM, Bradley WG: Central pontine myelinolysis: Two cases with associated electrolyte disturbance. Q J Med 179:373, 1976.

58. Walters G, Monks PJW, Chitty K: Meta-bolic disturbance due to villous papilloma of the rectum. Br J Surg 47:177, 1959.

59. Warren SE, Mitas JA, Swardlin AHR: Hy-pernatremia in hepatic failure. JAMA 243:1257, 1980.

60. Wasterlain CG, Posner JB: Cerebral edema in water intoxication. I. Clinical and chem-ical observations. Arch Neurol 19:71, 1968.

61. Wasterlain CG, Torack RM: Cerebral edema in water intoxication. II. An ultra-structural study. Arch Neurol 19:79, 1968.

62. Weizman Z, Goitein K, Amit Y, et al: Combined treatment of severe hyponatre-mia due to inappropriate antidiuretic hor-mone secretion. Pediatrics 69:610, 1982.

63. Welti W: Delirium with low serum so-dium. Arch Neurol Psychiat 76:559, 1956.

64. Wright DG, Laureno R, Victor M: Pontine and extrapontine myelinolysis. Brain 102:361, 1979.

65. Wynn V, Rob CG: Water intoxication: Dif-ferential diagnosis of the hypotonic syn-dromes. Lancet 1:587, 1954.

# The Case for Rapid Correction

Gary D. Dubois, M.D.
Allen I. Arieff, M.D.

## ETIOLOGY AND PATHOGENESIS OF HYPONATREMIA

Hyponatremia may be either acute or chronic, and total body water may be either high, low, or normal. The pathophysiology of the different types has been discussed in several review articles,[24,41,48] and lists of its causes often span several pages. In general, nine major etiologic groups may be defined depending on both the patient's volume status, and the underlying causes. If there is extracellular fluid (ECF) volume depletion, losses of fluid can be either (a) renal or (b) extrarenal. Hyponatremia can then occur when the patient ingests hypotonic fluid. If the ECF volume is clinically judged to be normal or only modestly decreased, hyponatremia is probably related to either (c) hormone deficiency (hypothyroidism, Addison's Disease), (d) hormone excess (antidiuretic hormone), (e) drugs which inhibit the ability of the kidney to excrete water, or (f) postsurgical nonosmotic stimuli to retain water. If the ECF volume is expanded, hyponatremia is usually associated with (g) hepatic cirrhosis, nephrotic syndrome, or congestive heart failure, or (h) acute or chronic renal failure. In a more simplistic sense, hyponatremia is almost always associated with dilution, as it is nearly impossible to lose body fluid (such as urine, diarrhea, emesis) which is

hypertonic with respect to the plasma sodium. (i) Acute water intoxication is an extreme case of dilution, where there is administration of water (usually as intravenous 280 mmol/L glucose in water) at a time when there is impairment in the ability of the kidney to excrete water.

Any discussion of the therapy of hyponatremia must include both the underlying cause, as well as the duration, of the hyponatremia. In many types of hyponatremia, therapy must be primarily directed at the underlying disease state. Even with very low levels of plasma sodium, volume expanded patients with hepatic cirrhosis, congestive heart failure, or nephrotic syndrome will probably not derive benefit from treatment with hypertonic NaCl. In such patients, there is probably a primary stimulus for renal retention of sodium and water.[41] Patients with extrarenal losses or redistribution of body fluid (diarrhea, emesis, third space) may respond with elevations of plasma antidiuretic hormone (ADH). When such individuals then ingest hypotonic fluid, they may retain water and develop hyponatremia. Such a sequence frequently occurs after surgery, and affected individuals may benefit from treatment with hypertonic NaCl.[42,53,55] In clinical practice, hyponatremia is frequently observed following surgery. Increased ADH activity may be due to volume depletion secondary to blood loss, as well as various combinations of emesis, nasogastric suction, prior diuretic administration, and decreased dietary sodium intake, or other nonosmotic stimuli, such as pain, anxiety, or fear. When postsurgical patients are given predominantly hypotonic fluids, hyponatremia may occur, which may be fatal.[3,22,42,53] Another group of patients who may develop acute symptomatic hyponatremia are those with the syndrome of inappropriate secretion of antidiuretic hormone (SIADH) who ingest or are given large quantities of water.[20] Such patients are often symptomatic from their hyponatremia, and therapy with hypertonic NaCl must be considered.

In patients who have hormone deficiencies which may predispose to hyponatremia (hypothyroidism, adrenal insufficiency), treatment should be directed primarily at the underlying disorder.[30] If the hyponatremia is symptomatic, NaCl should be administered along with the appropriate replacement hormone, and in myxedema or Addison's disease, 154 mmol/L NaCl is usually sufficient, since the plasma sodium is rarely below 125 mmol/L, and therapy with hypertonic NaCl is rarely required.

There are a vast number of pharmacologic agents which interfere with the ability of the kidney to excrete a water load. Several review articles have elucidated these drugs.[24,33,40] Included are large numbers of sedatives, hypnotics, analgesics, oral hypoglycemic agents, tranquilizers, antidepressants, antipsychotic agents, narcotics, and antineoplastic drugs. Hyponatremia associated with these agents may be acute, is often symptomatic, and may require treatment with hypertonic NaCl. Hyponatremia in association with these drugs occurs when patients ingest (or are given) water in excess of the ability of the kidney to excrete it. Such a sequence is actually quite common among psychotic patients who are taking some of the above agents.[5,10,21,38] Se-

vere water intoxication may also occur in psychotic individuals who are not taking such drugs.[17,26,37,52]

Postsurgical water intoxication is actually both quite common and preventable, and the pathogenesis will now be reviewed. During the era (1940–1960) when the fluid of choice for postsurgical intravenous therapy was primarily 280 mmol/L dextrose and water, a number of reports emphasized the risk of symptomatic water intoxication postoperatively.[16,42,53,55] Initial symptoms consisted of lethargy or agitation with weakness and disorientation. Sixty-four percent of patients experienced convulsions, the majority occurring within 2 days of surgery, and 50 percent manifested coma. The mean age was 67 years old (38 to 88 years old) suggesting that older patients are at greater risk.

The mean serum sodium was 114 mmol/L (range 94 to 126) in 30 patients who had neurologic manifestations. Factors found to predispose to postoperative water intoxication were older age, a long extensive operation, preoperative sodium depletion, postoperative oliguria (even without development of azotemia) and the use of up to 4 L of salt-free intravenous solutions per day during and after the operation.

Several factors which often occur postoperatively act to prevent normal free-water excretion. If hypotonic fluid intake exceeds solute and water losses, hyponatremia will occur. The degree of hyponatremia can be accurately accounted for by assessment of intake, output, and insensible losses in most patients.[54] However, balance studies in the setting of severe hyponatremia (below 114 mmol/L) may actually underestimate the true fall in serum sodium by up to 50 percent. In a number of published series of postoperative hyponatremia, the decrement in serum sodium concentration is far greater than would be predicted from records of intake and output.[6,42,55]

Osmotic regulation of ADH secretion is overridden by nonosmotic stimuli for ADH release in the postoperative period. Such stimuli include pain, anxiety, and a decrease in effective ECF volume which is related to fluid sequestration in traumatized tissue. Postoperative oliguria and urinary hyperosmolality can be partially corrected in many but not all patients by the administration of sodium-containing solution.[51] These serve to expand the decreased effective ECF volume and replace external solute losses.[35,51] Water excretion will increase, but hypotonic urine seldom becomes hypotonic until later in the postoperative period (in some cases it takes as long as 12 days). Therefore, despite initiation of a diuresis with saline administration, excessive water loads will still produce hyponatremia and should thus be avoided.

# TREATMENT OF HYPONATREMIA: RELATED FACTORS AND UNDERLYING PRINCIPLES

In general then, there are four classes of patients in whom the decision to treat hyponatremia "rapidly" or "slowly" must be made. These include: (a) The patient who has the syndrome of inappropriate secretion of ADH and has symptomatic hyponatremia; (b) the patient who has symptomatic hyponatremia secondary to water intoxication and either has substantial psychosis[17,37,38] or is taking drugs which limit the ability of the kidney to excrete water,[33] or both; (c) postsurgical patients who have symptomatic hyponatremia, usually due to nonosmotic stimuli to

ADH secretion[40] combined with administration of free water;[6,22,42,53,55] (d) elderly patients who are taking thiazide or thiazide-like diuretics and manifest an idiosyncratic reaction which leads to symptomatic hyponatremia. Such patients develop nausea and emesis and lose both sodium and potassium in the urine such that the hyponatremia is largely due to urinary loss of cation.[4] Such patients may also ingest large quantities of water.[5,8,12,18,23] It is recognized that in virtually any patient with symptomatic hyponatremia, therapy with hypertonic NaCl may have to be considered. Nonetheless, the aforementioned four groups will encompass most such patients encountered in clinical practice.

It should be emphasized that even in the four groups mentioned, hyponatremia per se is not in and of itself a reason to treat with hypertonic NaCl. Patients with serum sodium below 125 mmol/L who are asymptomatic generally do well when treated with water restriction or intravenous 154 mmol/L NaCl.[3] However, patients who are symptomatic and have serum sodium concentrations below 120 mmol/L should probably be treated with hypertonic NaCl. The reasons for such therapy will be elucidated.

The treatment of symptomatic hyponatremia has undergone cyclic oscillations over the past 70 years. Mengoli[31] has analyzed the fluctuation in preferred postoperative fluid management and has shown an alternating preference for saline versus water (280 mmol/L glucose). Similarly, the treatment of symptomatic hyponatremia has oscillated between hypertonic NaCl versus no treatment (water restriction). Recently, it has been suggested that treatment of symptomatic hyponatremia with hypertonic NaCl may lead to a rare neurological disorder called central pontine myelinolysis (CPM). A description of CPM, its presumed pathogenesis, and any possible relationship to hyponatremia may shed some light on this association.

### Does Hyponatremia or Its Correction Cause Central Pontine Myelinolysis?

**Clinical Studies.** Central pontine myelinolysis was first described in 1959,[1] in patients who were both alcoholic and malnourished. The lesion involved the center of the basis pontis and often extended from midbrain to nerves in the lower pons. Most medullary sheaths were destroyed within the area of the lesion. The destruction of myelin involved all tracts, regardless of site of origin, termination, or function. However, in contrast to the complete destruction of myelin, the axis cylinders, nerve cells, and blood vessels were relatively well preserved. For detailed descriptions of the pathology, the reader is referred to several reviews.[1,39,47] Apparently, there are a large number of reported cases where extrapontine lesions are present which differ from those lesions present in the pons.[50] Extrapontine demyelinating lesions may frequently be anoxic in nature, and may not be related to CPM. The clinical characteristics of CPM may be quite variable and among patients with documented CPM the clinical manifestations may be minimal to absent.[11,19,46] In the original description,[1] patients had flaccid quadriplegia, facial weakness, inability to speak and swallow, and impaired response to painful stimuli. Facial and tongue weakness were thought to be pseudobulbar phenomena. The symptoms apparently vary according to the extent of the lesion, and in some cases, small lesions in the mid-pons may give rise to minimal symptomatology.[11] At the present time, over 170 cases have been described. At least 60 percent have a history of alcoholism and the remainder have a variety of severe debilitating medical illness, including cancer, lymphoma, leukemia, sepsis, and severe malnutrition. An association with hyponatremia has been noted by several investigators, but this association is by no means universal.[50] Messert and associates[32] reviewed 110 cases of CPM and of these, only 20 (18 percent) had hyponatremia (defined in this review as a serum sodium below 128 mmol/L). In another review of 62 patients with CPM,[9] 23 patients (37 percent) had hyponatremia. Thus, the majority of patients with CPM do not have hyponatremia. It must be mentioned that many patients with CPM have had underlying diseases (such as cirrhosis) which were also commonly associated with hyponatremia. Of the 110 cases reviewed by Messert,[32] six actually had hypernatremia.

It has also been suggested that CPM may be somehow associated with the "overly rapid" treatment of hyponatremia.[34,47] The data in humans that might suggest such a relationship are somewhat scanty. In the 110 patients reviewed by Messert and associates,[32] although 18 percent had hyponatremia, only four of the 110 had a history of "rapid" correction of the hyponatremia, while none of 62 patients (37 percent had hyponatremia) reviewed by Burcar and associates[9] had been so treated. In another study,[47] two patients had their serum sodium concentration elevated from a mean of 100 mmol/L to 131 mmol/L over 3½ case days, a mean rate of increase only 0.4 mmol/L each hour. By either current standards, or those of 15 to 30 years ago, such a rate of correction is actually quite slow.[3,5,6,20,53] Furthermore, both of these patients had plasma sodium of 100 mmol/L. Preliminary data from our laboratory[16] show that rabbits with serum sodium concentration below 110 mmol/L have a mortality of 81 percent and in dogs with a similar degree of hyponatremia, mortality is at least 63 percent.[28] Thus the patients described by Tomlinson et al.[47] may have died from the hyponatremia per se, and

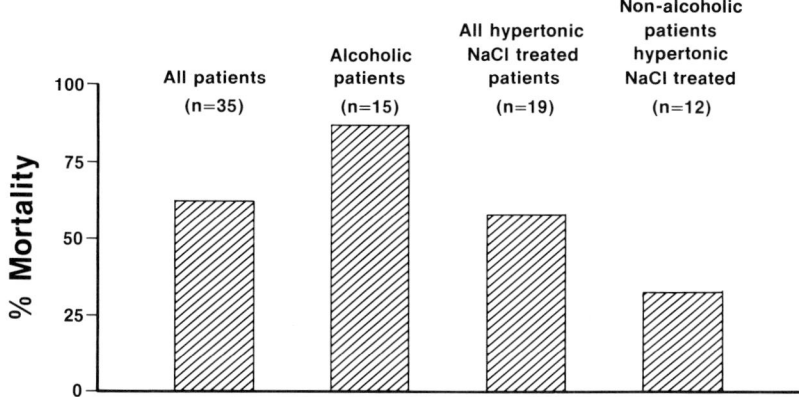

**Fig. 11-7.** This figure shows the mortality for patients whose serum sodium concentration was 105 mM or less. The overall mortality was 63 percent but among alcoholic and cachectic subjects, the mortality was 86 percent. Among relatively healthy subjects who were not alcoholic and cachectic, did not have debilitating medical illness, and were treated with hypertonic NaCl, the mortality was 33 percent. Data were taken from references 3, 4, 5, 7, 9, 14, 17, 22, 23, 26, 29, 34, 37, 38, 42, 44, 47, 50, 55.

had CPM for other reasons. Norenberg and associates reviewed the records of 12 patients with CPM.[34] Only nine of 12 had been hyponatremic, and virtually all had either chronic alcoholism or another condition frequently associated with CPM. In 11 of 12, the serum sodium concentration had been elevated to hypernatremic levels (range of 147 to 160 mM). In contrast to a "control" group who also had hyponatremia but was not treated with hypertonic NaCl, four of 12 patients had serum Na below 102 mM, a condition in which survival is infrequent whatever the therapy (Fig. 11-7;[14,22,29,37,42,47]). In the patients with CPM, and those who had "hyponatremia" without CPM, eight of 21 either did not have levels of hyponatremia which might have required hypertonic NaCl therapy (serum sodium of 120 mM or less), or were never corrected to a serum sodium level above 128 mM. Among the remaining 13 patients (seven with CPM; six without CPM), the time required to raise serum sodium above 128 mM was not different. In seven patients with CPM it was (± S.D.) 1.7 ± 1.3 days, versus

the value of 2.0 ± 1.4 days in six patients without CPM (NS). Thus, the evidence that "overly rapid" correction of hyponatremia might have led to the CPM observed in these patients is minimal. However, the study suggests that elevation of serum sodium concentration in alcoholic/malnourished patients to hypernatremic levels may predispose to CPM.

In summary, CPM is a demyelinating lesion of the pons which was initially described in alcoholic and/or malnourished individuals.[1] Subsequently, it has been described in over 170 patients, virtually all of whom either had some chronic debilitating medical illness, were malnourished, were chronic alcoholics, or some combination thereof. The symptoms of CPM range from a fulminent neurological picture with quadriplegia, inability to swallow and other pseudobulbar phenomena[1,47] to an almost asymptomatic clinical picture with incidental findings at autopsy.[19,46] A positive clinical diagnosis is very difficult, with a diagnostic accuracy which may be as low as 2 percent.[19] A distinct minority of patients with CPM have had hyponatremia,[9,32] many have in fact been hypernatremic,[32,34] and less than 4 percent have had "overly rapid" correction of hyponatremia with hypertonic NaCl. Thus, in clinical studies available at this time, the association between CPM and either hyponatremia or its therapy must be regarded as unproven. The relevant animal studies will now be reviewed.

**Animal Studies.** There are several studies in laboratory animals where the relationships among hyponatremia, its therapy, and the possible development of CPM have been investigated. In one study, Kleinschmidt-DeMasters and Norenberg[25] made rats acutely hyponatremic with subcutaneous vasopressin (10 units/kg) and intraperitoneal 140 mM glucose (5 percent body weight) both administered five times over 72 hours. Mean serum sodium concentration ($\pm$ S.D.) fell from 139 $\pm$ 3 to 106 $\pm$ 12 mM. Animals then were given 1000 mM NaCl (20 ml/kg) twice in 24 hours, and survivors were killed after 8 to 10 days. Mean serum sodium concentration rose from 106 to 152 mM in about 25 hours. During this interval, the rats lost 26 percent of body weight. Control animals were also made hyponatremic (plasma sodium 100 $\pm$ 4 mM) and "self-corrected" to 136 $\pm$ 4 mM in five days. Demyelinating lesions were found only in rats treated with hypertonic (5.8 percent) NaCl. The lesions did not occur in the pons, but did occur in eight other parts of the brain.

In evaluating the aforementioned study, it must be pointed out that rats which developed demyelinating lesion were "corrected" to grossly hypernatremic levels (152 mM) while controls were only corrected to 136 mM. Also, the substantial weight loss (26 percent of body weight) indicates marked cachexia, and a possible predilection to develop CPM. Control hyponatremic rats who did not develop CPM had their serum sodium concentrations corrected only to 136 mM rather than 152 mM. In a preliminary study,[5] hy-

ponatremic rats (serum sodium = 110 mM) had their serum Na increased to 132 mM with hypertonic NaCl. None developed CPM. Thus, it appears that elevation of serum sodium concentration to hypernatremic levels against a background of cachexia may lead to CPM, while correction to 130 to 140 mM does not. To assume otherwise is to ascribe some "toxic" properties to hypertonic NaCl, for which the evidence in man is quite dubious (see Figs. 11-8,11-9). In both dogs and rats, infusion of hypertonic NaCl to normal animals did not result in CPM.[25,28]

In another study, Laureno[28] produced hyponatremia (serum sodium below 120 mM) in mongrel dogs (mean weight 16kg). The dogs were given daily vasopressin in oil 2.5 – 3.1 units/kg daily, as well as 2000 ml (13 percent body weight) of intraperitoneal water. In 60 dogs, four days of such a regimen produced a mortality of 63 percent, with a mean ($\pm$ S.D.) serum sodium in 16 survivors of 108 $\pm$ 14 mM. Six dogs (serum sodium 101 $\pm$ 5mM) were sacrificed and studied after four days of water and vasopressin —none had CPM. Sixteen dogs received 514 mM NaCl, 50 to 200 ml over 6 hours plus water restriction. Five dogs improved neurologically and did not have CPM, while five deteriorated neurologically and had either CPM (four dogs) or extrapontine myelinolysis (one dog). There are several rather striking differences, in that the four dogs who developed CPM had, prior to therapy, a serum Na of 100 $\pm$ 4 mM, while the six without CPM had serum sodium of 121 $\pm$ 14 mM (p < .05). Five of six with myelinolysis were "corrected" to hypertonic (serum sodium 142–157 mM) levels. From a preliminary publication, it is clear that the dogs were severely malnourished, as is often the case in patients who develop CPM. Dogs who were sacrificed after four days of water intoxication did not have time to develop the lesions of CPM.

One must also consider the possible

**Fig. 11-8.** This figure compares the mortality of symptomatic hyponatremia (serum sodium of 120 mM or less) among patients who were treated "rapidly" with hypertonic NaCl such that serum sodium concentration was increased at a mean rate of 2 mmol/L/hr, versus patients who were treated "slowly" (with fluid restriction, isotonic NaCl, or small quantities of hypertonic NaCl) such that serum sodium concentration was increased at a rate of less than 0.6 mmol/L/hr. In some of the "slowly" treated patients, serum sodium concentration was never increased above 128 mM. For an explanation of where the rates for "rapid" versus "slow" correction were derived, see text. Data are from references, 6, 26, 29, 44, 53, 55 for "rapid" correction) and 3, 4, 34, 36, 45, 47 for "slow" correction.

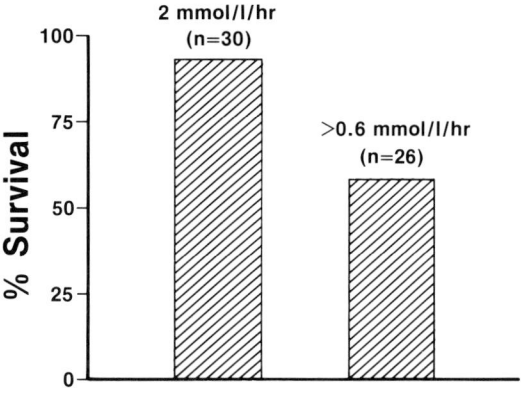

effects of truly massive doses of vasopressin in both animal studies.[25,28] Animals were given either 2.5 to 3.1 or 20 units/kg/day of vasopressin, equivalent to 150 to 1200 units in a 60 kg human. The usual maintenance dose in man is 10 to 30 units/day. Vasopressin is a very potent vasoconstrictive agent, and such massive doses may lead to cerebral vasoconstriction, which could be increased by subsequent fluid retention. In fact, all the demyelinating lesions seen in the rats were extrapontine, which are often associated with hypoxia.[50]

Overall then, the animal studies suggest that elevation of very low (below 105 mM) plasma sodium concentration to hypernatremic levels (above 140 mmol) with hypertonic NaCl, when superimposed upon a background of malnutrition plus massive vasopressin administration, may induce demyelinating lesions. How such studies relate to more modest correction of plasma sodium concentration to subnormal levels (approximately 130 mM) in reasonably healthy subjects who have not received massive doses of vasopressin is unclear.

## Effects of Hyponatremia on the Central Nervous System

Having reviewed CPM and its possible relationship to hyponatremia, we will

**Fig. 11-9.** This figure shows the survival of symptomatic hyponatremia (serum sodium concentration of 120 mM or less among patients who were treated with hypertonic NaCl in two different eras (1973–1982 and 1951–1965). Among all patients so treated, the mean rate of increase in serum sodium concentration was 2 mmol/L/hr. Patients with a history of alcoholism and/or cachexia are not included. The overall survival for all patients excedes 90 percent and no patient developed central pontine myelinolysis. Data were taken from references 3, 4, 5, 6, 20, 38, 26, 29, 44, 53, 55.

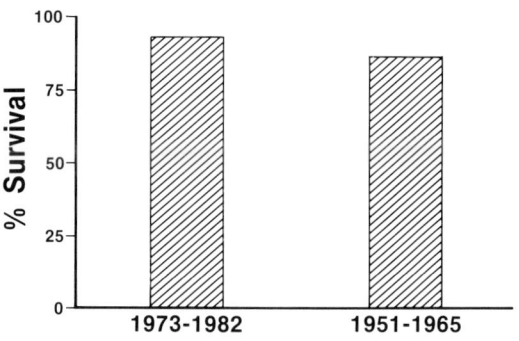

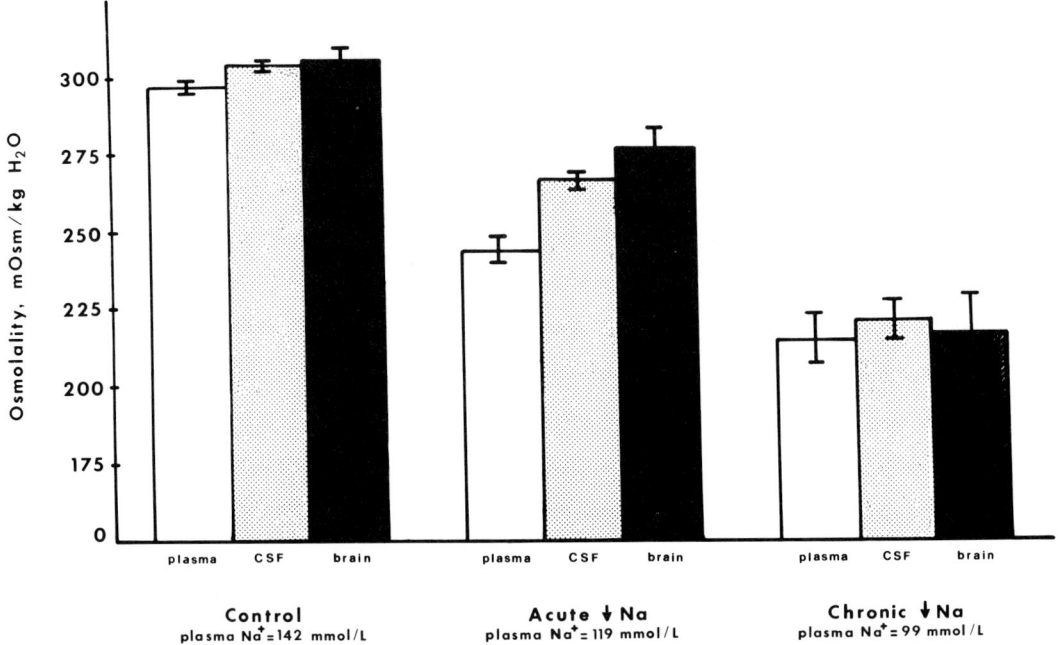

**Fig. 11-10.** This figure shows osmolalities of plasma, cerebrospinal fluid (CSF) and brain (cerebral cortex) in normal rabbits and those with acute hyponatremia. Rapid lowering of serum sodium concentration induces and osmotic gradient between brain and blood which favors the movement of water into the brain. In chonic hyponatremia, osmolalities of plasma, CSF and brain are not significantly different. (From Alfrey AC, Miller NL, Butkus D: Evaluation of body magnesium stores. J Lab Clin Med 84:153, 1974).

briefly review the effects of hyponatremia on the central nervous system. This will enable us to have a better understanding of the possible effects of therapy, without considering a possible complicating effect of CPM. Much of the literature relating to effects of hyponatremia on brain water and electrolytes has been recently summarized.[13] The results are variable, depending on the animal model studied and level of plasma sodium concentration reached. In general, with acute water intoxication, an osmotic gradient is induced where brain osmolality exceeds that of plasma, resulting in a gradient which favors movement of water into the brain (Fig. 11-10). The more acute the hyponatremia, the more pronounced the gain of brain water. When plasma sodium concentration is lowered to 119 mM in two hours, there is a 17 percent increase in brain water. With the same degree of hyponatremia in three and a half days, there is only a 7 percent increase in brain water. Even after 17 days with serum sodium of 99 mM, brain water is still 7 percent above control values (Fig. 11-11). The brain adapts to chronic hyponatremia by lowering its cellular osmolality. This is accomplished by a loss of electrolytes[3] and perhaps amino acids as well. Even after only two hours of hyponatremia, there is some loss of brain content of sodium, potassium, and chloride, while after 3½ days to 2½ weeks of hyponatremia, the loss of electrolytes is almost identical to the observed decrement in brain osmolality.[3] Thus, survival in acute hyponatremia depends on the ability of the brain to lower its intracellular osmolality by extruding electrolytes, rather than gaining water, the latter of course can lead to brain swelling and herniation.[3] In patients with hyponatremia, it can be assumed that the brain cell content of sodium, potassium and chloride is low and brain water is modestly elevated. The possible effects of any therapy must be evaluated against such a background.

Experimentally, the brain, in contrast to other tissues, does not behave as a perfect osmometer. In both hyper- and hypoosmolar states, the brain will gain or lose less water than will other tissues, such as skeletal muscle.[15] In fact, an osmotic gradient of at least 20 mOsm/kg between plasma and brain appears to be necessary to promote an acute net loss or gain of water from the brain.[2] Thus, treatment of hyponatremia with water restriction or infusion of 154 mM NaCl would not be expected to acutely shrink an already swollen brain. When confronted with a patient who has acute hyponatremia, brain edema and threatened herniation, these principles must be considered.

# CLINICAL OUTCOME OF THERAPY

## Effect of Alcoholism/Malnutrition on Mortality

In considering the general concepts underlying the treatment of symptomatic hyponatremia, certain principles seem pertinent. It must be borne in mind that alcoholic and cachectic subjects probably represent a special case. If one reviews the literature describing patients with symptomatic hyponatremia with serum sodium concentrations of 120 mM or less, most are represented by 144 cases in 29 articles. Of these patients, 36 had either chronic alcoholism, malnutrition, or cachexia and their mean (± S.D.) serum sodium was 109 ± 8 mM. The other 108

patients had essentially the same serum sodium concentration of 110 ± 8mM. However, mortality in the alcoholic and cachectic subjects was 67 percent, essentially twice that seen in the other patients (Fig. 11-12). The mortality of severe hyponatremia (serum sodium below 106 mM), was 86 percent in alcoholic subjects, versus only 33 percent in other patients. Thus, alcoholic and cachectic subjects have a hyponatremia-associated mortality which increases when lower values of serum sodium are achieved, whereas other patients may not (Figs. 11-7 and 11-12).

In general, relatively healthy patients with symptomatic hyponatremia (serum sodium of 120 mM or less) have a reported mortality of approximately 33 percent, whatever the therapy. Alcoholic and cachectic subjects have a mortality of approximately 67 percent when their mean plasma sodium concentration is 109 ± 8 mM; mortality increases to 86 percent when mean plasma sodium concentration is 105 mM or less (Fig. 11-7). Any effects of therapy must be considered against such a background.

## Mortality of Severe Hyponatremia and Effects of Treatment

With the foregoing in mind, the case for "slow" versus "rapid" correction of hyponatremia will now be considered. In general, many physicians do not employ hypertonic NaCl to treat symptomatic hyponatremia because of the presumed hazards of circulatory overload. At the present time, it would appear that the major argument for "slow" correction of symptomatic hyponatremia is the possible development of CPM. Although a possible association between hyponatremia and CPM had been suggested in the 1960s (see references 3,5,6,7,9 in Messert et al.), it was a report by Tomlinson, Pierides, and Bradley[47] that strongly suggested that

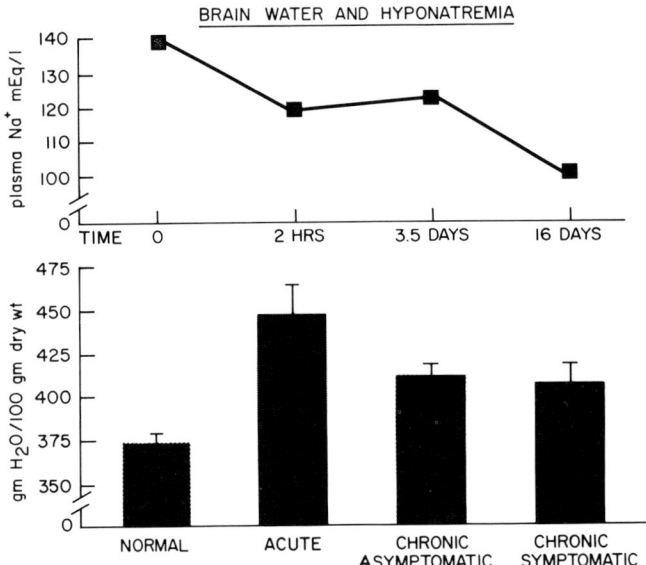

BRAIN WATER AND HYPONATREMIA

**Fig. 11-11.** This figure compares serum sodium concentration with brain water content and the resultant symptomatology. In rabbits with acute hyponatremia, serum sodium is 119 mM, there is brain edema, and all animals develop seizures and died. With the same serum sodium concentration induced over 3.5 days, animals are not symptomatic, do not have seizures and brain water is much less. With chronic hyponatremia for 2.5 weeks, animals are symptomatic and brain water remains about 7 percent above control values. Data are from reference 3.

hypertonic (514 mM) NaCl given to a hyponatremic patient might somehow cause CPM. Their report described two women in their mid 50's with nausea and vomiting for 1½ to 3 weeks and a gradual onset of diminished sensorium. The serum sodium was 100 mM in both. Both received 514 mM NaCl (amounts are not given) and their serum sodium concentrations were raised to values in excess of 130 mM over a mean period of 3½ days. The duration of hyponatremia prior to therapy is not known, but could have been as long as five days. Both patients had their plasma sodium eventually corrected to a mean of 140 mM, and neither ever regained consciousness. They died after five weeks and seven months of coma and at autopsy, both had CPM. In analyzing these cases, it appears likely that both patients eventually died due to brain damage from their hyponatremia. As shown in Figure 11-7 among all patients with serum sodium concentrations below 105 mM, regardless of therapy, the overall mortality is 63 percent. These data represent a nearly complete literature review of 35 cases from 20 articles. Among the 13 patients who survived, eight were treated with hypertonic NaCl, one with isotonic NaCl, one with 50 percent glucose, one with fluid restriction and in two, treatment is not known. Among the 22 patients who died, 12 were not treated with hypertonic NaCl while ten received hypertonic NaCl. Among the eight survivors treated with hypertonic NaCl, all were corrected faster than those reported by Tomlinson et al.[47] Thus, a plasma sodium concentration below 105 mmol carries a mortality of 63 percent whatever the therapy, and among 18 such patients treated with hypertonic NaCl, the 58 percent mortality reflects, if anything, a slight reduction. Perhaps more significant is the fact that few if any patients who were not alcoholics and/or malnourished, developed autopsy proven CPM, even though they were rapidly treated with hypertonic NaCl.[4,5,17,22,23,26,29,37,38,44,55] In light of the aforementioned, there appears to be little if any rationale for thinking that in man, rapid treatment of a serum sodium concentration of 105 mM or less with hypertonic NaCl may lead to CPM, as long as the serum sodium concentration is not elevated to hyperatremic levels. Rather, survival is rare unless treatment with hypertonic NaCl is rapidly instituted, while in alcoholic subjects

**Fig. 11-12.** This figure shows the overall mortality for patients with symptomatic hyponatremia whose serum sodium concentration was 120 mM or less. There are 114 cases from 29 articles. The mean serum sodium concentration was 109 mM. Of these 114 cases, 36 patients had either alcoholism or other debilitating medical illness and their mean serum sodium concentration was 109 mM. The mortality was 67 percent in alcoholic and/or cachectic subjects, versus only 33 percent in the other patients. (Data were taken from references 3, 4, 5, 6, 7, 8, 9, 12, 14, 17, 20, 22, 22a, 23, 26, 29, 32, 34, 36, 37, 38, 42, 44, 45, 47, 50, 52, 53, 55).

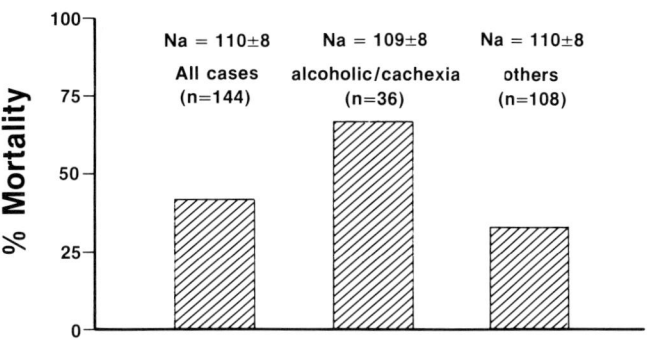

whose serum sodium is 105 mM or less, the overall mortality is 86 percent whatever the therapy.[7,9,14,22a,32,34] In fact, among 12 patients with serum sodium of 105 mM or less who were not alcoholic or malnourished and were treated with hypertonic NaCl, survival was 67 percent. Thus, the two most important factors which determine survival in patients with serum sodium concentrations below 106 mM are the existence of alcoholism and/or malnutrition, and the institution of treatment with hypertonic NaCl. It could be that severe hyponatremia supreimposed upon a background of debilitating medical illness makes the occurrence of CPM more likely, but even this is unclear. It does appear, however, that elevation of serum sodium to hypernatremic levels (above 140 mM) in alcoholic and malnourished subjects may lead to CPM.[34,47] Animal studies also suggest such a sequence.[25]

## Rapid Treatment of Symptomatic Hyponatremia: Past and Present

Having ascertained that rapid correction of severe (serum sodium of 105 mM or less) hyponatremia to about 130 mM

not only does not lead to CPM but, in fact, is probably necessary for survival, we will now examine the case for rapid correction of less severe symptomatic hyponatremia. The definition of "slow" versus "rapid" correction of hyponatremia has to be somewhat arbitrary. Discounting abstracts and single case reports, if one examines five large series of hyponatremic nonalcoholic patients published in the decade 1973 to 1982, there are 30 well studied patients with symptomatic hyponatremia and serum sodium concentrations ($\pm$ S.D.) of 111 $\pm$ 8mM.[3-5,20,38] In the aforementioned five studies, the serum sodium was increased by a mean rate of 1.9 mmol/L/hr, 2.4 mmol/L/hr, 1.8 mmol/L/hr, 0.7 mmol/L/hr and 1.1 mmol/L/hr, respectively, with a mean rate of correction for the 30 patients of 1.9 $\pm$ 0.6 mmol/L/hr. In all 30 patients, correction was halted when serum sodium was between 123 and 135 mM, with a mean correction to 130 mM. The survival among these 30 patients was 93 percent, and the therapy is the most rapid rate of correction described in the world's literature. Among the 30 patients, none manifested any symptoms of CPM. If one then examines the older literature for the 15 year period 1951 to 1965, a similar picture emerges. Discounting abstracts and single case reports, there are at least 35 well studied patients in seven series.[6,26,29,42,44,55] Serum sodium concentration ($\pm$ S.D.) was 109 $\pm$ 11 mM and none of the patients had conditions which predisposed to CPM. The details are less abundant in the older case reports, so we have selected only those cases where adequate information is available. Among 21 of 35 patients from 1951 to 1965 who were treated with hypertonic NaCl, survival was 86 percent overall, which compares favorably to the 93 percent survival recorded in the period 1973 to 1982. Treatment data in the seven series of patients are often incomplete, but good records are available on the rate of correction for 13 patients in six series.[6,26,29,44,53,55] Among these 13 patients, survival was 85 percent, virtually the same as in the group as a whole. The mean rate of increase in serum sodium concentration was 2.0 $\pm$ 1.7 mmol/L/hr for the time required to increase ($\pm$ S.D.) serum sodium concentration from 109 $\pm$ 11 to 130 mM. No patient manifested symptoms suggestive of CPM. Thus, "rapid" correction of symptomatic hyponatremia with hypertonic NaCl at a rate of 2 mmol/L/hr resulted in a survival of 85 percent to 93 percent in two different eras (1951–1965 and 1973–1982). Such data provide overwhelming evidence that rapid correction of symptomatic hyponatremia in nonalcoholic patients (serum sodium concentrations ranging from 84–120 mM) to 130 mM does not, per se, result in CPM.

For the 30 patients with symptomatic hyponatremia in the 1973 to 1982 decade who were corrected "rapidly," the mean $\pm$ 2 S.D. rate of correction was 0.7 to 3.4 mmol/L/hr. Using these figures, we will arbitrarily define "slow" correction of hyponatremia as a rate of 0.6 mmol/L/hr or less. Applying such criteria, it is difficult to find patients who were so treated

in the literature. We have used only those reports where: reasonably complete treatment data are available; patient's initial serum sodium concentration was below 120 mM; the rate of correction to above 125 mM was less than 0.7 mmol/L/hr; patients did not have cirrhosis, congestive heart failure, or Addison's Disease; series were published in the decade 1973 to 1982. There were 32 patients in six series[3,4,34,45,47] whose mean ($\pm$ S.D.) serum sodium concentration was 111 $\pm$ 6 mM. Six of the 32 were alcoholic and all had CPM at autopsy. The overall mortality was 50 percent and among the 26 patients who were not alcoholic, the mortality was 42 percent. in Figure 11-8, we have compared the mortality in nonalcoholic patients who were studied over the same decade (1973–1982), had identical serum sodium concentrations (111 mM) and were treated either "rapidly" (1.9 $\pm$ 0.7 mmol/L/hr or "slowly" (below 0.7 mmol/L/hr). The survival is 93 percent in the "rapidly" treated group, versus 58 percent in those treated "slowly." Central pontine myelinolysis occurred only in alcoholic and malnourished subjects.

## SUMMARY

These data serve to define "slow" versus "rapid" treatment of hyponatremia in symptomatic patients who have: (a) serum sodium concentrations below 120 mM; (b) symptomatic hyponatremia due to any of four general catagories which include syndrome of inappropriate ADH (SIADH), acute water intoxication associated with psychosis or certain drugs, postsurgical patients with water intoxication, thiazide or thiazide-like diuretics. Alcoholic or malnourished subjects with symptomatic hyponatremia seem to represent a special case and should be treated cautiously. The mortality among such patients is high, and may bear little relationship to therapy. As clearly shown in Figures 11-8, 11-9 for nonalcoholics rapid treatment of symptomatic hyponatremia offers the best hope for patient survival.

In general then, the treatment of symptomatic hyponatremia (serum sodium concentrations of 120 mM or less) can be summarized: principles apply only to the four conditions previously enumerated. Such patients should be treated with hypertonic (514 mM) NaCl at a rate of infusion such that serum sodium concentration is raised at a rate of 2 mmol/L/hr until a serum sodium concentration of 125 to 130 mM is achieved. At that time hypertonic NaCl should be discontinued. This regimen may have to be modified in patients with severe renal or cardiac disease. Because of the possible dangers of CPM, the serum sodium concentration should never be increased to hypertonic levels and indeed, should not be elevated acutely above 135 mM. In patients who have symptomatic hyponatremia and have SIADH, serum sodium concentration should be raised at the same rate using a combination of 514 mM NaCl and intravenous furosemide.[20] Such a regimen has been shown to increase survival in patients with symptomatic hyponatremia from an overall value of 58 percent to a value above 95 percent (Fig. 11-9) and has not been shown to produce CPM in either patients or laboratory animals.

# REFERENCES

1. Adams RD, Victor M, Mancall EL: Central pontine myelinolysis: A hitherto undescribed disease occurring in alcoholic and malnourished patients. Arch Neurol Psychiat 81:154, 1959.
2. Arieff, AI, Kleeman CR, Keushkerian A, et al: Brain tissue osmolality: Method of determination and variations in hyper- and hypo-osmolar states. J Lab Clin Med 79:334, 1972.
3. Arieff AI, Llach F, Massry SG: Neurological manifestations and morbidity of hyponatremia: Correlation with brain water and electrolytes. Medicine 55:121, 1976.
4. Ashraf N, Locksley R, Arieff AI: Thiazide-induced hyponatremia associated with death or neurologic damage in outpatients. Am J Med 70:1163, 1981.
5. Ayus JC, Olivero JJ, Frommer JP: Rapid correction of severe hyponatremia with intravenous hypertonic saline solution. Am J Med 72:43, 1982.
5a. Ayus JC, Krothapalli R, Pace E, et al: Safety of rapid correction of severe hyponatremia in Sprague-Dawley rats. Kidney Int 23:117, 1983.
6. Bartholomew LG, Scholz DA: Reversible postoperative neurological symptoms: Report of five cases secondary to water intoxication and sodium depletion. JAMA 162:22, 1956.
7. Berry K, Olszewski J: Central pontine myelinolysis: A case report. Neurology 13:531, 1963.
8. Beresford, HR: Polydipsia, hydrochlorothiazide and water intoxication. JAMA 214:879, 1956.
9. Burcar PJ, Norenberg MD, Yarnell PR: Hyponatremia and central pontine myelinolysis. Neurology 27:223, 1977.
10. Cadnapaphornchai P, Taher S, McDonald FD: Syndrome of inappropriate antidiuretic hormone secretion in chronic schizophrenia. Kidney Int 14:647, 1978.
11. Chason JL, Landers JW, Gonzales JE: Central pontine myelinolysis. J Neurol Neurosurg Psychiat 27:317, 1964.
12. Conger JD, McIntyre JA, Jacoby WJ: Central pontine myelinolysis associated with inappropriate antidiuretic hormone secretion. Am J Med 47:813, 1969.
13. Covey CM, Arieff AI: Disorders of sodium and water metabolism and their effects on the central nervous system. p. 212. In Brenner, BM, Stein JH, Eds: Contemporary Issues in Nephrology. Vol I. New York, Churchill Livingstone, 1978.
14. Demanet JC, Bonnyns M, Stevens-Rocmans C: Coma due to water intoxication in beer drinkers. Lancet 2:1115, 1971.
15. Dila CJ, Pappius HM: Cerebral water and electrolytes: An experimental model of

inappropriate secretion of antidiuretic hormone. Arch Neurol 26:85, 1972.

16. Dubois GD, Leach WJ, Arieff AI: Central pontine myelinolysis and hyponatremia. Clin Res 31:98A, 1983.

17. Dubovsky SL, Grabon S, Berl T, Schrier RW: Syndrome of inappropriate secretion of antidiuretic hormone with exacerbated psychosis. Ann Intern Med 79:551, 1973.

18. Fichman MP, Vorherr H, Kleeman CR, et al: Diuretic-induced hyponatremia. Ann Intern Med 75:853, 1971.

19. Goebel HH, Herman-Ben Zur P: Central pontine myelinolysis: A clinical and pathological study of 10 cases. Brain 95:495, 1972.

20. Hantman D, Rossier B, Zohlman R, et al: Rapid correction of hyponatremia in the syndrome of inappropriate secretion of antidiuretic hormone. Ann Intern Med 78:870, 1973.

21. Hariprasad MK, Eisinger RP, Padmanabhan CS, et al: Reset osmostat associated with hyponatremia and dementia in psychotic patients. Kidney Int 11:653, 1978.

22. Helwig FC, Schultz CB, Curry DE: Water intoxication: Report of a fatal case with clinical, pathological and experimental studies. JAMA 104:1569, 1935.

22a. Hilden T, Svendsen TL: Electrolyte disturbances in beer drinkers. Lancet 2:245, 1975.

23. Kennedy RM, Early LE: Profound hyponatremia resulting from a thiazide-induced decrease in urinary diluting capacity in a patient with primary polydipsia. N Engl J Med 202:1185, 1970.

24. Kleeman CR: Hypo-osmolar syndromes secondary to impaired water excretion. Ann Rev Med 21:259, 1970.

25. Kleinschmidt-DeMasters BK, Norenberg MD: Rapid correction of hyponatremia causes demyelination: Relation to central pontine myelinosis. Science 211:1068, 1981.

26. Langgard H, Smith WO: Self-induced water intoxication without predisposing illness. N Engl J Med 266:378, 1962.

27. Laureno R: Experimental pontine and extrapontine myelinolysis. Trans Am Neurol Assoc 105:354, 1980.

28. Laureno R: Central pontine myelinolysis following rapid correction of hyponatremia. Ann Neurol 13:232, 1983.

29. Lipsmeyer E, Ackerman GL: Irreversible brain damage after water intoxication. JAMA 196:286, 1966.

30. Macaron C, Famuyiwa O: Hyponatremia of hypothyroidism. Arch Intern Med 138:820, 1978.

31. Mengoli LR: Excerpts from the history of postoperative fluid therapy. Am J Surg 121:311, 1971.

32. Messert B, Orrison WW, Hawkins MJ, et al: Central pontine myelinolysis. Neurology 29:147, 1979.

33. Miller M, Moses A: Drug-induced states of impaired water excretion. Kidney Int 10:96, 1976.

34. Norenberg MD, Leslie KO, Robertson AS: Association between rise in serum sodium and central myelinolysis. Ann Neurol 11: 128, 1982.

35. Randall RE, Papper S: Mechanism of postoperative limitation in sodium excretion: The role of extracellular fluid volume and of adrenal cortical activity, J Clin Invest 37:1628, 1958.

36. Raskind M: Psychosis, polydipsia, and water intoxication: Report of a fatal case. Arch Gen Psychiatry 30:112, 1974.

37. Rendell M, McGrane D, Cuesta M: Fatal compulsive water drinking. JAMA 240: 2557, 1978.

38. Rosenbaum JF, Rothman JS, Murray GB: Psychosis and water intoxication. J Clin Psychiatry 40:287, 1979.

39. Schneck SA: Central pontine myelinolysis. In Minckler J. Ed: Pathology of the Nervous System. Vol I. New York, McGraw-Hill Book, 1968, p 859.

40. Schrier RW, Berl T: Nonosmolar factors affecting renal water excretion. N Engl J Med 292:81, 1975.

41. Schrier RW, Berl T: Disorders of water metabolism. In Schrier RW, Ed: Renal and Electrolyte Disorders. 2nd ed. Boston, Little, Brown, Boston, 1980, p 1.

42. Scott JC, Welch JS, Berman IB: Water intoxication and sodium depletion in surgical patients. Obstet Gynecol 26:168, 1965.

43. Stormont JM, Waterhouse C: The genesis of hyponatremia associated with marked

overhydration and water intoxication. Circulation 24:191, 1961.

44. Swanson AG, Iseri OA: Acute encephalopathy due to water intoxication. N Engl J Med 258:831, 1958.

45. Telfer RB, Miller EM: Central pontine myelinolysis following hyponatremia, demonstrated by computerized tomography. Ann Neurol 6:455, 1979.

46. Tihen WS: Central pontine myelinolysis and Rosenthal fibers of the brainstem. Neurology 22:710, 1972.

47. Tomlinson BE, Pierides AM, Bradley WG: Central pontine myelinolysis. Q J Med 65:373, 1976.

48. Weitzman R, Kleeman CR: Water metabolism and the neurohypophyseal hormones: Hypo-osmolar syndromes. In Maxwell MH, Kleeman CR, Eds: Clinical Disorders of Fluid and Electrolyte Metabolism. New York, McGraw-Hill, 1980, p 615.

49. Wiederholt WC, Kobayashi RM, Stockard JJ, et al: Central pontine myelinolysis: A clinical reappraisal. Arch Neurol 34:220, 1977.

50. Wright DG, Laureno R, Victor M: Pontine and extrapontine myelinolysis. Brain 102:361, 1979.

51. Wright HK, Gann DS: Correction of defect in free water excretion in postoperative patients by extracellular fluid volume expansion. Ann Surg 158:70, 1963.

52. Wright R: Overdosing on water. p. 46, Newsweek, Mar 14, 1977.

53. Wynn V, Rob CG: Water intoxication. Lancet 1:587, 1954.

54. Wynn V, Houghton BJ: Observations in man upon the osmotic behaviour of the body cells after trauma. Q J Med 26:375, 1957.

55. Zimmerman B, Wangensteen OH: Observation on water intoxication in surgical patients. Surgery 31:654, 1952.

# 12

# The Role of High-Dose Steroids in Nephritic Syndromes

# The Case for a More Conservative Approach

## Richard J. Glassock, M.D.

## INTRODUCTION

As with any debate, it is helpful to carefully define the territorial limits of the topic before launching into a discussion of the merits of one's particular point of view. In this context, I will define *"high-dose" steroids* as the administration of glucocorticoids, as methylprednisolone, in individual doses equal to or greater than 15 mg/kg to either adults or children. This form of treatment is also known as "pulse" or "megadose" therapy. Courses of treatment usually consist of an intravenous infusion of methylprednisolone lasting 30 minutes to several hours and repeating the "pulse" daily for every other day for 3 to 7 times. The usual total dose of methylprednisolone administered to adults over a course of "pulse" therapy is 3 to 10 g, averaging about 6 g. Following completion of the course, oral glucocorticoids are often continued at approximately 1 to 2 mg/kg on alternate days for variable lengths of time depending upon the clinical response. In some circumstances (e.g., multisystem disease and necrotizing vasculitis), oral cytotoxic or cytostatic drugs such as cyclophosphamide or azathioprine are added to the oral glucocorticoid regimen.

For the purpose of this discussion, *nephritic syndromes* will encompass those primary and multisystem disorders in which glomerular inflammation leads to depression of the glomerular filtration rate and increased excretion rates of pro-

tein and erythrocytes. The individual pathologic entities encompassed by this definition which will be discussed here include crescentic glomerulonephritis, membranoproliferative glomerulonephritis, lupus nephritis, and systemic necrotizing vasculitis.

One overriding characteristic of the available information bearing on the question posed in this debate is that prospective, randomized controlled studies of the safety and efficacy of "high-dose" glucocorticoid therapeutic regimens as compared to lower oral prednisone treatment are not presently available for the nephritic syndromes. The analyses must, therefore, be confined to examination of the clinical course of patients treated with "high-dose" glucocorticoids (as defined above) compared to historical controls from the literature or compared to patients from the same center who for one reason or another (often unspecified) were untreated or who received other modalities of therapy. Although the lack of prospective and randomized studies considerably complicates the analysis and renders any conclusion, either favoring therapy or denying its effectiveness, unquestionably suspect, this should not dissuade us from attempting to evaluate the reported claims of efficacy in an attempt to sharpen the focus of the debate. We must be mindful of the fact that the literature reports in and of themselves tend to be the results of a selection process in that unfavorable outcomes or evidence of a

lack of efficacy of newly proposed therapeutic strategies often surface only many
years after the initial claims of "significant
benefits." Furthermore, the literature is
replete with examples of "successful"
treatment regimens based on small numbers of cases which were followed for relatively brief periods of times which after
more prolonged follow-up became much
less impressive in terms of overall effectiveness. Short-term follow-up studies often must rely on endpoints of dubious or
unproven value for the identification of
long-term reversal of disease processes.
For example, one might question whether
a reported 30 percent increase in endogenous creatinine clearance over baseline
pretreatment values will ultimately be
translated into long-term freedom from
the necessity for regular dialysis treatment.

## THE RATIONALE OF HIGH-DOSE GLUCOCORTICOID THERAPY

The notion that high-dose glucocorticoid therapy might be of value in the
treatment of renal disease was originally
derived from clinical experiences in renal
allograft recipients. Bell and coworkers[2]
reported in an uncontrolled study that
1.0 g boluses of intravenous methylprednisolone repeated three times over 4 to 5
days reversed 86 percent of the initial rejection episodes in renal allograft recipients. This early experience lead to rapid
and uncritical acceptance of a "pulse" regimen into many transplant programs.
Years later, several randomized and prospective studies have failed to clearly
demonstrate any superiority of "pulse"
therapy in the reversal of renal allograft
rejection as compared to oral prednisone given in doses of 3 to 4 mg/kg/day
for similar periods of time.[1,9,21,27,28,34,39,40]
Some studies even suggested an adverse
effect of high-dose glucocorticoids on re-

nal morphology and patient survival, particularly when intravenous methylprednisolone dosages in excess of 5 g were used.
Furthermore, sudden death due to cardiac
arrythmias have been reported in association with bolus methylprednisolone therapy in renal allograft recipients.[33]

Since *oral prednisone* is rapidly absorbed and efficiently converted to the
metabolically active *prednisolone*,[19,32] there
is no theoretic advantage of the use of intravenous prednisolone in these circumstances. The half-life of prednisolone in
the circulation is relatively short (usually
180 to 240 minutes) and with very high
doses steriod binding sites on serum albumin and transcortin are undoubtedly saturated giving rise to high levels of free
prednisolone.[18,22] According to pharmacokinetic studies carried out in children,
peak plasma prednisolone levels of about
100 µg/dl would be predicted to be obtained by a dose of 3 mg/kg of oral
prednisone.[22] The metabolic clearance rate
of prednisolone averages about 80 L/day
and tends to increase to 100 L/day or
above as the dose administered is increased, probably by affecting the ratio of
bound to unbound fraction and the volume of distribution.[18,22,32] The freely dif-
fusable, unbound fraction of predno-
solone is likely responsible for the
intracellular events accounting for the
antiinflammatory and antiproliferative effects of glucocorticoids.[20,23,26] These effects are believed to underly the putative
beneficial effect of steriods on glomerulonephritic diseases. Since many of these
actions do not display a clear-cut dose-dependent relationship,[14,16] it is difficult to
envision how 15 mg/kg or more of intravenous methylprednisolone would produce a more dramatic effect than 3 to 4
mg/kg or oral prednisone,[14] unless a population of cells and/or mediators resistant
to levels of free prednisolone readily obtained by oral prednisone doses of 3 to 4
mg/kg participate in disease processes responsible for nephritic syndromes.

The effects of glucocorticoid on aspects of the inflammatory process and immunological systems are many and varied and the mechanisms by which glucocorticoids beneficially alter disease states are not entirely understood. In the context of these putative beneficial effects on glomerulonephritis, several points can be summarized and emphasized. Glucocorticoids result in transient T-lymphocytopenia, largely the result of redistribution of pools of T-lymphocytes into tissue sites and later because of an antiproliferative effect.[11,17] The thymus undergoes involution and T-lymphocyte dependent areas of lymph nodes become atrophic. Monocytes are particularly vulnerable to the action of glucocorticoids whereas polymorphonuclear leukocytes are relatively resistant.[24] Monocyte chemotaxis is greatly reduced and the secretion of monokines may be impaired.[11,16,43] The differential effects of glucocorticoids on monocytes and polymorphonuclear leukocytes may underly their putative beneficial effects in glomerulonephritis, as some glomerulonephritic lesions seem to be highly dependent on monocyte infiltration.[24,30] Within inflammatory cells, glucocorticoids bind to nuclear receptors and rapidly induce changes in chromatin structure.[26] New RNA and cellular protein synthesis is stimulated. One of the glucocorticoid stimulated proteins (macrocortin) has potent phospholipase $A_2$ inhibiting properties.[3,23] Thus, one of the major antiinflammatory effects of glucocorticoids may be mediated by a reduction in arachidonic acid availability through the phospholipase inhibiting action of the glucocorticoid-dependent macrocortin. Inhibition of the local production of arachidonic acid metabolites (prostaglandins, leukotrienes) might be expected to have dramatic effects on permeability, vasomotor reactivity, and local immunologic function. Finally, glucocorticoids may stabilize lysosome membranes and inhibit the release of lysosomal hydrolases and proteinases, thus limiting local structural damage by these intracellular enzymes.[20] Notwithstanding these effects of glucocorticoids, it bears repeating that there is a paucity of information supporting the notion that differences exist in the ability of glucocorticoids to induce these changes across the dose ranges encompassed by "high-dose" versus conventional dose glucocorticoid therapy.[16] A recent editorial discussing the merits of "high-dose" glucocorticoid therapy in collagen-vascular diseases stated that "studies do not, however, make a case for huge doses since no *dose-related* response could be seen between 80 mg and 1000 mg intravenously or between 1 g and 3 g "pulses."[14]

Thus, the clinical usage of pulses of high-dose glucocorticoids is based on empiric observations rather than a rational formulation soundly based on fundamental differences in the antiinflammatory or antiproliferative effects of "high-dose" intravenous versus conventional doses of oral glucocorticoids. The initial postulated benefits of "high-dose" glucocorticoid therapy in renal allotransplantation has not stood up to careful examination in that oral glucocorticoids in doses of 3-4 mg/kg are approximately equivalent to intravenous pulse methyprednisolone. With this background information calling into question the putative benefits of a "high-dose" glucocorticoid regimen, it would be worthwhile at this point to review the reports of efficacy of high-dose methylprednisolone in nephritic syndromes.

## STUDIES OF "HIGH-DOSE" GLUCOCORTICOID THERAPY IN NEPHRITIC SYNDROMES

### Crescentic Glomerulonephritis

Several reports describing small series of anecdotal uncontrolled experiences with the use of "pulse" therapy in crescentic glomerulonephritis have appeared in recent years.[4-8,12,37,38,44] Cole and colleagues[12] used 30 mg/kg "pulses" of intravenous methyprednisolone on each of six alternate days in eight pediatric cases of "severe" proliferative glomerulonephritis. Five patients had idiopathic crescentic glomerulonephritis of varying severity and three had membranoproliferative glomerulonephritis with recent deterioration of renal function. Short-term follow-up observations indicated improvement in glomerular filtration rate (GFR), particularly among those patients with a short duration of disease before starting therapy. O'Neill, Etheridge, and Bloomer[37] treated 10 adult patients with idiopathic crescentic glomerulonephritis with 1.0 g of methyprednisolone intravenously on a daily basis for seven days, followed by oral prednisone. Four of the cases "improved" with a decline of serum creatinine of 50 percent or more. Responsiveness was associated with a short duration of symptoms, normal blood pressure, and a relative lack of interstitial fibrosis or glomerulosclerosis on initial renal biopsy. Most patients had over 80 percent of the glomeruli involved with crescents unassociated with extensive immunoglobulin deposits in the glomerular capillaries or mesangium. Bolton and Couser[7] reported on nine adult cases treated with 1.0 g of methylprednisolone intravenously for three doses followed by oral prednisone. All patients were presumed to have idiopathic crescentic glomerulonephritis, and the majority were oliguric and requiring dialysis. Six of the nine patients noted improved renal function with average serum creatinine concentrations falling from 10.6 mg/dl to 2.2 mg/dl within 1 to 2 months of starting treatment. Responsive patients were largely those with the relative absence of deposits in glomeruli on initial biopsy. Oredugba and coworkers[38] reported on five adult cases with idiopathic

crescentic glomerulonephritis treated with 1.0 g of methylprednisolone for five consecutive days. Average serum creatinine concentration fell from 7.4 mg/dl to 2.4 mg/dl within four weeks of starting therapy. One patient died of cryptococcal meningitis. Bruns and colleagues[8] treated nine adults with crescentic glomerulonephritis with 30 mg/kg boluses of methylprednisolone repeated 4 to 11 times. Average serum creatinine concentration declined from 6.5 mg/dl to 3.7 mg/dl over three months. Seven of the nine patients remained alive with stable renal function at the end of one year of follow-up. This group of patients also received bi-monthly cyclophosphamide and oral glucocorticoids for 3 to 7 months. Rose, Cole, and Robson[44] reported again on the use of 30 mg/kg "pulses" of intravenous methylprednisolone every other day for up to three doses in children with "severe" proliferative glomerulonephritis including seven with idiopathic crescentic glomerulonephritis. Short-term improvement in GFR was noted in most instances. Bolton,[6] in a review of the cumulative experience of a group of collaborative investigators in Virginia, reported the only body of information in which patients *not* receiving high-dose glucocorticoids were concomitantly analyzed. Patients receiving 30 mg/kg methylprednisolone daily for every day for three doses were compared to patients receiving other types of treatment, including lower doses of oral prednisone. Among a total of 13 patients with idiopathic crescentic glomerulonephritis secondary to antiglomerular basement membrane antibody disease, five of whom did not receive high-dose glucocorticoid therapy, only one patient noted improvement in renal function. On the other hand, 9 of 10 patients with idiopathic crescentic glomerulonephritis in which granular or scanty deposits of immunoglobulin were found upon immunofluorescence study of renal biopsy experienced improved renal function with "high-dose" glucocorticoid therapy. Only two of nine patients treated with conventional doses (i.e., 1 to 2 mg/kg/day) of oral prednisone experienced similar degrees of improvement. Overall, 55 percent of oliguric patients noted improvement in GFR and exhibited a diuresis with "high-dose" glucocorticoid therapy. There was no correlation noted between the extent of crescentic involvement of glomeruli and the likelihood of improvement. Glomerular sclerosis (greater than 30 percent of glomeruli demonstrating global sclerosis) was not uniformly indicative of a poor prognosis. Approximately 75 percent of improved cases exhibited stable renal function over variable periods of follow-up.

If one takes these anecdotal studies at their face value, it would indicate that a favorable short-term response, defined in terms of improving GFR, can be expected in about 80 percent of patients with idiopathic crescentic glomerulonephritis, *not* due to antiglomerular basement membrane antibody mediated disease when a "high-dose" regimen of glucocorticoids is employed early in the course of rapidly progressive disease. Responsiveness may be sustained during continued oral prednisone therapy with or without combined cytotoxic drugs. Most patients who exhibit an initial response will be left with residual disease as denoted by persistently elevated serum creatinine and proteinuria. Infections, primarily of a pulmonary nature, are not common and lethal infections are unusual. The short-term (i.e., 6 month) mortality is low.

It is important to emphasize that no direct comparisons have been made with a group receiving lower doses of oral glucocorticoids (e.g., less than 3 mg/kg of prednisone) although in the studies mentioned above some patients had received prior steroid therapy and presumably deteriorated. A putative beneficial effect of

therapy can be correlated with short duration of disease, absence of extensive interstitial fibrosis and glomerular sclerosis and the absence of extensive granular immunoglobulin deposits in glomeruli. The need for dialysis and the extent of crescentic involvement on initial biopsies are poor predictors of response. When this experience is compared with historical controls or with untreated or less vigorously treated non-randomized controls, the initial response rate approaching 80 percent is indeed impressive. Most studies of patients with crescentic glomerulonephritis, presumably comparable to the treated cases described above, managed with more conventional doses of oral glucocorticoids (3 mg/kg of prednisone or less) have enjoyed only about a 20 to 30 percent survival without the need for dialysis for at least 6 months. An improved outcome in conventionally or conservatively treated patients has been noted on occasion in younger patients and in those where infectious causes of crescentic glomerulonephritis were likely. Of course, without concurrent controls it cannot be stated with certainty that the observed response rate is indeed a function of the aggressive high-dose glucocorticoid regimen employed or whether lower doses of oral glucocorticoids would have been equally effective as has been proven to be the case in therapy for acute renal allograft rejection.[9,21,27,28,34,39,40] Furthermore, the role of the inherent selection of case material in the apparently improved outcome will remain a matter of speculation. Prospective, direct, case-by-case comparisons of different therapeutic regimens seems unlikely to ever be possible, since crescentic glomerulonephritis is a relatively rare condition and the necessity of stratification of cases according to age, duration of illness, underlying immunopathogenetic mechanisms, and evidence of irreversible renal injury would seem to impose formidable obstacles for the design of a successful randomized controlled study. Therefore, it seems reasonable until further data is available to recommend "high-dose" glucocorticoid treatment only for a select group of patients. These might include those children or adults who present with rapidly progressive renal failure over a short time span, say 3 months or less; who have documented extensive crescentic glomerulonephritis (greater than 50 percent of glomeruli involved) with circumferential crescents in the absence of a identifiable infectious or multisystem disease; who have documented by immunofluorescence either heavy granular or scanty glomerular IgG deposits and who lack unequivocal evidence of irreversible disease (e.g., bilateral renal atrophy, extensive global glomerular sclerosis or interstitial fibrosis and tubular atrophy). Using such strict criteria, it is estimated that fewer than one in three patients with idiopathic crescentic glomerulonephritis would receive "pulse" glucocorticoid therapy. The remainder could either continue untreated or be considered candidates for other forms of experimental therapy which are beyond the scope of the present discussion. For example, the group with idiopathic crescentic glomerulonephritis secondary to antiglomerular basement membrane antibody production could be considered excellent candidates for combined oral glucocorticoid-cytotoxic-plasma exchange therapy, providing they had not yet advanced to the point of requiring dialysis treatment.

The mechanism of the putative beneficial effect of glucocorticoids in this small group of highly select patients remains unknown, but based on current concepts of the pathogenesis of crescentic disease, it could be due to an effect of glucocorticoids on monocyte accumulation in glomeruli or upon the ability of monocytes to secrete lymphokines, manufacture arachidonic acid metabolites, secrete lysosomal enzymes, or express procoagulant activ-

ity. The overall risks and long-term benefits of such an approach must equally remain uncertain. For the present, pulmonary and meningeal infection with opportunistic organisms remains the main threat, probably due to an effect of glucocorticoids on pulmonary and tissue macrophages. The prevalence of lethal infectious complications over the short-term is likely to be low, that is, in the vicinity of 10 percent or less, if the total dose of methylprednisolone is kept to under 5 to 7 g. However, with repeated courses or more protracted therapy, a much higher and unacceptable complication rate is likely to ensue. Since few patients will experience a complete remission of disease and since the extent of damage to the remaining nephron population is likely to be quite heterogeneous, the late progression of disease by nonimmunologic mechanisms remains a distinct possibility (see Meyer, Anderson, Brenner, this volume). I have personally seen at least three patients who, after what appeared to be a satisfactory response to initial therapy, develop slowly progressive disease accompanied by heavy proteinuria and progressive glomerulosclerosis unresponsive to all therapeutic modalities.

## Other Primary Proliferative Glomerulonephritides

The role of high dose methylprednisolone in the management of other primary proliferative glomerulonephritides has not yet been established. Although transient increases in GFR may accompany their use in *membranoproliferative glomerulonephritis* particularly with evidence of recent progressively declining GFR, the potential hazards of such an approach have not been well-defined.[6,44] Dangerous exacerbations of high blood pressure may occur with "high-dose" glucocorticoid therapy in this disease. Reduction in the levels of transcortin and albumin in nephrotic patients with primary proliferative glomerulonephritis may greatly increase peak free prednisolone levels and also concomitantly increase metabolic clearance rate.[18] Much further study is required before "high-dose" methylprednisolone can be added to the already limited therapeutic armamentarium available in the treatment of membranoproliferative glomerulonephritis.

Finally, based on uncontrolled observations Ponticelli and coworkers[41] have suggested that "pulse" methylprednisolone may be of value in stabilizing the course of *frequently relapsing minimal change disease* with nephrotic syndrome. Pulse methylprednisolone will uniformly induce a prompt remission of proteinuria in patients with minimal change disease who have previously demonstrated their responsiveness to oral prednisone. Subsequent relapses may be less frequent than expected in patients receiving intravenous methylprednisolone in high dosage. In fact, only two of eleven cases so treated subsequently relapsed within 6 months and retreatment of these relapsing patients induced remissions lasting 6 months or more. However, in this group of patients oral glucocorticoids were continued for six months in gradually decreasing doses following "high-dose" intravenous methylprednisolone. Thus, oral glucocorticoids probably contributed to the relative freedom from relapses. A randomized controlled trial of intravenous methylprednisolone therapy in frequently relapsing patients with minimal change disease will be needed to validate this interesting finding.

## Multisystem Diseases

Only two multisystem diseases, namely, *lupus nephritis* and *systemic necrotizing vasculitis*, have been studied to any appreciable extent concerning possible responsiveness to high-dose glucocorticoid therapy. In this context, it is quite possible that some of the patients studied as examples of idiopathic crescentic glomerulonephritis may have in fact represented *"forme fruste"* of necrotizing vasculitis as many of the former had symptoms suggesting that multiorgan disease was present (e.g., fever, myalgia, arthralgias) yet pathologic definition of extraglomerular vasculitis was lacking.

Cathcart et al.[10] were the first to suggest that patients with *diffuse proliferative lupus glomerulonephritis* with declining GFR might experience improvement in both renal function parameters and serologic indices of disease activity following high-dose methylprednisolone treatment. This anecdote involving seven patients was rapidly followed by additional reports involving one to several patients purporting beneficial effects on both renal function and extrarenal manifestation of disease even if "conventional" doses of oral prednisone had failed to control disease activity.[13–15,25,29,31,35,42] The putative beneficial effects of therapy often occurred rapidly. Levels of antibody to native DNA decreased, serum concentrations of C3 and C4 rose and in one study a dramatic decline on the circulating levels of immune complexes was noted. Despite the uncontrolled and anecdotal nature of these reports, high-dose pulse methylprednisolone therapy became widely utilized in the treatment of severe diffuse proliferative lupus nephritis. Recently, Kimberly and colleagues[29] have clarified the situation somewhat by providing detailed description of the response to "high-dose" methylprednisolone therapy in 34 patients of systemic lupus erythematosus with nephritis. In contradistinction to earlier reports, a response, defined as a decrease in serum creatinine concentration of greater than 20 percent of the baseline value by two months, was by no means universal. In fact, by this definition, only 35 percent (12 of 34) of patients responded. The responder group tended to have a shorter duration of deteriorating renal function and parameters of active serologic disease. *Sustained* improvement was noted in only 60 percent of those who responded for at least 6 months. The proteinuria was not consistently diminished.

Similarly Isenberg, Morrow, and Snaith[25] in a recent study noted sustained improvements in only seven of 20 (35 percent) ambulatory patients with SLE treated with pulses of methylprednisolone. Thus, in a very select population of patients with SLE, "high-dose" methylprednisolone, therapy may provide temporary benefits not unlike those observed in the treatment of allograft rejection. In fact, many parallels exist between "high-dose" methylprednisolone treatment of lupus nephritis and allograft rejection; both are expressions of an ongoing disease and in both monocytes and macrophages may participate importantly in the pathogenesis of the lesions. A major question remains concerning the necessity for high-dose intravenous therapy since oral glucocorticoids in doses of 3 to 4 mg/kg/day might be expected to produce similar results. Patients with SLE may be at especially high risk of infectious complications because of prior prolonged glucocorticoid therapy, concomitant use of cytotoxic agents and the presence of underlying defects in cellular and humoral immunity and in the activity of the mononuclear phagocyte system. Thus, the relative merits of less intensive oral glucocorticoid therapy versus "high-dose" methylprednisolone or plasma exchange (see Kincaid-Smith, this volume) in the management of severe diffuse proliferative lupus glomerulonephritis remains to be determined.

Few patients with *systemic necrotizing vasculitis* have been treated with "high-dose" intravenous methylprednisolone.[5,36] Improvement has been noted in nearly all reported instances. Whether the efficacy and safety of this approach is superior to the use of more conventional doses of oral prednisone combined with cyclophosphamide remains to be determined. At the present state of our understanding, it would appear that a combined therapeutic approach involving oral prednisone in doses of 1 to 2 mg/kg/day combined with an alkylating agent, preferably cyclophosphamide, is the most overall dependable therapeutic regimen. Pulses of methylprednisolone may yet find a place in the management of patient with severe exacerbations of disease accompanied by immediate life threatening organ dysfunction, such as acute renal failure or massive pulmonary hemorrhage.

## SUMMARY AND CONCLUSIONS

The available current evidence provides reasonable, but limited, support for the selective use of high-dose methylprednisolone in certain clinical situations involving glomerulonephritis. These include: (1) rapidly progressive renal failure developing as a result of idiopathic crescentic glomerulonephritis accompanied by granular or scanty immunoglobulin deposits in the glomerular capillaries or mesangium and a relatively brief duration of illness without evidence of "irreversible" morphologic changes in glomeruli or tubulointerstitial areas; (2) diffuse proliferative lupus glomerulonephritis of recent onset showing acute deterioration of renal function in the presence of serological parameters indicating disease activity (e.g., high levels of circulating immune complexes, low C3/C4 concentrations, high levels of antinative DNA antibody); (3) systemic necrotizing vasculitis with life threatening renal or extrarenal involvement. Similar degrees of improvement might be expected to occur with lower doses of oral prednisone (i.e., 3 to 4 mg/kg/day) but this has not yet been determined by randomized, prospective studies. However, in view of current evidence derived from experience in the treatment of renal allograft rejection, *milligram* doses of oral prednisone might be equally effective as *gram* doses of intravenous methylprednisolone. Much further study is required before "high-dose" intravenous methylprednisolone can be added to the therapeutic armamentarium for other diffuse proliferative glomerulonephrities such as membranoproliferative glomerulonephritis for the management of patients of frequently relapsing nephrotic syndrome secondary to minimal change disease, or for the treatment of the life threatening extrarenal complications of systemic lupus erythematosus.

# REFERENCES

1. Alarcon-Zurita A, Ladefoged J: Treatment of acute allograft rejection with high doses of corticosteroids. Kidney Int 9:351, 1976.
2. Bell PRF, Calman KC, Wood RFM, et al: Reversal of acute clinical and experimental organ rejection using large doses of intravenous prednisolone. Lancet 1:876, 1971.
3. Blackwell GJ, Carnuccio R, DiRosa M, et al: Macrocortin: A polypeptide causing the anti-phospholipase effect of glucocorticoids. Nature 287:147, 1980.
4. Bolton WK: Pulse methylprednisolone therapy (Rx) of idiopathic acute crescentic rapidly progressive glomerulnephritis (AC-RPGN). Abstracts of the American Society of Nephrology, 13A, 1980.
5. Bolton WK: Pulse methylprednisolone therapy of polyarteritis nodosa (PAN) acute crescentic rapidly progressive glomerulonephritis (AC-RPGN). Abstracts of the American Society of Nephrology, 18A, 1981.
6. Bolton WK: Pulse methylprednisolone therapy of rapidly progressive glomerulonephritis. Cont Nephrol 3:213, 1981.
7. Bolton WK, Couser WG: Intravenous pulse methylprednisolone therapy of acute crescentic rapidly progressive glomerulonephritis. Am J Med 66:495, 1979.
8. Bruns FJ, Fraley DS, Adler S, et al: Megadose methylprednisolone versus plasmapheresis in treatment of rapidly progressive glomerulonephritis (RPGN). Abstracts of the American Society of Nephrology. 14A, 1980.
9. Burleson RL, Marbarger PD, Jermanovich N: A prospective study of methylprednisolone and prednisone as immunosuppressive agents in clinical renal transplantation. Transplant Proc 13:339, 1981.
10. Cathcart ES, Scheinberg MA, Idelson BA, et al: Beneficial effects of methylprednisolone "pulse" therapy in diffuse proliferative lupus nephritis. Lancet, 1:163, 1976.
11. Cheigh JS, Stenzel KH, Riggio RR, et al: Effects of intravenous methylprednisolone on mixed lymphocyte cultures in normal humans. Transplant Proc 7:31, 1975.
12. Cole BR, Brocklebank JT, Kienstra RA, et al: "Pulse" methylprednisolone therapy in the treatment of severe glomerulonephritis. J Pediatr 88:307, 1976.
13. Dosa S, Mallick NP, Lawler W, et al: The treatment of lupus nephritis by methylprednisolone pulse therapy. J Postgrad Med 54:628, 1978.
14. Editorial: Prednisolone pulses in collagen diseases: Grammes or milligrammes. Lancet 1:280, 1983.
15. Eyanson S, Passo MH, Aldo-Benson MA, et al: Methylprednisolone pulse therapy for non-renal lupus erythematosus. Ann Rheum Dis 39:377, 1980.
16. Fan PT, Yu DTY, Clements PJ, et al: Effect of corticosteroids on human immune response: Comparison of one and three daily 1 gm. intravenous pulses of methylprednisolone. J Lab Clin Med 91:625, 1978.
17. Fauci AS: Corticosteroids and circulating lymphocytes. Transplant Proc 8:37, 1975.
18. Frey FJ, Frey BM: Altered prednisolone kinetics in patients with the nephrotic syndrome. Nephron 32:45, 1982.
19. Gambertoglio J, Frey F, Birnbaum J, et al: Comparison of the bioavailability of oral prednisone and prednisolone in kidney transplant patients. Kidney Int 19:266, 1981.

20. Goldstein IM: Effect of steroids on lysosomes. Transplant Proc 7:21, 1975.
21. Gray D, Shepherd H, Daar A, et al: Oral versus intravenous high dose steroid treatment of renal allograft rejection. The big shot or not? Lancet 1:117, 1978.
22. Green OC, Winter RJ, Kawahara FS, et al: Pharmacokinetic studies of prednisolone in children. J Pediatr 93:299, 1978.
23. Hirata F, Schiffmann E, Venkatasubramanian K, et al: A phospholipase $A_2$ inhibitory protein in rabbit neutrophils induced by glucocorticoids. Proc Natl Acad Sci 77: 2533, 1980.
24. Holdsworth, S, Bellomo R: Differential effects of steroids on leucocyte mediated glomerulonephritis in the rabbit. Abstracts of the American Society of Nephrology, 90A, 1982.
25. Isenberg DA, Morrow WJW, Snaith ML: Methylprednisolone pulse therapy in the treatment of systemic lupus erythematosus. Ann Rheum Dis 41:347, 1982.
26. Johnson LK, Lan NC, Baxter JD: Stimulation and inhibition of cellular functions by glucocorticoids. Correlations with rapid influences on chromatin structure. J Biol Chem 254:7785, 1979.
27. Kauffman HM, Sampson D, Fox PS, et al: High dose (bolus) intravenous methylprednisolone at the time of kidney homotransplantation. Ann Surg 186:631, 1977.
28. Kauffman HM, Stromstad SA, Sampson D, et al: Randomized steroid therapy of human kidney transplant rejection. Transplant Proc 11:36, 1979.
29. Kimberly RP, Lockshin MO, Sherman RL, et al: High dose intravenous methylprednisolone pulse therapy in systemic lupus erythematosus. Am J Med, 70:817, 1981.
30. Leibowich SJ, Ross R: A macrophage-dependent factor that stimulates the proliferation of fibroblasts in vitro. Am J Pathol 84:501, 1976.
31. Levinsky RJ Cameron JS, Soothill JF: Serum immune complexes and disease activity in lupus nephritis. Lancet 1:567, 1977.
32. Meickle AW, Weed JA, Tyler FH: Kinetics and interconversion of prednisolone and prednisone studied with new radioimmunoassays. J Clin Endocrinol Metab 41:717, 1975.
33. McDougal BA, Whittier FC, Cross DE: Sudden death after bolus steroid therapy for acute rejection. Transplant Proc 8:493, 1976.
34. Mussche MM, Ringoir SMG, Lameire NN: High intravenous doses of methylprednisolone for acute cadaveric renal allograft rejection. Nephron 16:287, 1976.
35. Nebout T, Sobel A, Lagrue G: Intravenous methylprednisolone pulses in diffuse proliferative lupus nephritis. Lancet 1:909, 1977.
36. Neild GH, Lee HA: Methylprednisolone pulse therapy in the treatment of polyarteritis nodosa. Postgrad Med 53:382, 1977.
37. O'Neill WM Jr, Etheridge WB, Bloomer HA: High dose corticosteroids. Their use in treating idiopathic rapidly progressive glomerulonephritis. Arch Intern Med 139:514, 1979.
38. Oredugba O, Mazumbar DC, Meyer JS, et al: Pulse methylprednisolone therapy in idiopathic rapidly progressive glomerulonephritis. Ann Intern Med 92:504, 1980.
39. Orta-Siba N, Chantler C, Benick M, et al: Comparison of high dose intravenous methylprednisolone with low dose oral prednisone in acute renal allograft rejection in children. Br Med J 285:258, 1982.
40. Park GD, Bartucci M, Smith MC: High versus low dose methylprednisolone (MP) for acute rejection episodes in renal transplantation. Kidney Int 21:298, 1982.
41. Ponticelli C, Imbasciati E, Case N, et al: Intravenous methylprednisolone in minimal change nephrotic syndrome. Br Med J 280:685, 1980.
42. Ponticelli C, Tarantino A, Pioltelli P, et al: High dose methylprednisolone pulses in active lupus nephritis. Lancet 1:1063, 1977.
43. Rinehart JJ, Balcerzak SP, Sagone AL, et al: Effects of corticosteroids on human monocyte function. J Clin Invest 54:1337, 1974.
44. Rose GM, Cole BR, Robson AM: The treatment of severe glomerulopathies in children using high dose intravenous methylprednisolone pulses. Am J Kid Dis 1:148, 1981.
45. Tremann JA, Agodoa LCY, Cooper TP, et al: The adverse effect of high dose steroids on renal autografts and homografts. Surgery 79:370, 1976.

# The Case for Aggressive Use

## W. Kline Bolton, M.D.

## INTRODUCTION

In 1914, Volhard and Fahr[175] described a clinicopathologic entity characterized by a rapid decrease in kidney function with associated growth of the cells lining Bowman's capsule. Three decades later, in his classic treatise on postinfectious nephritis, Ellis[58] observed that a certain subset of patients developed proliferation of Bowman's capsule with extensive crescent formation and appeared to have a worse prognosis than other patients. A number of those patients had proliferation of the capsule without evidence of significant tuftal proliferation. Attention was first brought to the distinct clinicopathologic entity of rapidly progressive glomerulonephritis (RPGN) by Bacani et al. in 1968.[6] These investigators described eight patients with a very rapid clinical course from onset to uremia and death over a period of weeks or months. Renal biopsy demonstrated extensive cellular crescent formation which progressed to glomerular obsolescence at autopsy. Six of the patients appeared to have no predisposing disease, one had a preceding infection and one appeared to have a vasculitis. The renal biopsies of two patients were examined by immunofluorescence, a novel approach at that time; one had linear deposits of IgG along the glomerular basement membrane (GBM).

Since these first descriptions a large number of patients with several different syndromes described loosely as RPGN have been reported in both the pediatric and adult literature, and from many countries throughout the world. The early descriptions of RPGN were based upon light microscopic and clinical observations alone, and are certainly to be forgiven if patients with different etiologies with one clinical presentation were lumped together. In the last 10 to 15 years, however, immunofluorescence and ultrastructural analysis has been readily available and use of these techniques, along with light microscopic examination of renal biopsies, would probably have greatly diminished the morass of confusion and multiplicity of meanings that have been applied to the entity of acute crescentic rapidly progressive glomerulonephritis (AC-RPGN). This paper will attempt to sort out and assess the course and effect of therapy on the major types of RPGN.

## TERMINOLOGY AND CLASSIFICATION

The term *rapidly progressive glomerulonephritis* describes the clinical course of patients and by no means indicates what histologic lesion will be present. Through common usage, this is often equated with crescentic nephritis,[77,151,159] but this is an inappropriate association. RPGN is best described as any type of glomerulonephritis which is associated with a rapid decline in renal function.[28,29,69,70] This may be defined as a documented halving of re-

The author is indebted to the members of the Charlottesville Collaborative Study Group, who continue to participate in the study of pulse methylprednisolone therapy in patients with rapidly progressive nephritis as described in this report.

nal function as assessed by creatinine clearance or by serum creatinine increase over a period of three months or less, associated with a histologic diagnosis of glomerulonephritis.[28,29] If crescents are present, then the term "crescentic" or "acute crescentic" glomerulonephritis may be applied. However, the finding of crescents and glomerulonephritis does not always dictate that the patient will have a clinically rapidly progressive course, and the two terms should not be used interchangeably.[41,179] The term glomerulonephritis will be used in this chapter to describe any glomerular process with an increased number of endogenous cells, or an increase in the cellular matrix or cytoplasm, or an infiltration of the glomerulus or its associated structures with exogenous cells. Thus, any increase in size or number of endothelial, mesangial, or epithelial cells fits the description of glomerulonephritis. Also, any process associated with exudative changes, such as postinfectious nephritis, in which there is an infiltration of polymorphonuclear leukocytes may be included. In other situations, it is now becoming increasingly more evident that other cells, such as monocytes or macrophages, may infiltrate the glomerulus.[4,5,22,109,120,123] An exception to the term would be those toxic entities associated with swelling or proliferation of the endothelial cells per se, such as toxemia of pregnancy. When crescents are present, the degree of their formation may be assessed in a variety of ways. These may be defined in terms of the circumference of the crescent, the number of layers of cells present, whether the crescents are cellular or fibrous, and the percentage of glomeruli containing crescents. Inasmuch as many glomeruli are sectioned in a noncoronal plane, the limitation of crescents to either circumferential or to a specific percentate of the glomerulus may be fraught with bias. While some investigators use 50 to 60 percent or more

crescents for the term AC-RPGN, our experience indicates that patients with much less crescent formation by light microscopy may have similar clinical courses to those with more crescents.[27,28,161] Thus, we have selected 20 percent or more crescents per section as significant.[27,29] In view of the foregoing considerations, many classifications of RPGN are possible. The classifications that will be used in this discussion will encompass a number of the standard and accepted categories for RPGN based upon etiologic considerations,[15,47,69] but will also depart from general classifications in several ways as will be described more fully in the section on pathogenetic mechanisms. The schema to be used is listed in Table 12-1. In this classification, RPGN is considered as a clinical syndrome and is classified into true RPGN with glomerulonephritis and "pseudo-RPGN" that is characterized by a similar clinical picture but lacks glomerulonephritis. In those patients with glomerulonephritis, the process has been further subdivided according to presumed etiologic factors, as (1) granular glomerular deposits, assumed to be immune complex disease, (2) antibodies deposited along the GBM, and (3) no-immunoglobulin-deposit (NID) nephritis, which is designated as a cell mediated immune process. All are associated with crescent formation by light and immunofluorescence microscopy. In the first category of granular glomerular deposits, a number of important postinfectious or infection-associated processes leading to RPGN have been clearly described. Endocapillary proliferation is listed here, indicating that it may occur as a sequel to well documented infectious diseases, and to act as a reminder that any time endocapillary proliferation is present, a postinfectious process should be sought. The other entities on this list, bacterial endocarditis, suppurative infections and shunt nephritis, are all well known causes of glomerulonephritis which occasionally follow a rapidly progressive course. The second category includes glomerulonephrides with granular glomerular deposits but without infection. These disorders are simply classified by the presence or absence of systemic manifestations. A large number of the systemic diseases are vasculitic or vasculitic-associated syndromes. The others are not associated with documented vasculitis and include malignancies and a variety of other processes. Certainly, systemic lupus erythematosus (SLE) may be associated with vasculitis from deposition of soluble complexes, but is listed as "nonvasculitic" in that the most common presentation is in this latter category. The section 1.B.ii is classified as nonsystemic rather than as primary glomerulonephritis, as used in other classifications.[47,69] This latter term is probably improper nomenclature since all of the diseases listed as primary, or isolated to the kidney, actually represent some type of systemic disease in which only the kidney is clinically affected. Further evidence that these are truly systemic diseases is provided by the fact that all of them have been shown to recur in transplanted kidneys.[101,125,144,152,180] The idiopathic variety of RPGN with granular deposits is subclassified on the basis of endocapillary proliferation. The prognoses of the entities may differ[78,100] and the etiology may also be different. It is entirely possible that the endocapillary nephritis in this last category may be the same or quite similar to the endocapillary proliferation category listed under postinfectious nephritis.

The second category of glomerulonephritis is that associated with antibodies along the GBM. This classically includes Goodpasture's syndrome, some forms of membranous nephropathy, the idiopathic variety which is, for practical purposes, identical to Goodpasture's syndrome but without overt pulmonary hemorrhage, and polyarteritis nodosa (PAN). The latter

category may also be found in the first grouping of granular glomerular deposits, but is associated in a significant number of cases with linear deposits of IgG and complement along the GBM and with the clinical course described below which appears essentially the same as anti-GBM mediated RPGN. The third category of glomerulonephritis is termed *idiopathic cell mediated*. The rationales for the two inclusions in this category are several and will be listed only briefly. First, the histologic findings are identical to the other types of RPGN described previously, but without immunoglobulin deposition. Second, the process responds to therapy like other cell-mediated entities. Third, there are experimental animal models of purely cell-mediated glomerulonephritis. PAN once again can appear in this category with proven vasculitis by biopsy, but without the presence of either anti-GBM antibodies in the circulation or along the GBM, and without any granular glomerular deposits. The basis for classification into these three categories will be further addressed in the section on pathogenetic mechanisms.

It is important to observe that the majority of the processes listed in Table 12-1 as clinical RPGN associated with glomerulonephritis actually have crescents as part of their histopathology and this is the genesis of the commonly held concept that AC-RPGN is equivalent to RPGN, which is not correct. Certain of these processes, especially those with endocapillary proliferation or membranoproliferative nephritis (MPGN), manifest the clinical course of RPGN but glomeruli have either no crescents or less than 20 percent crescents. This distinction needs to be observed in consideration of series in which the natural course of the disease and the effect of treatment is assessed.

The second category, "pseudo-RPGN" describes a variety of more or less common syndromes which will have the

**Table 12-1.** Classification of Clinical RPGN

I. *Clinical RPGN with Glomerulonephritis*
1. Granular glomerular deposits
   A. Postinfectious
      i) Endocapillary proliferation
      ii) Subacute bacterial endocarditis
      iii) Suppurative infections
      iv) Shunt nephrit s
   B. Noninfectious
      i) Systemic
         a) Vasculitis
            • Polyarteritis nodosa
            • Henoch-Schoenlein purpura
            • Wegener's granulomatosis
            • Behçet's syndrome
            • Relapsing polychondritis
         b) Nonvasculitic
            • Malignancy
            • Mixed cryoglobulinemia
            • Systemic lupus erythematosus
            • Alport's syndrome
            • C-3 nephritic factor
      ii) Nonsystemic
         a) Membranoproliferative
         b) IgG-IgA nephropathy
         c) Membranous nephropathy
         d) Idiopathic—with endocapillary proliferation
                    —without endocapillary proliferation
2. Anti-GBM antibodies on GBM
   A. Goodpasture's syndrome
   B. Membranous nephropathy
   C. Polyarteritis nodosa
   D. Idiopathic
3. Idiopathic cell mediated
   A. No immunoglobulin deposit disease
   B. Polyarteritis nodosa
II. *Pseudo-RPGN*
1. Acute intersitital nephritis
2. Acute tubular necrosis
3. Scleroderma
4. Malignant hypertension
5. Light chain nephropathy
6. Thrombotic thrombocytopenia purpura
7. Hemolytic uremic syndrome
8. Renal vein thrombosis
9. Renal artery obstruction

Data from references 13,47,52,53,69,70,74,82,85,93,122,129, 134,141,142.

same clinical presentation as RPGN with glomerulonephritis. In other words, each of the two groups may be associated with a rapid decrease in renal function of 50 percent or more within three months duration, a urinary sediment that is suggestive of glomerulonephritis such as proteinuria, hematuria, red and white cell casts, and in some cases the development of oligoanuria. As can be seen from Table 12-1, without dwelling further on part II,

it is critical to have a histologic diagnosis to define the underlying pathologic process and to ascertain whether or not a glomerulonephritis is present.

# PROGNOSIS OF IDIOPATHIC AC-RPGN

The emphasis of this chapter will be upon the effect of therapy, especially

**Table 12-2.** Overall Prognosis in Patients with Clinical RPGN

| Series | Ref | Year | # Pts | Stable or improved | % | DD | Anti-GBM # | Anti-GBM DD |
|---|---|---|---|---|---|---|---|---|
| Berlyne[a] | 19 | 1963 | 8 | 0 | 0 | 8 | | |
| Bacani | 6 | 1968 | 8 | 0 | 0 | 8 | 1 | 1 |
| Leonard[a] | 100 | 1970 | 29 | 11 | 38 | 18 | | |
| Lewis[a] | 103 | 1971 | 7 | 0 | 0 | 7 | 6 | 6 |
| Sonsino[ab] | 158 | 1972 | 31 | 13 | 42 | 18 | 0 | 0 |
| Striker | 162 | 1972 | 63 | 11 | 17 | 52 | | |
| Arieff | 2 | 1972 | 6 | 3 | 50 | 3 | | |
| Olsen[a] | 133 | 1974 | 59 | 0 | 0 | 59 | 3 | 3 |
| Jenson[a] | 86 | 1974 | 10 | 3 | 30 | 7 | | |
| Brown[ac] | 35 | 1974 | 16 | 10 | 62 | 6 | | |
| Whitworth | 179 | 1976 | 17 | 0 | 0 | 17 | 3 | 3 |
| Suc | 163 | 1976 | 14 | 3 | 21 | 11 | | |
| Beirne | 15 | 1977 | 40 | 11 | 28 | 29 | 29 | 24 |
| McLeish[ab] | 115 | 1978 | 42 | 6 | 14 | 36 | 8 | 7 |
| Morrin[a] | 124 | 1978 | 29 | 10 | 34 | 19 | 3 | 3 |
| Stilmant | 161 | 1979 | 9 | 4 | 44 | 5 | 1 | 1 |
| Nakamoto[ac] | 127 | 1979 | 24 | 11 | 46 | 13 | 1 | 1 |
| Ogg[ac] | 132 | 1981 | 39 | 17 | 44 | 22 | 3 | 3 |
| Cohen[ab] | 43 | 1981 | 36 | 5 | 14 | 31 | 9 | 9 |
| Dash[ab] | 51 | 1982 | 34 | 6 | 18 | 28 | | |
| Total | | | 521 | 124 (24%) | | 397 (76%) | | |
| Corrected for GBM | | | 454 | 117 (26%) | | 337 (74%) | 67 | 61 (91%) |

[c]Quadruple therapy.
[b]Excluding lost to follow-up.
[a]Mixed—poststreptococcal, SLE, Henoch-Schönlein purpura, polyarteritis nodosa, some noncrescentic and Wegener's granulomatosis.

high-dose steroids, on the nephritic syndromes. This requires a knowledge of the natural course of a disease and/or its course with other therapy. The severity of an illness, its prognosis, knowledge of its pathogenesis, and the relationship between its specific therapy and outcome can usually be ascertained by the number of types of therapy that have been applied to the entity. The plethora of therapeutic modalities used for RPGN should amply illustrate this. A variety of immunosuppressive agents have been used, including prednisone, azathiaprine, cyclophosphamide, chlorambucil and nitrogen mustard, numerous anticoagulants and antiplatelet agents, such as heparin, warfarin, arvin, dipyridamole, aspirin, cyproheptadine, sulfinpyrazone, and antiprostaglandin agents, such as indomethacin.[47,69] Nonetheless, the grim prognosis that was defined by the earliest studies of RPGN

and by the vivid descriptions of Bacani et al.[6] have continued to pertain throughout the last several decades. Table 12-2 provides a summary of a number of series describing patients with clinical RPGN, most of whom had AC-RPGN. These series are listed in chronological order to detect any trends that might be apparent with changes in overall support techniques and include all patients, either treated or untreated, with the exception of those treated with two recent modalities, pulse methylprednisolone and plasma exchange. Where possible, patients who were lost to follow-up have been excluded. Assessment of the course of disease and response to treatment in this extremely heterogeneous group of patients is difficult because of the inclusion of many processes under the same heading, lack of specific information on each patient, and failure to perform elec-

tron and immunofluorescence microscopy. Nonetheless, each series was carefully examined and the diagnoses
determined, if possible. Publications by
the same investigative groups were compared to previous reports, and only the
most recent utilized if each contained
some of the same patients. Single case reports were not included. Each series is
marked as to whether it consisted solely
of AC-RPGN patients of the idiopathic variety as defined in this chapter, or if they
contained patients with other entities
such as SLE, Henoch-Schönlein purpura,
PAN, Wegener's granulomatosis, and
noncrescentic glomerulonephritis. Of 521
patients reported since 1963, 124 (24 percent) were stable or improved, essentially
all with treatment, and 397 (76 percent) either died, were on dialysis, were transplanted, or had severe impairment of renal function (death or dialysis, DD). Most
series contained mixed patients and no
improvement related to technological advances were apparent. It is important to
note that in some series, excellent data on
individual patients or diseases are provided and will be addressed later in the
chapter. Where possible, patients with
anti-GBM disease have been separated
out for evaluation, as will be explained
later. As noted in the last two columns, of
67 patients with anti-GBM disease, 61
progressed to death or dialysis (91 percent). When those patients with anti-GBM
disease are corrected from the totals of
overall prognosis, 454 patients remain, of
whom 117 were stable or improved and
337 (74 percent) were dead or on dialysis.

This illustrates one of the major problems in assessing the reported series of
RPGN and its natural course or response
to therapy, that is, many different clinical
entities have been grouped and reported
together. One of the most strenuously opposed inclusions classically has been that
of postinfectious or, specifically, poststreptococcal RPGN. As is well docu-

mented, poststreptococcal nephritis has
an excellent prognosis in children and
even those with oligoanuric renal failure
or vasculitis do well with supportive therapy.[84,169] Despite this adage, increasing
evidence suggests that some children
with crescentic poststreptococcal nephritis
do not do as well as has previously been
reported,[1,8,9,50] and it seems obvious that
adults with postinfectious nephritis do
less well than children. Table 12-3 summarizes seven series of adult patients
with postinfectious oliguric acute renal
failure, irrespective of percent of crescents
present. Of 56 adult patients, 25 (45 percent) progressed to end-stage renal disease with little or no recovery. This is a
considerably better prognosis than that of
anti-GBM disease or RPGN (Table 12-2),
but is based on patients both *with* and
*without* crescents. Table 12-4 examines series in which adequate information is
available to determine the effect of crescent formation, again defined as 20 percent or more crescents. In these 9 series,
47 individuals had significant crescents,
some with and some without oliguria,
and of these, 24 (51 percent) progressed
to end-stage renal disease or death and 49
percent were stable or improved. These
patients were treated by supportive methods in some cases, and by immunosuppressive and cytotoxic agents in others.
Thus, even though the prognosis in poststreptococcal nephritis with crescents in
adults is not good, it is considerably better than the overall prognosis for RPGN.
A significant bias could thus be introduced into evaluation of the natural history of AC-RPGN in series containing
poststreptococcal nephritis. Table 12-5 addresses this by examining those series in
which it was possible to exclude patients
with probable poststreptococcal nephritis.
Other diagnoses and some patients without crescents may be included, but
patients with known postinfectious nephritis were not. Also included for

**Table 12-3.** Prognosis in Post infectious Oliguric ARF in Adult Patients

| Series | Ref | Year | # Pts | DD | % |
|--------|-----|------|-------|-----|-----|
| Harrison | 75 | 1964 | 13 | 6 | 46 |
| Nakamoto | 128 | 1965 | 2 | 0 | 0 |
| Lemieux | 99 | 1967 | 9 | 6 | 67 |
| Leonard | 100 | 1970 | 10 | 3 | 30 |
| Schreiner | 155 | 1972 | 12 | 4 | 25 |
| Baldwin | 8 | 1974 | 9 | 5 | 55 |
| Ogg | 132 | 1981 | 1 | 1 | |
| Total | | | 56 | 25 | 45 |

comparison are those patients in which it was possible to determine if anti-GBM disease was present. From 1968 to 1981, 244 patients were assessed, of whom 177 (73 percent) proceeded to death or dialysis. Twenty-seven percent were better and only two percent appeared to improve spontaneously in the absence of therapy. In those patients with oliguria, 88 percent progressed to death or dialysis. Once again, the percentage of anti-GBM patients proceeding to death or dialysis was 91 percent. If the series is corrected for patients with anti-GBM disease, the prognosis improves somewhat, with 67 percent proceeding to death or dialysis and 33 percent improving or stabilizing. Examination of the series indicates that three studies weigh heavily toward a good response—those of Nakamoto, Brown, and Ogg. All three used quadruple therapy consisting of corticosteroids, anticoagulants, antiplatelet agents, and cytotoxic drugs. The other series were either untreated or used a variety of agents in different combinations. Therefore, to attempt to assess this factor on prognosis, the last line is corrected for quadruple therapy. Of those patients remaining, 151 were treated with conventional methods excluding quadruple therapy, plasma exchange, or pulse methylprednisolone. One hundred fifteen of these proceeded to death or dialysis (76 percent) and 36 were better (24 percent). Thus, exclusion of patients with poststreptococcal nephritis with oliguric renal failure and/or crescents, considering standard immunosuppressive and other types of therapy, changes the prognosis from 74 percent death or dialysis to 76 percent death or dialysis, not significantly different. This may indicate that fewer postinfectious patients with severe progressive disease were included.

Critical information about patients with true idiopathic AC-RPGN is more difficult to obtain. Table 12-6 lists a se-

**Table 12-4.** Prognosis in Proliferative GN in Patients with Significant Crescents[a]

| Series | Ref | Year | # Pts | DD | Better |
|--------|-----|------|-------|-----|--------|
| Lee | 97 | 1966 | 2 | 2 | 0 |
| Lemieux | 99 | 1967 | 6 | 3 | 3 |
| Leonard | 100 | 1970 | 4 | 2 | 2 |
| Sonsino | 158 | 1972 | 11 | 2 | 9 |
| Baldwin | 8 | 1974 | 7 | 6 | 1 |
| Brown | 35 | 1974 | 1 | 1 | 0 |
| Morrin | 124 | 1978 | 12 | 6 | 6 |
| Nakamoto | 127 | 1979 | 2 | 1 | 1 |
| Ogg | 132 | 1981 | 2 | 1 | 1 |
| Total | | | 47 | 24 (51%) | 23 (49%) |

[a]Treated by conventional methods or untreated.

**Table 12-5.** AG-RPGN Prognosis[a]

| Series | Ref | Year | # Pts | Oliguric | Oliguric DD | DD | Better | Better | Anti-GBM # | Anti-GBM DD |
|---|---|---|---|---|---|---|---|---|---|---|
| Bacani | 6 | 1968 | 8 | 4 | 4 | 8 | 0 | 0 | 1 | 1 |
| Leonard[b] | 100 | 1970 | 16 | 16 | 16 | 16 | 0 | 0 | | |
| Lewis | 103 | 1971 | 7 | 6 | 6 | 7 | 0 | 0 | 6 | 6 |
| Sonsino[b] | 158 | 1972 | 20 | 12 | 12 | 16 | 4 | 0 | 0 | 0 |
| Arieff | 2 | 1972 | 6 | 6 | 3 | 3 | 3 | 0 | | |
| Brown[c] | 35 | 1974 | 15[c] | 6 | 6 | 6 | 9 | 0 | | |
| Jenson | 86 | 1974 | 7 | 7 | 4 | 4 | 3 | 0 | | |
| Suc | 163 | 1976 | 14 | 11 | 11 | 11 | 3 | 0 | | |
| Whitworth[b] | 179 | 1976 | 17 | 10 | 10 | 17 | 0 | 0 | 3 | 3 |
| Beirne | 15 | 1977 | 40 | ? | — | 29 | 11 | 2 | 29 | 24 |
| Morrin[b] | 124 | 1978 | 17 | 11 | 5 | 9 | 8 | 2→HD | 3 | 3 |
| Nakamoto[aad] | 127 | 1979 | 14 / 8[c] | | | 11 / 3[b] | 3 / 5[c] | 0 | 1 | 1 |
| Stilmant[d] | 161 | 1979 | 9 | 5 | 5 | 5 | 4 | 0 | | |
| Cohen | 43 | 1981 | 15 | — | — | 13 | 2 | — | 9 | 9 |
| Ogg[c] | 132 | 1981 | 15 / 16[c] | 15 / 4[c] | 14 / 4[c] | 15 / 4[a] | 0 / 12[c] | 0 / 0[b] | 2[c] | 2[c] |
| Totals | | | 244 | 113 | 100 (88%) | 177 (73%) | 67 (27%) | 4 (2%) | 54 | 49 (91%) |
| Total corrected for anti-GBM | | | 190 | | 128 (67%) | 62 (33%) | | | | |
| Total corrected for quadruple therapy | | | 151 | | 115 (76%) | 36 (24%) | | | | |

[a]Excludes plasma exchanged and pulsed patients.
[b]Quadruple therapy
[c]Excludes probable poststrept. May contain other diagnoses and patients without crescents.
[d]Excludes pulsed patients.

lected compilation of series reporting AC-RPGN which provides the most information about the natural course of the disease with conventional therapy. Only those series are included in which it was possible to ascertain the findings by immunofluorescence and light microscopy, and the specific histologic diagnosis. In this table, any patient with anti-GBM is excluded, as are patients with any etiology of RPGN as listed in Table 12-1 except for idiopathic immune complex and idiopathic NID. No patients treated by quadruple therapy, plasma exchange, or pulse therapy are included. Patients who were not treated, or treated with other agents including cytotoxics, prednisone, heparin, etc. have been included. Of 239 patients in the seven series, 70 fit the criteria for idiopathic non-anti-GBM AC-RPGN and, of these, 57 (81 percent) progressed to death or dialysis regardless of any type of therapy. This compilation probably represents the most accurate estimation of the prognosis of idiopathic AC-RPGN, excluding those patients with Henoch-Schönlein purpura, SLE, Wegener's granulomatosis, PAN, poststreptococcal nephritis, noncrescentic nephritis, MPGN, acute proliferative nephritis, and endocapillary proliferative nephritis which are commonly included in the other series.

Many of the original series of investigators reporting the prognosis and effect of therapy on RPGN included a significant number of patients with anti-GBM disease (Tables 12-2 and 12-5). In our first report of the beneficial effects of pulse methylprednisolone, we also included one patient with anti-GBM disease in our series of nine patients treated.[29] This individual did not respond. Through the years, as we have accumulated more pa-

**Table 12-6.** Idiopathic AC-RPGN Prognosis

| Series | Ref | Year | Total Pts | Idiopathic AC-RPGN[a] | DD | Better |
|---|---|---|---|---|---|---|
| Lewis | 103 | 1971 | 7 | 1 | 1 | 0 |
| Sonsino | 158 | 1972 | 31 | 20 | 16 | 4 |
| Whitworth | 179 | 1976 | 60 | 14 | 14 | 0 |
| Beirne | 15 | 1977 | 40 | 11 | 5 | 6 |
| Nakamoto[b] | 127 | 1979 | 24 | 4 | 3 | 1 |
| Ogg[b] | 132 | 1981 | 39 | 9 | 9 | 0 |
| Cohen | 43 | 1981 | 38 | 11 | 9 | 2 |
| Total | | | 239 | 70 | 57 (81%) | 13 (19%) |

[a]Excluding anti-GBM.
[b]Excluding quadruple therapy.

tients, it has become apparent that those patients with anti-GBM disease respond differently to therapy than those with either presumed immune complex or NID-RPGN. This information is documented in the literature and with diligent searching the overall poor prognosis of anti-GBM mediated AC-RPGN is obvious (Table 12-7). Some of these patients had anti-GBM disease associated with pulmonary hemorrhage, considered Goodpasture's syndrome, but for present purposes are included in the series. In the 12 series reviewed in Table 12-7 it was possible to ascertain which patients had deposits of antibody along the GBM in a linear fashion and/or had circulating antibodies within the serum. Patients in whom this could not be clearly documented or in whom there was no way to correlate the histologic finding with the clinical course, were excluded. Patients were also excluded if treated with either pulse methylprednisolone or plasma exchange. Eighty-one patients thus far reported clearly fit the criteria of anti-GBM mediated AC-RPGN. Of these, 72 (89 percent) have responded to no type of therapy thus far offered, and only 11 percent have improved. Essentially no patients on dialysis or with oligoanuria at presentation have shown a beneficial response to therapy. Thus, idiopathic AC-RPGN would appear at best to have a 73 percent rate of progression to death or dialysis (Table 2)

when eclectic in nature, or as poor as 81 percent failure for pure granular or NID disease, to 91 percent failure for anti-GBM disease. There was obviously a need for more effective treatment.

# CHARLOTTESVILLE COLLABORATIVE STUDY EXPERIENCE WITH PULSE METHYLPREDNISO-LONE

The experience of the University of Virginia and collaborating institutions in studying the course and treatment of RPGN began in 1973. This marked the initiation of combined evaluation of tissue by immunofluorescence, electron and light microscopy. Since the fall of 1973, 1269 biopsies (Table 12-8) have been evaluated by these techniques at the University of Virginia. Excluded from the total number are biopsies of patients with kidney transplants. As can be seen from Table 12-8, of those nearly 1300 biopsies, 400 were histologically some type of glomerulonephritis by light microscopy. These can be further categorized on the basis of clinical, immunofluorescence, and ultrastructural findings. Crescentic glomerulonephritis comprised 90 of the 400 biopsies for a percentage of 22.5 of those patients

**Table 12-7.** Prognosis of Anti-GBM AC-RPGN[a]

| Series | Ref | Year | # Pts | DD | Better |
|--------|-----|------|-------|-----|--------|
| Bacani | 6 | 1968 | 1 | 1 | 0 |
| Lewis | 103 | 1971 | 6 | 6 | 0 |
| Olsen | 133 | 1974 | 3 | 3 | 0 |
| Whitworth | 179 | 1974 | 3 | 3 | 0 |
| Sissons | 157 | 1974 | 7 | 7 | 0 |
| Beirne | 15 | 1977 | 29 | 14 | 5 |
| McLeish | 115 | 1978 | 8 | 7 | 1 |
| Morrin | 124 | 1978 | 3 | 3 | 0 |
| Nakamoto | 127 | 1979 | 1 | 1 | 0 |
| Ogg | 132 | 1981 | 2 | 2 | 0 |
| Cohen | 43 | 1981 | 9 | 9 | 0 |
| Moore | 121 | 1982 | 9 | 6 | 3 |
| Total | | | 81 | 72 (89%) | 9 (11%) |

[a]Excluding pts pulsed with methylprednisolone or treated with plasma exchange.

with glomerulonephritis. This is 7.1 percent of the total number of biopsies evaluated during that period of time and is slightly higher than reported in other centers,[15,179] but includes documented PAN, proliferative nephritis and nonevaluable crescentic disease. Forty-seven idiopathic patients, six with PAN, and five with MPGN, met the RPGN criteria described below. Thus, about 4 to 5 percent of patients biopsied in this geographic region will have AC-RPGN of these five types. If only idiopathic AC-RPGN with acceptable tissue and clinical data are included, this group is 12 percent of glomerulonephritides and 3.7 percent of total biopsies. The patients considered in our University of

**Table 12-8.** University of Virginia Kidney Biopsy Profile 1973–1982

| Histologic Diagnosis | # Bx | % |
|----------------------|------|-----|
| Systemic lupus erythematosus | 65 | 16.2 |
| Berger's nephropathy | 40 | 10.0 |
| Henoch-Schönlein purpura | 17 | 4.2 |
| Membranoproliferative glomerulonephritis | 82 | 20.5 |
| Acute glomerulonephritis | 18 | 4.5 |
| Postinfectious | 26 | 6.5 |
| Focal glomerulonephritis | 40 | 10.0 |
| Mesangial hypercellularity | 12 | 3.0 |
| Crescentic glomerulonephritis | 90 | 22.5 |
| Vasculitis | 10 | 2.5 |
| Total | 400 | 99.9 |

Total biopsies = 1269
Total glomerulonephritis = 400 (31.5%)

Virginia collaborative experience are those who fit the diagnostic and clinical criteria established previously:[27,29,161] (1) adequate tissue for diagnosis examined by light, electron, and immunofluorescence microscopy, the latter to include staining with antisera to human IgG, IgA, IgE, IgM, Clq, C-3, alpha-2-macroglobulin, Tamm Horsfall protein, kappa, and lambda light chains, and fibrinogen,[23,25,30,32] (2) 20 percent or more crescents in the biopsy specimen, and (3) the clinical course of RPGN as previously described.[27,29] Beginning in 1976, patients with the clinical and histologic criteria for AC-RPGN were offered the opportunity to undergo pulse methylprednisolone therapy. Prior to that time, patients did not receive pulse therapy. Patients refusing pulse therapy after that time are included with the previous patients as controls. Pulse methylprednisolone therapy was administered as previously described,[28] 30 mg/kg body weight given intravenously over 20 minutes with monitoring of blood pressure. We made sure patients were volume replete, had not received diuretics in the previous three hours, and were not to receive diuretics for 24 hours following therapy. The maximum dose given at one time was three g. This was repeated every other day for a total of three doses and 48 hours after the last dose patients were begun on oral prednisone in an alternate day regimen as detailed in Table 12-9. Patients were considered to be adequately treated if they survived for six weeks or longer, since our experience has shown that, of patients who respond, more than 90 percent will respond within the first six weeks. Patients were considered to be improved or stable if the serum creatinine remained stable with severe histologic lesions or decreased by 30 percent or more, or if they were able to discontinue dialytic support. Most of the patients not given pulse therapy received a variety of agents including anticoagulants, steroids, and cytotoxic agents. Patients were excluded from the study if inadequate tissue was present to make a diagnosis, if any systemic disease was present (as defined in the Introduction), or if the degree of crescent formation was less than 20 percent. Patients with PAN or proliferative nephritis who were treated will be considered separately.

### Results of Therapy in Granular Glomerular and NID Types of AC-RPGN

Fourteen patients (30 percent of total idiopathic AC-RPGN, Table 12-10) have been diagnosed as having idiopathic AC-RPGN associated with granular deposits of immunoglobulins and/or complement and dense deposits by electron microscopy. Seven of these were treated with conventional therapy which consisted of prednisone, and one recieved a combination of cyclophosphamide, prednisone, and heparin (triple therapy). Seven other patients were treated with pulse methylprednisolone. Oliguria was present in three of five untreated patients and five of seven treated patients. The percent crescents was similar, 72 percent for unpulsed and 65 percent for pulsed patients. Two unpulsed patients showed improvement as defined above, one of whom received triple therapy. Six of seven patients required dialysis. One of the six was able to discontinue dialysis, the same patient treated with triple therapy. In contrast, six of seven patients receiving pulse therapy showed improvement and, of the three patients who required dialysis, two were able to discontinue it. The changes in serum creatinine and function in response to therapy are listed in the next to last column. Six of seven patients had serum creatinines greater than 6 mg/dl, and five of these responded to pulse. Patient number 13's serum creatinine was reduced by half in response to pulse therapy. Upon reactivation of his disease and hospitalization, he was found to have metastatic carcinoma of the lung and no therapy was instituted. He was allowed to succumb to uremia rather than to his malignancy. The other patients who improved have maintained stable renal function or died of nonrenal causes.

Sixteen patients (34 percent) fit the criteria for selection into the NID subtype of idiopathic AC-RPGN (Table 12-11). Two of these received conventional therapy with patient number 1 receiving prednisone plus heparin. The other 14 patients were pulsed and of those, 12 showed an improvement. Nine of the pulsed patients were on dialysis and of these, seven were

**Table 12-9.** Regimen for Administering Oral Prednisone Therapy

| Dose of Alternate Day Prednisone[a] | Months of therapy |
| --- | --- |
| 2 mg/kg | 0.5 |
| 1.75 mg/kg | 1.0 |
| 1.50 mg/kg | 3.0 |
| 1.25 mg/kg | 6.0 |
| 1 mg/kg | 6.0 |
| 0.75 mg/kg | 6.0 |
| 0.50 mg/kg | 6.0 |
| 0.25 mg/kg | 6.0 |
| 0.125 mg/kg | 12.0 |
| 0.0625 mg/kg | 12.0 |

[a]75% of dose for pts ≥60 years of age.

**Table 12-10.** Pulse Methylprednisolone Therapy of Granular Glomerular Type AC-RPGN

| Patient | Age | Sex | Oligoanuria | Crescents (%) | Pulse | Improved | HD | Off HD | Serum creatinine mg/dl and outcome | Follow-up (months) |
|---|---|---|---|---|---|---|---|---|---|---|
| 1 | 49 | M | – | 100 | – | – | + | – | DD | – |
| 2 | 57 | M | | 100 | – | – | + | – | DD | – |
| 3[a] | 63 | F | + | 50 | – | + | + | – | 21.0 → 6.5 | 86 |
| 4 | 69 | F | + | 50 | – | – | + | + | DD | – |
| 5 | 43 | M | – | 20 | – | + | – | + | 5.1 → 1.4 | 66 |
| 6 | 65 | M | + | 100 | – | – | + | – | DD | – |
| 7 | 16 | M | | 85 | – | – | + | 1 | DD | – |
| | 52 ± 7[b] | | 3/5 | 72 ± 12[b] | | 2 | 6 | | | |
| 8 | 87 | F | – | 100 | + | + | – | | 8.4 → 3.5 | 5[c] |
| 9 | 65 | F | – | 60 | + | + | – | | 4.6 → 1.3 | 47 |
| 10 | 56 | M | + | 30 | + | + | + | + | >10 → 1.3 | 22[c] |
| 11 | 64 | F | + | 75 | + | + | + | + | >10 → 1.3 | 30 |
| 12[d] | 59 | M | + | 57 | + | + | – | | 10.0 → 1.6 | 4 |
| 13 | 64 | M | + | 50 | + | + | – | | 10→5.2→10 | 2 |
| 14 | 78 | F | + | 80 | + | – | + | – | DD | – |
| | 68 ± 4[b] | | 5/7 | 65 ± 9[b] | 7 | 6 | 3 | 2 | | |

HD = Hemodialysis
DD = death or dialysis
[a] = Cyclophosphamide, prednisone & heparin
[b] = SEM
[c] = died of non-renal causes
[d] = 1 gm pulse
[e] = see text

**Table 12-11.** Pulse Methylprednisolone Therapy of NID-Type AC-RPGN

| Patient | Age | Sex | Oligoanuria | Crescents (%) | Pulse | Improved | HD | Off HD | Serum creatinine mg/dl and Outcome | Follow-up (months) |
|---|---|---|---|---|---|---|---|---|---|---|
| 1[a] | 55 | M | − | 100 | − | + | − | + | 3.6 → 1.3 | 87 |
| 2 | 64 | F | − | 22 | − | + | − | | 7.0 → 1.8 | 6 |
| | | | 0/2 | | | | | | | |
| 3 | 61 | M | + | 53 | + | + | + | + | 13.0 → 2.6 | 65 |
| 4 | 13 | F | − | 78 | + | + | − | + | 1.9 → 0.8 | 72 |
| 5 | 13 | F | − | 90 | + | − | + | − | DD | — |
| 6 | 59 | M | + | 60 | + | + | + | + | 18.0 → 3.6 | 62 |
| 7 | 64 | M | + | 100 | + | + | + | + | 17.0 → 3.1 | 19 |
| 8 | 50 | M | | 100 | + | + | + | + | 17.0 → 4.0 | 30 |
| 9 | 69 | M | | 50 | + | + | + | + | >10→3.0→7.8 | 24 |
| 10[b] | 70 | M | + | 70 | + | + | − | | 8.1→4.8→HD | 4 |
| 11[b] | 52 | M | + | 75 | + | + | + | + | 9.0 → 3.1 | 24 |
| 12[b] | 70 | M | − | 20 | + | − | + | − | DD | — |
| 13 | 52 | M | | 100 | + | − | − | | stable 3.2-3.0 | 2 |
| 14 | 54 | F | + | 100 | + | +[c] | + | + | 13.0 → 4.6 | 7 |
| 15 | 66 | M | | 40 | + | + | − | | 4.9 → 3.5 | 6 |
| 16 | 61 | M | | 50 | + | + | − | | 3.6 → 1.8 | 9 |
| | 54 ± 5[d] | | 6/9 | 70 ± 7[d] | 14 | 12 | 9 | 7 | | |

HD, Hemodialysis; DD, Death or dialysis,
[a] = Prednisone & heparin.
[b] = 1 g pulse.
[c] = See text.
[d] = SEM

able to discontinue it. Once again, the second to last column of Table 12-11 gives the change in serum creatinine from the time a patient was first seen to last follow up. Some patients with creatinines as high as 17 to 18 mg/dl had a response with return of creatinine to the range of 3 to 4 mg/dl. Ten of 14 patients had serum creatinines greater than 6.0 mg/dl and 8 of those 10 responded to therapy. Of the patients who have responded, one (number 10) has relapsed and was not retreated. He has gone on to require hemodialysis. One patient progressed from NID on the first biopsy to granular deposits two months later. Follow up time ranged from 2 to 72 months in pulsed patients.

Inasmuch as the percent crescents and response to therapy in the two groups of granular and NID type AC-RPGN were similar, they were combined. This helps to provide a clearer illustration of the effect of therapy on the natural course of the disease. This information is presented in Table 12-12. One of 6 patients with conventional therapy was able to discontinue dialysis with a total of 4 of 9 improved, compared to 9 of 12 patients treated with pulse methylprednisolone who were able to discontinue dialysis and 18 of 21 improved. These numbers are highly significant. It is also important to point out from Tables 12-10 and 12-11 that two of the patients treated with conventional therapy with good response had 20 percent crescents.

The influence of percent crescents and oliguria on the prognosis in pulsed patients is given in Table 12-13. The patients are considered in two categories: (1)

improved with therapy and (2) on dialysis and able to discontinue it. Eighty-six percent of the entire series showed improvement in function and 75 percent of those patients on dialysis were able to discontinue it. Since many series consider high numbers of crescents as a significant negative factor in prognosis and low numbers of crescents predicting a good response, we have separated our patients into categories of percent crescents. This gives a breakdown which should allow for comparison to other studies. The percent crescents are divided into categories of 20 to 39, 40 to 59, 60 to 79, and 80 to 100. The next column gives the grouping of 60 to 100 percent, which is used by a number of other investigators. The last column provides data on the influence of oligoanuria on pulse methylprednisolone therapy. One of two patients in the first category (20 to 39 percent crescents) was improved and the other was able to discontinue dialysis. In the group with 40 to 59 percent crescents, all six patients showed improvement and two of two on dialysis were able to discontinue it. In the group with 60 to 79 percent crescents, all six showed improvement and all three patients on dialysis discontinued that support. In the last category of 80 to 100 percent crescents, five of seven (71 percent) improved and three of five (60 percent) were able to discontinue dialysis. In the 60 to 100 percent crescent group, 11 of 13 patients (85 percent) showed improvement. Eight patients in this group were on dialysis and six (75 percent) were able to discontinue it. Eleven patients had documented oligoanuria and of these, 10 (91

**Table 12-12.** Response to Pulse Therapy Compared to Conventional Treatment in Granular and NID Types AC-RPGN

| Therapy | # Pts | HD | Off HD | Improved |
|---|---|---|---|---|
| Conventional | 9 | 6 | 1 | 4 |
| Pulse | 21 | 12 | 9 | 18[a] |

HD, hemodialysis.
[a] = p < .025.

**Table 12-13.** Influence of Percent Crescents and Oligoanuria on Prognosis in Pulsed Patients: Granular and NID Types

| Prognosis | All | Percent Crescents | | | | | Oligo-anuria |
| | | 20–39 | 40–59 | 60–79 | 80–100 | 60–100 | |
|---|---|---|---|---|---|---|---|
| Improved | 18/21 | 1/2 | 6/6 | 6/6 | 5/7 | 11/13 | 10/11 |
| | (86%) | (50%) | (100%) | (100%) | (71%) | (85%) | (91%) |
| HD/Off HD | 9/12 | 1/2 | 2/2 | 3/3 | 3/5 | 6/8 | 7/8 |
| | (75%) | (50%) | (100%) | (100%) | (60%) | (75%) | (88%) |

HD, hemodialysis.

percent) showed improvement. Of eight oligoanuric patients who were on dialysis, seven (88 percent) were able to discontinue it. Even if the figures are adjusted to account for improved patients who relapsed and progressed to death or dialysis without therapy or in spite of therapy (Tables 12-10, 12-11), 16 of 21 (76 percent) still had a good response to pulse after a mean time of 27 months (range 2 to 72 months). Repeat biopsies in six patients showed markedly decreased or absent interstitial infiltrates, smaller remnant fibrocellular crescents, and diminished staining for fibrin within crescents.

A summary of the reported experience with pulse therapy of idiopathic AC-RPGN is provided in Table 12-14. This table includes our study of 21 patients and excludes anti-GBM patients. The other series also excluded anti-GBM patients, as best as could be ascertained from examination of the literature. Forty-five patients were treated with several different pulse regimens and of those, 34 (76 percent) were improved. The improvement rate ranged from 40 percent in O'Neill's series with use of 1 gram per day for seven days to as high as 100 percent in five patients

reported by Oredugba. Our series, which is thus far the largest of pulse methylprednisolone therapy, has an improvement rate of 86 percent, which is slightly higher than that reported by Bruns et al.[36] using 30 mg/kg every other day for 4 to 11 doses.

## Results of Therapy with Anti-GBM AC-RPGN

Results of our experience with anti-GBM AC-RPGN are presented in Table 12-15. Seventeen patients (36 percent of total) have been studied thus far. Five of these had associated pulmonary hemorrhage. Five patients were treated with modes of therapy other than intravenous pulse methylprednisone alone and all five required dialytic support. None of the five improved or were able to discontinue dialysis. Crescents in these five averaged 94 percent. Twelve patients were treated with pulse methylprednisolone. Of these, only two have responded, patients 6 and 14. One of those patients had 25 percent crescents and the other had 50 percent crescents, neither was oliguric,

**Table 12-14.** Response of Idiopathic AC-RPGN to Pulse Therapy[a]

| Series | Ref | Year | # Pts | Type Pulse | Stable or Improved | |
| | | | | | (#) | (%) |
|---|---|---|---|---|---|---|
| O'Neill | 135 | 1979 | 10 | 1 g/day × 7 days | 4 | 40 |
| Oredugba | 137 | 1980 | 5 | 1 g/day × 5 days | 5 | 100 |
| Bruns | 36 | 1981 | 9 | 30 mg/kd qod × 4-11 doses | 7 | 78 |
| Bolton, present study | | | 21 | 30 mg/kg qod × 3 doses | 18 | 86 |
| Total | | | 45 | | 34 | 76 |

[a]Excluding anti-GBM patients.

**Table 12-15.** Pulse Methylprednisolone Therapy of Anti-GBM type AC-RPGN

| Patient | Age | Sex | Oligo-anuria | (%) Cresc | Pulse | Improved | HD | Off HD | Sr. cr, mg/dl and outcome |
|---|---|---|---|---|---|---|---|---|---|
| 1 | 55 | M | + | 100 | − | − | + | + | DD |
| 2[a] | 21 | M | + | 100 | − | − | + | − | DD |
| 3 | 64 | F | | 90 | − | − | + | − | DD |
| 4[a] | 61 | M | + | 80 | − | − | + | − | DD |
| 5 | 44 | M | + | 100 | − | − | + | − | DD |
| | $49 \pm 8^b$ | | 4 | $94 \pm 4^b$ | 5 | 0 | 5 | 0 | |
| 6 | 50 | M | − | 50 | + | + | − | − | Stable 1.1 (39 mo) |
| 7 | 42 | M | − | 24 | + | − | + | − | DD |
| 8 | 39 | F | + | 94 | + | − | + | − | DD |
| 9 | 55 | M | + | 95 | + | − | + | − | DD |
| 10 | 26 | F | − | 100 | + | − | + | − | DD |
| 11[a] | 31 | M | + | 100 | + | − | + | − | DD |
| 12 | 50 | F | + | 100 | + | − | + | − | DD |
| 13[a] | 43 | F | + | 95 | + | − | + | − | DD |
| 14 | 59 | F | − | 25 | + | + | − | − | 4.3→1.4 (36 mo) |
| 15 | 56 | M | + | 50 | + | − | + | − | DD |
| 16[a] | 53 | F | + | 35 | + | − | + | − | DD |
| 17 | 67 | F | | 50 | + | − | + | − | DD |
| | $48 \pm 3^b$ | | 7 | $68 \pm 9^b$ | 12 | 2 | 10 | 0 | |

*Note.* HD, hemodialysis.
[a]Goodpasture's syndrome.
[b]SEM.

and both had minimal degrees of renal failure on presentation. However, patient number 6 had severe proliferative changes on biopsy with a stable serum creatinine and has remained stable. Patient number 14 had a good response with serum creatinine decreasing from 4.3 to 1.4 mg/dl. The other 10 patients, 7 of whom were oligonanuric, have required dialytic support and none has been able to discontinue it. Thus, results of pulse therapy in this subgroup of idiopathic AC-RPGN are no better than other treatment modalities and indicate patients with a significant degree of renal dysfunction, with oligoanuria or requiring dialytic support, will not show response to therapy. Two of three patients with Goodpasture's syndrome had dramatic improvement in pulmonary function after pulse, even though renal function remained unaltered.

## PAN Associated with AC-RPGN

In the course of following and treating some of our patients with idiopathic AC-RPGN, it became apparent at autopsy or by histologic examination of tissue other than kidney that they actually had PAN. These patients have not been included in the groups described above, but are considered separately at this point. As Table 12-1 illustrates, patients who have PAN may present with any one of three idiopathic AC-RPGN subtypes histologically and by immunofluorescence microscopy. It is this author's opinion that there may be more patients with PAN who have not been detected by routine kidney biopsy. As can be seen from Table 12-16, 94 percent of PAN-AC-RPGN patients do not respond to therapy, and a significant bias would be entered into a series if it contained these cases. Table 12-17 shows the results of pulse therapy in three of six patients with the histologic diagnosis of PAN. The three patients who were not pulsed had the diagnosis made prior to the histologic diagnosis of AC-RPGN and were treated with dialytic support. The three patients treated with pulse therapy were incorrectly diagnosed as idiopathic AC-RPGN and treated accordingly. As

**Table 12-16.** Prognosis in Pan-AC-RPGN[a]

| Series | Ref | Date | # Pts | Therapy | Better | DD |
|--------|-----|------|-------|---------|--------|-----|
| Rose | 150 | 1957 | 16 | | | 16 |
| Harrison | 75 | 1964 | 11 | | | 11 |
| Ladefoged | 95 | 1969 | 2 | | | 2 |
| Lewis[b] | 103 | 1971 | 2 | | | 2 |
| Arieff[b] | 2 | 1972 | 1 | | | 1 |
| Brown[b] | 35 | 1974 | 2 | | | 2 |
| Olsen[b] | 133 | 1974 | 8 | | 1 | 7 |
| Sissons | 157 | 1974 | 1 | | | 1 |
| Kanfer | 89 | 1976 | 5 | | | 5 |
| Nakamoto[b] | 127 | 1979 | 4 | | | 4 |
| Wu | 184 | 1980 | 2 | Pred.,Az. | 1 | 1 |
| Thomashow | 165 | 1980 | 1 | | | 1 |
| Bolton[b] | 28 | 1981 | 4 | | | 4 |
| Ogg[b] | 132 | 1981 | 8 | Quad. | 2 | 6 |
| Bhuyan | 21 | 1982 | 2 | | | 2 |
| Totals | | | 69 | | 4 (6%) | 65 (94%) |

[a]Excluding plasma exchange and pulse methylprednisolone.
[b]Selected from AC-RPGN series.

can be seen from the table, all patients had many crescents and five of six required dialysis. None of the three patients with supportive therapy showed any return of function. All three pulsed patients responded and two were able to discontinue dialysis. Two patients had return of creatinine clearance to 30 ml/min and the third increased her creatinine clearance to 100 ml/min. One patient died of a myocardial infarction at 14 months unrelated to PAN and the second died of an intraabdominal bleed secondary to reactivation of PAN. Neither was treated with cyclophosphamide, only pulse methylprednisolone and prednisone. The third patient was treated with a small dose of cyclophosphamide (50 mg/day) for a short period of time and at the same interval received pulse methylprednisolone. She is

well three years after pulse with normal renal function.

## Membranoproliferative Glomerulonephritis

We have treated only a few patients with MPGN using pulse methylprednisolone (Table 12-18). Of the six patients in this group, five had the clinical course of RPGN as described previously. The sixth patient had a more prolonged course of greater than three months. As can be seen from the table, one of two patients requiring dialysis was able to discontinue it and was stable at 12 months. Five of the six patients showed improvement in renal function. Two of the patients who responded have slowly had a decrease in function, with one of them requiring dial-

**Table 12-17.** Pulse Therapy of PAN-AC-RPGN

| Patient | Age | Sex | Pulse | % Cresc | Ccr Course & Outcome | HD | Off HD | Follow up, months |
|---------|-----|-----|-------|---------|----------------------|-----|--------|-------------------|
| 1 | 72 | M | + | 50 | <10 → 30 | + | + | 14 |
| 2 | 64 | M | + | 100 | 15 → 30 | − | − | 4 |
| 3 | 63 | F | + | 50 | <10 → 100 | + | + | 36 |
| 4 | 70 | M | − | 90 | DD | + | − | — |
| 5 | 62 | M | − | 90 | DD | + | − | — |
| 6 | 60 | F | − | 50 | DD | + | − | — |

Ccr = creatinine clearance, ml/min
HD = hemodialysis

**Table 12-18.** Pulse Therapy of MPGN

| Patient | Age | Sex | Pulse | S.cr, mg/dl and Outcome | HD | Off HD | Improved | Follow up, months |
|---------|-----|-----|-------|-------------------------|----|--------|----------|-------------------|
| 1[a] | 59 | F | + | >10.0 → 1.9 | + | + | + | 12 |
| 2[a] | 39 | M | + | 2.6 → 1.6 | | | + | 42 |
| 3[a] | 43 | M | + | 3.3 → 1.3 | | | + | 42 |
| 4[a] | 42 | M | + | >10.0 → HD | + | − | − | — |
| 5[a] | 43 | M | + | 10→4.0→HD | | | + | 4 |
| 6 | 43 | F | + | 2.6→4.0→1.6 | | | + | 50 |

*Note.* HD, hemodialysis.
[a]Clinical RPGN.

ysis. The other, patient number 6, had slowly deteriorating function with a serum creatinine of 3.2 mg/dl after 50 months. Each of the six had proliferative glomerulonephritis and all had ultrastructural changes compatible with MPGN. All had active urinary sediments and proteinuria, and four of six had stable antecedent renal disease with documented normal function which entered a rapidly progressive course leading to the institution of pulse therapy. Crescents were less prevalent in this group, with only patient number 2 having 50 percent crescents and the remainder having less than 20 percent crescents.

## Influence of Glomerular Sclerosis on Response to Pulse Therapy

Since granular and NID types of AC-RPGN responded well to pulse therapy, regardless of the number of crescents, as opposed to the anti-GBM type AC-RPGN, we assessed the influence of glomerulosclerosis on response to therapy when biopsy specimens contained 20 percent or more obsolescent or sclerotic glomeruli (Table 12-19). The patients are divided into anti-GBM, granular deposits, and NID disease. There were a total of four anti-GBM, four granular and seven NID subtypes with 20 percent, or more sclerosis. All of the anti-GBM patients required dialysis and did not respond, with a degree of sclerosis of 25 to 50 percent. One of the four granular deposit patients required di-

alysis but was able to discontinue it, with a serum creatinine of 3.7 mg/dl despite 80 percent sclerosis. All four of the granular deposit patients showed improvement in renal function and their degree of sclerosis ranged from 20 to 80 percent. One patient stopped his medications after responding to therapy and went on to require dialysis. The other three maintained a good response in follow up periods from 19 to 47 months. Of the seven NID patients, six had a good response. One did not respond and required dialysis. One other patient, number 13, had a gradual decline in renal function over two years, while the other patients have maintained their function up to 72 months after initial pulse therapy. Four of the five on dialysis were able to discontinue that support. Thus, in the granular and NID subtypes, even though significant degrees of glomerular sclerosis were present on biopsy, patients responded well to therapy with decrease in serum creatinine which was maintained in most instances over prolonged periods of follow-up.

## Complications

Thus far, treatment of patients with high-dose pulse methylprednisolone and alternate day oral prednisone has resulted in no major complications. Patients have complained of a metallic taste, occasional nausea, arthralgias, muscle weakness, bright lights or other psychotropic effects after the infusion period, or occasional

**Table 12-19.** Pulse Therapy Response Related to Glomerular Sclerosis

| Patient | Type | % Obs/ Scler | S.cr, mg/dl and Outcome | HD/ Off | Stable, Improved | Most recent S.Cr, mg/dl | Follow up, months |
|---|---|---|---|---|---|---|---|
| 1 | a-GBM | 32 | HD | +/− | − | [a] | |
| 2 | a-GBM | 50 | HD | +/− | − | HD | |
| 3 | a-GBM | 25 | HD | +/− | − | HD | |
| 4 | a-GBM | 48 | HD | +/− | − | HD | |
| 5 | granular | 40 | 6.1 → 3.3 + | − | + | HD[b] | |
| 6 | granular | 20 | 4.6 → 1.3 + | − | + | 1.3 | 47 |
| 7 | granular | 80 | 16.6 → 3.7 | +/+ | + | 3.7 | 19 |
| 8 | granular | 50 | 3.3 → 2.3 | − | + | 3.5 | 36 |
| 9 | NID | 43 | 12.0 → 2.1 + | +/+ | + | 2.6 | 65 |
| 10 | NID | 20 | HD | +/− | − | HD | |
| 11 | NID | 20 | 18.2 → 3.6 | +/+ | + | 3.6 | 62 |
| 12 | NID | 50 | 1.9 → 0.9 | − | + | 1.0 | 72 |
| 13 | NID | 47 | 3.8 → 1.0 | − | + | 9.0 | 24 |
| 14 | NID | 90 | 12.0 → 5.4 | +/+ | + | 4.6 | 10 |
| 15 | NID | 50 | HD → 3.0 | +/+ | + | 3.0 | 24 |

*Note.* Obs, obsolescent; Scler, sclerosis; HD, hemodialysis.
[a]Died of nonrenal causes.
[b]Stopped medications.

discomfort at the site of infusion. One patient developed an arrhythmia, although that patient had a preexisting history of cardiac instability. None of the other patients developed decreased blood pressure or arrhythmia. Of the possible long term complications of alternate day steroids, we have seen the development of cataracts, cushingoid fascies, acne and hirsutism. The cushingoid side effects have been minimal, since therapy has been alternate day from the beginning. Our previous experience suggests that there will be approximately one major complication of therapy with prolonged alternate day high dose steroids for each 12 patient years of therapy.[23]

# COMPARISON OF PULSE METHYL-PREDNISOLONE TO OTHER THERAPY

Examination of previous tables assessing the course and prognosis of various types of AC-RPGN with conventional, quadruple or pulse therapy indicates that there are significant differences in response with different types of therapy. The most recent successful therapeutic technique for AC-RPGN is plasma exchange with immunosuppressives. This may be a particularly important innovation for patients with anti-GBM type glomerulonephritis.

## Non-Anti-GBM AC-RPGN

As previously discussed, the heterogeneity of patients categorized as AC-RPGN makes evaluation of various series more difficult. Table 12-20 examines the effect of plasma exchange and immunosuppression in five series of patients in whom it was possible to exclude anti-GBM disease. A number of other entities, including Berger's, Henoch-Schönlein purpura, PAN, and proliferative nephritis were included. Forty-three patients were evaluated and of these, 13 went on to death or dialysis for a 30 percent failure rate. Thirty (70 percent) were stable or improved. Where that information was available, as indicated in the last column, severe complications including infection and death were present in 11 of 37 patients (30 percent). These complications

**Table 12-20.** Plasma Exchange and Immunosuppression in Non-Anti-GBM RPGN[a]

| Series | Ref | Year | # Pts | DD | Stable/ Improved | Severe Complication |
|--------|-----|------|-------|-----|------------------|---------------------|
| Lockwood | 106 | 1977 | 8 | 3 | 5 | 2 |
| Becker | 14 | 1977 | 4 | 1 | 3 | ? |
| Asaba | 3 | 1980 | 2 | 1 | 1 | ? |
| Wing | 181 | 1980 | 7 | 1 | 6 | 5 |
| Thysell | 168 | 1982 | 22 | 3/7[b] | 19/15 | 4 |
| | | | 43 | 13 | 30 | 11/37[c] |
| | | | | (30%) | (70%) | (30%) |

[a]Includes Berger's, Henoch-Schönlein purpura, PAN, acute proliferative GN; excludes Wegener's and transplants.

[b]3 → immediate DD, 4 at variable times.

[c]Severe infection, death.

were greater in some series, such as that of Wing (5 complications in 7 patients), as opposed to Thysall (4 complications in 22 patients). The latter severe complication rate is still 18 percent. Table 12-21 uses previously cited series for quadruple, miscellaneous, and pulse therapy (including our study), and plasma exchange with immunosuppression. Also included are the "pure" idiopathic AC-RPGN as listed in Table 12-6. The miscellaneous therapy group includes mixed types of AC-RPGN, but excludes patients with postinfectious and anti-GBM nephritis. Twenty-nine percent of patients treated with quadruple therapy progressed to death or dialysis compared to 24 percent with pulse therapy and 30 percent with plasma exchange and immunosuppression. These values are all comparable. In contradistinction, 73 percent treated with miscellaneous therapy progressed to death or dialysis, and 81 percent of pure idiopathic AC-

RPGN patients failed. Thus, the improvement rate for quadruple, pulse, and plasma exchange therapy was comparable, with pulse therapy having a slightly greater rate of improvement (76 percent).

## Anti-GBM AC-RPGN

The results of plasma exchange in anti-GBM type AC-RPGN are given in Table 12-22. The results of 10 series other than case reports are presented. Seventy-five patients have been treated thus far and of these, 34 percent (45 percent) were improved. Forty-one proceeded to death or dialysis (55 percent). Of note is the fact that, of 22 patients with documented oligoanuria, none showed improvement. Comparative results of different therapy for anti-GBM nephritis are given in Table 12-23. Patients were treated with quadruple, pulse methylprednisolone, plasma exchange with immunosuppressives, and

**Table 12-21.** Comparison of Therapies for Non-Anti-GBM AC-RPGN[a]

| Treatment | # Pts | DD | Improved |
|-----------|-------|-----|----------|
| Quadruple therapy | 41 | 12 (29%) | 29 (71%) |
| Miscellaneous[b] | 123 | 90 (73%) | 33 (27%) |
| "Pure" idiopathic AC-RPGN | 70 | 57 (81%) | 13 (19%) |
| Pulse therapy | 45 | 11 (24%) | 34 (76%) |
| Plasma exchange and immunosuppression | 43 | 13 (30%) | 30 (70%)[c] |

[a] = Excluding postinfectious patients

[b] = Includes mixed AC-RPGN.

[c] = Severe complications of treatment—30% of patients.

*Note.* DD = Death or dialysis.

**Table 12-22.** Effect of Plasma Exchange on Anti-GBM AC-RPGN

| Series | Ref | Year | # Pts | Better | DD | Improved with Oliguria |
|--------|-----|------|-------|--------|-----|------------------------|
| Walker | 176 | 1977 | 4 | 2 | 2 | |
| Swainson | 164 | 1978 | 3 | 0 | 3 | |
| Johnson | 87 | 1978 | 4 | 2 | 2 | 0/1 |
| Erickson | 59 | 1979 | 5 | 3 | 2 | |
| McKenzie | 114 | 1979 | 4 | 3 | 1 | 0/1 |
| Munk | 126 | 1979 | 2 | 1[a] | 1 | |
| Asaba | 3 | 1980 | 2 | 1 | 1 | 0/1 |
| Peters | 140 | 1982 | 41 | 16 | 25 | 0/19 |
| Moore | 121 | 1982 | 8 | 6 | 2 | ? |
| Thysell | 168 | 1982 | 2 | 0 | 2 | |
| Total | | | 75 | 34 (45%) | 41 (55%) | 0/22 |

[a]Negative anti-GBM antibody by RIA.

conventional therapy. Eighty-nine percent of patients treated with all types of therapy other than pulse or plasma exchange went on to death or dialysis, and 83 percent of pulsed patients required dialysis or died. Too little information is available to assess the effects of quadruple therapy, but none of three patients appears to have responded. In contrast, as shown in Table 12-22, 55 percent of patients treated with plasma exchange and immunosuppressives died, and 45 percent improved. This is significantly better than miscellaneous, pulse, or quadruple therapy. However, of note is the fact that no patient with oligoanuria responded to plasma exchange and immunosuppressive therapy, a phenomenon we noted in our series of patients treated with pulse therapy. In analyzing our series (Table 12-15), only four patients were not oligoanuric and of those, two responded to pulse methylprednisolone therapy. Thus, 50 percent of nonoligoanuric patients who were not on dialysis

responded, compared to the 50 percent response for plasma exchange and immunosuppressives. However, the very small number of nonoligoanuric patients who were pulsed and responded makes it very difficult to draw any conclusions. As previously reported, [55] pulse therapy significantly ameliorated the grave pulmonary hemorrhage that is the hallmark of the Goodpasture variant of anti-GBM AC-RPGN.[18,33,145,146]

PAN-AC-RPGN: Utilization of corticosteroids has greatly improved the overall prognosis of patients with PAN.[68] The same cannot be said for PAN-AC-RPGN. Table 12-24 contains information in the same format as the previous comparison tables. Once again, patients are gleaned from the literature as listed in Table 12-16 and references 127, 130, 132, 135, and 168. The number of patients treated with either quadruple, pulse, or plasma exchange therapy is small compared to the number of patients treated with all other

**Table 12-23.** Comparison of Therapies for Anti-GBM AC-RPGN

| Treatment | # Pts | DD | Improved |
|-----------|-------|-----|----------|
| Quadruple | 3 | 3 (100%) | — |
| Miscellaneous | 81 | 72 (89%) | 9 (11%) |
| Pulse | 12 | 10 (83%) | 2 (17%) |
| Plasma exchange and immunosuppression | 75 | 41 (55%) | 34 (45%)[a] |

[a]None improved with oligoanuria.

**Table 12-24.** Comparison of Therapies for Pan-AC-RPGN

| Treatment | # Pts | DD | Better |
|---|---|---|---|
| Quadruple therapy | 6 | 5 (83%) | 1 (17%)[a] |
| Miscellaneous | 69 | 65 (94%) | 4 ( 6%) |
| Pulse | 4 | 0 | 4 (100%) |
| Plasma exchange and immunosuppression | 8 | 1 (12%) | 7 (88%)[a] |

[a]No response in oligoanuric patients.
[b]One serious complication.

modalities. One patient improved with quadruple therapy, 4 of 69 (6 percent) with all other types of miscellaneous therapy, 4 of 4 patients responded to pulse therapy (one of these had a relapse and died of an intraabdominal hemorrhage), and 7 of 8 patients treated with plasma exchange responded. Based on these small numbers, a combination of either pulse methylprednisolone or plasma exchange and immunosuppressives appears to give the best results for PAN-AC-RPGN. One serious complication in eight patients treated with immunosuppressive therapy and plasma exchange was noted, and no complications occurred with pulse methylprednisolone therapy.

## Membranoproliferative Glomerulonephritis

Minimal information is available about patients with MPGN who also fit the definition of RPGN. It is clearly established that MPGN has a poor prognosis, especially in adults, with at least half the patients reaching end-stage disease between 6 and 11 years after diagnosis.[38,72,92,108,173] A number of these patients apparently have smoldering progressive disease which can enter an accelerated phase, and a few of them will present with de novo RPGN. The results of any type of therapy have been extremely poor, although high-dose alternate day oral prednisone appears to offer significant advantages in this entity if given over prolonged periods of time.[23,111] There is also little experience with pulse

methylprednisolone therapy of MPGN. Cole et al.[44] used it in three of their patients with proliferative nephritis who had documented membranoproliferative changes. Two of the three had a good response to therapy and the other progressed to dialysis. In our series, four of six patients, the same ratio, have been stable after pulse therapy, although one (patient number 6) has slowly progressive deteriorating renal function and one discontinued dialysis. If minimal information is available regarding pulse therapy of MPGN-RPGN, less is available regarding plasma exchange and immunosuppression. While pulse therapy would appear to be beneficial in the two series reported, more patients with a bona fide RPGN will have to be examined before this can be clearly ascertained.

Thus, for the categories of idiopathic AC-RPGN, PAN-AC-RPGN, and MPG-RPGN, aggressive therapeutic intervention significantly alters the course of disese in all but anti-GBM disease. Although the number of patients in the anti-GBM pulse therapy group who were similar to those treated with plasma exchange is too small for comparison, the failure of patients to respond significantly suggests that pulse therapy is less efficacious than plasma exchange.

## PATHOGENESIS

Examination of the histologic subtypes and their response (or lack thereof) to therapy may provide information about their respective pathogeneses. As illustrated in Table 12-1, there are many processes which may result in the histologic entity of crescentic nephritis, most of which are associated with a rapidly progressive course. While some cases of acute crescentic nephritis are secondary to the diseases noted in Table 1, others, which the author has designated as idiopathic, are mediated by several presumably different pathogenetic mechanisms. These are by: (1) deposition of antibody along the basement membrane, (2) deposition of circulating soluble immune complexes within the glomerulus, or fixation of antibody to in situ antigens,[48] or (3) cell-mediated mechanisms.[45,66,112] Most patients with crescentic nephritis have certain common histologic features. These include a severe interstitial infiltrate with mononuclear cells which appear similar to monocytes and lymphocytes, multinucleated giant cells, both within the interstitium and the glomerulus, tubular increscences, defects in Bowman's capsule, gaps in the GBM, and a periglomerular fibrotic reaction.[22,61,88,117,133] The commonality of the histologic picture, regardless of the etiology, suggests that crescentic nephritis may represent the final common pathway of clinically and pathogenetically distinct variants. The interstitial reaction and course of the nephritis in these histologic entities are very similar to acute cell mediated allograft rejections of the kidney transplant.[28,29,47] In addition, the response of the disease process to the same treatment modality used to treat transplant rejection strongly implies that similar mechanisms may be involved. Figure 12-1 presents a proposed model for the pathogenesis of RPGN, whether it be of the acute crescentic variety or noncrescentic. The basic and original event would appear to be exposure of the individual to an antigen, resulting in initiation of an immune response. This immunization could occur against exogenous foreign antigens, or because of release of endogenous antigens which are normally sequestered and not available for immune recognition. It might also occur by exposure to self-antigens which have been altered by some mechanism, or by exogenous antigens which result in a hapten-like effect or by immunization via cross-reaction between exogenous and endogenous antigens. Cellular hypersensitivity to GBM antigen has been demonstrated in some patients with RPGN and there is an increase in cell mediated immunity to altered or fetal renal antigens in certain types of nephritis.[17,65,66,107,110,149,185] The strong propensity for glomerulonephritis to occur in individuals with altered immune states[156] and the association between crescentic nephritis and the elderly population[28,29,69,161] implicate an abnormality in immune status as a factor in the development of nephritis. Alteration in the ratio between helper and suppressor cells with senescence[139] or other lymphocyte abnormalities might render the individual more susceptible to immunization or allow forbidden clones to emerge, resulting in initiation of the disease process. The sequence of events that might follow immunization is probably strongly dependent upon genetic factors.[156] The ability to develop antibody to GBM in animals is a T-cell dependent phenomenon[24,26] and the antibody response to renal antigens is genetically influenced in mice with autoimmune glomerulotubular nephropathy.[138] Various types of renal disease have strong associations with HLA type[90,105,176] and this appears to be most important in anti-GBM mediated glomerulonephritis.[140] Teleologically, it is obvious that some patients, upon exposure to an antigen such as streptococcal antigen, will develop nephritis. Some will go on to more severe nephritis, while others will have no disease. It is probable that genetic factors, as they become better understood, will be shown to play an increasingly important role in the development of various types

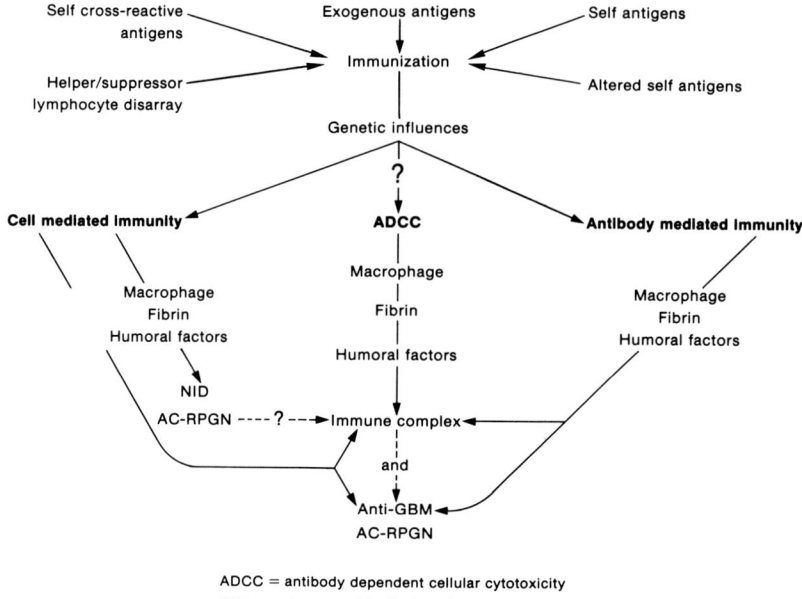

ADCC = antibody dependent cellular cytotoxicity
NID = no immunoglobulin deposit

**Fig. 12-1.** Proposed schema for pathogenetic mechanisms of RPGN. The presence of antibodies to GBM, immune complexes, and cell-mediated immunity to renal antigens have all been documented. Genetic influences have also been shown in certain subtypes. Macrophages, fibrin and humoral mediators have been demonstrated in various forms of human RPGN. Conversion from immune complex to anti-GBM type disease has been well documented, and probably NID to immune complex type. The participation and interaction of the three paths of the immune system illustrated here are partly hypothetical, but based upon current knowledge of human and experimental animal immune systems and renal diseases.

of glomerulonephritis. As postulated in Figure 12-1 after immunization by whatever mechanism occurs, and as modulated by numerous as yet unknown genetic factors, there will logically be formation of sensitized cells and antibodies to the immunizing antigen. These antibodies then deposit either as "immune complexes" by combining with antigen in the circulation or in situ antigens in the kidney.[46,48] They could presumably be attracted to endogenous constituents of the kidney or to implanted antigens. Curiously, antibody deposition always appears to be localized to the glomerulus or basement membrane structures. On the other hand, the cellular component in AC-RPGN is mostly in the crescents and interstitium, in obvious close apposition to the basement membranes. The reason cells are present is not clear, but they are presumably attracted by some mechanism such as antigens endogenous to the kidney, implanted in the kidney in cooperation with deposited antibody, or via unidentified released factors. The resultant humoral response with glomerular deposition of antibody and/or complexes may only be a marker of a concomitant cell mediated onslaught upon the kidney.[29,46] An increasingly persuasive amount of evidence points to the important role of cell mediated immunity in glomerulonephritis.[66,112,172] Macrophages have been identified in glomerulonephritis in the tufts, crescents and interstitium by light microscopy and histochemical stains,[109,120,123] and have been shown experimentally to be of bone marrow origin.[154] Macrophages have been identified by cell culture techniques to be present in large numbers in glomerular explants from patients with crescents and glomerulonephritis, but absent or considerably fewer in other individuals.[4,5] Tissue culture studies in experimental animal models demonstrate comparable results.[81,167] Experimentally, macrophages participate in glomerulonephritis, as shown by abrogation of proteinuria and proliferative changes in animals that receive antimacrophage antiserum or irradiation.[80,96,154] Furthermore, mononuclear cells have been clearly shown to be involved in serum sickness and nephrotoxic nephritis in experimental animals.[20,83,167] Cells, presumably of T-cell origin presensitized to glomerular bound antigens, will localize in the kidney where antigen has been previously fixed.[20,94] In addition, severe proliferative glomerulonephritis with crescents secondary to an intact cell-mediated immune system may be produced in chickens in the absence of any humoral immunity, indicating that humoral immunity is not required in all instances for the development of glomerulonephritis.[32,170] This latter model would appear to be analagous to the NID variety of AC-RPGN. In the same model, preservation of the humoral system with an intact cell-mediated immune system leads to a similar proliferative glomerulonephritis associated with antibody along the GBM.

Regardless of whether NID-type AC-RPGN is present, or nephritis associated with anti-GBM antibodies or immune complexes, the histologic lesion is always associated with proliferation of Bowman's capsule with an infiltration of monocytes and the presence within the crescent of copious amounts of fibrin. There seems to be little doubt that fibrinogen is involved in the development of crescents, and fibrin has been shown to pass across the GBM into Bowman's space to presumably be phagocytosed by macrophages or to attract macrophages into Bowman's space with formation of crescents.[117] It is quite obvious, however, that the mere presence of fibrin within Bowman's space, as may be found in numerous proteinuric states, is inadequate to elicit the formation of crescents per se, and that other factors must be involved. Exactly what these factors may be remains unexplained, but could well be prostaglandins, lymphokines, other cell products, or as yet undescribed mediators. As proposed in Figure 12-1, if cell-mediated immunity is the major arm of the immune system which is stimulated by a combination of the immunization and genetic factors, then NID-AC-RPGN may develop. On the other hand, if antibody to the basement membrane or immune complexes develops by activation of the humoral portion of the immune system, then presumably anti-GBM or immune complex type AC-RPGN is the consequence. Interchange between immune complex and anti-GBM disease, and between NID and immune complex types may rarely occur (dotted lines). Although it has been our experience that the two latter diseases remain distinct, we have now seen one patient in whom a repeat biopsy on reactivation clearly shows progression from an NID-type AC-RPGN to an immune complex type AC-RPGN over a period of a few months.

The proposed schema for the pathogenesis of AC-RPGN may help to explain the beneficial results of pulse methylprednisolone therapy. Large doses of steroidal agents result in leukopenia and impairment of mixed lymphocyte cultures.[40] There is depression of T-cell and B-cell function[37,64,178,182] and a marked monocytopenia with depressed macrophage function.[7,10,42,49,79,131,147,166] Other effects which might contribute to the results include prevention of leakage of lysosomal enzymes,[71] inhibition of fibroblasts and granulocyte function,[73,98] and depression of circulating immune complex levels in those patients in whom this might be a factor.[102,136] Large doses of methylprednisolone may also affect membrane permeability.[34] Their direct effects on renal blood flow and function are less likely to be involved.[54] Thus, pulse methylprednisolone might well be expected to have a beneficial effect on AC-RPGN mediated solely by steroid-sensitive cells, and in humorally mediated AC-RPGN in which steroid-sensitive-cell-mediated immunity plays an enhancing role. On the other hand, pulse methylprednisolone might not be expected to have a significant effect upon a pathogenetic process which relies either solely or in major part upon antibody-mediated damage, or which is also mediated by non-steroid-sensitive cells. The recurrence of anti-GBM antibodies on the GBM in kidney transplants, but usually without significant disease,[101,180] suggests the a priori need for some type of cellular cooperation present originally, but not at the time of the recurrence of transplant anti-GBM antibodies. The author would like to propose an interstitial process, analagous to acute cell-mediated rejection of kidney allografts. The interstitial infiltrate also responds histologically in the same manner as the allograft to appropriate therapy.[29] Thus, it seems reasonable that cell-mediated immunity is involved both in NID-type AC-RPGN and in antibody-mediated AC-RPGN. Whether that occurs as independent simultaneous activation of both the humoral and cellular immune systems, or by previously described mechanisms of interaction between antibodies and cell mediated immune systems, specifically antibody-dependent cellular cytotoxicity (ADCC) or a variant thereof, is not known. In Figure 12-1, the author postulates that cell-mediated immunity as a major factor may result in NID-type AC-RPGN, and antibody initiation as a major factor results in immune complex or anti-GBM disease, or cooperation in terms of ADCC may occur and produce either immune complex or anti-GBM disease. The difference in response to therapy and in prognosis between immune complex AC-RPGN and that mediated by anti-GBM antibody suggests that two different mechanisms are involved in their production. Since both immune complex and NID-type AC-RPGN appear to respond quite well to pulse methylprednisolone but anti-GBM disease does not, one might hypothesize that anti-GBM disease is mediated either mostly by the antibody itself, or by the antibody in cooperation with a steroid-resistant cell population while the other types are produced via steroid-sensitive cells alone or with complexes.[57] It is obvious that additional studies both in man and experimental animal models are needed to further delineate the pathogenetic mechanisms involved in the development of AC-RPGN and to clarify the relationship between some of the systemic diseases, such as PAN, which appear to produce an identical syndrome to certain types of idiopathic AC-RPGN. Figure 12-1 also suggests that both immune complex AC-RPGN and NID-type AC-RPGN are mediated by steroid-sensitive lymphocytes and macrophages, either with or without circulating soluble immune complexes, as opposed to anti-GBM-mediated AC-RPGN, which would be mediated either by antibodies or by antibodies in combination with steroid-insensitive lymphocytes. It is also possible that each of the mechanisms described above is dose related, in as much as pulse methylprednisolone might have a beneficial effect relatively far into the course of a cell-mediated process with minimal humoral component but may only have a beneficial effect early in the course of anti-GBM nephritis or if anti-GBM disease reactivates when immunosuppressives are already being used. This is suggested by the fact that the small number of anti-GBM patients who have benefited from pulse methylprednisolone are those with smaller degrees of crescents and lesser abnormalities in renal function. Unfortunately, the same rationale might hold for plasma exchange with immunosuppressive therapy, since none of the patients in a prospective randomized trial reported by Moore et al.[121] on dialysis with anti-GBM mediated RPGN were able to discontinue dialysis or showed any improvement. However, an encouraging finding was that, in patients randomly selected to receive plasma exchange, the number who benefited compared to the control group approached significance, indicating that early plasma exchange therapy with immunosuppressives might decrease the number of patients developing oligoanuric renal failure and requiring dialysis. No therapeutic modality is known which is as effective in anti-GBM disease in patients on dialysis as pulse methylprednisolone is in similar patients with either NID or immune complex type AC-RPGN. The proposed pathogenetic mechanism in Figure 12-1 would also explain the unique association of PAN-AC-RPGN with all three subtypes of idiopathic RPGN. The underlying pathogenetic process leading to PAN might then result in release of antigens and initiation of the sequence described in Figure 12-2 with development of idiopathic AC-RPGN along variable paths depending on yet unknown determining factors.

# DISCUSSION

Results of the review of the literature and the outcome of those series should clearly indicate the importance of a careful and thorough histologic and clinical diagnosis relative to the classification of patients with RPGN. As our understanding of the pathogenesis increases, there will be more subclassifiction and clarification of these entities. However, at the present time it is imperative that light, electron, and immunofluorescence microscopy, as well as serologic laboratory data, be analyzed to categorize patients as cleanly as is presently possible into separate types of AC-RPGN. The lumping of all patients with crescents who have a rapidly progressive clinical course into one group and then assessing the "natural course" of the process or the effect of therapy is unacceptable. Not only may patients be incorrectly treated according to the current state of the art, but development of the state of the art of appropriate and inappropriate treatments will be further delayed. It is clear in examining these diseases of known poor outcome that no therapy, or therapy with prednisone, anticoagulants, immunosuppressives, or other agents alone or in combinations of two or three, is ineffective. However, it is becoming increasingly evident for the NID and granular deposit types of AC-RPGN that several modes of therapy are effective. These are pulse methylprednisolone therapy, plasma exchange, or quadruple therapy as espoused by the British. Pulse methylprednisolone is not a new or unique treatment for patients with various types of severe systemic or organ-localized disease. It has been widely used in the treatment of cell-mediated renal transplant rejection[16,171,183] and in lung transplants,[174] and it was the histologic similarity between rejection and AC-RPGN that led to its use in our studies. One of the first applications to glomerulonephritis was that of Cathcart et al.[39] in which patients with diffuse proliferative lupus nephritis were treated with one gram dose of intravenous methylprednisolone. Since then, numerous reports of pulse therapy in SLE have been reported with the suggestion that prognosis of that disease is improved with this mode of therapy.[11,56,60,91,143] Pulse therapy has also been used in rheumatoid arthritis, ankylosing spondylitis, Wegener's granulomatosis, temporal arteritis and pulmonary hemorrhage.[55,67,76,104,116,118,119] The number of patients treated is small, and therefore, the results are difficult to interpret. Pulse did appear beneficial in many instances. Early reports of adverse reactions with death secondary to large doses of intravenous methylprednisolone were probably related to intravascular volume depletion with consequent hypotension and arrhythmias.[113] In our experience, administration of high-dose intravenous methylprednisolone very rapidly over only 20 minutes has not been associated with any serious side effects. In addition, in a high-risk population of more than 500 patients with acute myocardial infarction, there was no increased risk of arrhythmia or death in patients treated in the immediate postinfarction period with the same regimen used in our patients compared to a group of similar control patients not given intravenous methylprednisolone (personal communication, Craig Metz, Upjohn Company, Kalamazoo, Mich.). In examining our series and those in the literature, it appears that methylprednisolone 30 mg/kg, over 20 minutes by our regimen, is safe and more effective than other pulse regimens previously used, including 1 g daily for numerous doses. Our series contained four patients treated with 1 g rather than 30 mg/kg and, of these, half were eventually failures.[29] This is lower than the percentage of patients who responded well to pulse therapy overall and reconfirms the efficacy of the larger dose given as indicated. In addition to giving methylprednisolone rapidly in high doses, we give it on an alternate day schedule. We believe these three factors

are important in the beneficial effects with minimal complications. We do *not* give pulses as has been cited elsewhere.[70] Quadruple therapy has results similar to pulse therapy and appears to be a viable alternative, but requires the use of immunosuppressive agents with the inherent future risks of development of malignancy, and has a higher complication rate for infection and bleeding. Plasma exchange with immunosuppression also appears to have a proven beneficial effect. However, it is accompanied by a very high complication rate, especially in some series, and is quite expensive. It is this author's opinion, from our observations and those of others, that the use of pulse methylprednisolone is associated with a high rate of remission with minimal relapses and that this type of therapy is the least hazardous of those which have been shown to be effective.

The prognosis for anti-GBM disease, in contradistinction to the above types, is abysmal, regardless of any type of therapy thus far used. The results for pulse therapy in nonoligoanuric patients not on dialysis appear to be as good as plasma exchange with immunosuppression, but the latter offers the potential of preventing these patients from developing oligoanuria. Additional studies will be needed to clarify this. Pulse therapy appears to be quite effective in PAN-AC-RPGN in inducing a remission, but our series is small. One of three patients had a relapse and died of PAN complications. In view of wide experience in the treatment of PAN with cyclophosphamide,[63] it is probable that patients with documented PAN should receive pulse methylprednisolone in combination with cyclophosphamide. The results of treatment of MPGN are difficult to assess because of the heterogeneity of this group of patients. Nonetheless, in patients with the clinical course of RPGN or with numerous cellular crescents, our experience and that of others would suggest that pulse therapy is efficacious in arresting the disease process.

The author has not addressed the other subtypes of AC-RPGN in this chapter. Nonetheless, the documented literature experience of postinfectious RPGN with a 51 percent failure rate suggests that pulse therapy should be attempted in these patients as well. While one cannot dispute that 51 percent is a much better failure rate than the 85 or 95 percent for idiopathic and PAN types of AC-RPGN, this is still totally unacceptable and should be treated aggressively. The author has also not attempted to examine the arguments for or against the use of other therapeutic modalities for AC-RPGN since these are of little, if any, benefit. The rationale for their use from experimental animal models, and assessment of results in man, have been critically examined in a recent excellent review.[47] It should be remembered that patients treated by those modalities are included in this assessment of therapy as "conventional or no therapy."

No doubt there will continue to be controversy concerning the treatment of patients with severe progressive disease of the type described here. It should be obvious from a review of the literature that no or minimal treatment is an unacceptable alternative for these patients and that, with aggressive therapy, survival of the patient off dialysis and removal from dialysis is not only feasible but expected. The author, as well as others, would like to see prospective randomized trials performed to assess the effect of various treatments. However, a no-treatment control is an unacceptable ideal in a disease with such a high mortality rate, and neither the collaborating physicians in our study nor in those of other large centers are willing to have their patients undergo the risks of not receiving the apparently appropriate therapy. Although it could be argued that some of these patients may eventually develop slowly progressive end-stage disease that is unresponsive to any therapy, as we have seen on occasion, and therefore other modes of therapy should be tried, it is our experience that very few of these patients actually progress to end-stage disease. Perhaps a decade from now additional experience will contradict this concept, but we must also weigh the risks of more aggressive therapy and the chance that the patient may develop a life-threatening or fatal complication now or a decade later. The world's transplantation literature is replete with experience in treating patients with pulse methylprednisolone and oral prednisone. It seems unlikely that this therapy will be associated with increased risk of malignancy or other problems except as noted here. The same cannot be said for plasma exchange or immunosuppressive therapy. It is this author's opinion that these modalities should be used when pulse therapy has been shown to fail. It is our practice to repeat the kidney biopsy in any patient who has received pulse therapy and not responded by two months to reassess the need for change in therapy. In those patients with anti-GBM disease who continue to progress rapidly downhill despite pulse therapy, it is probable that more aggressive treatment such as plasma exchange and immunosuppression should be instituted immediately. Inasmuch as it is the physician's role to appropriately treat patients to the best of his ability and to offer them the greatest benefit with the least risk, pulse methylprednisolone seems to have a strong preference and to be the first treatment of choice for these devastating diseases.

Concentration upon the facts and figures, the pros and cons, and the "scientific data" sometimes obscures more important aspects of successful therapy of

RPGN. The ability of patients to stop dialytic support and return to normal lifestyles cannot be overemphasized as a beneficial effect, as the return of an individual to a useful life and a contributing member of society is a goal to be sought. These factors are difficult to measure, whereas the savings to society of the cost of dialysis and end-stage support is more tangible.[12,148] Using our experience with patients treated since 1976, the savings to society in this small series is nearly $2,000,000. The search for better therapeutic modalities with fewer side effects is laudable and to be encouraged; nonetheless, the mode of therapy that seems most efficacious should be used in the interim. At the present time, our recommendations are for pulse methylprednisolone therapy and alternate day prednisone according to the previously mentioned protocol for patients with both NID and granular deposit type AC-RPGN; for PAN-AC-RPGN, the same regimen with cyclophosphamide; and for anti-GBM mediated disease, a combination of pulse methylprednisolone and plasma exchange with immunosuppression, if response to pulse is not evident immediately. All are followed by alternate day high-dose oral prednisone. The beneficial effects on the disease as described in this chapter are undeniable; our lack of understanding of the mechanisms of disease production or of the way treatment exerts its beneficial effect do not in any way lessen the impact of therapy on the disease process. Those who doubt may continue to use other therapy and wait for a prospective controlled trial to confirm or deny the efficacy of more recent therapeutic approaches to the treatment of this devastating disease in any of its numerous forms. It is the consensus of the author and many other investigators that it is unconscionable to deny patients a therapy which is probably effective, based only upon the rigid criterion that "controlled trials must be done."

For now, pulse therapy appears to be the best there is relative to risk/benefit ratio and complications with an eye to the long term survival of patients. We await with interest modifications of this basic therapy which will improve its efficacy without loss of safety.

## SUMMARY

Acute crescentic rapidly progressive glomerulonephritis (AC-RPGN) is associated with an extremely poor prognosis with conventional therapy. Death or dialysis will result in about 51 percent of patients with documented postinfectious nephritis as the etiology, 81 percent with NID or granular deposit type of idiopathic AC-RPGN, 89 percent of anti-GBM mediated disease, and 94 percent with PAN-AC-RPGN. Many types of therapeutic intervention have been unsuccessful in the past. Use of intravenous pulse methylprednisolone, 30 mg/kg, dramatically alters the course of this disease. Eighty-six percent of patients with NID or granular type AC-RPGN in this study had a favorable response, and 75 percent of patients on hemodialysis were able to stop that support. Even after long-term follow-up, with some patients developing slowly progressive disease or needing to return to dialysis, 76 percent remained stable and off dialysis. Patients with anti-GBM disease responded poorly to pulse methylprednisolone with only those patients with fewer crescents and good urine output having a favorable response. A good response to therapy was also noted in patients with PAN-AC-RPGN and those with MPGN.

Reports of series of patients described as having RPGN were carefully evaluated for information regarding individual patients and their disease process. From this information, data were derived regarding the natural course of the disease, re-

**Table 12-25.** Summary of Effects of Therapy on AC-RPGN—Percent Improved

| Type | Conventional[a] | Quadruple | Plasma Exchange | Pulse |
|---|---|---|---|---|
| Idiopathic NID and granular | 19–27% | 71% | 70% | 76% |
| Anti-GBM | 11 | 0 | 45 | 17 |
| PAN | 6 | 17 | 88 | 75–100% |

[a]As defined in text.

sponse to conventional, pulse methylprednisolone, quadruple, and plasma exchange therapy. Data were derived from over 700 patients in the literature and from our own experience. Examination of conventional, quadruple, plasma exchange, and pulse therapy, as shown in the Table 12-25, clearly demonstrates that conventional therapy has little effect on the course of the diseases. Quadruple therapy, plasma exchange, and pulse therapies are similar for idiopathic NID and granular types, and plasma exchange and pulse therapies appear similar in efficacy for PAN. Plasma exchange may be the best method for anti-GBM disease. However, both plasma exchange and quadruple therapy are associated with higher risks and complications, and plasma exchange is extremely expensive. Pulse methylprednisolone therapy and long-term alternate day steroids have been associated with minimal side effects and complications.

It is now obvious that aggressive intervention in these devastating diseases will be successful in altering the natural course, and that several therapeutic modalities are comparable. However, pulse methylprednisolone and alternate day prednisone appear to be among the most effective, least expensive, and associated with fewer complications, and are indicated for any patient with crescents and the clinical course of RPGN as defined in the text. It seems unreasonable at this time with the information now available to deny patients aggressive therapy which

has a good probability of resulting in improvement of their disease process.

# ACKNOWLEDGMENTS

The author gratefully acknowledges the excellent compilative help of Jan Hill and Barbara Rogers. This work was supported in part by USPHS grant # AM 32530.

# REFERENCES

1. Anand SK, Trygstad CW, Sharma HM, et al: Extracapillary proliferative glomerulonephritis in children. Pediatrics 56:434, 1975.
2. Arieff AI, Pinggera WF: Rapidly progressive glomerulonephritis treated with anticoagulants. Arch Intern Med 129:77, 1972.
3. Asaba H, Rekola S, Bergstrand A, et al: Clinical trial of plasma exchange with a membrane filter in treatment of crescentic glomerulonephritis. Clin Nephrol 14:60, 1980.
4. Atkins RC, Glasgow EF, Holdsworth SR, et al: Tissue culture of isolated glomeruli from patients with glomerulonephritis. Kidney Int 17:515, 1980.
5. Atkins RC, Glasgow EF, Holdsworth SR, et al: The macrophage in human rapidly progressive glomerulonephritis. Lancet 1:830, 1976.
6. Bacani RA, Velasquez F, Kanter A, et al: Rapidly progressive (nonstreptococcal) glomerulonephritis. Ann Intern Med 69:463, 1968.
7. Bach JF, Duval D, Dardenne M, et al: The

effects of steroids on T-cells. Transplant Proc 7:25, 1975.

8. Baldwin DS, Gluck MC, Schacht RG, et al: The long-term course of poststreptococcal glomerulonephritis. Ann Intern Med 80:342, 1974.

9. Baldwin DS, Gluck MC, Schacht RG, et al: Long-term follow-up of poststreptococcal glomerulonephritis. In Kincaid-Smith P, Mathew TH, Becker EL, Eds: Perspectives in Nephrology and Hypertension. Vol. 1, part I. Glomerulonephritis: Morphology, Natural History, and Treatment. New York, Wiley, 1973, p 327.

10. Balow JF, Rosenthal AS: Glucocorticoid suppression of macrophage migration inhibitory factor. J Exp Med 137:1031, 1973.

11. Barron KS, Person DA, Brewer EJ Jr, et al: Pulse methylprednisolone therapy in diffuse proliferative lupus nephritis. J Pediat 101:137, 1982.

12. Baum M, Powell D, Calvin S, et al: Continuous ambulatory peritoneal dialysis in children: comparison with hemodialysis. N Engl J Med 307:1537, 1982.

13. Beaufils M, Morel-Maroger L, Sraer J.-D, et al: Acute renal failure of glomerular origin during visceral abscesses. N Engl J Med 295:185, 1976.

14. Becker GJ, D'Apice AJF, Walker RG, et al: Plasmapheresis in the treatment of glomerulonephritis. Med J Aust 2:693, 1977.

15. Beirne GJ, Wagnild JP, Zimmerman SW, et al: Idiopathic crescentic glomerulonephritis. Medicine 56:349, 1977.

16. Bell PRF, Calman KC, Wood RFM, et al: Reversal of acute clinical and experimental organ rejection using large doses of intravenous prednisolone. Lancet 1:876, 1971.

17. Bendixen G: Organ-specific inhibition of the invitro migration of leucocytes in human glomerulonephritis. Acta Med Scand 184:99, 1968.

18. Benoit FL, Rulon DB, Theil GB, et al: Goodpasture's syndrome. A clinicopathologic entity. Am J Med 34:424, 1964.

19. Berlyne GM, Baker SB deC: Acute anuric glomerulonephritis. Q J Med 33:105, 1964.

20. Bhan A, Schneeberger E, Collins A, et al: Evidence for a pathogenic role of a cell-mediated immune mechanism in experimental glomerulonephritis. J Exp Med 148:246, 1978.

21. Bhuyan UN, Dash SC, Srivastava RN, et al: Immunopathology, extent and course of glomerulonephritis with crescent formation. Clin Nephrol 18:280, 1982.

22. Bohman SO, Olsen S, Petersen VP: Glomerular ultrastructure in extracapillary glomerulonephritis. Acta Pathol Microbiol Scand [A] 82 suppl. 249,29–54, 1974.

23. Bolton WK, Atuk NO, Sturgill BC, et al: Therapy of the idiopathic nephrotic syndrome with alternate day steroids. Am J Med 62:60, 1977.

24. Bolton WK, Benton FR, Lobo PI: Requirement of functional T-cells in the production of autoimmune glomerulotubular nephropathy in mice. Clin Exp Immunol 33:474, 1978.

25. Bolton WK, Benton FR, Maclay JG, et al: Spontaneous glomerular sclerosis in aging Sprague-Dawley rats. I. Lesions associated with mesangial IgM deposits. Am J Pathol 85:277, 1976.

26. Bolton WK, Benton FR, Sturgill BC: Autoimmune glomerulotubular nephropathy in mice. Clin Exp Immunol 33:463, 1978.

27. Bolton WK, Charlottesville Collaborative Study: Pulse methylprednisolone therapy of polyarteritis nodosa acute crescentic rapidly progressive glomerulonephritis (Abstract). Proceedings of the 8th International Congress of Nephrology in Athens, Greece, June 1981, p 248.

28. Bolton WK, Charlottesville Collaborative Study: Pulse methylprednisolone therapy of rapidly progressive glomerulonephritis. In Schreiner GE, Ed: Controversies in Nephrology. Vol. 3. Nephrology Division, Georgetown University, Washington, DC, 1981, p 213.

29. Bolton WK, Couser WG: Intravenous pulse methylprednisolone therapy of acute crescentic rapidly progressive glomerulonephritis. Am J Med 66:495, 1979.

30. Bolton WK, Mesnard RM: New technique of kidney tissue processing for immunofluorescence microscopy: Formol sucrose/gum sucrose/paraffin (FSGSP). Lab Invest 47:206, 1982.

31. Bolton WK, Sturgill BC: Spontaneous glomerular sclerosis in aging Sprague-Dawley rats. II. Ultrastructural studies. Am J Pathol 98:339, 1980.

32. Bolton WK, Tucker FL, Sturgill BC: Experimental autoimmune glomerulonephritis in chickens. J Clin Lab Immunol 3:179, 1980.

33. Briggs WA, Johnson JP, Teichman S, et al: Antiglomerular basement membrane antibody mediated glomerulonephritis and Goodpasture's syndrome. Medicine 58:318, 1979.

34. Brigham KL, Bowers RE, McKeen CR: Methylprednisolone prevention of increased lung vascular permeability following endotoxemia in sheep. J Clin Invest 67:1103, 1981.

35. Brown CB, Turner D, Ogg CS, et al: Combined immunosuppression and anticoagulation in rapidly progressive glomerulonephritis. Lancet 2:1166, 1974.

36. Bruns FJ, Fraley DS, Adler S, et al: Megadose methylprednisolone versus plasmapheresis in treatment of rapidly progressive glomerulonephritis (Abstract). Kidney Int 19:121, 1981.

37. Butler W, Rossen R: Effects of corticosteroids on immunity in man. I. Decreased serum IgG concentration caused by 3 or 5 days of high doses of methylprednisolone. J Clin Invest 52:2629, 1973.

38. Cameron JS, Ogg CS, White RHR, et al: The clinical features and prognosis of patients with normocomplementemic mesangiocapillary glomerulonephritis. Clin Nephrol 1:7, 1973.

39. Cathcart E, Idelson B, Scheinburg M, et al: Beneficial effects of methylprednisolone "pulse" therapy in diffuse proliferative lupus nephritis. Lancet 1:163, 1976.

40. Cheigh JS, Stenzel KIJ, Riggio RR, et al: Effects of intravenous methylprednisolone on mixed lymphocyte cultures in normal humans. Transplant Proc 7:31, 1975.

41. Churg J, Morita T, Suzuki Y: Glomerulonephritis with fibrin and crescent formation. In Kincaid-Smith P, Mathew TH, Becker EL, Ed: Glomerulonephritis: Morphology, Natural History, and Treatment. New York, Wiley, 1973, p 677.

42. Claman HN, Moorhead JW, Brenner WH: Corticosteroids and lymphoid cells in vitro. I. Hydrocortisone lysis of human, guinea pig and mouse thymous cells. J Lab Clin Med 78:499, 1971.

43. Cohen AH, Border WA, Shankel E, et al: Crescentic glomerulonephritis: Immune vs nonimmune mechanisms. Am J Nephrol 1:78, 1981.

44. Cole BR, Brocklebank JT, Kienstra RA, et al: "Pulse" methylprednisolone therapy in the treatment of severe glomerulonephritis. J Pediat 88:307, 1976.

45. Cotran R: Monocytes, proliferation and glomerulonephritis (Editorial). J Lab Clin Med 92:837, 1978.

46. Couser W: What are circulating immune complexes doing in glomerulonephritis? (Editorial) N Engl J Med 300:1230, 1981.

47. Couser WG: Idiopathic rapidly progressive glomerulonephritis. Am J Nephrol 2:57, 1982.

48. Couser W, Salant D: In situ immune complex formation and glomerular injury (Editorial review). Kidney Int 17:1, 1980.

49. Craddock CG, Winkelstein A, Matsuyuki Y, et al: The immune response to foreign red blood cells and the participation of short-lived lymphocytes. J Exp Med 125:1149, 1967.

50. Cunningham RJ III, Gilfoil M, Cavallo T, et al: Rapidly progressive glomerulonephritis in children: A report of thirteen cases and a review of the literature. Pediat Res 14:128, 1980.

51 Dash SC, Malhotra KK, Sharma RK, et al: Spectrum of rapidly progressive (crescentic) glomerulonephritis in northern India. Nephron 30:45, 1982.

52. Davis CA, McAdams AJ, Wyatt RJ, et al: Indiopathic rapidly progressive glomerulonephritis with C3 nephritic factor and hypocomplementemia. J Pediat 94:559, 1979.

53. Davson J, Ball J, Platt R: The kidney in periarteritis nodosa. Q J Med 17:175, 1948.

54. DeBermudez L, Hayslett JP: Effect of methylprednisolone on renal function and the zonal distribution of blood flow in the rat. Circ Res 31:44, 1972.

55. deTorrente A, Popovtzer MM, Guggen-

heim SJ, et al: Serious pulmonary hemorrhage, glomerulonephritis and massive steroid therapy. Ann Intern Med 83:218, 1975.

56. Dosa S, Cairns SA, Lawler W, et al: The treatment of lupus nephritis by methylprednisolone pulse therapy. Postgrad Med J 54:628, 1978.

57. Dumble LJ, MacDonald IM, Kincaid-Smith P, et al: Correlation between ADCC resistance to *in-vitro* steroid and allograft failure. Transplant Proc 13:1569, 1981.

58. Ellis A: Natural history of Bright's disease. Clinical, histological and experimental observations. Lancet 1:1, 1942.

59. Erickson SB, Kurtz SB, Donadio JV Jr, et al: Use of combined plasmapheresis and immunosuppression in the treatment of Goodpasture's syndrome. Mayo Clin Proc 54:714, 1979.

60. Eyanson S, Passo MH, Aldo-Benson MA, et al: Methylprednisolone pulse therapy for nonrenal lupus erythematosus. Ann Rheum Dis 39:377, 1980.

61. Faarup P, Norgaard T, Elling F, et al: Structural changes in kidneys of patients with oliguric extracapillary glomerulonephritis during immunosuppressive therapy. Acta Pathol Microbiol Scand [A] 86:409, 1978.

62. Fauci AS, Haynes BF, Katz P, et al: Wegener's granulomatosis: prospective clinical and therapeutic experience with 85 patients for 21 years. Ann Intern Med 98:76, 1983.

63. Fauci AS, Katz P, Haynes BF, et al: Cyclophosphamide therapy of severe systemic necrotizing vasculitis. N Engl J Med 301:235, 1979.

64. Fauci AS, Murakami T, Brandon DD, et al: Mechanisms of corticosteroid action on lymphocyte subpopulations. VI. Lack of correlation between glucocorticosteroid receptors and the differential effects of glucocorticosteroids on T-cell subpopulations. Cell Immunol 49:43, 1980.

65. Fillit HM, Read SE, Sherman RL, et al: Cellular reactivity to altered glomerular basement membrane in glomerulonephritis. N Engl J Med 298:861, 1978.

66. Fillit HM, Zabriskie JB: Cellular immunity in glomerulonephritis. Am J Pathol 109:227, 1982.

67. Forster PJG, Grindulis KA, Neumann V, et al: High-dose intravenous methylprednisolone in rheumatoid arthritis. Ann Rheum Dis 41:444, 1982.

68. Frohnert PP, Sheps SG: Long-term follow-up study of periarteritis nodosa. Am J Med 43:8, 1967.

69. Glassock R: A clinical and immunopathologic dissection of rapidly progressive glomerulonephritis. Nephron 22:253, 1978.

70. Glassock R, Cohen A, Bennett C, et al: Primary glomerular diseases. In Brenner BM, Rector FC: The Kidney. 2nd Ed. Vol. 2, W.B. Saunders Company, Philadelphia, 1981, p 1351.

71. Goldstein IM: Effect of steroids on lysosomes. Transplant Proc 7:21, 1975.

72. Habib R, Kleinknecht C, Gubler MC, et al: Idiopathic membranoproliferative glomerulonephritis in children. Report of 105 cases. Clin Nephrol 1:194, 1973.

73. Hammerschmidt DE, White JG, Craddock PR, et al: Corticosteroids inhibit complement-induced granulocyte aggregation. J Clin Invest 63:798, 1979.

74. Harris JP, Rakowski TA, Argy WP Jr, et al: Alport's syndrome presenting as crescentic glomerulonephritis: A report of two siblings. Clin Nephrol 10:245, 1978.

75. Harrison CV, Loughridge LW, Milne MD: Acute oliguric renal failure in acute glomerulonephritis and polyarteritis nodosa. Q J Med 33:39, 1964.

76. Harrison HL, Linshaw MA, Lindsley CB, et al: Bolus corticosteroids and cyclophosphamide for initial treatment of Wegener's granulomatosis. JAMA 244:1599, 1980.

77. Heptinstall RH: Rapidly progressive glomerulonephritis. In Heptinstall RH: Pathology of the Kidney. 2nd Ed. Boston, Little, Brown, 1974, p 371.

78. Hinglais N, Garcia-Torres R, Kleinknecht D: Long-term prognosis in acute glomerulonephritis. The predictive value of early clinical and pathologic features observed in 65 patients. Am J Med 56:52, 1974.

79. Hirschberg H, Hirschberg T, Nousiainen

H, et al: The effects of corticosteroids on the antigen presenting properties of human monocytes and endothelial cells. Clin Immunol Immunopathol 23:577, 1982.

80. Holdsworth S, Neale T, Wilson C: Abrogation of macrophage dependent injury in experimental glomerulonephritis in the rabbit. Use of an anti-macrophage serum. J Clin Invest 68:686, 1981.

81. Holdsworth SR, Thomson NM, Glasgow EF, et al: Tissue culture of isolated glomeruli in experimental crescentic glomerulonephritis. J Exp Med 147:98, 1978.

82. Hopper J, Biava C, Naughton C: Glomerular extracapillary proliferation (crescentic glomerulonephritis) associated with non-renal malignancies. Kidney Int 10:554, 1976.

83. Hunsicker L, Shearer T, Plattner S, et al: The role of monocytes in serum sickness nephritis. J Exp Med 150:413, 1979.

84. Ingelfinger JR, McCluskey RT, Schneeberger EE, et al: Necrotizing arteritis in acute poststreptococcal glomerulonephritis—report of a recovered case. J Pediat 91:228, 1977.

85. Jennette JC, Lamanna RW, Burnette JP, et al: Concurrent antiglomerular basement membrane antibody and immune complex mediated glomerulonephritis. Am J Clin Pathol 78:381, 1982.

86. Jensen H, Olgaard K, Faarup P: Successful immunosuppressive treatment of oliguric extracapillary glomerulonephritis. Acta Med Scand 196:383, 1974.

87. Johnson JP, Whitman W, Briggs WA, et al: Plasmapheresis and immunosuppressive agents in antibasement membrane antibody-induced Goodpasture's syndrome. Am J Med 64:354, 1978.

88. Kalowski S, McKay DG, Howes EL Jr, et al: Multinucleated giant cells in antiglomerular basement membrane antibody-induced glomerulonephritis. Nephron 16:415, 1976.

89. Kanfer A, Sraer JD, Feintuch MJ, et al: Insuffisance renale aigue au cours de la periarterite noueuse. La Nouvelle Presse Medicale 5:1883, 1976.

90. Kashiwabara H, Shishido H, Tomura S, et al: Strong association between IgA ne-

phropathy and HLA-DR4 antigen. Kidney Int 22:377, 1982.

91. Kimberly RP, Lockshin MD, Sherman RL et al: High-dose intravenous methylprednisolone pulse therapy in systemic lupus erythematosus. Am J Med 70:817, 1981.

92. Kincaid-Smith P: The natural history and treatment of mesangiocapillary glomerulonephritis. In Kincaid-Smith P, Mathew TH, Becker EL, Eds: Glomerulonephritis: Morphology, Natural History, and Treatment. New York, Wiley, 1973, p 591.

93. Klassen J, Elwood C, Grossberg AL, et al: Evolution of membranous nephropathy into anti-glomerular-basement-membrane glomerulonephritis. N Engl J Med 290:1340, 1974.

94. Kreisberg J, Wayne D, Karnovsky M: Rapid and focal loss of negative charge associated with mononuclear cell infiltration early in nephrotoxic serum nephritis. Kidney Int 16:290, 1979.

95. Ladefoged J, Nielsen B, Raaschou F, et al: Acute anuria due to polyarteritis nodosa. Am J Med 46:827, 1969.

96. Lavelle KJ, Durland BD, Yum MN: The effect of antimacrophage antiserum on immune complex glomerulonephritis. J Lab Clin Med 98:195, 1981.

97. Lee HA, Stirling G, Sharpstone P: Acute glomerulonephritis in middle-aged and elderly patients. Br Med J 2:1361, 1966.

98. Leibovich SJ, Ross R: A macrophage dependent factor that stimulates the proliferation of fibroblasts in vitro. Am J Pathol 84:501, 1976.

99. Lemieux G, Cuvelier AA, Lefebvre R: The clinical spectrum of renal insufficiency during acute glomerulonephritis in the adult. Canad Med Assoc J 96:1129, 1967.

100. Leonard CD, Nagle RB, Striker GE, et al: Acute glomerulonephritis with prolonged oliguria. An analysis of 29 cases. Ann Intern Med 73:703, 1970.

101. Lerner RA, Glassock RJ, Dixon FJ: The role of anti-glomerular basement membrane antibody in the pathogenesis of human glomerulonephritis. J Exp Med 126:989, 1967.

102. Levinsky RJ, Cameron JS, Soothill JF: Serum immune complexes and disease ac-

tivity in lupus nephritis. Lancet 1:564, 1977.

103. Lesis EJ, Cavallo T, Harrington JT, et al: An immunopathologic study of rapidly progressive glomerulonephritis in the adult. Human Pathol 2:185, 1971.

104. Liebling MR, Leib E, McLaughlin K, et al: Pulse methylprednisolone in rheumatoid arthritis. A double-blind cross-over trial. Ann Intern Med 94:21, 1981.

105. Lippman SM, Arnett FC, Conley CL, et al: Genetic factors predisposing to auto-immune diseases. Autoimmune hemolytic anemia, chronic thrombocytopenic purpura, and systemic lupus erythematosus. Am J Med 73:827, 1982.

106. Lockwood CM, Pinching AJ, Sweny P, et al: Plasma-exchange and immunosuppression in the treatment of fulminating immune-complex crescentic nephritis. Lancet 1:63, 1977.

107. Macanovic M, Evans DJ, Peters DK: Allergic response to glomerular basement membrane in patients with glomerulonephritis. Lancet 2:207, 1972.

108. Magil AB, Price JDE, Bower G, et al: Membranoproliferative glomerulonephritis type 1: Comparison of natural history in children and adults. Clin Nephrol 11:239, 1979.

109. Magil AB, Wadsworth LD, Loewen M: Monocytes and human renal glomerular disease: A quantitative evaluation. Lab Invest 44:27, 1981.

110. Mahieu P, Dardenne M, Bach J: Detection of humoral and cell-mediated immunity to kidney basement membranes in human renal diseases. Am J Med 53:185, 1972.

111. McAdams AJ, McEnery PT, West CD: Mesangiocapillary glomerulonephritis: Changes in glomerular morphology with long-term alternate-day prednisone therapy. J Pediat 86:23, 1975.

112. McCluskey RT, Bhan AK: Cell-mediated mechanisms in renal disease. Kidney Int 21: suppl. 11, S6-S12, 1982.

113. McDougal BA, Whittier FC, Cross DE: Sudden death after bolus steroid therapy for acute rejection. Transplant Proc 8:493, 1976.

114. McKenzie PE, Taylor AE, Woodroffe AJ,

et al: Plasmapheresis in glomerulonephritis. Clin Nephrol 12:97, 1979.

115. McLeish KR, Yum MN, Luft FC: Rapidly progressive glomerulonephritis in adults: Clinical and histologic correlations. Clin Nephrol 10:43, 1978.

116. Miller JJ III: Prolonged use of large intravenous steroid pulses in the rheumatic diseases of children. Pediatrics 65:989, 1980.

117. Min KW, Györkey F, Györkey P, et al: The morphogenesis of glomerular crescents in rapidly progressive glomerulonephritis. Kidney Int 5:47, 1974.

118. Mintz G, Enriquez RD, Mercado U, et al: Intravenous methylprednisolone pulse therapy in severe ankylosing spondylitis. Arth Rheum 24:734, 1981.

119. Model DG: Reversal of blindness in temporal arteritis with methylprednisolone (Letter). Lancet 1:340, 1978.

120. Monga G, Mazzucco G, di Belgiojoso GB, et al: The presence and possible role of monocyte infiltration in human chronic proliferative glomerulonephrides. Am J Pathol 94:271, 1979.

121. Moore J, Johnson JP, Bohan L, et al: Therapy of anti-glomerular basement membrane antibody disease: A prospective study (Abstract). 15th Annual Meeting of the American Society of Nephrology, 1982, p 103A.

122. Moorthy AV, Zimmerman SW, Burkholder PM, et al: Association of crescentic glomerulonephritis with membranous glomerulonephropathy: A report of three cases. Clin Nephrol 6:319, 1976.

123. Morita T, Suzuki Y, Churg J: Structure and development of the glomerular crescent. Am J Pathol 72:349, 1973.

124. Morrin PAF, Hinglais N, Nabarra B, et al: Rapidly progressive glomerulonephritis. A clinical and pathologic study. Am J Med 65:446, 1978.

125. Morzycka M, Crocker BP, Seigler HF: Evaluation of recurrent glomerulonephritis in kidney allografts. Am J Med 72:588, 1982.

126. Munk ZM, Scamene E: Goodpasture's syndrome—effects of plasmapheresis. Clin Exp Immunol 36:244, 1979.

127. Nakamoto Y, Dohi K, Fujioka M, et al:

Combined anticoagulant and immuno-suppressive treatment in rapidly progressive glomerulonephritis (RPGN). A long-term follow-up study. Jap J Med 18:210, 1979.

128. Nakamoto S, Dunea G, Kolff WJ, et al: Treatment of oliguric glomerulonephritis with dialysis and steroids. Ann Intern Med 63:359, 1965.

129. Neild GH, Cameron JS, Lessor MH, et al: Relapsing polychondritis with crescentic glomerulonephritis. Br Med J 1:743, 1978.

130. Neild GH, Lee HA: Methylprednisolone pulse therapy in the treatment of polyarteritis nodosa. Postgrad Med J 53:382, 1977.

131. Novak E, Stubbs SS, Seckman CE, et al: Effects of a single large intravenous dose of methylprednisolone sodium succinate. Clin Pharm Ther 11:711, 1970.

132. Ogg CS, Neild GH, Cameron JS, et al: Is rapidly progressive glomerulonephritis treatable? In Schreiner GE, Ed: Controversies in Nephrology. Vol. 3. Nephrology Division, Georgetown University, Washington, DC, 1981, p 201.

133. Olsen S: Extracapillary glomerulonephritis: A semiquantitative light-microscopical study of 59 patients. Acta Pathol Microbiol Scand Sect A, 82: suppl. 249, 7–19, 1974.

134. Olsson PJ, Gaffney E, Alexander RW, et al: Proliferative glomerulonephritis with crescent formation in Behçet's syndrome. Arch Intern Med 140:713, 1980.

135. O'Neill WM Jr, Etheridge WB, Bloomer HA: High-dose corticosteroids. Their use in treating idiopathic rapidly progressive glomerulonephritis. Arch Intern Med 139:514, 1979.

136. Ooi YM, Ooi BS, Vallota EN, et al: Circulating immune complexes after renal transplantation. Correlation of increased $^{125}$I-Clq binding activity with acute rejection characterized by fibrin deposition in the kidney. J Clin Invest 60:611, 1977.

137. Oredugba O, Mazumdar DC, Meyers JS, et al: Pulse methylprednisolone therapy in idiopathic, rapidly progressive glomerulonephritis. Ann Intern Med 92:504, 1980.

138. O'Reilly JP, Bolton WK: Importance of genetics in the development of autoimmune glomerulotubular nephropathy in mice. Kidney Int 19:188, 1981.

139. Pahwa SG, Pahwa RN, Good RA: Decreased in vitro humoral immune responses in aged humans. J Clin Invest 67:1094, 1981.

140. Peters DK, Rees AJ, Lockwood CM, et al: Treatment and prognosis in antibasement membrane antibody-mediated nephritis. Transplant Proc 14:513, 1982.

141. Petzel RA, Brown DC, Staley NA, et al: Crescentic glomerulonephritis and renal failure associated with malignant lymphoma. Am J Clin Pathol 71:728, 1979.

142. Pollak V, Mendoza N: Rapidly progressive glomerulonephritis. Med Clin North Am 55:1397, 1971.

143. Ponticelli C, Zucchelli P, Banfi G, et al: Treatment of diffuse proliferative lupus nephritis by intravenous high-dose methylprednisolone. Q J Med 51:16, 1982.

144. Posborg Petersen V, Olsen S, Kissmeyer-Nielsen F, et al: Transmission of glomerulonephritis from host to human kidney allotransplant. N Engl J Med 275:1269, 1966.

145. Poskitt TR: Immunologic and electron microscopic studies in Goodpasture's syndrome. Am J Med 49:250, 1970.

146. Proskey AJ, Weatherbee L, Easterling RE, et al: Goodpasture's syndrome. A report of five cases and review of the literature. Am J Med 48:162, 1970.

147. Rinehart J, Balcerzak S, Sagone A, et al: Effects of corticosteroids on human monocyte function. J Clin Invest 54:1337, 1974.

148. Roberts SD, Maxwell DR, Gross TL: Cost-effective care of end-stage renal disease: A billion dollar question. Ann Intern Med 92:243, 1980.

149. Rocklin R, Lewis E, David J: Invitro evidence for cellular hypersensitivity to glomerular-basement-membrane antigens in human glomerulonephritis. N Engl J Med 283:497, 1970.

150. Rose GA: The natural history of polyarteritis. Br Med J 2:1148, 1957.

151. Rosen S: Crescentic glomerulonephritis. Occurrence, mechanisms, and prognosis.

In Sommers S, Ed: Pathology Annual. Appleton Century Crofts, New York, 1975, p 37.

152. Rosenfeld J, Levi J, Robson M, et al: Fulminatingly progressive recurrent glomerulonephritis in a renal allograft. Am J Med 49:563, 1970.

153. Sambhi MP, Weil MH, Udhoji VN: Acute pharmacodynamic effects of glucocorticoids. Circulation 31:523, 1965.

154. Schreiner G, Cotran R, Pardo V, et al: A mononuclear cell component in experimental immunological glomerulonephritis. J Exp Med 147:369, 1978.

155. Schreiner GE, Rakowski TA, Argy WP: Natural history of oliguric glomerulonephritis. In Kincaid-Smith P, Mathew HT, Becker EL, Eds: Glomerulonephritis: Morphology, Natural History, and Treatment. New York, Wiley, 1973, p 711.

156. Schur PH, Carpenter CB: Host and genetic factors contributing to immunologic renal disease. In Wilson CB, Brenner BM, Stein JH, Eds: Immunologic Mechanisms of Renal Disease. Vol. 3. New York, Churchill Livingstone, 1979, p 144.

157. Sissons JGP, Evans DJ, Peters DK, et al: Glomerulonephritis associated with antibody to glomerular basement membrane. Br Med J 4:11, 1974.

158. Sonsino E, Nabarra B, Kazatchkine M, et al: Extracapillary proliferative glomerulonephritis so-called malignant glomerulonephritis. In Hamburger J, Crosnier J, Maxwell MH, Eds: Advances in Nephrology. Vol. 2. Chicago, Year Book Medical Pub 1972, p 121.

159. Spargo B, Ordonez N, Ringus J: The differential diagnosis of crescentic glomerulonephritis. The pathology of specific lesions with prognostic implications. Human Pathol 8:187. 1977.

160. Stejskal J, Pirani CL, Okada M, et al: Discontinuities (gaps) of the glomerular capillary wall and basement membrane in renal disease. Lab Invest 28:149, 1973.

161. Stilmant MM, Bolton WK, Sturgill BC, et al: Crescentic glomerulonephritis without immune deposits: Clinicopathologic features. Kidney Int 15:184, 1979.

162. Striker GE, Cutler RE, Huang TW, et al: Renal failure, glomerulonephritis, and glomerular epithelial cell hyperplasia. In Kincaid-Smith P, Mathew TH, Becker EL, Eds: Glomerulonephritis: Morphology, Natural History and Treatment. New York, Wiley, 1973, p 657.

163. Suc JM, Durand D, Conte J, et al: The use of heparin in the treatment of idiopathic rapidly progressive glomerulonephritis. Clin Nephrol 5:9, 1976.

164. Swainson CP, Robson JS, Urbaniak SJ, et al: Treatment of Goodpasture's disease by plasma exchange and immunosuppression. Clin Exp Immunol 32:233, 1978.

165. Thomashow BM, Felton CP, Navarro C: Diffuse intrapulmonary hemorrhage, renal failure and a systemic vasculitis. A case report and review of the literature. Am J Med 68:299, 1980.

166. Thompson J, vanFurth R: The effect of glucocorticosteroids on the kinetics of mononuclear phagocytes. J Exp Med 131:429, 1970.

167. Thomson N, Holdsworth S, Glasgow E, et al: The macrophage in the development of experimental crescentic glomerulonephritis. Studies using tissue culture and electron microscopy. Am J Pathol 94:233, 1979.

168. Thysell H, Bygren P, Bengtsson U, et al: Immunosuppression and the additive effect of plasma exchange in treatment of rapidly progressive glomerulonephritis. Acta Med Scand 212:107, 1982.

169. Travis LB, Dodge WF, Beathard GA, et al: Acute glomerulonephritis in children. A review of the natural history with emphasis on prognosis. Clin Nephrol 1:169, 1973.

170. Tucker FL, Sturgill BC, Bolton WK: Cell mediated immunity in the pathogenesis of experimental autoimmune glomerulonephritis in chickens. Clin Res 30:359, 1982.

171. Turcotte JG, Feduska NJ, Carpenter EW, et al: Rejection crises in human renal transplant recipients: Control with high dose methylprednisolone therapy. Arch Surg 105:230, 1972.

172. Unanue E, Schreiner G, Cotran R: A role of mononuclear phagocytes in immunologically induced glomerulonephritis. In Cummings NB, Michael AF, Wilson CB,

Eds: Immune Mechanisms in Renal Disease. New York, Plenum Press, 1982.

173. Vargas RA, Thomson KJ, Wilson D, et al: Mesangiocapillary glomerulonephritis with dense "deposits" in the basement membranes of the kidney. Clin Nephrol 5:73, 1976.

174. Veith FJ, Koerner SK, Attai LA, et al: Single-lung transplantation in emphysema. Lancet 1:1138, 1972.

175. Volhard F, Fahr T: Die brightische Nierenkrankheit. Berlin, Springer, 1914.

176. Walker RG, D'Apice AJF, Becker GJ, et al: Plasmapheresis in Goodpasture's syndrome with renal failure. Med J Aust 1:875, 1977.

177. Webel ML, Donadio JV, Woods JE, et al: Effects of large dose of methylprednisolone on renal function. J Lab Clin Med 80:765, 1972.

178. Webel ML, Ritts RE Jr, Taswell HF, et al: Cellular immunity after intravenous administration of methylprednisolone. J Lab Clin Med 83:383, 1974.

179. Whitworth JA, Morel-Maroger L, Mignon F, et al: The significance of extracapillary proliferation. Clinicopathological review of 60 patients. Nephron 16:1, 1976.

180. Wilson CB, Dixon FJ: Antiglomerular basement membrane antibody-induced glomerulonephritis. Kidney Int 3:74, 1973.

181. Wing WJ, Bruns FJ, Fraley DS, et al: Infectious complications with plasmapheresis in rapidly progressive glomerulonephritis. JAMA 244:2423, 1980.

182. Wong LG, Colburn KK, Kacena A, et al: Effect of methylprednisolone on the production of neutrophil migration inhibition factor by T-lymphocytes (NIF-T). Immunopharmacology 3:179, 1981.

183. Woods JE, Anderson CF, DeWeerd JH, et al: High-dosage intravenously administered methylprednisolone in renal transplantation. JAMA 223:896, 1973.

184. Wu MJ, Rajaram R, Shelp WD, et al: Vasculitis in Goodpasture's syndrome. Arch Pathol Lab Med 104:300, 1980.

185. Zabriskie J, Lewshenia R, Moller G, et al: Lymphocyte responses to streptococcal antigens in glomerulonephritic patients. Science 168:1105, 1970.

# 13

# The Role of Plasmapheresis in the Nephritic Syndromes

# The Case for Plasmapheresis

Priscilla Kincaid-Smith, M.D., D.Sc.
Rowan G. Walker, M.B., B.S.

## INTRODUCTION

Glomerulonephritis is a common disease, present in some one to two percent of the population. In the great majority of cases the only manifestations of glomerulonephritis are the urine abnormalities. Even at a tertiary referral level in a teaching hospital department of nephrology, 50 percent of patients diagnosed as having glomerulonephritis on renal biopsy have urine abnormalities alone with no symptoms or signs, and some of those asymptomatic patients have serious and potentially progressive glomerulonephritis.

Patients who exhibit isolated proteinuria often have a benign long-term course[74] and the best indication of an active glomerular lesion which may progress rapidly is the degree of microscopic hematuria. When $> 10^5$ glomerular red cells/ml are present in the urine a high percentage of patients will have one of the more serious forms of glomerulonephritis.[27] When there are $> 10^6$ glomerular red cells/ml of urine the renal biopsy is likely to show crescents. Crescents were observed in 70 percent of adults with mesangial IgA nephropathy when the urinary red cell count exceeded $10^6$/ml.[5] When macroscopic hematuria is present, 100 percent of patients with mesangial IgA nephropathy show crescents.[4,5] It is likely that in other forms of glomerulonephritis $> 10^6$ urinary red cells/ml is also indicative of the presence of crescents, but this has not yet been carefully analyzed.

At a community level, the only means of detecting crescentic glomerulonephritis in asymptomatic patients is with initial chemical "dip-stick" testing for hematuria followed by careful quantitation of glomerular red cells on urine microscopy[27] and proceeding to renal biopsy when indicated. The application of such testing at a community level could greatly increase the detection number of patients with crescentic glomerulonephritis before progression to end-stage renal failure has occurred.

Although only 12.5 percent of patients with diffuse crescentic glomerulonephritis are asymptomatic, 57 percent of those with focal and segmental proliferative glomerulonephritis and crescents are asymptomatic. Many of these patients may remain undetected until all glomeruli are sclerosed and irreversible end-stage renal failure has developed. Even in patients with the most fulminating form of crescentic glomerulonephritis, namely, Goodpasture's syndrome or antiglomerular basement membrane antibody glomerulonephritis, symptoms may be relatively nonspecific.

One clinical feature seen in almost every patient with diffuse crescents is macroscopic hematuria. Even if the patient has not noticed macroscopic hematuria it is usually apparent to a doctor and a urine specimen on microscopy will show $> 10^7$ red cells/ml. Very prompt recognition of this feature and early referral are essential, as a patient may progress from 50 percent to 100 percent crescents over a few days and destruction of glomeruli by crescents is very rapid. Once anuria has developed crescentic lesions are irreversible.

Most nephrologists have rather negative views on the treatment of glomerulonephritis, despite the fact that even in chronic progressive lesions, such as membranous glomerulonephritis, recent controlled trials show benefit in the treated groups.[17]

The form of glomerulonephritis in which treatment has had the most promising results is also the one in which the prognosis is worst in untreated cases, namely crescentic glomerulonephritis (Table 13-1).

Because the prognosis of crescentic glomerulonephritis is so poor in untreated cases (and even in those treated with steroids and azathioprine) we have for some years used active treatment in these patients, particularly when > 50 percent of glomeruli are involved with crescents. In 1968,[46] we proposed that the addition of anticoagulants and antiplatelet agents to immunosuppressive and normal regimens greatly improved the prognosis in this form of glomerulonephritis.

The "Melbourne cocktail," as combined anticoagulant, antiplatelet, and immunosuppression was termed, was taken up with some enthusiasm by Cameron's group[10,13,15] but was little used by other groups. We continued to use this treatment regimen until plasmapheresis became available in 1976.

Our overall results of using the Melbourne cocktail in patients with crescents in 80 to 100 percent of glomeruli were reported in 1979[44] and are shown in Fig. 13-1. They compare favorably with some early results using plasmapheresis[3,45,54,87] and indeed are still as good as the overall results we have achieved using plasmapheresis over the past 7 years; these results are discussed in this chapter. For the reasons outlined by Cameron et al.[14,15] it

seems unlikely that this treatment regimen will even be analyzed in a controlled trial, particularly now that plasmapheresis is available.

Our experience with these two methods of treatment is quite extensive, and although the results of treating serious crescentic glomerulonephritis are similar[44] there is no doubt that it is easier to carry out plasmapheresis. The likelihood of the complication of hemorrhage,[40] particularly in patients who have had recent renal biopsies, is less using plasmapheresis combined with immunosuppression and antiplatelet agents than it is using heparin combined with immunosuppression and antiplatelet agents.

# GOODPASTURE'S SYNDROME AND ANTIGLOMERULAR BASEMENT MEMBRANE ANTIBODY NEPHRITIS

Within the category of crescentic glomerulonephritis the group for whom plasma exchange was first suggested as a method of treatment was Goodpasture's syndrome.[50,53] Goodpasture's syndrome, including antiglomerular basement membrane antibody nephritis without lung involvement, is the group most widely accepted as sharing benefit from plasma exchange and currently the combination of immunosuppression and plasmapheresis[33,53,47,87] is considered the treatment of choice in this condition.

Although the spectrum of severity of disease in Goodpasture's and antiglomerular basement membrane antibody nephritis is extremely wide[61] the renal prognosis appears to depend on the severity of the underlying renal pathology and extent of obliterative crescent formation,[9,61,90] which can be predicted to some

**Table 13-1.** Renal "Survival" of Untreated Crescentic Glomerulonephritis

| Author | Reference No. | % Crescents | Number of patients studied | Renal "Survival" (%) |
|---|---|---|---|---|
| Sonsino et al. | 81 | 60%–100% | 20[a,b] | 5 (25%) Δ |
| Cameron & Ogg | 12 | 70%–100% | 22[a,b,d] | 5 (23%) † |
| Whitworth et al. | 89 | 80%–100% | 31[a,b,c,d] | 11 (35%) Δ |
| Mathew & Kincaid-Smith | 57 | 50%–100% | 33[a,b,c,d] | 9 (27%) * |

Note. Most patients untreated but some patients were treated with cytotoxics[a], steroids[b], antiplatelet agents[c], anticoagulants[d], or combinations of these therapies. Sufficient renal function to sustain life at 6 months †, up to 2 years Δ, for an unspecified period*.

degree from the intensity of the clinical signs and symptoms.[9] The overall prognosis of Goodpasture's syndrome was generally considered to be extremely poor[6,71] and achieving remission in cases *with* renal failure was virtually unrecorded prior to the use of plasmapheresis.[66] Remission had previously only occurred in patients *without* renal failure by using various combinations of steroids, anticoagulants, immunosuppression, and bilateral nephrectomy.[26,80]

The introduction of plasmapheresis to treatment regimens for Goodpasture's syndrome was associated with numerous observations of a dramatic reversal of fulminating pulmonary hemorrhage.[24,38,53] So impressive was this response that the use of bilateral nephrectomy to control pulmonary hemorrhage in Goodpasture's syndrome[80] has now almost entirely been abandoned.

In addition to the effect of plasmapheresis on pulmonary hemorrhage of Goodpasture's syndrome, many reports have documented improvement and/or

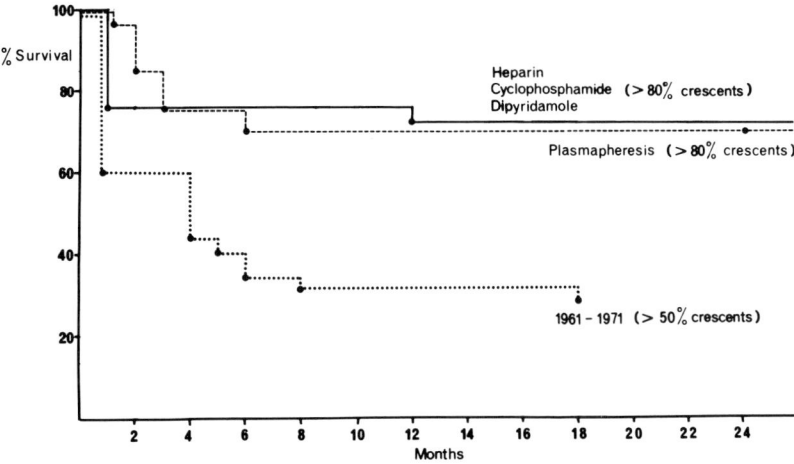

**Fig. 13-1.** Renal "survival" (sufficient renal function to sustain life), of patients with crescentic nephritis treated with 'Melbourne Cocktail' (·–·) compared with early results using plasmapheresis (·····) (Kincaid-Smith 1979, Ref. No. 44). Note also the comparison with renal 'survival' of patients with crescentic nephritis prior to the use of either 'Melbourne Cocktail' or plasmapheresis (····) (Mathew & Kincaid-Smith 1973, Ref. No. 57).

stabilization of renal function[1,9,11,24,25,28,47,58,65,75] in both Goodpasture's syndrome and antiglomerular basement membrane antibody nephritis, provided anuria was not a feature of presentation. In some reports, in which documentation of improved renal function has occurred, evidence of healing of the histological process has also been obtained[75,87,88] in which the initial biopsies have shown high percentages of glomeruli involved with crescents and subsequent biopsies have shown only focal mesangial proliferative changes and glomerulosclerosis.

Further evidence that plasmapheresis favorably alters the natural history of Goodpasture's syndrome or antiglomerular basement membrane antibody nephritis is suggested from the observations that the clinical situation may rapidly deteriorate upon early withdrawal of the plasmapheresis therapy.[28,56,59,87] Such cases are not necessarily associated with high levels of circulating antiglomerular basement membrane antibodies at the time of withdrawal of plasmapheresis. However, reinstituting plasmapheresis in such instances may be associated with rapid reversal of deteriorating renal function and/or improvement of renal function.[1,87]

The prompt initiation of plasmapheresis early in the disease course has been emphasized by several authors as critical to inducing a satisfactory response to the therapy[1,9,38,87] If delays in institution of plasmapheresis therapy until severe oliguria or anuria have occurred, a particularly poor prognosis may be anticipated.[47,53,87]

The duration of plasmapheresis therapy required has not clearly been determined. Relapses in the clinical situation up to 2 years[1] following withdrawal of plasmapheresis therapy have occurred even though circulating antiglomerular basement membrane antibody levels were low at the time of withdrawal.[1] For patients with Goodpasture's syndrome and antiglomerular basement membrane nephritis the duration of plasmapheresis needs to be sufficient to allow the natural resolution of the disease process which includes the cessation of antibasement membrane antibody production to occur.[90] The rebound of high antibody titers demonstrable in animal studies[8] may be prevented, at least in part, by the concomitant use of immunosuppressive agents[21] but others have argued that immunosuppressive therapy as an adjunct to plasmapheresis may not be necessary because antiglomerular basement membrane antibody production is a self-limiting process.[65]

Although it has been suggested that the spectrum of severity of clinical disease and of renal histopathology are a function of antiglomerular basement membrane antibody production, the mechanisms by which plasmapheresis produces a beneficial effect in these patients is not clearly established. Levels of circulating antibodies usually decrease rapidly[11,24,84] within days/weeks but the levels of circulating antibodies are not always well correlated with either pulmonary hemorrhage[53] or activity of the nephritis. Other factors which may be important include decrease in primary immune reactants and mediators of inflammation and of tissue injury such as complement and fibrinogen.[20,23,40,41,45]

The present anecdotal evidence favoring the use of plasmapheresis in Goodpasture's syndrome and antiglomerular basement membrane antibody nephritis has been criticized on the basis that no controlled prospective trials have ever been undertaken.[20] The view of the authors is that the rarity of the severest forms of this condition, its heterogeneity in terms of etiology and its undoubted poor prognosis without treatment[6,71] make it unlikely that any satisfactory controlled study could ever be undertaken.[24] The weight of evidence (albeit anecdotal)

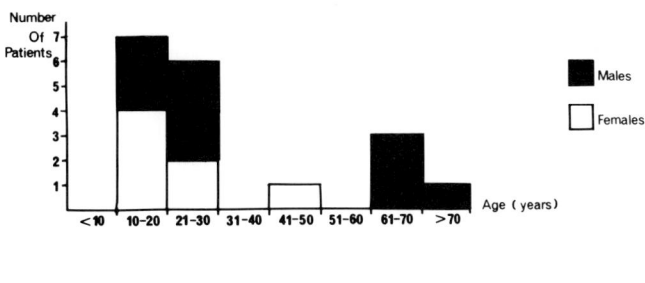

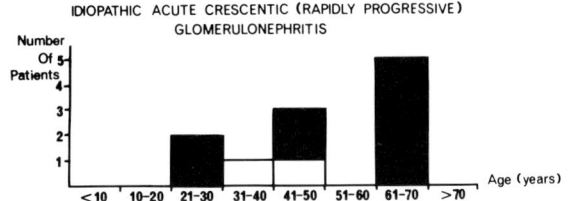

**Fig. 13-2.** Patients with either Goodpasture's syndrome/antiglomerular basement membrane (GBM) antibody nephritis and idiopathic acute crescentic (rapidly progressive) glomerulonephritis related to sex and age.

suggesting such a markedly improved prognosis in Goodpasture's syndrome and antiglomerular basement membrane antibody nephritis since the introduction of plasmapheresis is so great that to withhold plasmapheresis therapy in these patients seems ethically indefensible.

Since the introduction of plasmapheresis we have treated (Appendix) 18 patients with documented circulating antiglomerular basement membrane antibody and immunofluorescent studies showing linear IgG along glomerular basement membranes (i.e., Goodpasture's syndrome or antiglomerular basement membrane antibody nephritis). The details of the age, sex, and percentage of crescents in nonsclerosed glomeruli (Appendix) of these patients is demonstrated in Figs. 13-2 and 13-3. The percentage of crescents in nonsclerosed glomeruli varied from 9 to 100 percent (median 68).

In analyzing the results of therapy with plasmapheresis, the most important prognostic feature in the group was anuria. None of the three patients who were anuric at presentation showed any recovery of renal function. All three required dialysis and all died, one of uncontrolled pulmonary hemorrhage, and two of septicemia, two weeks and one month after

plasmapheresis therapy commenced. The renal biopsies in each case showed circumferential crescents in all glomeruli.

Of the patients who were oliguric on

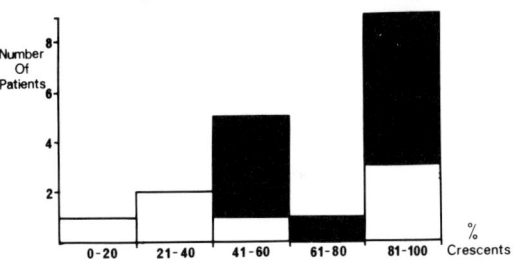

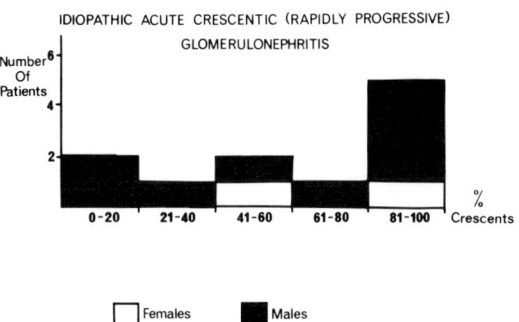

**Fig. 13-3.** Patients with either Goodpasture's syndrome/antiglomerular basement membrane (GBM) antibody nephritis and idiopathic acute crescentic (rapidly progressive) glomerulonephritis related to sex and percentage (%) of crescents in nonsclerosed glomeruli (Appendix).

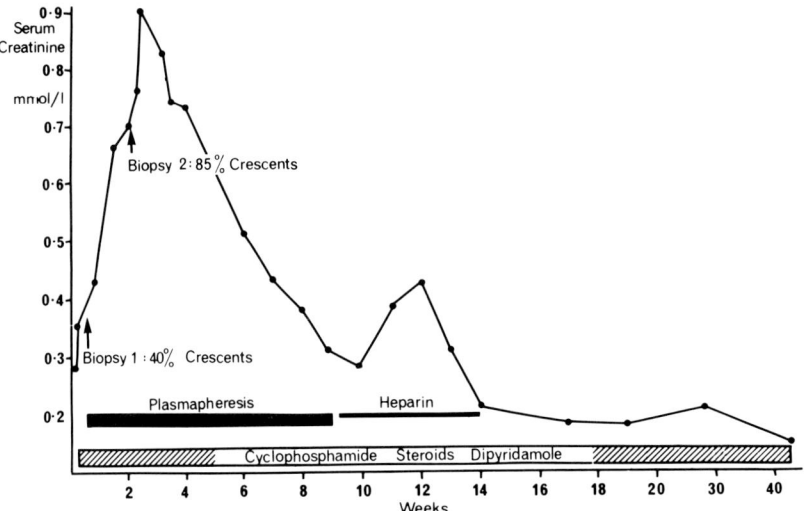

**Fig. 13-4.** A 21-year-old female with crescentic antiglomerular basement membrane (GBM) antibody nephritis treated with plasmapheresis. A second renal biopsy 2 weeks after the first showed an increase in % crescents despite the therapy. This illustrates the fulminant nature of anti-GBM nephritis and the need to institute plasmapheresis therapy promptly. Creatinine: multiply mmol/L by 11.3 to convert to mg/dl.

admission (< 750 ml of urine in 24 hours), all but one showed a response to treatment by plasmapheresis with improvement in urine output and fall in serum creatinine levels. In the one patient who failed to respond, not only were crescents present in 100 percent of glomeruli, but there were circumferential crescents in 87 percent of glomeruli. Five other oliguric patients showed crescents in 58 to 97 percent of nonsclerosed glomeruli and all of these oliguric patients showed an improvement in urine output and serum creatinine levels over periods of 3 weeks to 3 months of plasmapheresis therapy. This is a critical group in whom early withdrawal of treatment may lead to rapid destruction of remaining glomeruli by continuing crescent formation. In such patients the percentage of crescents may increase even after plasmapheresis and other therapy has commenced (Fig. 13-4). The need to carefully monitor such patients daily urine output, urinary red cell

excretion and serum creatinine levels cannot be overemphasized.

In some patients subsequent renal biopsies may be necessary. The renal biopsy shows whether deterioration or failure to improve is due to further crescent formation or to a form of acute tubular necrosis which occasionally occurs and accompanies the macroscopic hematuria.

One patient in this group died of cryptococcal meningitis three months after presentation [serum creatinine at presentation, 0.96 mmol/L (10.8 mg/dl)] when renal function had shown substantial improvement [serum creatinine 0.26 mmol/L (2.9 mg/dl)]. This infection must clearly be regarded as a complication of his treatment.

The four other oliguric patients are alive with functioning kidneys, 5 months, 10 months, 1 year and 2½ years after plasmapheresis. The extent of crescentic lesions is not really reflected by the serum creatinine level at follow up. Two of these

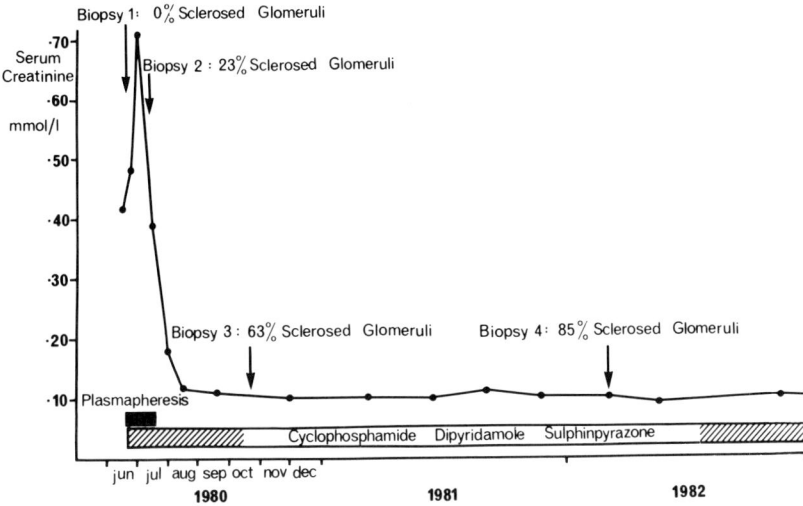

**Fig. 13-5.** A 19-year-old female with crescentic antiglomerular basement membrane (GBM) antibody nephritis who had 97% crescents on original biopsy (biopsy 1). Subsequent biopsies up to 2 years (biopsies 2, 3, and 4) showed progressive increases in the number of sclerosing/sclerosed glomeruli (Appendix). Despite severe glomerular destruction, renal function remains relatively stable. Creatinine: multiply mmol/L by 11.3 to convert to mg/dl.

patients had later renal biopsies up to two years after the acute episodes. The latest renal biopsies in both cases showed > 65 percent of glomeruli were sclerosed or sclerosing despite serum creatinine levels of 0.20 and 0.10 mmol/L, respectively. The long-term outcome in such patients must remain in some doubt because of the extensive glomerular destruction. However, in the patient with the longest follow-up (Fig. 13-5), the renal function appears to be quite stable. If the course of the experimental subtotal nephrectomy model[64,69,83] applies in such patients some deterioration might be expected in the future.

The six patients with crescents involving 9 to 55 percent of glomeruli all showed improvement in renal function. One patient died of uncontrollable pulmonary hemorrhage associated with a probable cytomegalovirus infection 3 weeks after presentation. Another patient died from acute myocardial infarction three

months after presentation. The other four patients are well after 2 years, 3½ years, 5¼ years, and 6½ years of follow-up.

Three patients with 60, 85, and 100 percent of crescents probably had plasmapheresis therapy stopped too early. All showed some initial response to therapy followed by deterioration which was treated by a second course of plasmapheresis after an interval of 2 weeks to 3 months. The renal biopsy had deteriorated in each case over the period and there was no response to the second course of plasmapheresis in two cases. The third case responded to the second course of plasmapheresis but failed to respond to a third course.[87]

The overall results of plasmapheresis therapy in this group of patients show that nine have improved or have stable renal function, eight patients are dead and one patient is on maintenance hemodialysis. When viewed in relation to the presentation with oliguria and anuria, and the renal biopsy findings, these results are very promising.

Anuric patients do not respond to plasmapheresis and biopsies show diffuse circumferential crescents in 90 to 100 percent of nonsclerosed glomeruli. Patients with oliguria usually have over 80 percent of glomeruli involved with crescents and require very careful management in relation to the initial biopsy and may require repeat biopsy.

All our oliguric patients except one responded in terms of improvement in renal function and resolution of the acute crescents. Two patients responded slowly and required 3 months of plasmapheresis and gradual reduction in frequency of the exchanges of plasma and other medication, but the medium term results in this group are very encouraging in spite of the diffuse crescentic lesions demonstrated in their renal biopsies.

We attributed poor results in three patients to early withdrawal of plasmapheresis. In two cases our own inexperience about the need to continue treatment for longer periods was probably relevant and in the third patient noncompliance was the major factor leading to early cessation of plasmapheresis therapy.

In the Goodpasture's syndrome–antiglomerular basement membrane antibody nephritis group as a whole, the renal biopsy had an excellent predictive value. Sclerosed glomeruli and those with circumferential crescents do not recover.

# IDIOPATHIC ACUTE CRESCENTIC (RAPIDLY PROGRESSIVE) GLOMERULONEPHRITIS

Another group of crescentic nephritides with a poor prognosis is idiopathic acute crescentic (rapidly progressive) glomerulonephritis.[2,7,32,48,49,60] A recent literature review of 339 cases of idiopathic acute crescentic (rapidly progressive) glomerulonephritis, prior to plasmapheresis therapy, showed that only 27 percent of patients have sufficient renal function to sustain life at two years.[19] The disease has a particularly poor outlook if 60 to 70 percent of glomeruli on renal biopsy show enveloping crescents.[22]

The role of plasmapheresis in the treatment of this condition is less well established. There are far fewer reports than for Goodpasture's syndrome. The heterogeneity of the pathology and etiology in idiopathic acute crescentic (rapidly progressive) glomerulonephritis has made the establishment of any particular treatment regimen virtually impossible by means of a controlled trial.

Several reports have suggested a good response[1,34,68,70,79,88] to plasmapheresis but the most significant experience in treating idiopathic acute crescent glomerulonephritis by this method has been reported by our own group.[3,20,78] In a study by Russ and d'Apice,[78] 22 of 24 patients with crescentic nephritis including 10 patients with idiopathic acute glomerulonephritis had improvement or stabilization of renal function attributable at least in part, to the plasmapheresis therapy.

In nearly all the cases reported, various combinations of immunosuppressive agents, anticoagulants and antiplatelet agents have been used in combination with plasmapheresis. It has therefore not been possible to determine whether results obtained represent an improvement due to plasmapheresis because similar good results have been obtained using combinations of immunosuppression and anticoagulation alone.[14,15]

It has been argued that in various forms of rapidly progressive glomerulonephritis (including idiopathic), the benefits of plasmapheresis therapy are less likely to occur in patients without demonstrable circulating immune complexes.[51,52] Many patients with idiopathic acute crescentic (rapidly progressive) glomerulonephritis fall into this category.[82] A satisfactory response to plasmapheresis therapy, however, has occurred in some cases of idiopathic acute crescentic (rapidly progressive) glomerulonephritis without circulating immune complexes,[78,79] suggesting that mechanisms apart from removal of circulating immune complexes may be important in producing a beneficial effect.

The usually acute onset and rapid progression in Goodpasture's syndrome means that the number of already sclerosed glomeruli tends to be lower and the confusion with chronic glomerulonephritis does not arise. In our own series, only one patient in the Goodpasture's syndrome group showed > 50 percent of sclerosed glomeruli on the initial biopsy. This was a young man without lung hemorrhage in whom the diagnosis had been missed over a five week period.

In the idiopathic group, all but one patient showed some sclerosed glomeruli. To make this a comparably acute group for comparison with those patients with Goodpasture's syndrome and antiglomerular basement membrane antibody nephritis, patients with known previous impairment of renal function or with sclerosis in more than 50 percent of glomeruli were excluded as having chronic disease. There were eleven patients remaining in this group and the details of age, sex and distribution of percentage of glomeruli involved with crescents, are demonstrated in Figs. 13-2 and 13-3. The percentage of crescents in nonsclerosed glomeruli varied from 12 to 100 percent (median 75).

In spite of the fact that the percentage of crescents in nonsclerosed glomeruli were similar in the two groups (Fig. 13-3) and the preplasmapheresis serum creatinine levels were also similar, the peak serum creatinine levels tended to be higher than preplasmapheresis serum creatinine

levels in patients with Goodpasture's syndrome or antiglomerular basement membrane antibody nephritis (paired t test, $p < 0.05$), whereas the preplasmapheresis and peak serum creatinine levels were similar in the idiopathic acute crescentic (rapidly progressive) glomerulonephritis group (Fig. 13-6). Only 1 of 11 patients in the idiopathic group showed continuing deterioration in renal function, once plasmapheresis therapy had commenced, whereas 11 of 17 of the Goodpasture's group showed initial deterioration of renal function on plasmapheresis before any improvement occurred ($p = .0046$, Fisher's Exact Test). These observations highlight the severity and fulminant nature of Goodpasture's syndrome and antiglomerular basement membrane antibody nephritis compared with other forms of crescentic nephritis.

The overall results of plasmapheresis therapy in the treatment of the idiopathic acute crescentic (rapidly progressive) glomerulonephritis group are very encouraging. Eight of the eleven patients are well with improved and stable renal function 3 months to 5 years after cessation of the plasmapheresis therapy. Despite the high percentage of sclerosed glomeruli and crescents in nonsclerosed glomeruli on initial biopsy, seven of these eight patients have serum creatinine levels $< 0.25$ mmol/L at the most recent follow-up.

One patient who was virtually anuric at presentation (30 ml of urine in 24 hours) and who had circumferential crescents in 100 percent of nonsclerosed glomeruli, failed to show any response to plasmapheresis treatment and was placed on maintenance hemodialysis. The two remaining patients died early in the disease course. One patient, a 47-year-old man, died from an acute gastrointestinal hemorrhage (duodenal ulcer) one week after plasmapheresis had commenced. The other patient, a 67-year-old man died

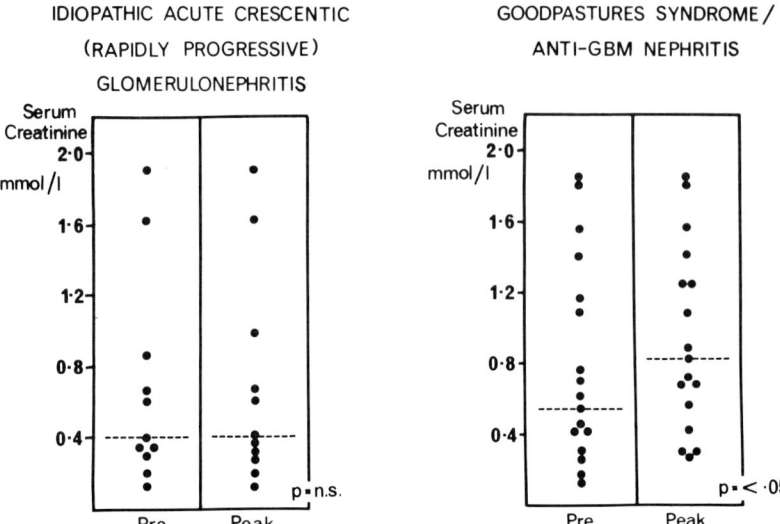

**Fig. 13-6.** Comparison between serum creatinine levels prior (pre) to plasmapheresis therapy and maximum serum creatinine levels (peak) on treatment for 11 patients with idiopathic acute crescentic (rapidly progressive) glomerulonephritis and 17 patients with Goodpasture's syndrome/antiglomerular basement membrane (GBM) antibody nephritis (--- = median value, n.s. = not significant). Creatinine: multiply mmol/L by 11.3 to convert to mg/dl.

from cardiorespiratory failure and septicemia.

## SYSTEMIC LUPUS ERYTHEMATOSUS WITH RENAL INVOLVEMENT

In the treatment of systemic lupus, there are theoretical reasons to anticipate that plasmapheresis therapy might influence the course of the disease.[35,36] The removal of circulating immune complexes and mediators of tissue inflammation and injury, has been demonstrated to occur with plasmapheresis.[72,76] Such effects are known to facilitate immune reticuloendothelial function.[30,35] However, reports of actual treatment of systemic lupus with renal involvement by plasmapheresis suggest that the results of this therapy are quite variable. Nearly all studies have been uncontrolled and treatment has generally been directed at acute disease presentations or acute exacerbations of the disease.[37,58,62,72,76,85,93]

Verrier-Jones and colleagues extended preliminary observations to report a favorable response to plasmapheresis in 14 patients with systemic lupus.[85,86] Of the eight patients studied that appeared to respond to the plasmapheresis therapy, seven had renal involvement but only one had crescentic disease. McKenzie and colleagues[58] reported improved or stabilized renal function in three of four patients with systemic lupus and crescentic glomerulonephritis but Sanz Guajardo and colleagues[79] found no benefit from plasmapheresis in three similar patients treated by plasmapheresis. Lockwood and colleagues report on six cases of systemic lupus with renal involvement and four showed improvement in renal function.[52]

In a pilot study, six patients with systemic lupus and diffuse proliferative glomerulonephritis were treated with chronic monthly plasma exchange, steroids, and immunosuppression for up to 2 years and early results suggested better preservation of renal function compared with control patients treated with steroids and immunosuppression alone.[16]

The benefits of plasmapheresis in systemic lupus erythematosus and renal involvement do not appear to be significantly greater than those of conventional therapy and the response to plasmapheresis is clearly quite unpredictable. The risk of infection in this group appears to be higher than corresponding groups of immunologically mediated renal diseases undergoing such therapy.[18]

Our own results in lupus nephritis using standard treatment with steroids have been excellent.[67] So much so that we have not needed to use plasmapheresis for acute lupus nephritis presenting with diffuse acute glomerular lesions and crescents. An occasional patient with severe active lupus nephritis, diffuse crescents, and severely impaired renal function may respond quite dramatically to treatment with steroids, azathioprine and antiplatelet and anticoagulant treatment.[42,43] We have not seen a patient with diffuse crescents and severely impaired renal function due to lupus nephritis since plasmapheresis therapy has been available.

No patient in our Renal Unit has progressed to end-stage renal failure in lupus nephritis in over 20 years experience with the exception of one 20-year-old woman who of her own accord ceased her steroid and azathioprine treatment when she had normal renal function. She returned some 3 months later with severe cerebral lupus and end-stage renal failure.

We have treated 11 female patients aged 16 to 53 years with lupus nephritis and crescents in 25 to 89 percent of glomeruli by plasmapheresis. In only one patient have we tried prolonged treatment with weekly plasma exchange and this patient died of an acute myocardial infarction after 3 months of therapy.

Apart from the above two patients, all are well 7 months to 5 years after cessation of plasmapheresis.

It is perhaps easiest to see the effect of plasmapheresis in those patients who have been relatively resistant to conventional treatment. One such patient, a 20-year-old woman, had a renal biopsy showing 89 percent of glomeruli involved with crescents and a serum creatinine of 0.14 mmol/L (1.6 mg/dl) after energetic treatment with steroids, azathioprine and cyclophosphamide. She was treated by plasmapheresis for 3 months, and during plasmapheresis, steroids were continued at a dose of 60 mg/day, and azathioprine at a dose of 100 mg/day. Her renal function improved and eventually stabilized and 4 years later her serum creatinine is 0.07 mmol/L (0.79 mg/dl).

The course of one patient who stopped steroids of her own accord, is charted in Fig. 13-7. She returned in apparent end-stage renal failure with 70 percent of glomeruli sclerosed and crescents in 75 percent of the remaining glomeruli, but responded well to plasmapheresis given in combination with prednisolone and azathioprine. Her serum creatinine fell from a peak of 0.79 mmol/L (8.9 mg/dl) to 0.26 mmol/L (2.9 mg/dl) and appears stable 6 months later.

In these two patients, plasmapheresis therapy appears to have produced benefit which may not have occurred with standard treatment. In most of the other patients, in spite of good clinical outcome, it is difficult to argue that plasmapheresis achieved more than the standard treat-

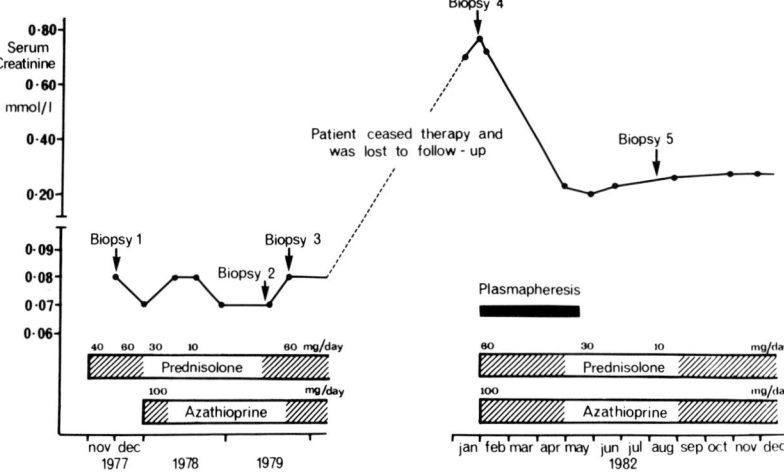

**Fig. 13-7.** A 20-year-old female with systemic lupus and a renal biopsy (biopsy 1) showing active mesangial proliferative glomerulonephritis with focal and segmental lesions including crescents, fibrin thrombi and wire loops. Proliferative lesions were less marked (biopsy 2) following treatment with steroids and azathioprine and the histopathology resolved, showing mild mesangial proliferative and membranous changes (biopsy 3). The patient re-presented 2 years after having stopped her therapy with an advanced proliferative glomerulonephritis (biopsy 4) with extensive crescents and glomerular destruction by sclerosis. Following plasmapheresis and reintroduction of prednisolone and azathioprine therapy there was a dramatic resolution of active proliferative change (biopsy 5) but with marked tubular atrophy and interstitial fibrosis consistent with glomerular loss due to sclerosis. Creatinine: multiply mmol/L by 11.3 to convert to mg/dl.

ment. One such case is illustrated in Fig. 13-8.

## MICROSCOPIC POLYARTERITIS AND WEGENER'S GRANULOMATOSIS

The use of plasmapheresis in other vasculitic processes, such as microscopic polyarteritis and Wegener's granulomatosis, has only infrequently been documented. In one study of 14 patients with nonlupus rapidly progressive nephritis, 7 had Wegener's granulomatosis and 6 had microscopic polyarteritis.[52] Four had crescentic nephritis. Of the 13 patients, 10 showed an improvement in renal function following plasmapheresis and 2 showed stabilization of renal function. One patient with Wegener's granulomatosis who was anuric at presentation failed to respond to the plasmapheresis therapy. Three of these patients (one with Wegener's granulomatosis and two with microscopic polyarteritis) subsequently died of opportunistic infection.

The study of Russ and d'Apice[78] of six patients with Wegener's granulomatosis and three patients with microscopic polyarteritis, all with crescentic glomerulonephritis and treated with plasmapheresis and immunosuppression, forms the basis of the experience reported here.

A group of patients with Wegener's

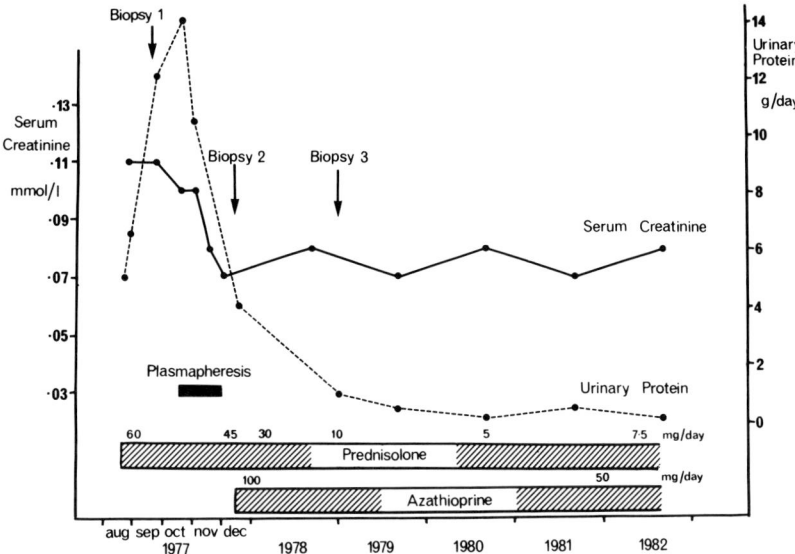

**Fig. 13-8.** A 16-year-old female with systemic lupus and severe diffuse proliferative glomerulonephritis with crescents (biopsy 1) and patchy mesangiocapillary and membranous changes in capillary walls which dramatically resolved (biopsy 2) with a decrease in urinary protein excretion and improvement and stabilization of renal function following steroids, azathioprine and plasmapheresis. Further renal biopsy (biopsy 3) showed virtually inactive disease with complete resolution of mesangiocapillary and membranous changes.

granulomatosis treated by plasmapheresis includes six males aged 23 to 68 years, and the acute nature of the glomerular lesion contrasts with the idiopathic acute crescentic group but is similar to the Goodpasture's group. Seven percent of glomeruli from one man, aged 66, were sclerosed while 50 percent from another patient, aged 68, showed similar changes. More than 60 percent of glomeruli from all patients had crescents and, 80 to 100 percent of glomeruli had crescents in four of the six patients. All patients had nasopharyngeal and renal lesions and in two patients the acute lesions recurred when cyclophosphamide was discontinued. The second episode in both these patients failed to respond and the patient required maintenance hemodialysis. Three patients are well with improved renal function 26 months to 5 years after cessation of plas-

mapheresis. As in the Goodpasture's syndrome group, we almost certainly discontinued treatment too early in one patient. A second course of plasmapheresis was commenced later, but no response occurred and the patient was transferred to maintenance hemodialysis and has since had a successful renal allograft.

In four patients with crescentic glomerulonephritis a diagnosis of polyarteritis was based on histological evidence of arteritis. Renal biopsies from these patients, one woman and three men, showed crescents in 29, 60, 67, and 69 percent of nonsclerosed glomeruli. Renal function improved initially in all patients after plasmapheresis therapy commenced. One patient, an 80-year-old man, died of pneumonia 3 days after plasmapheresis therapy was discontinued. Two patients are well with improved renal function 1 to

2 years later and one showed stabilization of impaired renal function but died of gastrointestinal hemorrhage 6 years later.

## DIFFUSE MESANGIOCAPILLARY GLOMERULONE-PHRITIS

We have also used intermittent plasmapheresis therapy in a variety of patients with mesangiocapillary glomerulonephritis.

A group in whom plasmapheresis was intended to reverse acute histological lesions includes five patients (four males, one female) aged 9 to 60 years. All five of these patients had the recent onset of acute mesangiocapillary glomerulonephritis. Crescents were present in 4 to 68 percent of glomeruli. In two patients, mesangiocapillary lesions appeared to resolve following plasmapheresis therapy and have not recurred.[20] Both of these patients are well with improved renal function five and six years after treatment. Features of the renal biopsies from these patients are shown in Fig. 13-9. In one patient, a 9-year-old girl, there was little apparent clinical histological improvement in the mesangiocapillary glomerulonephritis after three months of plasmapheresis therapy.

In one patient, an acute exudative lesion was associated with the mesangiocapillary lesions and resolved after plasmapheresis therapy. Over the same period, the leukocyte count in the urine, which had been raised over a 2-year period prior to plasmapheresis therapy, decreased to the normal range and this leukocyturia has not recurred.

The final patient simultaneously developed mesangiocapillary glomerulonephritis and documented sarcoidosis. His renal function, which had been deterior-ating, stabilized and had not deteriorated by the last follow-up, 12 months later.

We have also used plasmapheresis therapy as a "last ditch" or "final measure" procedure in three other patients with chronic mesangiocapillary glomerulonephritis, approaching end-stage renal failure. There was no apparent benefit from the plasmapheresis therapy in these three cases.

## PROGRESSIVE IDIOPATHIC FOCAL AND SEGMENTAL PROLIFERATIVE GLOMERULONE-PHRITIS

Renal biopsies, the clinical course, or both, in eight patients with idiopathic focal and segmental proliferative glomerulonephritis suggested chronic progressive disease, but crescents were still present. We used plasmapheresis therapy in these patients in an attempt to slow the rate of deterioration towards end-stage renal failure. This group of patients includes four males and four females aged 19 to 29 years.

Some of these patients had apparent end-stage renal failure when treatment was first attempted with plasmapheresis. In one such patient, significant improvement in renal function occurred in spite of having 83 percent of his glomeruli sclerosed. In one patient plasmapheresis treatment over only three weeks resulted in no apparent benefit. In the third patient, treatment over 12 months maintained a stable clinical and biochemical course, but when plasmapheresis therapy ceased, she rapidly deteriorated to end-stage renal failure. Her progress is shown in Fig. 13-10.

Although it is preferable to the patient, it is doubtful whether the use of plasmapheresis used in the way described in the previous patient over a long period is justified as a means of maintaining the patient in stable chronic renal failure.

Four of the remaining five patients have relatively stable, but impaired, renal function 8 months, 15 months, 18 months and 6 years after cessation of plasmapheresis. The final patient has deteriorated to end-stage renal failure and maintenance hemodialysis despite two further periods of plasmapheresis therapy.

## CRESCENTIC GLOMERULONE-PHRITIS FOLLOWING RENAL TRANSPLANTATION

In two patients, one a 65-year-old woman and the other a 53-year-old man, we have observed development of de novo idiopathic acute crescentic glomerulonephritis in renal allografts. Both patients were oliguric (urine volume < 750 ml/day) and both developed rapid deterioration in renal function. Institution of plasmapheresis in both cases was associated with rapid restoration of renal function to the levels observed prior to development of the crescentic glomerulonephritis. One of these cases was reported in detail previously.[78]

## CRESCENTIC GLOMERULONE-PHRITIS SUPERIMPOSED ON DIFFUSE MEMBRANOUS GLOMERULONE-PHRITIS

This is a rare occurrence. One man, aged 62, with rheumatoid arthritis in whom membranous glomerulonephritis had been documented on a previous renal biopsy, developed macroscopic hematuria and diffuse crescents affecting 88 percent of glomeruli. Plasmapheresis achieved a rapid response and renal function is unimpaired and stable four years later. Another man, aged 61, presented with macroscopic hematuria and rapidly deteriorating renal function and was found to have advanced membranous glomerulonephritis with sclerosis in 80 percent of glomeruli and crescents in 17 percent of the remaining glomeruli. Plasmapheresis was associated with stabilization of renal function and there has been no further deterioration over a period of 16 months of follow-up.

## CONCLUSIONS AND OVERVIEW OF PLASMAPHERESIS

Plasmapheresis probably offers little benefit over the results achieved by our group[44] and by Cameron's group[15] using steroids, immunosuppressive drugs, antiplatelet and anticoagulant agents in treating crescentic glomerulonephritis. However, plasmapheresis, in our experience, has been far easier to use and associated with fewer hemorrhagic complications.

As might be anticipated, infectious complications that occur seem to affect the elderly and debilitated patients. Vigorous plasmapheresis therapy is associated, in some studies, with an increased incidence of opportunistic infections.[91] Other studies have found no increase in infection rates (especially in patients with antiglomerular basement antibody glomerulonephritis) beyond that found in other immunosuppressed patients.[18] In such instances, the level of uremia and dosage of prednisolone appear to be more important determinants of the incidence of infection than the number of exchanges

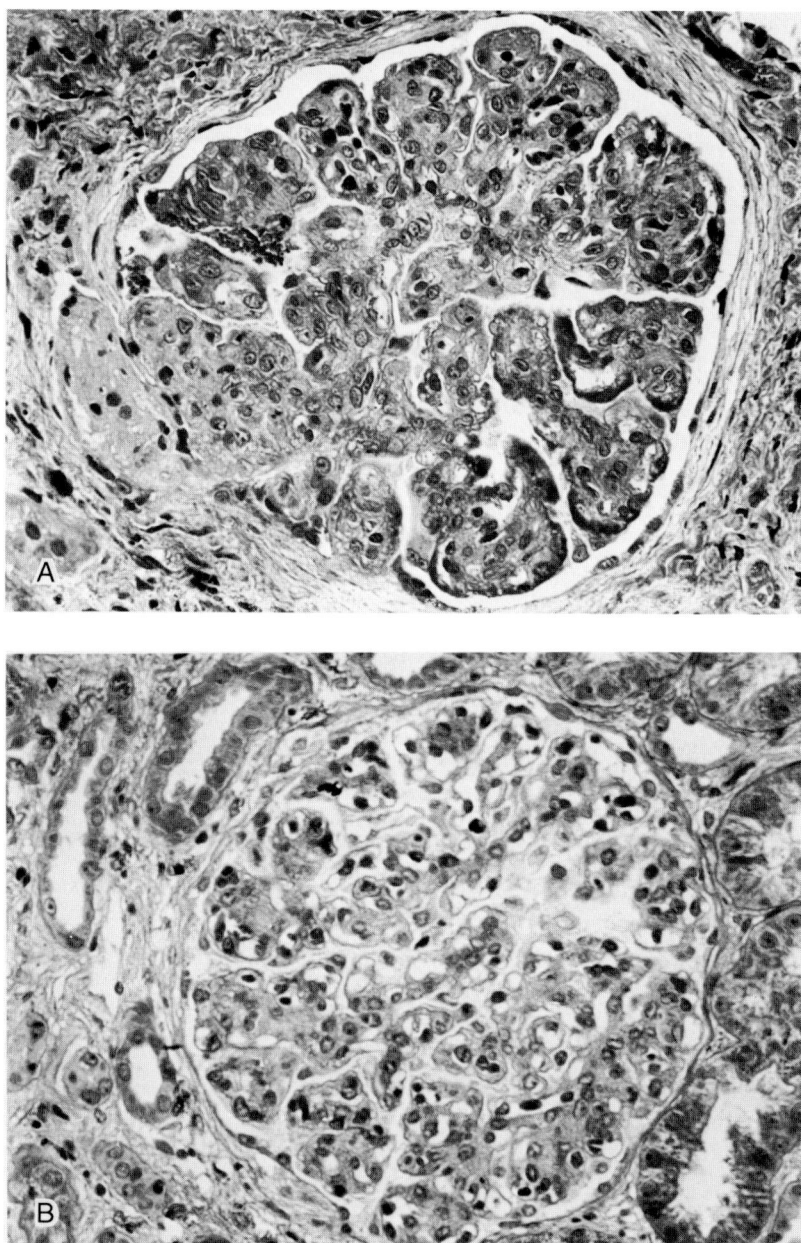

**Fig. 13-9.** Representative glomerulus (A) of a patient with severe mes-angiocapillary glomerulonephritis with extensive fibrin deposits and sub-endothelial deposits. Following plasmapheresis (B) virtual complete reso-lution of fibrin deposits and marked reduction of subendothelial deposits occurred.

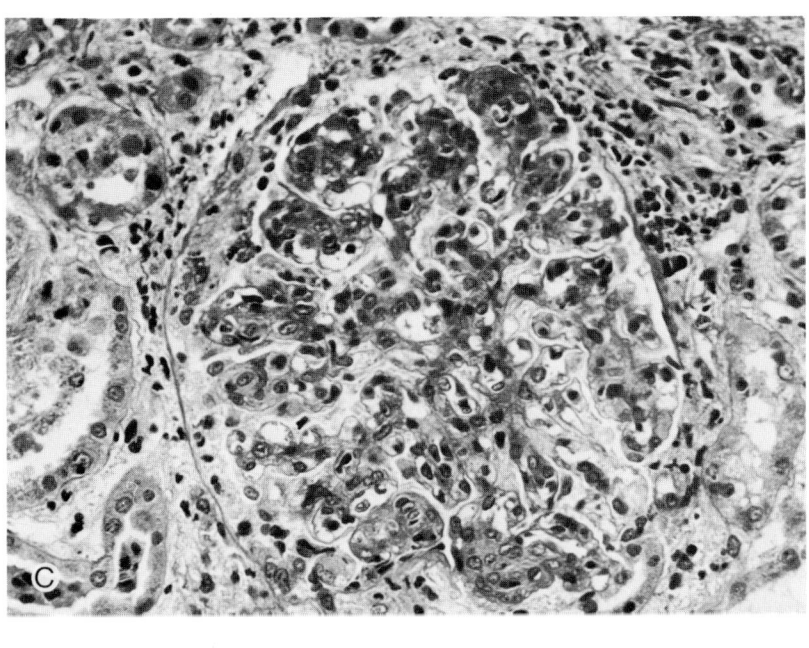

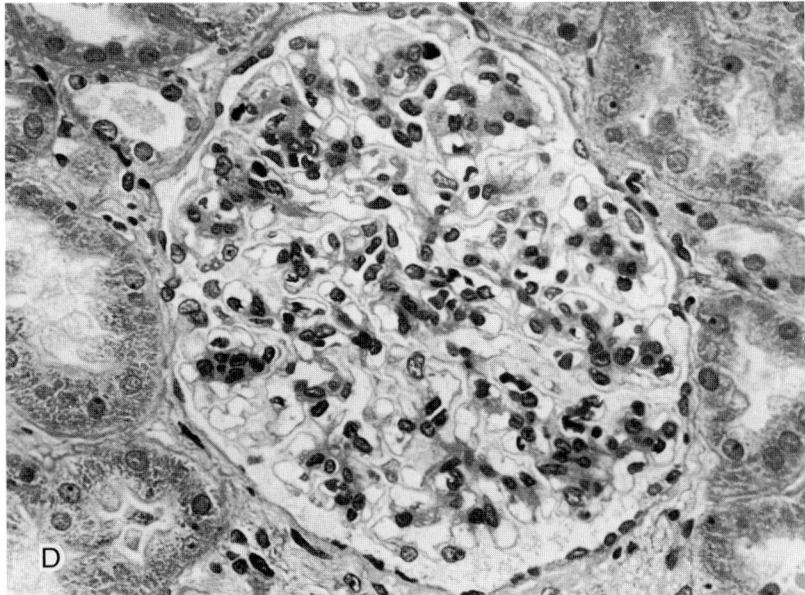

**Fig. 13-9 (cont.)**   (C) From another patient with severe mesangiocapillary glomerulonephritis with crescents and extensive subendothelial deposits. Dramatic resolution of these histological features (D) followed plasmapheresis.

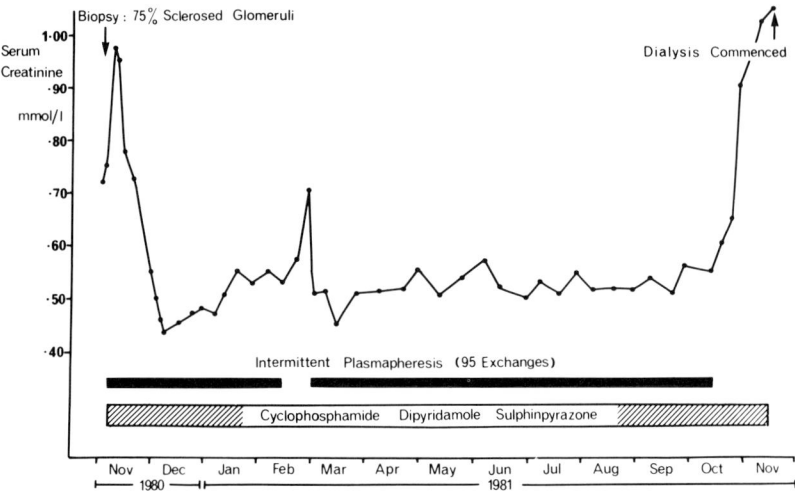

**Fig. 13-10.**  The clinical course of a 22-year-old female with idiopathic focal and segmental proliferative glomerulonephritis and extensive glomerular sclerosis on renal biopsy is shown. The patient was near end stage renal failure [peak serum creatinine 0.98 mmol/L (11.1 mg/dl)] but was maintained in stable condition for over 12 months by intermittent plasmapheresis therapy before commencing maintenance dialysis soon after plasmapheresis therapy was discontinued. Creatinine: multiply mmol/L by 11.3 to convert to mg/dl.

during the period of treatment with plasmapheresis.[18]

Based on our experience with plasmapheresis, we believe that in virtually all patients who have glomeruli which are capable of function—that is, that are not sclerosed or obliterated by circumferential crescents—clinical improvement in renal function occurs and usually occurs promptly after starting treatment. Occasional patients with antiglomerular basement membrane antibody glomerulonephritis will develop more crescents while on treatment (Fig. 13-4) but biopsies after plasmapheresis have generally shown disappearance of crescents. The percentage of sclerosed glomeruli or segmentally scarred glomeruli is high in follow-up biopsies, but excellent return of renal function is seen even when a high percentage of glomeruli are sclerosed.

In patients with documented circulating antiglomerular basement membrane antibody and linear IgG staining on fluorescent microscopy, it is possible to withdraw all medication after the acute episode. In three patients, followed for more than five years, no recurrence of disease has occurred and one of these patients has recently had a successful pregnancy.

Patients with idiopathic acute crescentic (rapidly progressive) glomerulonephritis and diffuse crescents are a less homogenous group. They have more sclerosed glomeruli before treatment is commenced and do not show the dramatic response to treatment that the Goodpasture's syndrome–antiglomerular basement membrane antibody glomerulonephritis group, demonstrate. Crescentic glomerulonephritis complicating Wegener's granulomatosis, microscopic polyarteritis, systemic lupus, membranous glomerulonephritis, and occurring after renal transplantation will all respond to plasmapheresis when combined with steroids, immunosuppression, antiplatelet agents and anticoagulation (Appendix).

In polyarteritis, which often responds to steroids,[31,77] in Wegener's granulomatosis, which may have an excellent response to cyclophosphamide,[73,92] and in lupus erythematosus, in which conventional treatment is usually successful,[43,67] there is perhaps less argument for using plasmapheresis and certainly more justification for a controlled trial.[39]

In chronic glomerulonephritis with crescents in some glomeruli, results are often disappointing, but have, in our experience, occasionally been rewarding. Some cases of mesangiocapillary glomerulonephritis appear to resolve during plasmapheresis therapy.

Perhaps the most important conclusions that the nephrologist should draw from this review of plasmapheresis therapy are:

1. The renal biopsy provides an excellent guide to the likelihood of response to plasmapheresis therapy. Sclerosed or sclerosing glomeruli and circumferential crescents cannot be made to function with plasmapheresis or any other method of treatment.

2. Valuable time is often lost after the onset of symptoms and before referral for a renal biopsy. Macroscopic hematuria due to glomerular red cells should be regarded as a medical emergency. Such hematuria usually means crescentic disease and only a renal biopsy can determine the extent and severity of the underlying lesion.

3. The only clinical feature which is of prognostic value in patients with crescentic glomerulonephritis is anuria. Severely oliguric patients often respond to plasmapheresis therapy provided treatment is instituted promptly.

## APPENDIX

Plasmapheresis therapy in this study was performed with an Aminco Celltrifuge.* The number of exchanges of plasma varied from 4 to 95 with a median number of 13 exchanges. The duration of a single period of plasmapheresis therapy varied from five days up to one year.

A single plasmapheresis usually consisted of an exchange of 4 L of plasma but some patients had volumes of 3 L and 2 L exchanged. Exchanges were usually performed on a daily basis for 3 to 5 days and then on alternate days and subsequently with decreasing frequency depending on the clinical situation.

Stable plasma protein solution (SPPS, Commonwealth Serum Laboratories, Melbourne) was the standard replacement fluid for the pheresed plasma but some patients received concentrated albumin (Commonwealth Serum Laboratories, Melbourne) in Hartman's solution because of a mild reaction to SPPS.

Drug therapy was used in all patients during and following the period of plasmapheresis. Various combinations of prednisolone (dosage 60 mg/day), cyclophosphamide (1 to 2 mg/kg/day) azathioprine (1 to 2 mg/kg/day), sulphinpyrazone (400 to 800 mg/day) and dipyridamole (100 to 400 mg/day) were used. In some patients, additional long-term therapy was given with warfarin (adjusted according to prothrombin efficiency) and in a few patients, brief periods of therapy with heparin (adjusted according to partial thromboplastin time) was also used.

Vascular access for plasmapheresis was usually achieved by a forearm arteriovenous shunt but patients given prolonged courses of plasmapheresis had access created with arteriovenous fistulas.

Renal needle biopsies were obtained percutaneously. Tissue was processed for light microscopy, fluorescent microscopy, and electron microscopy by conventional techniques. The percentage of sclerosed

*One patient plasmapheresed manually.[87]

glomeruli was determined by dividing the number of glomeruli exhibiting sclerosis by the total number of glomeruli in the biopsy. The percentage of glomeruli showing crescents in this study is the number of glomeruli exhibiting crescents as a percentage of those glomeruli that are *not* sclerosed, i.e.,

$$100 \times \frac{\text{glomeruli with crescents}}{(\text{Total glomeruli}) - (\text{sclerosed glomeruli})}$$

# REFERENCES

1. Adler S, Bruns FJ, Fraley DS, et al: Rapidly progressive glomerulonephritis: Relapse after prolonged remission. Arch Intern Med 141:852, 1981.
2. Bacani R, Velasquez F, Kanter A, et al: Rapidly progressive (non-streptococcal) glomerulonephritis. Ann Intern Med 69:463, 1968.
3. Becker GJ, d'Apice AJ, Walker RG, et al: Plasmapheresis in the treatment of glomerulonephritis. Med J Aust 2:693, 1977.
4. Bennett WM, Kincaid-Smith P: Macroscopic hematuria in mesangial IgA nephrology: Clinicopathologic correlation. Aust NZ J Med 12:341, 1982.
5. Bennett WM, Kincaid-Smith P: Macroscopic haematuria in mesangial IgA nephropathy: correlation with glomerular crescents and renal disfunction. Kidney Int, 23:393, 1983.
6. Benoit FL, Rulon DB, Theil GB, et al: Goodpasture's Syndrome: A clinicopathologic entity. Am J Med 37:424, 1964.
7. Berlyne G, Baker S: Acute anuric glomerulonephritis. Q J Med 33:105, 1964.
8. Branda RF, Moldow CF, McCullough JJ, et al: Plasma exchange in the treatment of immune disease. Transfusion 15:570, 1975.
9. Briggs WA, Johnson JP, Teichman S, et al: Antiglomerular basement membrane antibody-mediated glomerulonephritis and Goodpasture's syndrome. Medicine (Baltimore) 58:348, 1979.
10. Brown C, Wilson D, Turner D, et al: Combined immunosuppression and anticoagulation in rapidly progressive glomerulonephritis. Lancet 2:1166, 1974.
11. Bruns FJ, Stachura I, Adler S, et al: Effect of early plasmapheresis and immunosuppressive therapy on natural history of antiglomerular basement membrane glomerulonephritis: report of a 22-month follow-up. Arch Intern Med 139:372, 1979.
12. Cameron JS, Ogg C: Rapidly progressive glomerulonephritis with extensive crescents. In Kincaid-Smith P, Mathew T, Becker G, Eds: Glomerulonephritis: Morphology, Natural History and Treatment. Vol. 2. Wiley, New York, 1973, p 735.
13. Cameron JS, Gill D, Turner D, et al: Combined immunosuppression and anticoagulation in rapidly progressive glomerulonephritis. Lancet 2:923, 1975.
14. Cameron JS: Treatment of glomerulonephritis by drugs. Br Med J 1:1457, 1977.
15. Cameron JS: The treatment of severe glomerulonephritis with combined immunosuppression and anticoagulation. In Barcelo R, Bergeron M, Carrere S, et al, Eds: Proceedings VIIth International Congress Nephrology. Les Presses de l'Universite de Montreal, Montreal. Karger, Basel, 1978.
16. Clark WF, Lindsay RM, Cattran DC, et al: Monthly plasmapheresis for systemic lupus erythematosus with diffuse proliferative glomerulonephritis: a pilot study. CMA Journal 125:171, 1981.
17. Coggins CH, Pinn V, Glassock RT et al: A controlled study of short-term prednisone treatment in adults with membranous nephropathy. Collaborative study of the adult idiopathic nephrotic syndrome. N Engl J Med 301:1301, 1979.
18. Cohen J, Pinching AJ, Rees AJ, et al: Infection and immunosuppression. Q J Med 201:1, 1982.
19. Couser WG: Idiopathic rapidly progressive glomerulonephritis. Am J Nephrol 2:57, 1982.
20. d'Apice ATF Kincaid-Smith P: Plasma exchange in the treatment of glomerulonephritis. In Kincaid-Smith P, d'Apice A, At-

kins R, Eds: Progress in Glomerulonephritis. Wiley, New York, 1979, p 371.

21. Editorial: Plasmapheresis. Br Med J 1:1011, 1978.
22. Editorial: Plasmapheresis and severe glomerulonephritis. Br Med J 1:434, 1979.
23. Editorial: Plasmapheresis and immunosuppression. Lancet 1:1113, 1976.
24. Erickson SB, Kurtz SB, Donadio JV, et al: Use of combined plasmapheresis and immunosuppression in the treatment of Goodpasture's syndrome. Mayo Clin Proc 54:714, 1979.
25. Espinosa-Mellendez E, Forbes RD, Hollomby DJ, et al: Goodpasture's syndrome treated with plasmapheresis. Report of a case. Arch Intern Med 140:542, 1980.
26. Fairley KF, Kincaid-Smith P: Goodpasture's syndrome. Br Med J 2:1646, 1961.
27. Fairley KF, Birch DF: Haematuria: A simple method for identifying glomerular bleeding. Kidney Int 21:105, 1982.
28. Finch RA, Rustky EA, McGowan E, et al: Treatment of Goodpasture's syndrome with immunosuppression and plasmapheresis. South Med J 72:1288, 1979.
29. Friedman EA: Plasmapheresis for rapidly progressive glomerulonephritis: the mystique of dramatic intervention. JAMA 244:2446, 1980.
30. Frank MM, Hamburger MI, Lawley TJ, et al: Defective reticuloendothelial system Fc-receptor function in systemic lupus erythematosus. N Engl J Med 300:518, 1979.
31. Frohnert PP, Sheps SG: Long term follow-up study of periarteritis nodosa. Am J Med 43:8, 1967.
32. Glassock RJ: A clinical and immunopathologic dissection of rapidly progressive glomerulonephritis. Nephrology 22:253, 1978.
33. Glassock RJ, Cohen A, Bennett C, et al: Primary glomerular diseases. In Brenner BM, Rector FC, Jr, Eds: The Kidney. 2nd Ed. Saunders, Philadelphia, 1981, p 1351.
34. Harmer D, Finn R, Goldsmith JH, et al: Plasmapheresis in fulminating crescentic nephritis. Lancet 1:679, 1979.
35. Hughes GR: Plasma exchange (plasmapheresis). Agents Actions 7:62, 1980.
36. Hughes GR: Systemic lupus erythematosus: Treatment and prognosis. Br Med J 2:1019, 1979.

37. Isbister JP, Ralston M, Hayes JM, et al: Fulminant lupus pneumonitis with acute renal failure and RBC aplasia. Successful management with plasmapheresis and immunosuppression. Arch Intern Med 141:1081, 1981.
38. Johnson JP, Whitman W, Briggs WA, et al: Plasmapheresis and immunosuppressive agents in antibasement membrane antibody-induced Goodpasture's syndrome. Am J Med 64:354, 1978.
39. Jones JV: Plasmapheresis: A great economy in the use of horses. N Engl J Med 297:1173, 1977.
40. Keller AJ, Chirnside A, Urbaniak SJ: Coagulation abnormalities produced by plasma exchange on the cell separator with special reference to fibrinogen and platelet levels. Br J Haematol 42:593, 1979.
41. Keller AJ, Urbaniak SJ: Intensive plasma exchange on the cell separator: Effects on serum immunoglobulins and complement components. Br J Haematol 38:531, 1978.
42. Kincaid-Smith P: The prevention of renal failure. In Villarreal H, Ed: Proceedings of the Fifth International Congress of Nephrology. Vol. 3. Karger, Basel, 1974.
43. Kincaid-Smith P: Lupus nephritis. In Kincaid-Smith P, Ed: The Kidney. A Clinicopathological Study. Blackwell Scientific Publications, Oxford, 1975, p 329.
44. Kincaid-Smith P: The treatment of glomerulonephritis. In Oshima K, Yoshitoshi Y, Hatano M, Eds: Proceedings of the First Asian Pacific Congress of Nephrology. Secretariat of the First Asian Pacific Congress of Nephrology, Tokyo, 1979, p 1.
45. Kincaid-Smith P, d'Apice AJF: Plasmapheresis in rapidly progressive glomerulonephritis. Am J Med 65:654, 1978.
46. Kincaid-Smith P, Saker B, Fairley K: Anticoagulants in "irreversible" acute renal failure. Lancet 2:1360, 1968.
47. Lang CH, Brown DC, Staley N, et al: Goodpasture's syndrome treated with immunosuppression and plasma exchange. Arch Intern Med 137:1076, 1977.
48. Leonard C, Nagle R, Striker G, et al: Acute glomerulonephritis with prolonged oliguria. Ann Intern Med 73:703, 1970.
49. Lewis E, Cavallo T, Harrington J, et al: An immunopathologic study of rapidly pro-

gressive glomerulonephritis in the adult. Hum Pathol 2:185, 1971.

50. Lockwood CM, Boulton-Jones JH, Lowenthal RM, et al: Recovery from Goodpasture's syndrome after immunosuppressive treatment and plasmapheresis. Brit. Med J 2:252, 1975.

51. Lockwood C, Peters DK: Plasma exchange in glomerulonephritis and related vasculitides. Ann Rev Med 31:167, 1980.

52. Lockwood C, Pussell B, Wilson C, et al: Plasma exchange in nephritis. In Hamburger J, Crosnier J, Grunfeld J-P, et al, Eds: Advances in Nephrology. Vol. 8. Year-Book, Chicago, 1979, p 383.

53. Lockwood CM, Rees AJ, Pearson TA, et al: Immunosuppression and plasma-exchange in the treatment of Goodpasture's syndrome. Lancet 1:711, 1976.

54. Lockwood CM, Rees AJ, Pinching AJ, et al: Plasma-exchange and immunosuppression in the treatment of fulminating immune-complex crescentic nephritis. Lancet 1:63, 1977.

55. Lockwood CM, Worlledge S, Nicholas A, et al: Reversal of impaired splenic function in patients with nephritis or vasculitis (or both) by plasma exchange. N Engl J Med 300:524, 1979.

56. Martini A, Binda S, Mariani G, et al: Goodpasture's syndrome in a child: Natural history and effect of treatment. Acta Paediatr Scand 70:435, 1981.

57. Mathew T, Kincaid-Smith P: Severe fibrin and crescent glomerulonephritis. Clinical and morphologic aspects of 33 patients. In Kincaid-Smith P, Mathew T, Becker E, Eds. Glomerulonephritis: Morphology, Natural History and Treatment. Wiley, New York, 1973, p 727.

58. McKenzie PE, Taylor AE, Woodroffe AJ, et al: Plasmapheresis in glomerulonephritis. Clin Nephrol 12:97, 1979.

59. McLeish KR, Maxwell DR, Luft FC: Failure of plasma exchange and immunosuppression to improve renal function in Goodpasture's syndrome. Clin Nephrol 10:71, 1978.

60. McLeish K, Yum M, Luft F: Rapidly progressive glomerulonephritis in adults. Clinical and histologic correlations. Clin Nephrol 19:43, 1978.

61. McPhaull JJ, Jr, Mullins JD: Glomerulonephritis mediated by antibody to glomerulobasement membrane. J Clin Invest 47:351, 1976.

62. Moran CJ, Parry HF, Mowbray J, et al: Plasmapheresis in systemic lupus erythematosus. Br Med J 1:1573, 1977.

63. Morrin P, Hingalis N, Nabarra B, et al: Rapidly progressive glomerulonephritis. A clinical and pathologic study. Am J Med 65:446, 1978.

64. Morrison AB: Experimentally induced chronic renal insufficiency in the rat. Lab Invest 11:321, 1962.

65. Munk ZM, Skamene E: Goodpasture's syndrome—effects of plasmapheresis. Clin Exp Immunol 36:244, 1979.

66. Munro JE, Geddes AM, Lamb WL: Goodpasture's syndrome: Survival after acute renal failure. Br Med J 4:95, 1967.

67. Nanra RS, Kincaid-Smith P: Lupus nephritis: clinical course in relation to treatment. In Kincaid-Smith P, Mathew TH, Becker E, Eds: Glomerulonephritis: Morphology, Natural History and Treatment. Wiley, New York, 1973, Part II, p 1193.

68. Neilson EG, Phillips SM, Agus Z: Plasmapheresis in fulminating crescentic nephritis. Lancet 1:264, 1980.

69. Platt R, Roscoe MH, Smith FW: Experimental renal failure. Clin Sci 11:217, 1952.

70. Praga M, Mijares R, Ellosegui A, et al: Rapidly progressive glomerular disease treated with plasmapheresis. Med Clin (Barc) 77:33, 1981.

71. Proskey A, Weatherbee L, Easterling R, et al: Goodpasture's syndrome. A report of 5 cases and review of the literature. Am J Med 48:162, 1970.

72. Pussell BA, Lockwood CM, Scott DM, et al: Value of immune complex assays in diagnosis and management. Lancet 2:359, 1978.

73. Reza MJ, Dornfeld L, Goldberg LS, et al: Wegener's granulomatosis: Long term follow-up of patients treated with cyclophosphamide. Arthritis Rheum 18:501, 1975.

74. Robinson PR: Nephrology Forum. Isolated proteinuria in asymptomatic patients. Kidney Int 18:385, 1980.

75. Rosenblatt SG, Knight W, Bannayan GA, et al: Treatment of Goodpasture's syn-

drome with plasmapheresis. A case report and review of the literature. Am J Med 66:689, 1979.

76. Rossen RD, Hersh EM, Sharp JJ, et al: Effect of plasma exchange on circulating immune complexes and antibody formation in patients treated with cyclophosphamide and prednisolone. Am J Med 63:674, 1977.

77. Rupe CE: Treatment of polyarteritis nodosa and related arteritis. Mod Treat 3:1280, 1966.

78. Russ GR, d'Apice AJF: Plasma exchange and immunosuppression in crescentic glomerulonephritis. In Zurukzoglu W, Papadimitriou M, Pyrpasopoulos M, et al, Eds. Proceedings of the Eighth International Congress of Nephrology, University Studio Thessaloniki. Karger, Basel, 1981, p 667.

79. Sanz Guajardo D, Barbolla ML, Fernandez J, et al: Plasmapheresis in the treatment of extracapillary glomerulonephritis. Med Clin (Barc) 74:337, 1980.

80. Siegel RR: The basis of pulmonary disease resolution after nephrectomy in Goodpasture's syndrome. Am J Med Sci 259:201, 1970.

81. Sonsino E, Nabarra B, Kazatchkine M, et al: Extracapillary proliferative glomerulonephritis, so-called malignant glomerulonephritis. In Hamburger J, Crosnier J, Maxwell MH, Eds: Advances in Nephrology. Vol. 2. Year Book, Chicago, 1972, p 121.

82. Stilmant M, Bolton WK, Sturgill B, et al: Crescentic glomerulonephritis without immune deposits. Clinicopathologic features. Kidney Int 15:184, 1979.

83. Sterner G: Experimental chronic renal failure in rats. Nephron 24:207, 1979.

84. Swainson C, Robson J, Urbaniak S, et al: Treatment of Goodpasture's disease by plasma exchange and immunosuppression. Clin Exp Immunol 32:233, 1978.

85. Verrier-Jones J, Cumming RH, Bacon PA, et al: Evidence for a therapeutic effect of plasmapheresis in patients with systemic lupus erythematosus. Q J Med 48:555, 1979.

86. Verrier-Jones J, Cumming RH, Bucknall RC, et al: Plasmapheresis in the management of acute systemic lupus? Lancet 1:709, 1976.

87. Walker RG, d'Apice AJF, Becker GJ, et al: Plasmapheresis in Goodpasture's syndrome with renal failure. Med J Aust 1:875, 1977.

88. Warren SE, Mitas JA, Golbus SM, et al: Recovery from rapidly progressive glomerulonephritis. Improvement after plasmapheresis and immunosuppression. Arch Intern Med 141:175, 1981.

89. Whitworth J, Morel-Maroger L, Mignon F, et al: The significance of extracapillary proliferation. Clinicopathological review of 60 patients. Nephron 16:1, 1976.

90. Wilson C, Dixon F: Anti-glomerular basement membrane antibody-induced glomerulonephritis. Kidney Int 3:74, 1973.

91. Wing EJ, Bruns FJ, Fraley DS, et al: Infectious complications with plasmapheresis in rapidly progressive glomerulonephritis. JAMA 244:2423, 1980.

92. Wolff SM, Fauci AS, Horn, RG, et al: Wegener's granulomatosis. Ann Intern Med 81:513, 1974.

93. Young DW, Thompson RA, Mackie PH: Plasmapheresis in hereditary angioneurotic edema and systemic lupus erythematosus. Arch Intern Med 140:127, 1980.

# Critical Assessment of Purported Benefits

## Eli A. Friedman, M.D.

I shall be content if those shall pronounce
my history useful who wish to be given a
view of events as they really happened, and
as they are very likely to repeat themselves.
                    Thucydides, Historia

## INTRODUCTION

Reluctance to adopt new potentially hazardous therapies for proliferative (crescentic) glomerulonephritis in the absence of objective evidence supporting their efficacy has been termed "a nihilistic view" by Lewis and Schwartz.[18] In their opinion, "Despite a multitude of conflicting reports, one would prefer to 'do something' rather than simply follow the natural course of a lesion characterized by a rapid and permanent decline in the glomerular filtration rate." Nephrologists were exposed to similar reasoning a decade ago, in the form of an enthusiastic report of the value of a "cocktail" containing cyclophosphamide, dipyridamole, and phenindione or sodium warfarin in arresting the course of membranoproliferative glomerulonephritis.[14] Kincaid-Smith found a highly significant greater survival, at 30 months, in 16 patients given the "cocktail" as compared with 13 patients who did not receive this form of treatment. I can recall the excitement inspired by this article[14] at Journal Club, when our renal fellows felt that an effective means of managing a formerly untreatable disorder was in hand. Unfortunately, a follow up, prospective, ran-domized trial of the "cocktail" conducted by the Australian Working Party in Glomerulonephritis, was unable to reach any firm conclusions. The trial was discontinued for want of enough patients. Only six patients entered the experimental group and 14 entered the nontreatment group. The investigators concluded that they were studying a spectrum of disorders and that a rational therapeutic protocol could not be devised until the diseases were further clarified.[37] A subsequent, independent controlled trial of cyclophosphamide, warfarin, and dipyridamole undertaken by the Metropolitan Toronto Glomerulonephritis Group was unable to detect any benefit of treatment after 18 months in 63 randomized adults with type I or II lesions.[4] Lewis and Schwartz collected the literature of agents or techniques purported to "do something" to reverse or arrest the course of proliferative glomerulonephritis.[18] Listed in Table 13-2 are those interventions judged in uncontrolled trials to be useful in glomerulonephritis.

## THE MYSTIQUE OF DRAMATIC INTERVENTION

Make haste and use all new remedies before
they loose their effectiveness.
                    Sir William Wythey Gull

Physicians other than nephrologists have responded to the compulsion to

**Table 13-2.** Regimens Found Effective for Proliferative Glomerulonephritis

| |
|---|
| 1. Adrenocorticosteroids[25] |
| 2. Azathioprine[22] |
| 3. Cyclophosphamide[38] |
| 4. Heparin[3] |
| 5. Oral anticoagulants and antiplatelet agents[2] |
| 6. Indomethacin[36] |
| 7. Antilymphocyte globulin[28] |
| 8. Bolus methylprednisolone[32] |
| 9. Plasmapheresis |
| 10. Combinations of (1) through (9) |

(Modified from Lewis EJ, Schwartz MM: Idiopathic crescentic glomerulonephritis. Sem Nephrol 2: 193–213, 1982.)

"do something" to serve their suffering or dying patients when established therapy was worthless and deterioration was evident. Listed in Table 13-3 are several "no value" regimens introduced since I entered medical school, with initial uncontrolled but magnificent results.

Overholt, for example, a superior thoracic surgeon, concerned over the "tyranny and cruelty" of asthma removed one or both carotid bodies from asthmatics who had intractable asthma ". . . which had not been relieved by desensitization, brochodilators, changes of climate, steroids, and other standard therapeutic methods. . . ."[26] In a 1962 JAMA paper detailing the effect of carotid body resection in 157 patients, Overholt reported that "Slightly over half of the patients were either dramatically or significantly improved."[27] Confirmation of any worth of carotid body removal for asthma, or later for emphysema, did not appear; the operation is no longer advised. Tonsillectomy,

performed 2 million times in "an average year" up to the 1960s may be the best illustration of medical intervention without a rational basis. Defenders of tonsillectomy went so far as to attribute ". . . the gradual improvement in the health of children in the United States." to this operation.[6] As recently as 1977, there were 414,000 tonsillectomies performed in America on children under the age of 15 years, each of these operations, though supposedly designed to do good, was in fact, an assault on the integrity of vital host immunologic defences undertaken for no good reason.

Machine-based therapies are especially likely to attract physicians frustrated by an inability to provide drug or conventional effective treatment to a failing patient. Owen H. Wangensteen was dissatisfied with usual ulcer management. He described his original and insightful investigations of the pathogenesis of peptic ulceration in the Alvarenga Prize Lec-

**Table 13-3.** Widely Utilized Medical Regimens Found to Be Worthless

| |
|---|
| 1) Colectomy or colon bypass for stasis[35] |
| 2) Tonsillectomy for respiratory infections[6] |
| 3) Carotid body resection for asthma[26] |
| 4) Intestinal bypass for morbid obesity[31] |
| 5) Gluing of fractures[10] |
| 6) Carotid body resection for emphysema[44] |
| 7) Internal mammary ligation for angina[9] |
| 8) Gastric freezing for peptic ulcer[41] |
| 9) Insulin coma for schizophrenia[1] |
| 10) Hemodialysis for schizophrenia[29] |

ture delivered before the College of Physicians of Philadelphia in 1949.[40] A decade later, based on the finding that systemic hypothermia at temperatures in the range of 10° to 14°C suspended gastric digestion in frogs, toads, snakes and the rat, Wangensteen developed a machine which would cause local hypothermia in the stomach of dog and man. After four years of trials of gastric freezing, Wangansteen concluded that he had established ". . . the validity of the thesis that local gastric cooling has a definite place in the management of massive gastric hemorrhage.[41] Gastric freezing machines (Swenko Company, Minneapolis) were purchased throughout the nation; at least 120 patients had their stomach mucosa frozen before intestinal perforations, recurrent ulcers, and persistent hemorrhage prompted discontinuance of this form of treatment.

Kidney doctors have not been immune to the allure of machines as solutions to difficult clinical problems. Stimulated by the outstanding success of hemodialysis as a life prolonging therapy in uremia, dialytic therapy has been employed in liver failure, malignancy, psychoses, and dermatologic disorders. Until prospective controlled studies showed that hemodialysis for chronic schizophrenia[29] was of no benefit, psychiatric services around the world were preparing to dialyze as many as 1 percent of the general population. Dermatologists were quick to join their colleagues in nephrology in extending dialytic therapy to psoriasis. First came case reports and multiple uncontrolled small series of psoriatic patients purportedly improved by dialysis. In 1983, however, the enthusiasm of both dermatologists and nephrologists has been diminished by their inability to reproduce earlier glowing reports of efficacy derived from inconstant protocols and uncontrolled experiments. Hanicki et al.

conclude that "Hemodialysis alone, is not a satisfactory method for treating patients with psoriasis." They then suggest that "peritoneal dialysis seems to have a beneficial effect."[10] It will probably take a decade for the last of the uncontrolled properitoneal dialysis reports to be digested.

## THE CASE FOR PLASMAPHERESIS IN PROLIFERATIVE GLOMERULOPATHIES

There are some patients whom we cannot help; there are none whom we cannot harm."

Bloomfield

Plasmapheresis theoretically could arrest the course of an immunological disease by (1) removing specific antibodies, immune complexes, antigens, complement components, or fibrinogen; (2) extracting mediators of the immune response; or (3) removing abnormal circulating immunosuppressive factors. Advocates of the salutory effects of plasmapheresis initiated a special journal (Plasma Therapy), which in its first issue described plasmapheresis-induced-improvement in systemic lupus erythematosus, Wegener's granulomatosus, polyarteritis, subacute bacterial endocarditis, cryoglobulinemia, cutaneous vasculitis, thrombotic thrombocytopenic purpura, transplant rejection, motor neuron disease, hypertension, Raynaud's disease, and asthma.[19] Additional disorders in which plasmapheresis has been found advantageous include sickle cell anemia,[15] rheumatoid arthritis,[34] myasthenia gravis,[11] fulminant hepatitis,[7] and disseminated cancer.[12] The third meeting of the International Society for Artificial Organs, in 1981, programmed 32 papers on plasmapheresis ranging from technical aspects,[13] to demonstration that plasmapheresis is "a valuable form of treatment" for essential cryoglobulinemia.[30]

How can nephrologists resist overt and subtle pressures to treat their nephritic patients by plasma exchange? Glassock has concluded that plasmapheresis ". . . appears to be an established form of therapy for rapidly progressive glomerulonephritis occurring in antiglomerular basement membrane antibody disease providing therapy is begun early. . . ."[8] He subsequently comments that "It is premature to assign a definitive role for plasmapheresis per se in the management of the immune complex mediated glomerulonephritides." A less restrained endorsement of plasma exchange therapy in "immunological diseases" was presented by Shiokawa and coworkers, who treated a total of 92 patients with a positive outcome, though "further studies will be needed, such as the double-blind test"[34] Representative of the glowing assessments of plasmapheresis in glomerulonephritis is the report of Chalopin et al. who treated six patients with IgA nephropathies and found that "The clinical syptoms have completely disappeared in three patients. . . . The fast and definitive disappearance of the crescents in two of these cases is especially interesting."[5] Echoing Glassock's endorsement of the great merit of plasma exchange in antiglomerular basement membrane disease is the view of Lockwood that "Now it is possible to talk in terms of a cure for many patients with autoantibody-mediated nephritis who have been treated by plasma exchange and immunosuppressive agents."[20] The problem with each of the pro-plasmapheresis studies to date is that: (1) they have been uncontrolled, (2) side effects and cost are barely mentioned, and (3) nearly all plasmapheresis treated patients simultaneously received one or more cytotoxic drugs, as well as corticosteroids. There is another side to the premature assessment.

# PROBLEMS IN THE UNIVERSAL ACCEPTANCE OF PLASMAPHERESIS

It is mandatory that we continue to be alert to the subtle hazards of each drug and procedure we employ, since we are adequately propagandized regarding the apparent and well-publicized benefits.

Moser[24]

Readers of this text seek guidance in the management of their patients with proliferative glomerulonephritis. The central issue requiring resolution is: Should plasmapheresis be considered a routine, or an investigational treatment for nephritis of probable immune origin? There are only three reasons for a physician to use any treatment. A preferred justification is that the treatment has been proven to be of value. Streptomycin for tuberculosis is an example of unquestioned efficacy. Second in importance as a rationale for a new therapy is the enrollment of a patient in a controlled study to determine whether or not the treatment is of value. Oncologists regularly test toxic chemotherapeutic drugs in prospective, controlled trials with this justification. Lastly, because medicine is an art as well as a science, and clinicians are humanitarians, is the justified administration of a drug or procedure when a patient is dying and the proposed therapy is worth the gamble in a nearly lost cause.

Subjecting plasmapheresis for proliferative glomerulonephritis to these criteria leads to the following inferences: (1) Plasmapheresis is not of proven value. McLeish et al. document the failure of intensive plasmapheresis, continued for a month, to reverse the course of renal failure in proliferative glomerulonephritis despite reduction in antiglomerular basement membrane antibody, IgG, and $C_3$.[21] Pertinent to the question of efficacy of plasmapheresis in renal disorders is the report by Morse and Pisciotto of its failure to favorably alter the course in two patients with diagnoses (thrombotic thrombocytopenic purpura, and light chain myeloma) benefited in prior studies.[23] More disturbing than failure to produce a positive response, is an adverse reaction to plasmapheresis exemplified by deterioration in clinical condition noted in all four patients treated by plasmapheresis for systemic lupus erythematosus, in a trial which actually found increased levels of circulating immune complexes following plasma exchange.[33] Most of the enthusiastic reports cited above hedge their conclusions with statements such as: "Further controlled trials are needed . . ."[33] or "A controlled trial of this regimen is urgently required."[8] (2)Plasmapheresis is not without risk. Wing and associates reported that in rapidly progressive glomerulonephritis, five of eight patients treated by plasmapheresis developed "life-threatening infections," a serious complication which occurred in only 2 of 21 patients with similar renal disease, treated with immunosuppressive drugs but not plasmapheresis.[43] (3) Plasmapheresis is expensive. After purchase of pheresis machinery ($20,000 ±), daily treatments as advocated by Lockwood[14] will in one month add (in Brooklyn) a charge of ($15,000 ±) to the patient's hospital bill. (4) Withholding plasmapheresis in progressive renal failure does not necessarily mean the death of the patient. Hemodialysis and kidney transplantation in younger uremic patients (those with the greatest attack rate for immune nephritis) will extend their life, in the majority, for at least a decade.

## PROPOSED ACTION PLAN

It usually requires a considerable time to determine with certainty the virtues of a new method of treatment and usually still longer to ascertain the harmful effects.

Blalock

Plasmapheresis should not be employed outside of an experimental protocol for the immediate future. An exception can be made for the severely stricken patient with pulmonary hemorrhage and antiglomerular basement membrane disease. Academicians should stimulate and collaborate in controlled trials of plasmapheresis for nephritic syndromes, providing that the cost of treatment is borne by research funds. As observed by Schlansky et al., "plasmapheresis can function as a powerful placebo with its elaborate machinery, high cost, and the constant attendance of nursing and medical staff during the procedure."[33] Nephrologists are vulnerable to what has been termed "Rushed judgement in uremia therapy,"[7] a conjecture derived from study of the phenomenal rate of acceptance of newly uremic patients to treatment with continuous ambulatory peritoneal dialysis (CAPD), and continuous cyclic peritoneal dialysis (CCPD). Neither peritoneal dialysis regimen has been prospectively evaluated against hemodialysis in a controlled manner. With the passasge of time following clinical usage of a regimen, the probability of initiating a controlled evaluation of its efficacy falls. Once a therapy is "generally adopted", like tonsillectomy in the 1950s, or CAPD in 1983, marketing pressures by manufacturers of machines or supplies, and the tendency of practicioners to employ treatments "proven by tradition", provide powerful forces resisting its discontinuance.

Clinicians responsible for the welfare of patients with immunologic renal diseases appreciate the necessity for prospective controlled trials of plasmapheresis. Proponents and doubters of plasma exchange will gladly trade fact for rhetoric. The facts may be forthcoming. One recent well devised study of plasmapheresis in lupus erythematosus conducted at the Clinical Center of the National Institutes of Health did not discern benefit for the therapy. The authors concluded that: ". . . we have been unable to demonstrate in a controlled, randomised study that plasma exchange produces significant improvements in the clinical manifestations of mild acute SLE. The study suggests that plasma exchange in SLE, particularly in mild states, should continue to be regarded as an investigational procedure."[42] It would be injudicious, and cost ineffective, to characterize plasmapheresis as an established therapy for any renal disease at this time.

# REFERENCES

1. Ackner B, Harris A, Lodham AJ: Insulin treatment of schizophrenia. A controlled study. Lancet 1:607, 1957.
2. Arieff AI, Pinggera WF: Rapidly progressive glomerulonephritis treated with anticoagulants. Arch Intern Med 129:77, 1972.
3. Cameron JS, Gill D, Turner DR, et al: Combined immunosuppression and anticoagulation in rapidly progressive glomerulonephritis. Lancet 2:923, 1975.
4. Cattran D, Charron R, Cardella C, et al: Controlled trial in mesangiocapillary glomerulonephritis (MCGN) (abstract). In Zurukzoglu W, Papadimitriou M, Sion M, et al, Eds: Eighth International Congress of Nephrology: Advances in Basic and Clinical Nephrology. Karger, Basel, 1981, p 287.
5. Chalopin JM, Rifle G, Tanter Y, Besancenot JF, Cabanna JF, Justrabo E: Treatment of IgA nephropathy by plasma exchanges alone. Artif Org 5:138, 1981.
6. Clein NW: Influence of tonsillectomy and adenoidectomy on children with special reference to the allergic implications on respiratory symptoms. Ann Allerg 10:568, 1952.
7. Friedman EA, Lundin AP, Butt KMH: Rushed judgement in uremia therapy. Artif Org 5:97, 1981.
8. Glassock RJ: Plasmapheresis: Is it useful? Contr Nephrol 1:291, 1979.
9. Glover RP, Kitchell JR, Davila JC, et al: Bilateral ligation of the internal mammary artery in the treatment of angina pectoris. Am J Cardiol :937, 1960.
10. Hanicki Z, Cichocki T, Klein A, et al: Dialysis for psoriasis—Preliminary remarks concerning mode of action. Arch Dermatol Res 271:401, 1981.
11. Howard JF, Jr, Sanders DB, Johns TR: The role of plasma exchange therapy in myasthenia gravis. Haemonetics Research Institute Advanced Component Seminar, Boston, 1978.
12. Israel L, Edelstein R, Mannoni P, et al: Plasmapheresis in patients with disseminated cancer. Plasma Ther 1:57, 1980.
13. Jones JV, McLeod BC: Development and assessment of systems for removal of plasma components. Artif Org 5:117, 1981.
14. Kincaid-Smith P: The treatment of chronic mesangiocapillary (membranoproliferative) glomerulonephritis with impaired renal function. Med J Aust 2:587, 1972.
15. Kleinman S, Thompson-Brenton R, Rifkind S, et al: Exchange red blood cell pheresis in the mangement of complications of sickle cell anemia. Haemonetics Research Institute Advanced Component Seminar, Boston, 1979.
16. Lambert EC: Medical Mistakes. Indiana University Press, Bloomington, 1978, p 40.
17. Lepore MJ, McKenna PJ, Martinez DB, et al: Fulminant hepatitis with coma successfully treated by plasmapheresis and hyperimmune Australia-antibody-rich plasma. Plasma Ther 1:49, 1979.
18. Lewis EJ, Schwartz MM: Idiopathic crescentic glomerulonephritis. Sem Nephrol 2:193, 1982.
19. Lockwood CM: Plasma-exchange: An overview. Plasma Ther 1:1, 1979.
20. Lockwood CM: Plasma exchange in anti-GBM nephritis. Artif Org 5:135, 1981.
21. McLeish KR, Maxwell DR, Luft FC: Failure of plasma exchange and immunosuppression to improve renal function in Goodpasture's syndrome. Clin Nephrol 10:71, 1978.
22. Michael AF, Vernier RL, Drummond KN, et al: Immunosuppressive therapy of

chronic renal disease. N Engl J Med 276:817, 1967.

23. Morse EE, Pisciotta PT: Therapeutic plasmapheresis in patients with renal disease. Ann Clin Lab Sci 11:361, 1981.

24. Moser RH: Diseases of Medical Progress: A Study of Iatrogenic Disease. Charles C Thomas, Publisher, Springfield, Ill, 1959.

25. Nakamoto S, Dunea G, Kolff WJ, et al: Treatment of oliguric glomerulonephritis with dialysis and steroids. Ann Intern Med 63:359, 1965.

26. Overholt RH: Pulmonary denervation and resection in asthmatic patients. Ann Allerg 17:534, 1959.

27. Overholt RH: Resection of carotid body (cervical glomectomy) for asthma. JAMA 180:91, 1962.

28. Pirofsky B, Reid RH, Bardana EJ Jr, et al: Antithymocyte antisera therapy in non-surgical immunologic disease. Transplant Proc 3:769, 1971.

29. Port FK, Kroll PD, Swartz RD: Clinical and research reports. Am J Psychiatr 135:743, 1978.

30. Pusey CD, Schifferli JA, Lockwood CM, et al: Use of plasma exchange in the management of mixed essential cryoglobulinemia. Artif Org 5:183, 1981.

31. Rand CSW, Kuldau JM, Robbins L: Surgery for obesity and marriage quality. JAMA 247:1419, 1982.

32. Rose GM, Cole BR, Robson AM: The treatment of severe glomerulopathies in children using high dose intravenous methylprednisolone pulses. Am J Kidney Dis 1:148, 1981.

33. Schlansky R, DeHoratius RJ, Pincus T, et al: Plasmapheresis in systemic lupus erythematosus. A cautionary note. Arthritis Rheum 24:49, 1981.

34. Shiokawa Y, Shiozawa K, Yamagata J, et al: Immune disease and plasma exchange therapy. Artif Org 5:152, 1981.

35. Smith JL: Sir Arbuthnot Lane, chronic intestinal stasis, and autointoxication. Am Intern Med 96:365, 1982.

36. Suc JM, Conte J, Conte M: Treatment of glomerulonephritis with indomethacine and heparin. In Kincaid-Smith P, Mathew TH, Becker EL, Eds: Glomerulonephritis: Morphology, Natural History and Treatment, New York, John Wiley and Sons, 1973, p 927.

37. Tiller DJ, Clarkson AR, Mathew T, et al: A prospective randomized trial in the use of cyclophosphamide, dipyridamole, and warfarin in membranous and mesangiocapillary glomerulonephritis. In Zurukzoglu W, Papadimitriou M, Sion M, et al, Eds: Eighth International Congress of Nephrology: Advances in Basic and Clinical Nephrology, Karger, Basel, 1981, p 345.

38. Urizar RE, Tinglof B, McIntosh R, et al: Immunosuppressive therapy of proliferative glomerulonephritis in children. Am J Dis Child 118:411, 1969.

39. Wallace DJ, Goldfinger D, Gatti R, et al: Plasmapheresis and lymphoplasmapheresis in the management of rheumatoid arthritis. Arthritis Rheum 221:703, 1979.

40. Wangensteen OH: An assessment of etiologic aspects of peptic ulcer and surgical therapy. Including obscure, massive acid-peptic linked hemorrhage, esophagitis and cardiospasm and their surgical relief. Trans & Studies, Coll of Phys of Phila 18:1, 1950.

41. Wangensteen OH, Peter ET, Bernstein EF, et al: Can physiological gastrectomy be achieved by gastric freezing? Ann Surg 156:579, 1962.

42. Wei N, Klippel JH, Huston DP, et al: Randomised trial of plasma exchange in mild systemic lupus erythematosus. Lancet 1:17, 1983.

43. Wing EJ, Bruns FJ, Fraley DS, et al: Infectious complications with plasmapheressis in rapidly progressive glomerulonephritis. JAMA 244:2423, 1980.

44. Winter B: Bilateral carotid body resection for asthma and emphysema. A new surgical approach without hypoventilation or baroreceptor dysfunction. Int Surg 57:458, 1972.

# 14

# Reflux Nephropathy

# The Case for Surgical Management

## Alan B. Retik, M.D.

## INTRODUCTION

Vesicoureteral reflux (VUR) is one of the most common abnormalities of the urinary tract and its management continues to be the source of major controversy. As with most other congenital abnormalities, the presentations of VUR vary and its treatment very often depends upon the severity of the abnormality. This paper will discuss a rationale for the management of such patients. Although the emphasis will be on the indications and results of surgery, I must immediately confess that most children with mild to moderate degrees of reflux can and should be handled nonoperatively at least initially.

## HISTORICAL ASPECTS

In 1924, Graves and Davidoff[14] demonstrated VUR in 86 percent of normal rabbits. Gruber[16] in 1929 showed experimentally that the intravesical ureter is short and the trigone is poorly developed in those animals susceptible to reflux. However, the significance of VUR was not truly appreciated until the early 1950s, when Hutch[21] demonstrated pyelonephritic scarring in patients with neurogenic bladder dysfunction and VUR.

## INCIDENCE

The incidence of VUR is 1 to 2 per 1000 population.[6,56] It is primarily a disorder of Caucasians, rarely being described in blacks.[25] It is five times more common in females than males, although this figure may be somewhat misleading because the short female urethra may predispose to urinary tract infection and thus to an increased investigation for and detection of reflux.

Although VUR is commonly thought of as a disorder primarily of childhood, it is not uncommonly seen in adults.[1,3,30] As increasing numbers of patients with end-stage renal failure become candidates for transplantation, investigation of the lower urinary tract has uncovered a significant incidence of previously undetected severe VUR. During the past few years, a number of authors[9,10,31,5,27,2,44,32,7,22] have suggested a polygenic mode of inheritance in which males require a greater number of predisposing genes.

## ETIOLOGY

Various studies have shown that reflux does not occur in the urinary tract of normal man.[23,24,28,34,35] Milder degrees of reflux have been observed in neonates with normal urinary tracts. However, this reflux has not been clinically significant and has invariably disappeared over a period of years.

A number of factors are responsible for the prevention of reflux in normal individuals. These include an oblique entry of the ureter into the bladder and an adequate length of the intramural ureter, especially of its submucosal segment. The ratio of the submucosal tunnel length to the ureteral diameter is the most important factor that determines the effectiveness of the valve mechanism. Adequate distal fixation to the normal trigone by the ureterotrigonal ligaments and good support from the bladder musculature are also important elements that contribute to the prevention of reflux. The prevention of reflux may be due to active muscle contraction or to passive valvular action. Both mechanisms probably are operative. Stephens and Lenaghan[48] stated that the active contraction of the longitudinal fibers crossing the roof of the intravesical ureter compresses the ureter and closes it after ureteral efflux has appeared. Most authors stress the length of the intravesical portion of the ureter as the most important factor in the prevention of reflux. With growth, there is maturation of the trigone, the submucosal ureter elongates, and the ratio between the submucosal tunnel length and ureteral diameter increases, making it less likely for reflux to occur.

A number of circumstances can compromise the valvular efficiency and result in VUR. Distal obstruction was originally considered to be the prime cause of reflux. We now know that most chidlren with reflux are not obstructed. More recently, urinary tract infection has been thought to be the cause of most cases of VUR. However, recent studies[15] have disproved this and have shown that reflux and urinary tract infection are independent variables that often coexist. It is possible that urinary tract infection with associated inflammation of the bladder wall and of the intravesicular segment of the ureter may sufficiently alter the structure of the ureteral–vesical junction as to permit transient, mild reflux in a few children with borderline anatomic abnormalities.

In the vast majority of children with VUR, a congenitally short or absent intravesical ureter and/or deficient muscular support of this segment are the primary factors responsible for reflux.

## CLINICAL FEATURES

Vesicoureteral reflux is most often detected in children who present with urinary tract infection. Many children have irritative symptoms such as frequency, urgency, and enuresis while some present with high fever and abdominal or back pain. Infants especially may be septic or may present with failure to thrive. A small but significant percentage of asymptomatic children have been found to have infected urine and VUR, or reflux and a sterile urine when investigated for other reasons.

Although reflux is often an incidental finding in the evaluation of children with urinary tract infections, severe reflux often predisposes to infection by leading to continuous residual urine in the bladder. Vesicoureteral reflux has been found in an increasing number of patients with chronic pyelonephritis. In our series of children,[54,55] with radiologic evidence of pyelonephritis, VUR was demonstrated by voiding cystourethrography in greater than 90 percent. In some of the remaining children, a definite anatomic abnormality of the ureteral orifice was seen cystoscopically, leading to the assumption that reflux had been present in the past and had subsided or that these orifices refluxed intermittently. These conclusions have been shared by others.[18,20,26,29,42,43,45–47,51,52] Between 30 and 60 percent of children with reflux exhibit radiologic signs of pyelonephritis.[47] It has been shown that the more severe the degree of reflux, the more likely is the patient to show progressive renal damage. Renal scarring may not become evident for up to two years following infection.

It is felt that renal scarring results

from the extension of reflux into the collecting tubules (intrarenal reflux) and from the associated urinary infection. It is also generally agreed that the appearance of fresh scars or the extension of established scars is very unusual in children with sterile reflux, in the absence of obstruction or neurogenic bladder dysfunction. Hodson[19] was able to produce intrarenal reflux with scarring in pigs with elevated intravesical pressures. Experimentally, it has been shown[38,39,50] that the areas of renal parenchyma susceptible to intrarenal reflux and subsequent scarring are drained by flat or concave papillae which occur predominantly in the polar regions of the kidney. Studies in the pig suggest that in the presence of infected urine, intrarenal reflux results in the development of scarring in less than 4 weeks.

It has been suggested that renal growth is inhibited in the presence of reflux.[29,40] In our series,[54,55] however, preoperative measurements of refluxing kidneys without pyelonephritis have not varied significantly from normal. Although reflux may inhibit renal growth in selected instances, very small kidneys with reflux alone and no pyelonephritic scarring more likely represent maldevelopment of the entire ureterorenal unit. Faulty development of the ureteral bud may account for an incompetent ureterovesical junction with hypoplasia and dysplasia of the renal parenchyma. It appears, therefore, that for reflux to cause impaired renal growth, it must be associated with infection leading to pyelonephritis.

## DIAGNOSIS AND EVALUATION

Most VUR is detected during the course of radiologic evaluation in children with urinary tract infections. Although the findings on the excretory urogram may lead one to suspect that VUR is present, the definitive diagnosis is made by the voiding cystourethrogram, which should be done while the subject is awake. We have traditionally employed the Dwoskin-Perlmutter Classification[11] to grade reflux from 1 (mild) to 4 (very severe). More recently, the International Classification (utilizing grades I–V), has become popular (Fig. 14-1). More severe grades of reflux are generally observed in the scarred kidneys of infants and younger children while more mild grades are found in older children, suggesting that VUR improves or ceases with time. This is so even among children with renal scarring and with dilitation of the upper

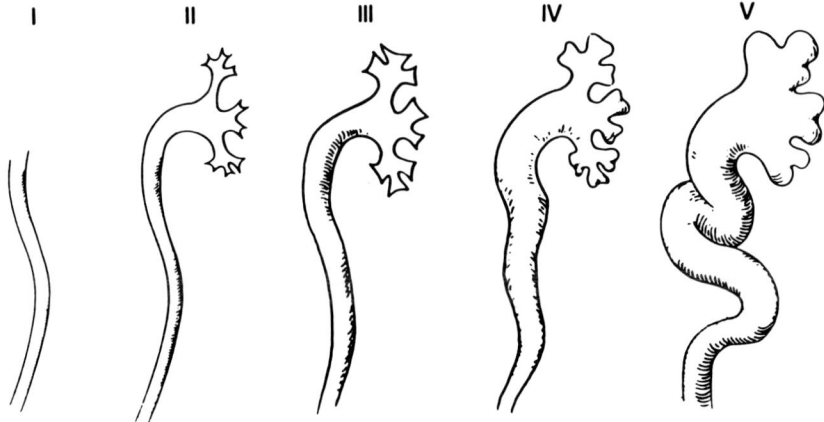

**Fig. 14-1.** International classification grades of reflux.

urinary tract. However, reflux is more likely to cease in milder grades and when kidneys are unscarred. Contrary to previous statements, the rate of disappearance of reflux appears to remain constant throughout childhood—being 20 to 30 percent within each 2-year period.[12,33] In our experience, virtually all grade 1/5 and approximately 70 percent of grade 2/5 reflux will eventually subside. This is probably an effect of maturation, the obliquity of the insertion of the ureter and hence, its intramural length and valvular competence increasing with skeletal growth. With greater degrees of reflux, there is less likelihood that disappearance will occur. Normand reported that reflux disappeared from only 41 percent of dilated ureters as compared to its eventual disappearance from more than 80 percent of nondilated ureters.[33] Some observers have noted that moderately severe reflux may subside over a period of years in the occasional patient, especially infants, with ureteral dilatation.[41]

## COMPLICATIONS OF VESICOURETERAL REFLUX

In addition to renal scarring, the most serious potential long-term complication of VUR is hypertension. Although the incidence of hypertension in patients with reflux nephropathy is not known, this complication might be more prevalent than renal scarring. It has been reported in as many as 20 percent of children with renal scars.[47] Many of the reported patients do not have renal failure. The etiology of hypertension in such instances is probably related to vascular lesions resulting in focal ischemia.[17,49] Elevated plasma renin levels have been observed in several children with hypertension and reflux nephropathy.[41]

In some children, severe VUR may cause some extreme tortuosity and kinking at the ureteropelvic junction, thus in effect producing a secondary ureteropelvic obstruction (Fig. 14-2). It is therefore important to obtain a voiding cystourethrogram in a child with ureteropelvic obstruction to ensure that surgery will be performed at the correct level of the ureter.

## THE MANAGEMENT OF PATIENTS WITH VESICOURETERAL REFLUX

The treatment of VUR must be individualized; factors such as: duration of disease, age of onset, number of infections and ease with which they are controlled should be considered in deciding whether surgery should be performed. It is generally agreed that reflux in the absence of infection in most children does not cause renal scarring. It has become apparent that most reflux unaccompanied by a dilatation of the urinary tract will subside with time. Therefore, most children with grade 3/5 reflux and less are placed on a nonoperative program initially. This consists of continuous low-dose antibiotic therapy, periodic urine cultures, and an excretory urogram, and radionuclide cystogram are obtained annually. Most of these children maintain a sterile urine, do well clinically, and ultimately will have discontinued antibiotics after reflux disappears. Therefore, there is little disagreement with regard to the initial management of children with the milder degrees of reflux. The controversy occurs with grades 4/5 and 5/5. Reflux has been reported to subside spontaneously in one large series in only 41 percent of such children, even after many years of observation.[12] It is also more difficult to maintain sterile urines in this group and

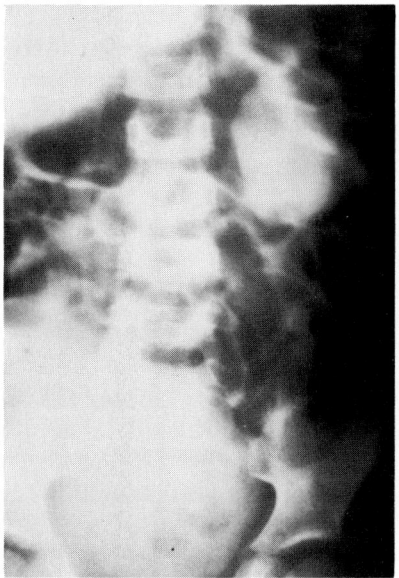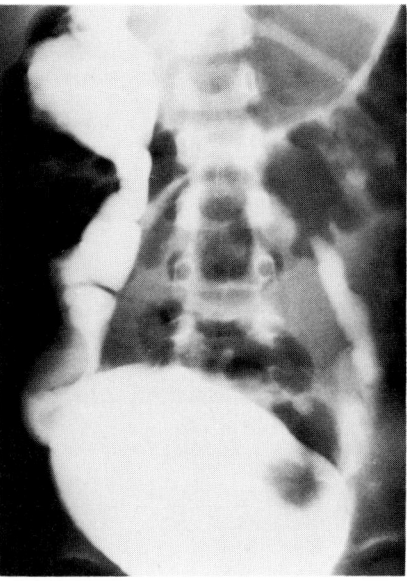

**Fig. 14-2.** Excretory urogram (left) and voiding cystourethrogram demonstrate severe left hydronephrosis due to kinking and tortuosity at ureteropelvic junction secondary to severe reflux. This child required a pyeloplasty as well as antireflux surgery.

secondary complications, for example, ureteropelvic obstruction, may also occur.

The indications for antireflux surgery that we have employed are:

1. Recurrent urinary tract infections despite adequate continuous antibiotics. This is the absolute indication for antireflux surgery and should pertain to children even with milder degrees of reflux.

2. Severe (grade 4/5 and grade 5/5) reflux especially with pyelonephritic changes (Fig. 14-3). This degree of reflux is unlikely to subside and the patient is already at risk for the development and progression of pyelonephritic scars.

3. Failure of renal growth on serial excretory urograms. Severe reflux has been implicated as a factor in the failure of kidneys to grow. Antireflux surgery has been reported to reverse such changes.[41]

4. Reflux persisting after full linear growth into puberty. It is unusual for VUR to subside after puberty. This is especially important when considering the relationship between reflux and pregnancy. Ureteral dilatation and increased bladder capacity are well recognized concomitants of pregnancy that may worsen preexisting reflux. The incidence of asymptomatic bacteriuria in pregnancy is 4 to 6 percent, approximately the same as in a population of similar nonpregnant women. Symptomatic pyelonephritis, however, occurs in 1 to 2 percent of pregnant women and is the most common renal complication of pregnancy. Twenty to 40 percent of women with symptomatic bacteriuria will develop symptomatic pyelonephritis unless treated successfully. While pyelonephritis may be harmful to the fetus, it has not been clearly established that asymptomatic bacteriuria is harmful.

One hundred women who had asymptomatic bacteriura during pregnancy were studied 4 to 6 months post-

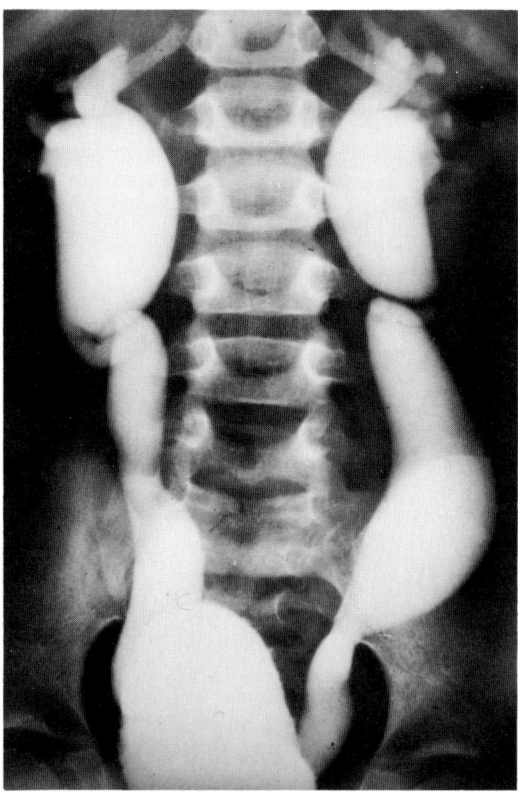

**Fig. 14-3.** Voiding cystourethrogram demonstrates severe (grade 4/5) reflux. The excretory urogram showed severe pyelonephritic scarring bilaterally.

partum.[53] The data demonstrated that women with reflux had an increased incidence of renal scarring, much more difficulty in clearing bacteriuria with antibiotics, and a higher incidence of bacteriuria postdelivery. These data suggest that women with bacteriuria and reflux should have the reflux corrected before pregnancy.

5. Patient noncompliance. An increasing number of children, for one reason or another, are not maintained on continuous antibiotics and subsequently have recurrent infections. They, therefore, do not adhere to the medical regimen and are at risk for the development of renal scarring. Surgery should be performed on this group of patients.

6. Persistent reflux with a congenital abnormality at the ureterovesical junction. It is unlikely for reflux to subside in the presence of an obvious anatomic abnormality at the ureteral orifice, e.g., for example, a Hutch or paraureteral saccule.

## SURGICAL PROCEDURES AND RESULTS

The purpose of surgery is to reimplant the ureter through a new submucosal tunnel in the bladder wall. This tunnel should be of sufficient length and appropriate placement between mucosa and detrusor, so that the mechanical requirements for a functioning flap valve are met, and it should be approximately five times the diameter of the ureter. In very dilated ureters it is necessary to narrow the caliber of the ureter to achieve an adequate tunnel and to permit more effective ureteral peristalsis.

A number of antireflux operations have been described.[8,13,36] (Fig. 14-4). The technical results of antireflux surgery are excellent and successes have been reported in 95 to 99 percent of cases. In our original series of children undergoing antireflux surgery, 223 were followed for periods ranging from 6 months to 7 years. Ureteral obstruction occurred in four children (1.2 percent) requiring reoperation in two. The obstruction in the remaining two patients was transient, being secondary to edema. Transient postoperative reflux was observed on the operated (ipsilateral) side in ten of the 242 ureters (3 percent), but spontaneously subsided in each case within one year. In 104 unilateral operations, 17 patients (16 percent) developed reflux on the nonoperated (contralateral) side. Within 1 year, this reflux stopped in all but two children, each of whom had demonstrated transient preoperative reflux. With increasing surgical

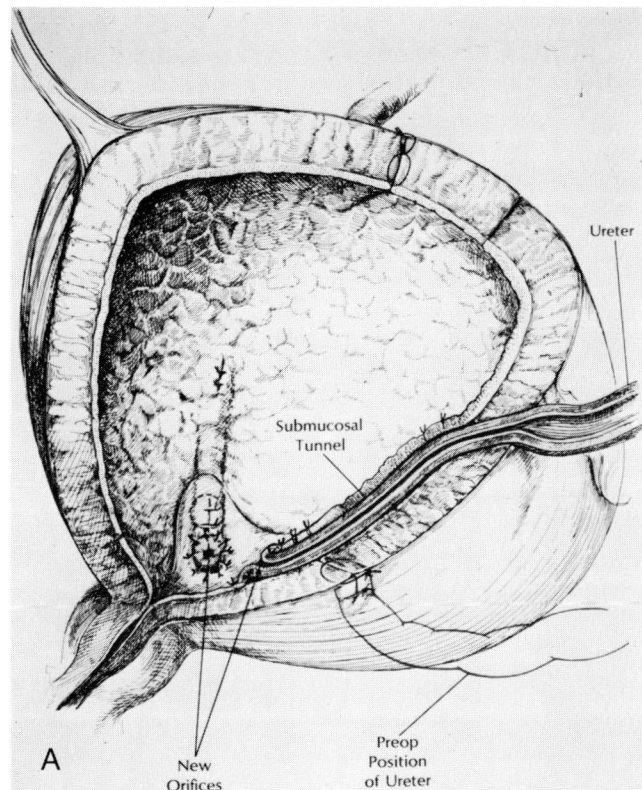

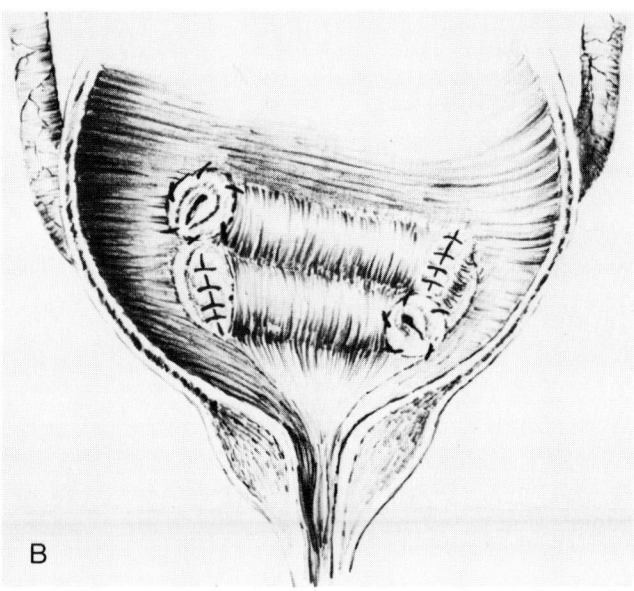

**Fig. 14-4** (A). Politano-Leadbetter operation (B). Cohen cross-trigonal procedure. Both procedures create longer submucosal tunnels.

experience, the results now are even better. Ureteral obstruction, persistent reflux and even transient contralateral reflux are rare.

Postoperative urinary infection occurred in 21 percent of the patients. There were only two boys in this group, each of whom was diagnosed clinically as having cystitis. The majority of postoperative infections occurred in girls (45 of 175 females), and as judged clinically, all but three (1.7 percent) were confined to the bladder. One-third of all postoperative infections occurred in the first 6 months while the child was still receiving antibiotics. With each infection there was less chance for development of subsequent infection. The incidence of postoperative infection was not influenced by the presence of pyelonephritis or hydronephrosis preoperatively. In addition, greater degrees of preoperative reflux did not predispose the patient to a higher incidence of postoperative infection.

The postoperative infection rate is generally reported to be between 10 and 30 percent. In this series, the incidence of infection after surgery was 21 percent and clinically confined to the bladder in the majority of cases. Boys rarely developed a postoperative infection. The protective effect of the longer male urethra probably accounts for this finding. Postoperative pyelonephritis is uncommon. Neither the severity of reflux, nor the preoperative presence of radiologic pyelonephritis, predisposes the patient to postoperative infection. It is felt that girls are reinfected because of anatomic and physiologic factors peculiar to the female lower urinary tract, rather than to the presence of old pyelonephritis. Abnormal flora in the vagina and introitus may also play a significant role in producing recurrent infection in girls.

We demonstrated that following successful antireflux surgery, kidneys grew at rates equal to or greater than expected normals.

Management of the severely pyelonephritic kidney associated with VUR can be a vexing problem. Whether one should remove the small kidney or reimplant its refluxing ureter has been left to the discretion of the individual urologist without the establishment of clear-cut guidelines upon which to base a decision. We consider a kidney to be salvageable if the differential renal scan reveals that the kidney in question provides at least 7 to 10 percent of the overall renal function. Bauer[59] followed 19 children with severe pyelonephritic scarring secondary to reflux and infection for periods of at least five years after surgical correction of reflux. The small kidneys in these children grew at a rate which paralleled expected normal, and this growth was independent of the degree of hypertrophy in the contralateral kidney or the size difference between each pair of renal units. The authors concluded that children with a small pyelonephritic kidney should undergo reimplantation rather than nephrectomy because of the recuperative powers of the growing kidney and its ability to become a potentially life-sustaining organ in the future.

## CONCLUSION

Although the majority of patients with VUR can be managed successfully without an operation, surgery most definitely plays a role in the management of patients with moderately severe and severe reflux. The technical surgical success rate is as high or perhaps higher than most commonly performed procedures. Successful surgery can help to eliminate the need for antibiotics, repeated radiologic investigation, clinical attacks of pyelonephritis and resultant renal scarring. Antireflux surgery may also decrease some of the complications of reflux such as secondary ureteropelvic obstruction, hypertension and the sequelae of urinary infection during and after pregnancy.

# REFERENCES

1. Amar AD, Singer B, Lewis R, et al: Vesico-ureteral reflux in adults: A twelve year study of 122 patients. Urology 3:184, 1974.
2. Amar AD: Familial vesico-ureteral reflux. J Urol 108:969, 1972.
3. Ambrose SS: Reflux pyelonephritis in adults secondary to congenital lesions of the ureteral orifice. J Urol 102:302, 1969.
4. Bauer SB, Willscher MK, Zammuto PJ, et al: The dilemma of the small pyelonephritic kidney associated with vesico-ureteral reflux. Urology 15:466, 1980.
5. Bredin HC, Winchester P, McGovern JH, et al: Family study of vesico-ureteral reflux. J Urol 113:623, 1975.
6. Burger RH, Smith C: Hereditary and familial vesico-ureteral reflux. J Urol 106:845, 1971.
7. Burger RH: A theory on the nature of transmission of congenital vesico-ureteral reflux. J Urol 108:249, 1972.
8. Cohen SJ: Ureterozystoneostomie. Eine neue antirefluxtecnik. A new technique for reflux prevention. Aktuelle Urologie 6:1, 1975.
9. De Vargas A, Evans K, Ransley P, et al: A family study of vesicouretric reflux. J Med Genet 15:85, 1978.
10. Dwoskin JY: Sibling uropathology. J Urol 115:726, 1976.
11. Dwoskin JY, Perlmutter AD: Vesico-ureteral reflux in children: A computerized review. J Urol 109:888, 1973.
12. Edwards D, Normand ICS, Prescod N, et al: Disappearance of vesico-ureteric reflux during long-term prophylaxis of urinary tract infection in children. Br Med J 2:285, 1977.
13. Glenn JF, Anderson EE: Distal tunnel ureteral implantation. J Urol 97:623, 1967.
14. Graves RC, Davidoff LM, II: Studies on the ureter and bladder with especial reference to regurgitation of the vesical of the contents. J Urol 12:93, 1924.
15. Gross GW, Lebowitz RL: Infection does not cause reflux. Am J Roentgenol 137:929, 1981.
16. Gruber CMI: A comparative study of the intravesical ureters in man and in experimental animals. J Urol 21:567, 1929.
17. Hicks CC, Woodward JR, Walton KW, et al: Hypertension as complication of vesico-ureteral reflux in children. Urology 7:587, 1976.
18. Hodson CJ: Obstructive atrophy of the kidney in children. Ann Radiol 10:273, 1967.
19. Hodson CJ, Maling TMJ, McManaman PH, et al: Reflux nephropathy. Kidney Int 8:550, 1975.
20. Hutch JA, Smith DR, Osborne R: Summary of pathogenesis of a new classification for urinary tract infections. J Urol 102:758, 1969.
21. Hutch JA: Vesico-ureteral reflux in the paraplegic: Cause and correction. J Urol 68:457, 1952.
22. Jenkins GR, Noe HN: Familial vesico-ureteral reflux: A prospective study. J Urol 128:774, 1982.
23. Jones BW, Headstream JW: Vesico-ureteral reflux in children. J Urol 80:114, 1958.
24. Kjellberg SR, Ericsson MO, Rudhe U: The Lower Urinary Tract in Childhood. Livingstone, Edinburgh, 1957.
25. Kunin CM, Deutsch R, Paquin A, Jr: Urinary tract infections in children: Epidemiologic, clinical and laboratory study. Medicine 43:91, 1964.
26. Lenaghan JD, Whitaker G, Johnson F, et al: The natural history of reflux and long-term effects of reflux on the kidney. J Urol 115:728, 1976.
27. Lewy PR, Belman AB: Familial occurrence of non-obstructive, non-infectious vesico-ureteral reflux with renal scarring. J Pediatr 86:851, 1975.
28. Lich R, Howerton LW, Good LS, et al: The uretro-vesical junction of the new born. J Urol 92:436, 1964.
29. Lyon RP: Renal arrest. J Urol 109:707, 1973.
30. McGovern JH, Marshall VF: Reflux and pyelonephritis in 35 adults. J Urol 101:668, 1969.
31. Middleton GW, Howards SS, Gillenwater JY: Sex-linked familial reflux. J Urol 114:36, 1975.
32. Mulcahy JJ, Kelalis PP, Strickler GB, et al: Familial vesico-ureteral reflux. J Urol 104:762, 1970.
33. Normand C, Smellie J: Vesico-ureteric reflux: A case for conservative management.

In Hodson J, Kincaid-Smith P, Eds: Nephropathy. Masson, New York, 1979, p 281.

34. Peters P, Johnson DE, Jackson JR: The incidence of vesico-ureteral reflux in the premature child. J Urol 97:259, 1967.

35. Politano VA: Uretero-vesical junction. J Urol 107:239, 1972.

36. Politano VA, Leadbetter WF: An operative technique for correction of vesico-ureteral reflux. J Urol 79:932, 1958.

37. Ransley PG: Vesico-ureteric reflux—the continuing surgical dilemma. Urology 12:246, 1978.

38. Ransley PG, Risdon RA: Reflux Nephropathy: The effects of anti-microbial therapy on the evolution of the early pyelonephritic scar. J Ped Nephrol Urol 1:1, 1981.

39. Ransley PG, Risdon RA: The renal papilla, intrarenal reflux and chronic pyelonephritis. In Hodson CJ, Kincaid-Smith P, Eds: Reflux Nephropathy. Masson, New York, 1979, p 126.

40. Redman JF, Scriber LJ, Bissad NK: Apparent failure of renal growth secondary to vesico-ureteral reflux. Urology 3:704, 1974.

41. Retik AB: Unpublished data.

42. Rolleston GL, Shannon FT, Utley WLF: Relationship of infantile vesico-ureteric reflux to renal damage. Br Med J 1:460, 1970.

43. Savage DCL, Wilson MI, Ross EM, et al: Asymptomatic bacteriuria in girl entrants to dundee primary school period. Br Med J 3:75, 1969.

44. Schmidt JD, Hawtrey CE, Flocks RH, et al: Vesico-ureteral reflux: an inherited lesion., JAMA 220:821, 1972.

45. Scott JES, Stansfield JM: Ureteric reflux and kidney scarring in children. Arch Dis Child 43:468, 1968.

46. Smellie J.M, Normand ICS: The clinical features and significance of urinary tract infection in childhood. Proc Soc Med 59:415, 1966.

47. Smellie JM, Edwards D, Hunter N, et al: Vesico-ureteric reflux and renal scarring. Kidney Int 8:565, 1975.

48. Stephens FD, Lenaghan D: The anatomical basis and dynamics of vesico-ureteric reflux. J Urol 87:669, 1962.

49. Stickler GB, Kelalis PP, Burke EC, et al: Primary interstitial nephritis with reflux—A cause of hypertension. J Dis Child 122:144, 1971.

50. Tamminen TE, Kaprio EA: The relation of the shape of renal papillae and of collecting duct openings to intrarenal reflux. Br J Urol 49:345, 1977.

51. Walker RD, Duckett J, Bartone F, et al: Screening school children for urologic disease. Section of urology, American Academy of Pediatrics. Pediatrics 60:329, 1977.

52. Williams DI: The ureter, the urologist, and the pediatrician. Proc R Soc Med 63:595, 1970.

53. Williams GI, Davies DKL, Evans KT, et al: Vesico-ureteral reflux in patients with bacteriuria in pregnancy. Lancet 2:1202, 1968.

54. Willscher MK, Bauer SB, Zammuto PJ, et al: Renal growth and urinary infection following anti-reflux surgery in infants and children. J Urol 115:722, 1976.

55. Willscher MK, Bauer SB, Zammuto PJ, et al: Infections of the urinary tract after anti-reflux surgery in infants and children. J Pediatr 89:743, 1976.

56. Zel G, Retik AB: Familial vesico-ureteral reflux. Urology 2:249, 1973.

# The Case for Medical Management

## Lawrence R. Freedman, M.D.

## A STATEMENT OF THE PROBLEM

Reflux nephropathy (RN), characterized radiologically by renal scars adjacent to clubbed calices, may be associated with slowing or arrest of renal growth and is often accompanied by varying degrees of vesicoureteral reflux (VUR). The term RN was introduced to distinguish those patients with renal scars associated with VUR from subjects with scars associated with other causes of renal papillary damage, for example, analgesic abuse, diabetes mellitus, sickle cell disorders. It is believed that VUR increases the susceptibility of the kidney to infection by facilitating the access of bacteria to vulnerable zones of the renal papilla. This latter process is referred to as intrarenal reflux. In addition, VUR may increase the susceptibility of the renal papilla to infection by pressure effects that may impair papillary circulation. Approximately one-third of children with urinary tract infection (UTI) have VUR and roughly one-third of these have RN.[35] Conversely, children in whom fresh renal scars have been detected have been found almost exclusively to have UTI and varying degrees of VUR.[31,35,40]

Affected children, first recognized by their UTI and subsequently discovered to have VUR, are very likely to have renal scars. The combination of findings (VUR and UTI) undoubtedly leads to mutilation of the kidney. It is presumed that progressive scarring eventually causes renal insufficiency but such progression has been only rarely observed.

Follow-up studies of children with RN has revealed hypertension to be a common complication, even prior to the development of renal insufficiency. Furthermore, children with RN have developed hypertension even when VUR has disappeared and subsequent UTI has been prevented. It follows that RN is generally considered to be an important cause of serious renal damage and hypertension and is currently the center of considerable interest—and controversy.

There is debate as to the appropriateness and usefulness of the term Reflux Nephropathy. The problem with the term is that it implies that VUR is always pathogenetically related to the development of the renal scarring. This implication has assumed increasing importance since it has been shown that VUR and renal scarring are not always causally related and conversely, since VUR may relapse and remit, the absence of VUR at the time the scar is detected does not absolve reflux as a factor in its pathogenesis.

Thus, any discussion of the management of RN depends critically on the prevailing view of whether VUR is a *necessary* factor in the pathogenesis of renal scarring. For example, there was a time in the United States when "urologists reimplanted any ureter that showed the slightest degree of VUR, with the result that surgery was carried out on far too many children."[36] Indeed, the question has been asked: What about those people who reflux intermittently such as the women with intermittent pyelonephritis, in whom we cannot demonstrate reflux? Should we be bold enough to take these people in and correct them anyhow?"[25]

In recent years, the surgical techniques which have been applied to most refluxing ureters have advanced to the point where success in curing VUR is highly predictable. On the other hand, clinical studies over the same time period demonstrated the frequency with which VUR disappears spontaneously (concomitant with suppression and eradication of UTI). It was also shown that severe VUR associated with RN is less amenable to successful surgical repair than those lesser degrees of VUR which pose only a minimal risk to the renal parenchyma.[5]

Today it is generally agreed that the mere presence of VUR is not an indication for its surgical repair. The question that remains unsettled is at what stage in the complex interrelations of RN, VUR, and UTI, surgical repair of reflux is indicated. The question has bearing not only on the few patients who might benefit from repair but also on the vast number, mostly children, subjected to the trauma and risks of investigative procedures currently deemed necessary for making the proper therapeutic decision.

The problem may be similar to many others which require determination of the point at which the treatment becomes a less acceptable danger than the disease itself. This is clearly illustrated by the therapy of hypertension where morbidity and mortality are linearly related to the degree of blood pressure elevation. No one disputes that benefit accrues from lowering the blood pressure from 180 to 150 mm Hg. The ratio of therapeutic gain to pharmacologic side effect is less likely to be as favorable, however, when an attempt is made to lower the pressure from 150 to 120 mm Hg. This dilemma exists with hypertension even though measurement of blood pressure is simple, the consequences of untreated disease well defined, and the drugs available relatively safe, effective, and easy to administer. The management of VUR is much more complex. There is dispute as to how to measure its presence and the methods available are invasive and not without risk. Furthermore, the consequences of VUR are not well defined and we do not have satisfactory methods for quantitating it. Finally, follow-up studies involve repetition of invasive procedures and recommended therapy may involve major surgery. The roots of controversy are not difficult to discern.

# VESICOURETERAL REFLUX: A DEFINITION

Vesicoureteral reflux is the retrograde movement of urine from bladder toward kidney via the ureter. The currently available evidence suggests that this is a normal concomitant of ureteral peristaltic activity.[33] Shapiro has presented the mathematical basis for this view[33] and Politano has placed substances such as charcoal and bacteria in the bladder and recovered them from the renal pelvis.[24] The clinical verification of this phenomenon is found in patients with pyelonephritis who, even when examined very soon after an acute infection, cannot be shown to have VUR by standard radiologic techniques. According to our current concepts of the pathogenesis of pyelonephritis, bacteria were delivered to the kidney from the bladder via the ureteral lumen. Thus, reflux of urine is sufficient to deliver bacteria to the kidney in numbers capable of producing acute pyelonephritis even in the absence of radiologically demonstrable VUR.

Since, at one extreme, VUR seems to be a normal concomitant of ureteral peristalsis and since, at the other extreme, there are unequivocal instances of patulous ureteral orifices with free reflux of urine into widely dilated ureters, the critical question is not whether someone does or does not have VUR, but rather, how much. Or, to pose the question in a different way, What amount of VUR increases the risk of renal damage sufficiently to accept the risks attending radiologic diagnosis and surgical repair?

VUR, detected by standard radiologic techniques, is classified according to whether radiopaque material ascends only to the lower ureter (Grade I), the renal pelvis (Grade II-during voiding only; Grade III-at rest), or if the dye-filled ureters and renal pelvis are dilated (Grade IV) (Fig. 14-5).[34] Other classification systems have been devised but they differ in detail and not in substance.[2] The essential point is that those forms of VUR associated with dilatation of the ureters and renal pelvis are considered to be the most severe.

There are several reasons why it is difficult to determine the amount of VUR beyond which surgical therapy offers a clear-cut therapeutic advantage. One of the major reasons is that there is no standard way of radiologically evaluating VUR despite the fact that the need for standardization was clearly recognized 25 years ago.[42] The factors which are known to influence the outcome of the search for VUR have been reviewed by Friedland.[10] These include:

1. Infants under one year of age have an easily distensible urinary tract with rapid return to normal when the cause of distention is removed.[10] Even a full bladder may be sufficient to distend the upper urinary tract in infants. Thus, it is likely that any grade of VUR will appear radiologically to be more severe in infants than

in adults. Similarly, any beneficial effect of therapy will appear to be more marked in infants.[10]

2. A large Foley catheter can irritate or distort the bladder trigone so as to provoke radiographically demonstrable VUR. Pulling on a catheter to assure occlusion of the urethra may also distort the trigone sufficiently to produce VUR.[10]

3. The higher the concentration and the lower the temperature of the contrast agent used for the voiding cystourethrogram (VCU), the more likely it is to irritate the bladder and produce reflux.[10]

4. The rate of instillation and volume of contrast medium used can influence the outcome of the test. Different authors, nevertheless, recommend different procedures.

5. The rate of urine flow is an important factor in determining the ease with which VUR can be demonstrated by VCU. For example, it has long been known that the administration of a diuretic agent could result in a normal VCU in patients previously demonstrated to have VUR under "standard" conditions.[6,23,42] This must be an important factor in examining the role of VUR in chronic renal insufficiency—obviously, the less the urine flow from a kidney the greater the likelihood of being able to demonstrate VUR by VCU. In other words, renal failure may be a "cause" of VUR.

6. The patient's position during the study as well as the use of anesthesia and sedation all influence the outcome of the VCU, in ways which are unpredictable.[10]

7. How many films should be taken during the VCU? What is the reproducibility of the test from one day to the next? In Friedland's experience there was significant variation on repeat testing.[10]

8. There is good evidence in experimental animals, corroborated by clinical observations, supporting the view that VUR may result from urinary tract infection.[11,20] It would be anticipated then that

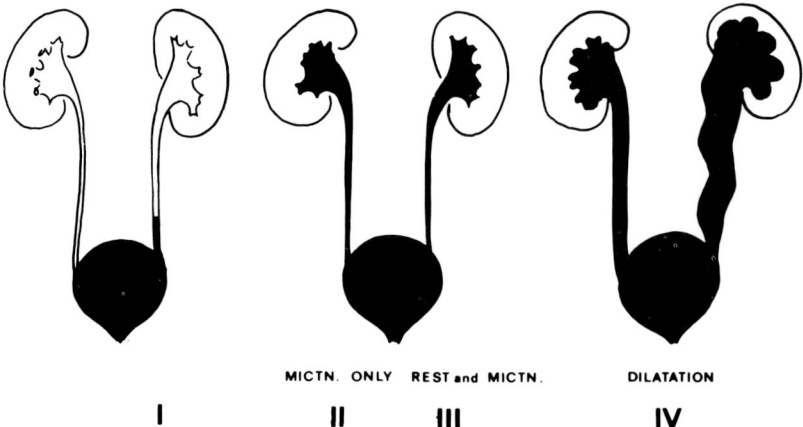

**Fig. 14-5.** Grades of reflux. Grade I, minimal; grades II and III reflux extending up to renal pelvis, grade II on voiding only and Grade II both at rest and during voiding; grade IV, including all ureteral and pelvic dilatation. (From Smellie J, Edwards D, Hunter N, et al: Vesico-ureteral reflux and renal scarring. Kidney Int 8:S65, 1975. Reprinted from Kidney International with permission.)

VUR would be common and easily demonstrable in subjects with UTI. The fact that one-third of children with UTI have VUR is consistent with this finding. Similarly, the fact that VUR disappears with time in the great majority of these children is further evidence in support of this view. Of course, since children mature with the passage of time, a role for maturation of the ureterovesical junction in the disappearance of VUR must also be considered.

It is clear that there are a sufficiently large number of factors influencing our ability to detect VUR. Standardization of the VCU technique must be agreed upon or we will never be able to rationally compare the results of studies in one hospital with those from another.

Finally, in addition to the lack of standardized techniques for the diagnosis of VUR there is also no agreement on what is meant by increased or decreased reflux. Does more reflux refer to the amount of fluid being transported from the bladder to the ureter or is it the transmission of higher pressures from the bladder to the kidney or has it to do with the width of the ureter? Clearly, without a precise definition of terms, the effort to determine the effects of VUR and its therapy, is bound to fail.

*In summary*, although it was once believed that all retrograde urinary reflux was abnormal, there is now good reason to suspect that small quantities of urine regularly ascend the ureter. The usual radiologic technique for demonstrating VUR employs an irritating substance as part of a procedure which is sufficiently traumatic to induce radiologically discernable VUR in persons considered normal. Furthermore, there is good evidence for the view that urinary infections induce VUR and yet it is by virtue of urinary infection that the great majority of children come to be investigated for VUR. Finally, there is no general agreement on the criteria for determining the amount of VUR to be considered significant or on the parameters essential to judging whether the reflux has increased or decreased.

# VUR AS A NORMAL DEVELOPMENTAL FINDING

Several important questions arise regarding the relationship of VUR to UTI in children: (1) VUR may be a fairly common finding in infants, and, as shown in many studies, declines in frequency with advancing age; (2) VUR may not be causally related to UTI and the prevalence of VUR in children with UTIs may not exceed that seen in a normal population; (3) VUR may be an independent abnormality which has its own natural history but which when combined with UTI represents a significant risk to the kidney.

The pathological nature of VUR has been emphasized by studies that failed to demonstrate reflux in normal neonates.[3] These studies are difficult to interpret, however, because of differences in technique, race, and age of the children examined. For example, Black children have about one-tenth the prevalence of VUR as compared with white children. Nevertheless, Bailey, in reviewing these studies, has concluded that VUR is likely to be demonstrable in only 0.4 to 1.8 percent of normal healthy children.[3]

Stamey and Winberg,[37,39] on the other hand, believe that there is good evidence in animals and man that reflux, although not demonstrable in the newborn, becomes very common as a spontaneous event or can be very easily provoked in the young child (50 to 60 percent of normal children up to one year of age). This finding decreases sharply with the passage of time, practically disappearing by three years of age. Winberg has suggested that there may be some maternal factor transferred to the newborn which prevents VUR. Thus, the presence of VUR in a young child may well be a normal finding and it may at least be postulated that UTI acts to unmask or exaggerate the nor-

mal tendency to VUR. In this formulation, VUR and UTI need not bear any causal relationship to each other, although the VUR may magnify the virulence of the infection. The transitory nature of the VUR was persuasively shown in one careful follow-up study of children with VUR and UTI.[35] Reflux disappeared in greater than 50 percent by 18 months after discovery and in 80 percent by the fourth year. Even severe degrees of VUR with dilated ureters have the capacity to return to normal with effective antibiotic therapy of the urinary infection.[20,35]

There is strong evidence to suggest that developmental abnormalities in the location and configuration of the ureteral orifices correlate with the finding of dysplastic and hypoplastic lesions in the kidney. These renal "scars" (better termed *zones of abnormal development*) are found in association with VUR (accompanied by displacement of ureteral orifices) and are consistent with aberrations in the development at each end of the embryonic ureteric bud. Such renal lesions are found in children without present or past history of UTI. Whereas it is always difficult to rule out the possibility of past unrecognized UTI, the prevailing view is that these renal scars are not due to VUR but are rather an associated developmental abnormality.[38] In Stephen's view, perhaps the majority of the "strange shapes and ureterocaliceal anomalies of reflux kidneys" are attributable to primary defects in the ureteric bud and mesenchyme.[38] These views were corroborated by an analysis of renal scars in neonates without UTI by Heale.[13] Finally, the familial association of VUR and RN in the absence of UTI lends added weight to the role of developmental abnormalities. Indeed, in one large series of children and adults with RN, approximately half the patients with renal failure were discovered fortuitously without any evidence of UTI at the time of study or in the past.[15]

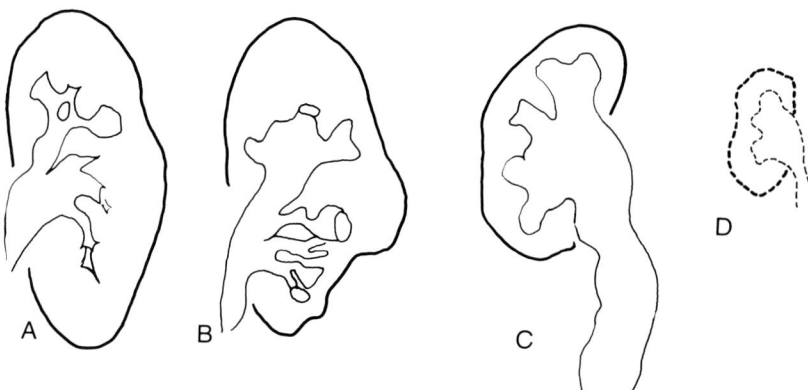

**Fig. 14-6** Types of renal scarring. (A) Mild scarring: not more than two scarred areas. (B) Severe scarring: more generalized, but some areas of normal tissue persist. (C) "Back-pressure" type: shows infective changes (irregular thinning of renal tissue) superimposed on the generalized calyceal deformity usually found in obstructive atrophy. (D) End-stage shrunken kidney, with little or no function. (From Smellie J, Edwards D, Hunter N, et al: Vesico-ureteral reflux and renal scarring. Kidney Int 8:S65, 1975. Reprinted from Kidney International with permission.)

*In summary*, there is suggestive evidence that a tendency toward VUR is a normal stage in the development of the young child and that this may be exaggerated by the presence of UTI. Ureteral reflux has been shown to spontaneously remit with advancing age.

There is very strong evidence to suggest that RN and VUR may be consequences of abnormal development of the ureteric bud. In these instances, there is no evidence that either VUR or UTI has a role in the pathogenesis of the renal lesion.

The radiologic changes that define RN are nonspecific, being produced by several disorders which may or may not be associated with VUR. Habib has therefore suggested that the term RN be dropped and the generic term *segmental corticopapillary scarring* be substituted.[12] When precise histologic criteria are applied, the specific diagnosis of dysplasia, pyelonephritis or segmental hypoplasia can then be made.[12]

## RENAL SCARRING IN CHILDREN

Although the characteristic lesion of RN is a discrete scar adjacent to a clubbed calyx, it is well known that VUR is found in association with other types of renal damage. Smellie and her colleagues have distinguished four types of renal "scarring" which they have encountered in their studies of children with UTI and VUR (Fig. 14-6).[34] The *typical discrete scar* is described as *mild* when there are not more than two scarred areas, or *severe*, when the scarring is more generalized but with the persistence of normal zones of renal parenchyma. In addition to these forms of scarring, is the *back-pressure* type, showing irregular zones of cortical thinning superimposed on the generalized caliceal dilatation seen in obstructive uropathy. Finally, there is the *end-stage kidney*, shrunken, without function, and indistinguishable from dysplastic and hypoplastic kidneys and perhaps from other etiologic entities.[34]

Careful observation of patients with different types of renal scars suggests that these are not necessarily stages of a progressive change but perhaps different lesions with different pathogeneses. Of course, if some of these scars are related to developmental abnormalities they might not be scars at all, but rather zones of arrested or abnormal development which are brought visibly to our attention by their contrast with normal adjacent renal tissue.

In the adult, the scars of RN, that is, segmental corticopapillary scarring (SCS), rarely develop anew or progress as a result of UTI, in the absence of abnormalities of the renal papilla.[7,8] Hodson has not seen new "pyelonephritic" scarring in adult kidneys despite follow-up periods of 10 to 15 years.[16]

Similarly, in children with urinary infections and renal scarring the vast majority of detected renal scars are already present at the initial investigation and it is not common to observe the development of new scars.

Thus, despite the intense interest in this subject, there have been very few reports documenting development of fresh scars in previously normal kidneys. Similarly, it is exceptionally rare to observe marked progression of renal scarring or to observe the insidious development of "back-pressure" or end-stage type kidneys in subjects initially found to have only mild scarring.[35]

Smellie and Normand have tabulated the reported instances of fresh renal scarring in previously normal kidneys and have been able to find approximately 100 cases.[35] The outstanding features of these cases are the almost invariable demonstration of VUR and UTI (although not necessarily at the time the scar is detected) and the fact that the majority of scars develop prior to 5 years of age. In addition, it is now well established that a scar may take up to two years to fully develop after an episode of UTI. Most importantly these authors "have seen no development or extension of renal scarring in 150 children with all grades of reflux which has persisted for two to ten years and in whom the urine had remained sterile during conservative management."[34] *In other words, there is no evidence in man that renal scars develop in the absence of urinary infection despite the persistence of even severe grades of VUR.*

Of course, children whose renal disease has advanced to the point of significant functional impairment or who develop hypertension may well undergo progressive deterioration of renal function even in the absence of UTI. The issue is completely unresolved as to whether repair of VUR in these children would decrease the risk of renal deterioration. In at least one instance, surgical correction of VUR did not prevent deterioration of renal function.[13]

There is considerable debate as to whether sterile VUR can produce renal scarring. Although this relationship was demonstrated in animals, experiments were carried out under conditions of very high intravesical pressure caused by urethral obstruction.[28,29] *In man, the overwhelming weight of evidence argues against sterile reflux as an important factor in the pathogenesis of renal scarring.*[14,35]

Certain curious clinical–pathologic correlations have been observed in the studies of RN. Follow-up studies have shown that hypertension occurred predominantly in girls.[17,18,35] On the other hand, the most severe grades of reflux detected in the investigation of UTI were in boys and were found at a very early age.[34] Furthermore, the "back-pressure" type of renal damage is found almost exclusively with the highest grades of VUR.[34] It should follow, therefore, that "back-pressure" renal damage would occur mostly in boys and would not be associated with hypertension. This prediction was borne out by the studies of Smellie and Normand who found blood pressure elevations to occur in children with all types of RN except the "back-pressure" type.[35]

Consistent with these studies are the data of Acton and Drew, who, in carrying out urologic studies on 160 neonates with UTI over a period of 5 years, detected 6 infants with Grade IV VUR—all boys.[1] Two of these infants died within a few months of the "sudden infant death syndrome" and a third infant died accidentally at age three. Radiologic and pathologic studies of these kidneys were consistent with the "back-pressure" type of renal damage.

In Winberg's study of infants and children with symptomatic UTI, renal scarring was found by intravenous pyelography with equal frequency in boys and girls. A finding consistent with the similar prevalence of urinary infection in both sexes during the first six months of life.[40,41] There is no description of the nature of these scars, nor of the frequency of different types of scarring at different ages.

*In summary*, there appear to be at least two types of renal "scarring" that can be distinguished at the present time. The "back-pressure" type of renal damage, found mainly in boys under one year of age (perhaps, predominantly under two months of age), which does not seem to be the forerunner of hypertension. This lesion does not seem to progress over a period of about 10 years of observation as long as renal insufficiency was not present at the outset, hypertension does not supervene, and the urine remains sterile.[35] Children, male or female, have not been noted to acquire this type of renal damage when it has not been present on the initial examination.

Focal, discrete renal "scarring" is that lesion which is seen to develop in children (mostly girls) with VUR who develop UTI. These lesions can be prevented if the urine is kept sterile, despite the persistence of VUR. It is the children with these "scars" that have been shown to become hypertensive on follow-up examination. There are probably several different types of lesions included in this group. It must be kept in mind that the great majority of scars are present when the children are first seen and that these scars are similar to the kinds of lesions detected in children who are seen initially because of high blood pressure in whom proteinuria is a more common finding than UTI. The histology of these lesions found in children with hypertension suggests the possibility that some of them are developmental in origin whereas others are acquired following UTI.[12]

End-stage kidneys might result from a wide variety of congenital and acquired disorders. Their development is so rarely observed and the histology of the renal lesion so difficult to interpret that little more can be said about the pathogenesis of these lesions at the present time.

## RESTATEMENT OF THE PROBLEM

It is evident that the attempt to identify the interrelationships between factors as dynamic as VUR, RN and UTI is an extraordinarily complex matter. Only now is it evident upon reviewing the literature that any study of this problem must take into account the following variables:

### Patient Population

Unequivocal evidence can be marshalled to show that the method by which patients are identified critically influences the outcome of any investigation. The earliest surveys of the nephropathic effects of UTI first investigated adult females and subsequently, the focus shifted to school children. In the overwhelming majority of subjects from both age groups, in whom renal damage was detected, the damage had occurred prior to the time of the initial investigation. Later studies of preschool children showed that the critical period of renal scarring occurred at yet an earlier age. Attention must now be focused on the newborn and the first year of life for it is here that the most severe grades of reflux are being detected along with serious renal disease.

Patterns of urinary infections change very rapidly in the infant. The first 2 months of life seem to be a particularly high risk period.[32,40] However, most studies of UTI in infancy do not attempt to separate out those infections beginning in the earliest months from those with later onsets.

Randolph designed studies to detect the first UTI in infants and demonstrated unequivocally that the majority will be missed if one simply investigates only ill-appearing infants.[26,27] Thus, any study of UTI and its consequences in children, must start with the newborn and cannot rely on conventional signs of illness to draw attention to the presence of infection.

## Technique for Performing VCU and Grading VUR

The need for standardizing the technical aspects of the VCU and for the grading system for VUR have been discussed in detail in an earlier section. The various grades of VUR carry different risks of complications and disappear at different rates with the passage of time. Furthermore, the age of the patient must be taken into consideration by the grading system since the distensibility of the urinary tract is much greater in infancy than in older children.

## Distinguishing the Different Types of Renal Scarring

There is enough information currently available to strongly suggest that the "back-pressure" type of renal damage has a pathogenesis distinct from that of discrete segmental corticopapillary scarring. The latter is in all likelihood, a nonspecific radiologic finding that may be produced by dysplasia, hypoplasia, atrophy, and infection and perhaps combinations of these processes. Smellie and Normand's classification of radiologically defined renal scars is quite useful. Follow-up studies are critical to recognize new and progressive renal scar formation.

## Consideration of VUR and Renal Scarring and UTI as Independent Variables

It is evident from the studies reviewed that there is sufficient uncertainty concerning the interrelationships among VUR, discrete segmental corticopapillary scarring and UTI that any analysis of pathogenesis, outcome and treatment should examine these factors as independent variables and thus avoid prejudicing the analysis. Unfortunately, there is not yet a satisfactory method for non-invasive screening for VUR. Patients with UTI and family members of patients with VUR and RN are usually the subjects screened for VUR. Since UTI is usually asymptomatic in the infant, it would seem worthwhile to apply the techniques developed by Randolph for his "urinary diary" to identify a population of infants who might have UTI.[26,27] Surely it is the first six months of life where the danger of renal damage is greatest and the signs and symptoms of UTI the most obscure.

# PATIENT MANAGEMENT

## Urinary Infections

Widely disparate views have been published regarding how aggressively one should pursue the diagnostic evaluation of the UTI in childhood. Friedland for example, has stated without equivocation that every infant or child should have a voiding cystourethrogram and an excretory urogram after the first urinary infection.[9] On the other hand, Moncrieff and Whitelow "suggest that cystography be deferred providing that the IVU is normal, until recurrent infections occur while under hospital care. . . ."[21] Thus, a physician can find justification for following any course that he feels comfortable with. I do not believe it is necessary or justified to perform an IVP and VCU on every child after his first UTI. I would proceed according to the following principles:

1. The overwhelming majority of urinary infections in children are not associated with any significant (i.e., detectable or repairable) abnormality of the urinary tract. A significant percentage of children with UTI will not have any recurrences of infection following prompt antibiotic treatment of the first infection.

2. Since there is a high frequency of congenital obstructive lesions in boys of all ages, they should have an IVP following the first detectable UTI.

3. Girls, with a normal physical examination and serum creatinine, whose UTI responds promptly to antibiotic treatment and whose urinary sediment is free of white blood cell casts, do not require radiologic procedures. Follow-up studies (urinalysis and urine culture) should be carried out weekly at first, monthly thereafter for a year, and perhaps annually thereafter for 5 to 10 years. An ultrasound of the abdomen might be useful to docu-

ment the presence of two kidneys and their size. If the child has a family history of urinary tract disease or if infection should recur, I would proceed with an IVP.

4. If there is no indication of an obstructive lesion by IVP and if the ureters are not dilated, I would not proceed with a voiding cystourethrogram in boys or girls. The procedure is not without physical risk and certainly not without psychological consequences in the child.[34]

It is well established that the presence of dilated ureters imparts the greatest risk of renal scarring to subjects with VUR. In most instances, this ureteral dilatation will be evident by IVP. I recognize that some instances of "severe" reflux and all instances of mild reflux, will not be detected by IVP, but this should not represent a risk to the patient since the great majority of refluxing ureters will stop refluxing spontaneously provided the urine remains sterile.

5. If there is evidence of renal scarring by IVP and the ureters are not dilated I would give the patient continuous low dose antibiotics to insure sterility of the urine and repeat the IVP after the urine has remained sterile for 2 years. It is this group of children in which it is essential to maintain a sterile urine continuously. These children have VUR and they require *continuous* antibiotic treatment. Recurrent infections treated intermittently allow scars to develop but new scar formation has not been reported in patients whose urine has remained sterile while on continuous antibiotics.[22]

6. If the IVP reveals dilated ureters in boys or girls, proceed with a VCU to rule out mechanical obstruction.

## Hypertension and Proteinuria

If a child is found to have hypertension or proteinuria, an IVP (and, of course, urine culture) should be performed.

## Indications for Antireflux Surgery

As mentioned earlier, it is technically possible to correct VUR; completely in mild and moderate grades but less predictably in more severe grades.[5] Yet it is the patient with severe VUR, renal scarring and recurrent UTI who is at greatest risk for progressive destruction of the kidney.[22] It is not known whether the progression of renal disease in children with "RN" will be favorably influenced by antireflux surgery. Similarly, it is not known whether children with hypertension and renal scarring and severe VUR would benefit from antireflux surgery.[30]

There are several studies attesting to the fact that the frequency of UTI is not influenced by successful antireflux surgery.[4] In addition, despite allusions to the possibility that pyelonephritis is less frequent after antireflux surgery, I know of no controlled studies which address this question.[19] Studies are in progress to evaluate the role of antireflux surgery in the management of patients with renal disease and hypertension possibly related to VUR.[30]

This discussion has focused on the problems of definition and epidemiology which will have to be taken into consideration in order to evaluate antireflux surgery. The major emphasis of this essay has been to point out that those children for whom antireflux surgery represents possible, not yet proven, beneficial therapy, are a very small percentage of the children we see with urinary infections. The principles of management of the vast majority of children with urinary tract infections should not be guided by the unsubstantiated hope of helping a very few Rather, the greatest attention should be directed to maintaining continuously sterile urine over prolonged periods of time in any infant or child with a known renal scar or with any degree of VUR. The maintenance of sterile urine is at the present time the only known method of preventing renal scarring in subjects with VUR.

# REFERENCES

1. Acton CM, Drew JH: Vesicoureteral reflux in the neonatal period. p 62, In Hodson J, Kincaid-Smith P, Eds: Reflux Nephropathy, Masson, New York, 1979, p 62.
2. Bailey RR: On overview of reflux nephropathy. P. 3. In Hodson J, Kincaid-Smith P, Eds: Reflux Nephropathy. Masson, New York, 1979.
3. Bailey RR: Vesicoureteral reflux in healthy infants and children. p 59, In Hodson J, Kincaid-Smith P, Eds: Reflux Nephropathy. Masson, New York, 1979, p 59.
4. Bauer SB, Willscher MK, Zammoto PJ, et al: Long-term results of antireflux surgery in children. In Hodson J, Kincaid-Smith P, Eds: Reflux Nephropathy, Masson, New York, 1979, p 287.
5. Colemen JW, McGovern JH: A 20-Year experience with pediatric ureteral reimplantation: Surgical results in 701 children. In Hodson J, Kincaid-Smith P, Eds: Reflux Nephropathy, Masson, New York, 1979, p 299.
6. Fairley KF: The effects of diuresis on vesicoureteral reflux. In Hodson J, Kincaid-Smith P, Eds: Reflux Nephropathy. Masson, New York, 1979, p 102.
7. Freedman LR: Natural history of urinary infection in adults. Kidney Int 8:S243, 1975.
8. Freedman LR: Interstitial renal inflammation, including pyelonephritis and urinary tract infection. In Early LE, Gottschalk CW, Eds: Strauss and Welt's Diseases of the Kidney. Little, Brown, Boston, 1979, p 817.
9. Friedland GW: Recurrent urinary tract infections in infants and children. Radiol Clin N Am 15:19, 1977.
10. Friedland GW: The voiding cystourethrogram: An unreliable examination. In Hodson J, Kincaid-Smith P, Eds: Reflux Nephropathy. Masson, New York, 1979, p 91.

11. Friedland GW: Post reimplantation renal scarring. In Hodson J, Kincaid-Smith P, Eds: Reflux Nephropathy. Masson, New York, 1979, p 323.

12. Habib R: Pathology of renal segmental corticopapillary scarring in children with hypertension: The concept of segmental hypoplasia. In Hodson J, Kincaid-Smith P, Eds: Reflux Nephropathy. Masson, New York, 1979, p 220.

13. Heale WF: Age of presentation and pathogenesis of reflux nephropathy. In Hodson J, Kincaid-Smith P, Eds: Reflux Nephropathy. Masson, New York, 1979, p 140.

14. Heale WF, Ferguson RS: The pathogenesis of renal scarring in children. In Kass EH, Brumfitt W, Eds: Infections of the Urinary Tract. The University of Chicago Press, Chicago, 1975, p 202.

15. Heale WF, Shannon FT, Utley WLF, et al: Familial and hereditary reflux nephropathy. In Hodson J, Kincaid-Smith P, Eds: Reflux Nephropathy. Masson, New York, 1979, p 48.

16. Hodson CJ: The effects of disturbance of flow on the kidney. J Inf Dis 120:54, 1969.

17. Holland N: Reflux nephropathy and hypertension. In Hodson J, Kincaid-Smith P, Eds: Reflux Nephropathy. Masson, New York, 1979, p 257.

18. Holland NH, Kotchen T, Bhathena D: Hypertension in children with chronic pyelonephritis. Kidney Int 8:S243, 1975.

19. Hutch JA, Miller E, Hinman F Jr: Vesicoureteral reflux. Am J Med 34:338, 1963.

20. Michie AJ: Chronic pyelonephritis mimicking ureteral obstruction. Ped Clin N Am 6:1117, 1959.

21. Moncrieff MW, Whitelaw R: Value of cystography in urinary tract infections. Arch Dis Child 51:893, 1976.

22. Normand CS, Smellie JM: Vesicoureteral reflux: The case for conservative management. In Hodson J, Kincaid-Smith P, Eds: Reflux Nephropathy. Masson, New York, 1979, p 281.

23. Paquin AJ, Zinner NR, Arbuckle LD: Mechanical factors influencing the demonstrability of vesicoureteral reflux. Am J Surg 107:492, 1964.

24. Politano VA: Discussion. 132, In Proceedings of a Workshop on Ureteral Reflux in Children. National Academy of Sciences-National Research Council, Washington, D.C., 1967, p 132.

25. Politano VA: Discussion. In Hodson J, Kincaid-Smith P, Eds: Reflux Nephropathy. Masson, New York, 1979, p 208.

26. Randolph MF, Morris KE, Gould EB: The first urinary tract infection in the female infant. J Pediatr 86:342, 1975.

27. Randolph MF, Woods SE, Klauber GJ: Bacteriuria in infancy: Home screening for early detection of UTI. In Hodson J, Kincaid-Smith P, Eds: Reflux Nephropathy. Masson, New York, 1979, p 70.

28. Ransley PB, Risdon RA: Reflux and renal scarring. Br J Radiol Suppl 14, 1978.

29. Ransley PG, Risdon RA: The renal papilla, intrarenal reflux and chronic pyelonephritis. In Hodson J, Kincaid-Smith P, Eds: Reflux Nephropathy. Masson, New York, 1979, p 126.

30. Report of the International Reflux Study Committee Medical versus surgical treatment of primary vesicoureteral reflux. Pediatrics 67:392, 1981.

31. Rolleston GL, Shannon RT, Utley WLF: Follow-up of vesico-ureteral reflux in the newborn. Kidney Int 8:S59, 1975.

32. Shannon FT: The significance and management of vesico-ureteric reflux in infancy. Part 1. Clinical aspects. In Renal infection and Renal Scarring, Kincaid-Smith P, Fairley KF, Eds: Mercedes Publishing Services, Melbourne, 1970.

33. Shapiro AH: Pumping and retrograde diffusion in peristaltic waves. In Proceedings of a Workshop on Ureteral Reflux in Children, National Academy of Sciences-National Research Council, Washington, D.C., 1967, p 109–126.

34. Smellie J, Edwards D, Hunter N, et al: Vesico-ureteric reflux and renal scarring. Kidney Int 8:S65, 1975.

35. Smellie JM, Normand ICS: Reflux nephropathy in childhood. In Hodson J, Kincaid-Smith P, Eds: Reflux Nephropathy. Masson, New York, 1979, p 14.

36. Stamey TA: Discussion. In Hodson J, Kincaid-Smith P, Eds: Reflux Nephropathy. Masson, New York, 1979, p 83.

37. Stamey TA: Pathogenesis and Treatment of Urinary Tract Infections. Williams and Wilkins, Baltimore, 1980.

38. Stephens FD: Cystoscopic appearances of the ureteric orifices associated with reflux nephropathy. In Hodson J, Kincaid-Smith P, Eds: Reflux Nephropathy. Masson, New York, 1979, p 119.

39. Winberg J: Discussion. In Hodson J, Kincaid-Smith P, Eds: Reflux Nephropathy. Masson, New York, 1979, p 115.

40. Winberg J, Bollgren I, Källenius G, et al: Clinical pyelonephritis and focal renal scarring. Ped Clin N Am 29:801, 1982.

41. Winberg J, Bergström T, Jacobsson B: Morbidity, age and sex distribution, recurrences and renal scarring in symptomatic urinary tract infection in childhood. Kidney Int. 8:S101, 1975.

42. Winter CC: Vesicoureteral Reflux and its Treatment. Appleton-Century-Crofts, New York, 1969, p 36.

# 15

# 1,25-Dihydroxycholecalciferol in Patients with Renal Failure

# The Case Against Its Prophylactic Use

## Ulrich Binswanger, M.D.

## INTRODUCTION

One striking epidemiologic aspect of renal bone disease is its geographic variability. Symptomatic osteodystrophy occurs in less than 5 percent of patients in Switzerland, in up to 25 percent in Germany[59] and appeared in a most disabling form in dialysis patients in Newcastle upon Tyne, England.[40] Since data from the United States originate in part from centers investigating bone disease using histologic techniques, case selection will likely bias the conclusions drawn.

Our experience in Switzerland indicates that bone disease complicating progressive renal failure and that complicating dialysis therapy of up to 10 years duration, is not a major problem. We, therefore, do not feel compelled to change our fundamental approach in treating chronic renal failure. Additional improvement would be rather difficult to document, and side effects associated with new and minimally effective treatment might compromise the favorable results heretofore obtained.

In approaching the issues related to treating renal osteodystrophy, we will first review the main pathogenetic factors underlying metabolic bone disease. Secondly, we will characterize our own patients with respect to these pathogenetic factors. Thirdly, we will review our own experience and that of others with regard to the use of 1,25-dihydroxycholecalciferol (1,25 $(OH)_2D_3$) in the prophylaxis and direct therapy of renal osteodystrophy. Finally, arguments against the indiscriminate use of 1,25 $(OH)_2D_3$ will be presented.

## PATHOPHYSIOLOGY OF RENAL OSTEODYSTROPHY

Increased concentrations of immunoreactive parathyroid hormone (iPTH) develop as an early consequence of disturbed calcium and phosphorus metabolism in renal failure.[3,9,58] We have shown that PTH levels measured with C-terminal sensitive assays, increase earlier and achieve higher levels than when estimated by N-terminal assays (Fig. 15-1). These data are in accord with the view that the C-terminal assay measures both the intact hormone and its immunologically reactive fragments that accumulate in renal failure.[24] Hypocalcemia is frequently, but not always, identified as the prime stimulus for PTH secretion (Fig. 15-2). Serum calcium concentrations are most often normal but may be low in early progressive chronic renal failure.[29,41] The serum phosphorus level increases normally with dietary loading,[50,60] but hyperphosphatemia is more protracted in patients with renal failure due to their diminished phosphaturia.[49] Serum inorganic phosphorus concentration is often in-

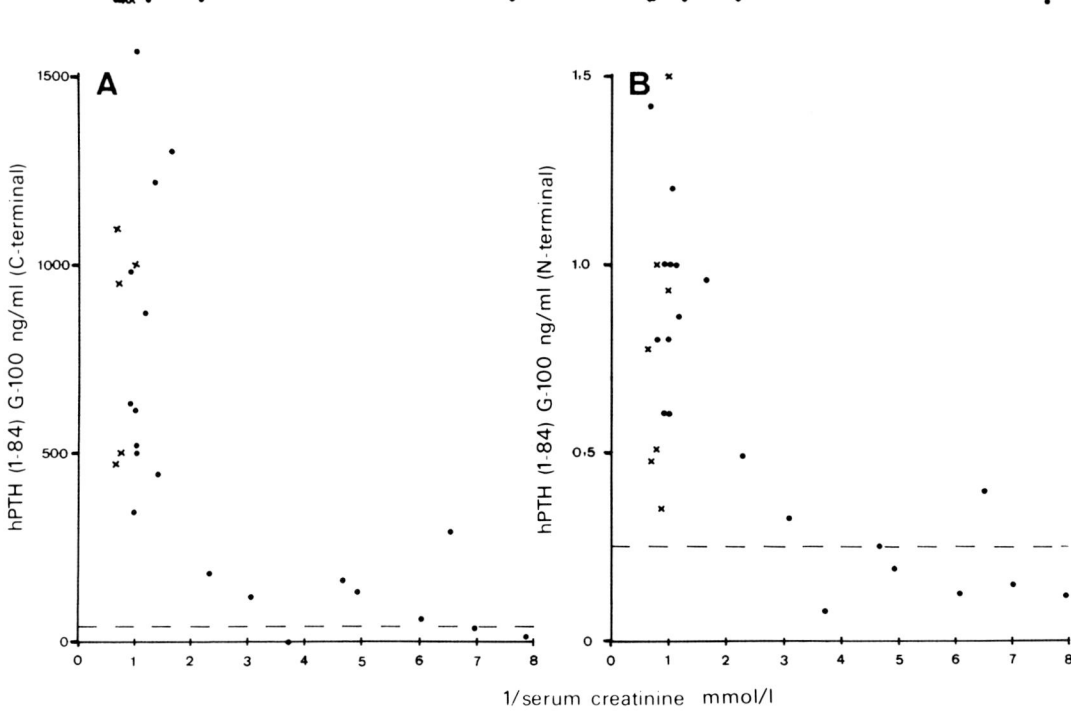

**Fig. 15-1.** Relationship between serum immunoreactive parathyroid hormone and 1/serum creatinine concentration in stable renal insufficiency. (●, without; ×, with hemodialysis treatment.)

creased in late renal failure (Fig. 15-3) and during hemodialysis treatment when iPTH levels are markedly elevated.[3,9,58] Others have shown, and we have confirmed (Fig. 15-4),[9] that these high hormone levels are correlated with the serum concentration of inorganic phosphorus.[32] Hyperphosphatemia might also be partially responsible for the PTH resistance of bone seen in chronic renal failure.[56] This contrasts with the hyperparathyoidism of early renal failure[68] where no correlation was found betwen PTH levels and serum ionized calcium concentrations (Fig. 15-2), nor was a correlation found between serum phosphorus and ionized calcium concentrations (Fig. 15-5).[9] PTH levels may be normalized by inducing a slight elevation of serum ionized calcium concentration (Fig. 15-6). Intestinal calcium absorption was found to be low,[7,20,46] even in early re-

nal failure.[7,46] In certain cases, PTH levels were found to be elevated despite normal serum calcium concentrations. This observation highlights the skeletal resistance to the action of PTH.[50] Normocalcemia is maintained therefore, only at the expense of increased plasma hormone levels. Early skeletal resistance to endogenous PTH was demonstrated in azotemic patients by infusion tests with EDTA which resulted in delayed recovery from hypocalcemia despite higher iPTH levels in comparision to normal controls.[43] It has been demonstrated that skeletal resistance can be improved by $1,25 (OH)_2D_3$ treatment or by dietary phosphorus restriction.[13,44] The latter is seldom indicated before the endogenous creatinine clearance is reduced to values below 30 ml/min (Fig. 15-3).

The osteodystrophy of early renal failure, diagnosed by quantitative bone

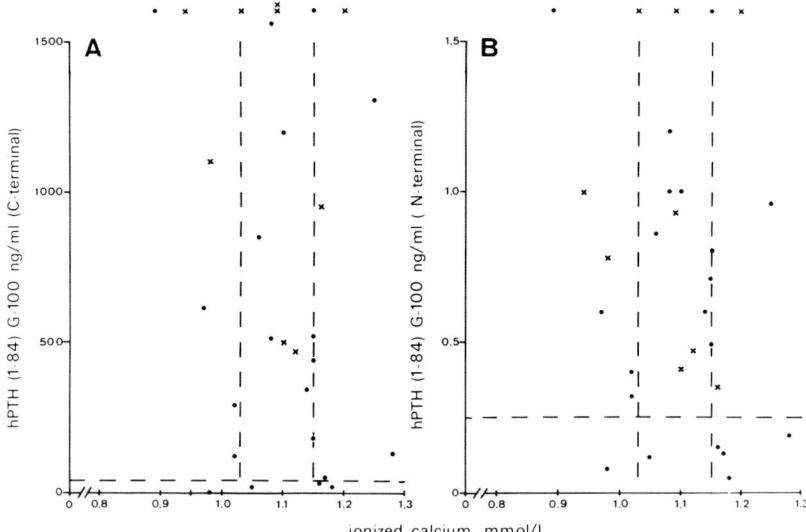

**Fig. 15-2.** Relationship between serum concentrations of PTH and ionized calcium in patients with stable renal insufficiency of variable degree.

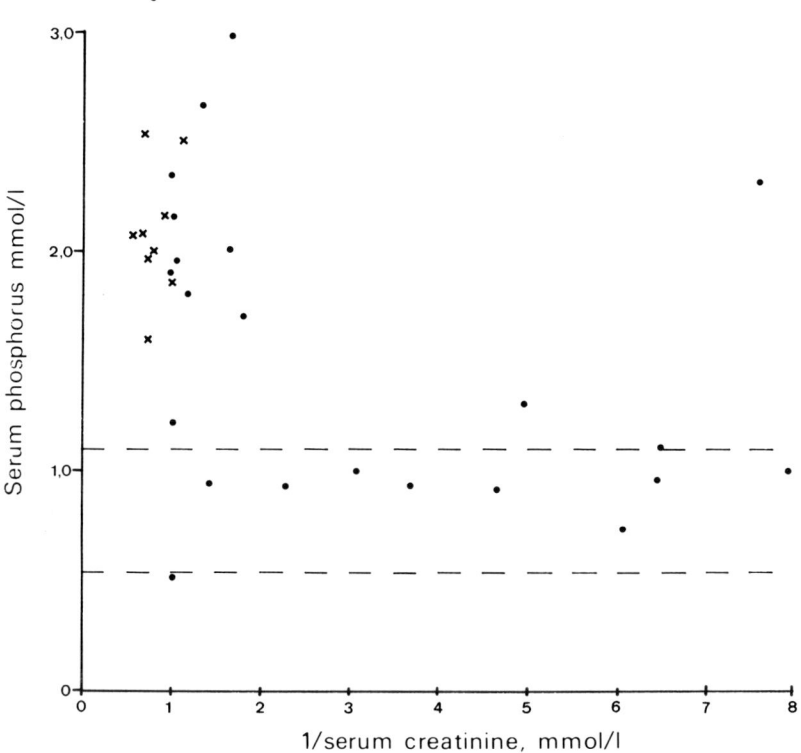

**Fig. 15-3.** Relationship between 1/serum creatinine concentration and inorganic phosphorus concentration in stable renal failure. (●, without; ×, with hemodialysis treatment.)

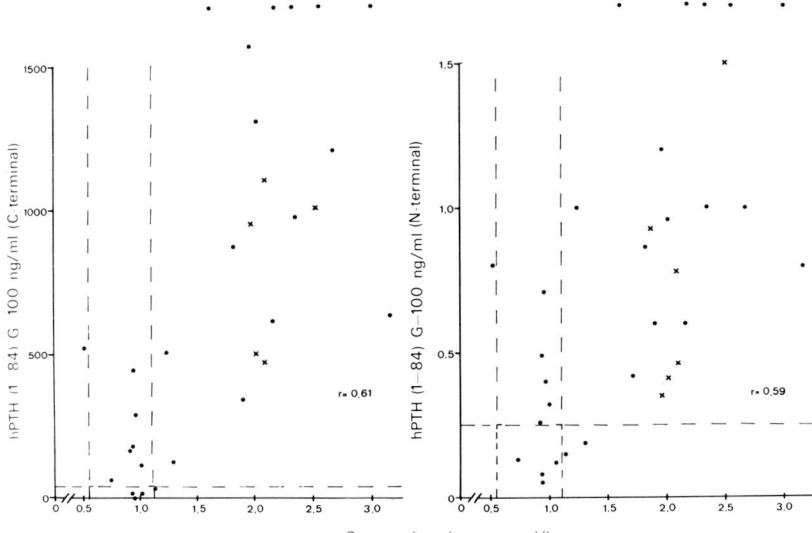

**Fig. 15-4.** Relationship between serum concentrations of phosphorus and PTH in patients with variable severity of stable renal insufficiency. (●, without; ×, with hemodialysis treatment.)

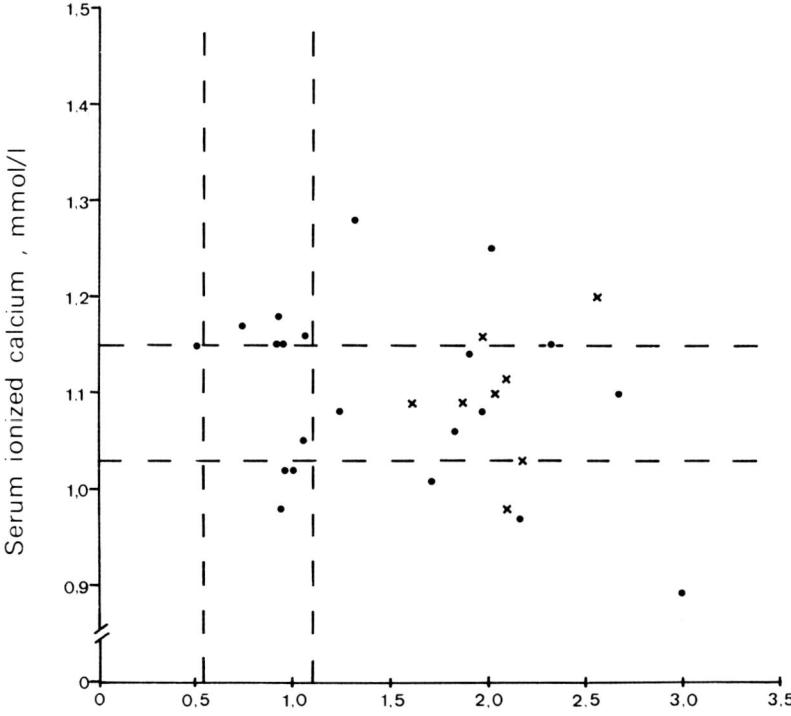

**Fig. 15-5.** Relationship between serum phosphorus and ionized calcium concentrations in stable renal failure. Dashed lines indicate this normal range. (●, without; ×, with hemodialysis treatment.)

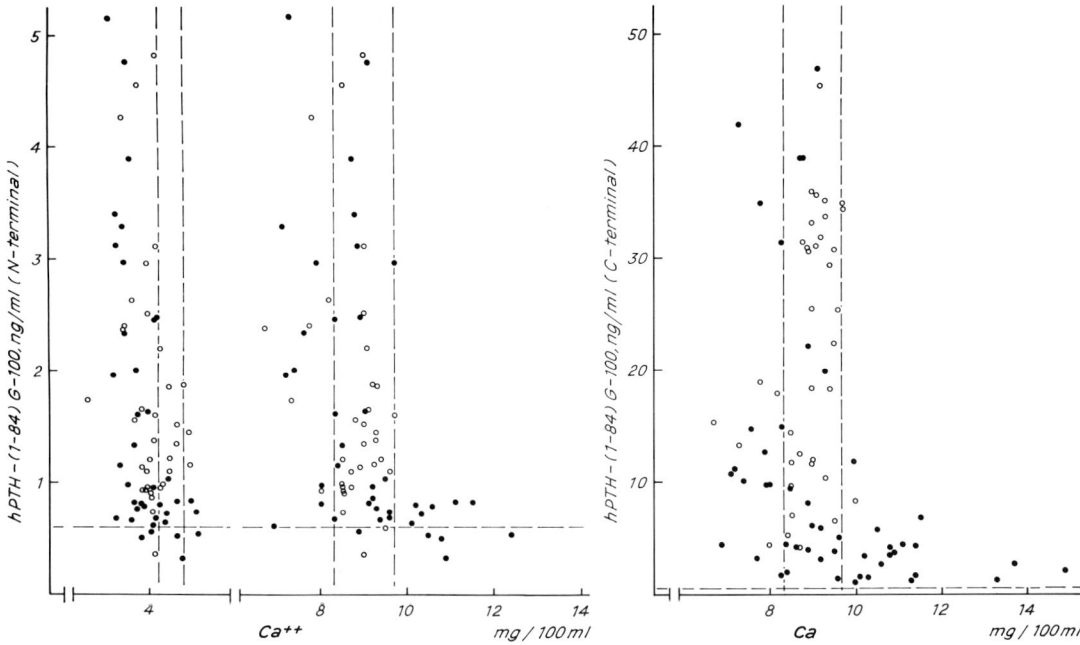

**Fig. 15-6.** N-terminal (left) and C-terminal (right) immunoreactive parathyroid hormone as related to ionized (ca$^{2+}$) and total (ca) serum calcium concentration. (○, without; ●, during 1,25 (OH)$_2$D$_3$ treatment.) (From Binswanger U, Fischer JA, Iselin H, et al: 1,25-dihydroxycholecalciferol treatment of clinically asymptomatic renal osteodystrophy. Min Electrol Metab 2: 103, 1979.)

histology, is primarily caused by hyperparathyroidism.[6,38,47] This lesion consists of increased bone resorption as evidenced by an expansion of the resorbing surface, and an increase in the number of osteoclasts. A "mixed-lesion" is diagnosed when a moderate degree of osteomalacia complicates hyperparathyroidism. Osteomalacia is defined as a decreased mineralization rate resulting in increased osteoid volume with normal or slightly depressed rates of matrix formation. This lesion occurs at later stages of renal failure and can only be diagnosed by tetracycline labeling.[46] Tetracycline is taken up by the "mineralization front", that is, that zone interfacing between osteoid and mineralized bone. Bone biopsied after giving two doses of antibiotic, several weeks apart, will show two distinct bands of fluorescent tetracycline. The distance between the bands, reflective of newly mineralized

bone, when factored by the time between antibiotic doses, yields an estimate of the rate of appositional bone growth.

As our understanding of vitamin D metabolism increased, so increased our hopes that therapy with appropriate metabolites of the vitamin might be helpful in treating renal bone disease. The most promising metabolite was thought to be 1,25 (OH)$_2$D$_3$ since it actively promoted intestinal calcium absorption as well as bone resorption. Its direct effect on bone mineralization, however, has since been questioned.[10]

Vitamin D depletion is an unusual complication of renal failure except in patients adhering to an extremely strict protein-deficient diet. The deficiency is most easily recognized by low circulating levels of the hepatic metabolite of vitamin D$_3$, 25-hydroxycholecalciferol 25(OH)D$_3$.[33] Urinary loss of this metabolite in nephrotic syndrome can also result in low serum levels.[62] Replacement therapy might well be indicated under such conditions.

Serum 1,25 $(OH)_2D_3$ is either normal or slightly elevated in early renal failure and indeed was found to be low but measurable even in anephric patients.[34,42,66] This finding suggests that extrarenal production of 1,25 $(OH)_2D_3$ occurs. Most interestingly, bone cells from normal humans have been shown to produce this metabolite.[37] These cells also produce 24,25-dihydroxycholecalciferol [24,25 $(OH)_2D_3$], a metabolite which like 1,25 $(OH)_2D_3$ is primarily produced in the kidney. It was shown *in vitro* that addition of either metabolite could suppress its own synthesis while increasing that of the other metabolite. These findings suggest that bone cell levels of vitamin D metabolites might be of equal or even more importance than their serum values.

It has repeatedly been shown that 1,25 $(OH)_2D_3$ treatment can increase intestinal calcium absorption in uremia,[8,13,20] elevate serum calcium levels,[8,13] depress PTH concentration,[8,54] and improve bone histology, especially those bony changes related to hyperparathyroidism.[48] The improvement of osteomalacia, however, was much less impressive. Indeed, cases of pure osteomalacia with low bone turnover have proven especially resistant to therapy. Vitamin D in the latter circumstance, rapidly created hypercalcemia without changing bone histology.[36] High circulating aluminum levels were sometimes found in patients with pure osteomalacia and the metal tended to collect at the mineralization front.[2,11,39]

The cause of hyperparathyroidism in early renal failure is not always clear, since hypocalcemia is sometimes absent. The idea of treating azotemic hyperparathyrodism with a generous amount of dietary calcium stems from the finding that absolute absorption can be increased despite depressed fractional absorption.

Since calcium is the most potent regulator of PTH secretion, it follows that a calcium-rich diet could suppress hormone secretion. Hyperparathyroidism, as is well known, is a major but not sole contributing factor to the maintenance of a normal serum phosphorus concentration in renal failure.[12,71] Surprisingly, however, hypophosphatemia is sometimes observed in renal failure.[66] Finding "normal" or only slightly elevated 1,25 $(OH)_2D_3$ levels might be interpreted as inappropriately low values since the accompanying hyperparathyroidism should stimulate the metabolite's appearance by activating the renal 1α-hydroxylase system which produces 1,25 $(OH)_2D_3$.

Since ample amounts of 1,25 $(OH)_2D_3$ are circulating in early renal failure, we see no compelling reason to further increase blood levels by treating patients with this vitamin. Indeed, such untoward side effects as feedback supression of endogenous 1,25 $(OH)_2D_3$ synthesis[31] or excessive intestinal absorption of calcium and phosphorus[14] may occur. A direct inhibitory effect of 1,25 $(OH)_2D_3$ on PTH secretion may also occur but needs further confirmation.[17]

We believe therefore, that theoretically, there is little reason to use 1,25 $(OH)_2D_3$ in early renal insufficiency. The same results can be obtained by adquately increasing dietary calcium and controlling hyperphosphatemia.

Late renal failure is accompanied by marked bony changes.[23] These changes consist of mixed lesions or pure forms of osteitis fibrosa from hyperparathyroidism or pure osteomalacia from any of several causes, that is, disturbances of vitamin D availability, lack of certain metabolites, accumulation of magnesium, or the effects of various toxins or acidosis.[16] Serum calcium and 1,25 $(OH)_2D_3$ levels[34] are low while the inorganic phosphorus concentration and iPTH[38,58] levels are often markedly elevated. Therapy with 1,25

(OH)$_2$D$_3$ will increase serum calcium concentrations and thereby depress the level of iPTH in the blood.[8,54]

Intestinal phosphorus uptake is also increased by the activated vitamin[14] and makes it mandatory for physicians to restrict dietary phosphorus and/or prescribe phosphate binders, that is, aluminum hydroxide. The question of whether 1,25 (OH)$_2$D$_3$ directly affects bone mineralization is a matter of some debate.[10] Some experimental observations negate any beneficial effect of 1,25 (OH)$_2$D$_3$ on the mineralization process while others suggest that the metabolite may in fact inhibit mineralization.[4]

We are therefore inclined to raise serum calcium concentration to control hyperparathyroidism not by giving 1,25 (OH)$_2$D$_3$, but rather by decreasing the inorganic phosphorus in the diet, giving phosphate binders and eventually by using ketoanalogues of amino acids.[30] Furthermore, osteomalacia should be prevented by maintaining a reasonably high bone turnover and by avoidance of certain toxins.[39] In cases where dietary vitamin D depletion occurs or where anticonvulsant therapy or nephrotic syndrome interferes with vitamin D metabolism, 25(OH)D$_3$ supplementation might be indicated.

## OUR OWN EXPERIENCES WITHOUT PROPHYLACTIC USE OF 1,25 (OH)$_2$D$_3$

Our patients with advanced renal failure are treated conservatively, receiving only antihypertensive drugs and antibiotics where indicated. Protein restriction is withheld until the creatinine clearance is approximately 20 ml/min. Aluminum hydroxide and/or dietary phosphorus restriction are also added at this time.

Oral calcium supplements are given only when hypocalcemia is persistent. Calcium carbonate is used when it is necessary to correct acidosis; otherwise calcium gluconate is given because of better patient compliance. Dietary histories revealed that our patients had a calcium intake that ranged between 0.5 and 0.7 g/day. Another 50 to 70 mg of calcium is provided with every liter of drinking water. We do not routinely prescribe vitamin D$_3$ or its metabolites to our patients.

On hemodialysis, our patients ingest a diet restricted of potassium and phosphate but otherwise normal, and as indicated, they continue to take phosphate binders. The dialysate calcium ranges from 1.80 to 1.85 mmol/L resulting in elevated total and ionized blood calcium levels at the end of treatment (Fig. 15-7). No peroral calcium supplements are given between dialyses.

Biochemical characterization of a randomly chosen group of patients receiving ambulatory conservative care and those on hemodialysis revealed that control of the serum phosphorus concentration was by no means ideal. When serum creatinine levels reach 0.5 mmol/L (5.7 mg/dl), serum phosphorus concentration has usually tripled (Fig. 15-3). No correlation was found between serum phosphorus and ionized calcium concentrations (Fig. 15-5). The ionized calcium is also not related to the prevailing iPTH concentration as estimated by C-terminal or N-terminal assay systems (Fig. 15-2). However, a rather close correlation can be established between serum phosphorus concentration and iPTH (Fig. 15-4). It was found that iPTH was increased at similar elevations of serum creatinine that initiated hyperphosphatemia (Fig. 15-3). A partial correlation study was performed to define the relationship between serum PTH, creatinine and phosphorus concentrations (Table 15-1). From these data it can be deduced that the single most important

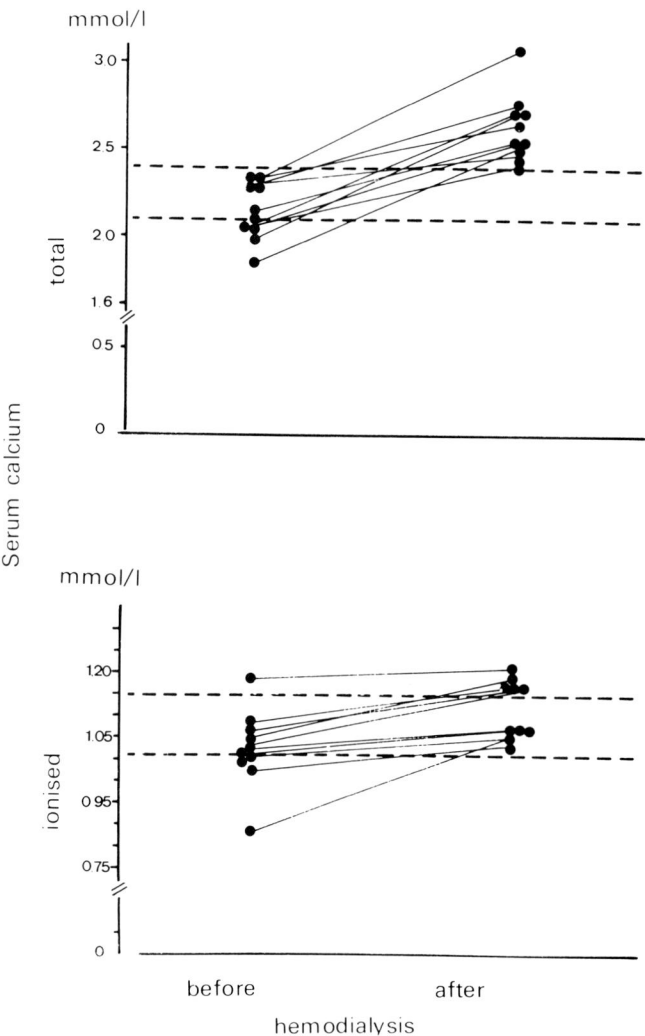

**Fig. 15-7.** Total and ionized serum calcium concentration before and after 5 hours of hemodialysis treatment. Dialysate calcium 1.80 mmol/L. (From Binswanger U, Fischer JA, Iselin H, et al: 1,25-dehydroxycholecalciferol treatment of clinically asymptomatic renal osteodystrophy. Min Electrol Lab 2:103, 1979.)

factor related to iPTH is the serum phosphorus concentration. Although documentation of the vitamin D status of our patients is incomplete, since they ingest a liberal diet, it may be assumed that vitamin D depletion is a rare finding. Serum levels of 1,25 $(OH)_2D_3$ and 24,25 $(OH)_2D_3$ are generally found to be low in end-stage renal disease. These assumptions have been validated by measurements sporadically made throughout the course of renal failure (courtesy Dr. U. Trechsel, Bern).

Bone histology[6,8] revealed mixtures of osteitis fibrosa and osteomalacia in most of our patients. Single cases with predominant hyperparathyroid and osteomalacic lesions were rare. All patients biopsied were asymptomatic.

Serum fluoride levels are elevated due to fluoridation of the table salt in Switzerland. Magnesium concentrations are also greater than normal.

Under these conditions we observed symptomatic bone disease in less than 5 percent of our patients and when it occurs, it is seen most often in patients on hemodialysis. Two-thirds of these cases show osteofibrosis which is treated by subtotal parathyroidectomy. The remain-

**Table 15-1.** Correlations and Partial Correlations between Serum Concentrations of PTH, Creatinine, and Phosphorus

|  |  | Correlation |  | Partial correlation |  |
|---|---|---|---|---|---|
| C-terminal | PTH—Creat | 0.30 | PTH—Creat (Phosph) | 0.03 |
| Essay | PTH—Phosph | 0.61 | PTH—Phosph (Creat) | 0.56 |
|  | Creat—Phosph | 0.53 | Creat—Phosph (PTH) | 0.47 |
| N-terminal | PTH—Creat | 0.57 | PTH—Creat (Phosph) | 0.38 |
| Essay | PTH—Phosph | 0.59 | PTH—Phosph (Creat) | 0.41 |
|  | Creat—Phosph | 0.53 | Creat—Phosph (PTH) | 0.29 |

ing one-third of symptomatic patients exhibit clinical and histologic signs of osteomalacia. Treatment of this lesion is much more difficult; however, in some cases it seems to respond to therapy with 25 (OH)D$_3$. Our experience with this metabolite is too limited however to critically evaluate its efficacy.

# REVIEW OF THE LITERATURE ON THERAPEUTIC AND PREVENTIVE TREATMENT OF EARLY AND LATE RENAL BONE DISEASE BY 1,25 (OH)$_2$D$_3$

## Early Renal Failure

Data on therapy of early renal osteodystrophy with 1,25 (OH)$_2$D$_3$ is lacking. This is not surprising since symptomatic bone disease at this stage is rare and therefore therapy is usually not considered.

There is one uncontrolled trial of prophylactic therapy with 1,25 (OH)$_2$D$_3$ in three patients suffering from early renal failure.[35] Their creatinine clearances were 32 to 51 ml/min, serum calcium was low-normal in two patients, serum phosphorus was normal in all three patients, and PTH was modestly elevated in two patients.[35] After treatment with 0.5 µg/day 1,25 (OH)$_2$D$_3$ for 6 months, serum cal-

cium concentration increased and iPTH decreased while the serum phosphorus level remained normal. Improvement of a mixed-type bone lesion was documented by quantitative histology.

A second controlled prophylactic trial compared therapy with 1,25 (OH)$_2$D$_3$ with that of vitamin D$_3$ plus 0.5 g of supplemental calcium, in 18 patients with slightly more severe renal failure than seen in the above study.[18] Serum calcium concentration increased in those treated with 1,25 (OH)$_2$D$_3$ and their iPTH levels simultaneously decreased. Hypercalcemia occurred in seven of the eight patients so treated. The serum phosphorus concentration remained in the normal range. A more rapid decrease in creatinine clearance was noted during the six months of 1,25 (OH)$_2$D$_3$ therapy, which, we believe, is most probably due to the hypercalcemia.

## Late Renal Failure

Herein follows a summary of clinical studies designed to assess the effectiveness of 1,25 (OH)$_2$D$_3$ therapy of renal osteodystrophy. Indications for therapy varied between the studies, but most patients were selected on the basis of bone pain, fractures, and biochemical or radiological abnormalities. Bone pain responded, often dramatically, and disability was commonly improved.[21] Hypercalcemia, usually of short duration, was frequent, occurring either soon after the onset of vitamin therapy or later with long-term treatment. Hyperphosphatemia required prescription of phosphate binders when higher doses of 1,25 $(OH)_2D_3$ were used. Two distinct groups with renal osteodystrophy proved resistant to the effects of vitamin D. Patients presenting with osteomalacia and low circulating iPTH levels[36] and those with aluminum-related osteomalacia, were not helped by therapy. These groups have drawn considerable attention and interest and more work must be done to clarify the basis of their resistance.

Investigators reviewing bone biopsies generally agree that signs of hyperparathyroidism are ameliorated by 1,25 $(OH)_2D_3$ treatment.[1,48,54] This view is in accord with measurements showing that serum hormone levels decrease as serum calcium concentrations rise. There is currently no evidence to prove that iPTH suppression is caused by the direct effects of 1,25 $(OH)_2D_3$ on the parathyroid glands. Mixed-type bone disease is ameliorated by active vitamin D therapy. There is evidence, however, showing that osteomalacia, especially when occurring in its pure form with reduced bone turnover, is not helped by 1,25 $(OH)_2D_3$ therapy.[11,36,39] It should be noted that some of these otherwise resistant osteomalacic subjects seem to respond to treatment with 1,25 and 24,25 $(OH)_2D_3$.[64] Furthermore, aluminum-associated osteomalacia seems to be improved by desferrioxamine without changing the aluminum content of bone.[15]

For as yet unclear reasons, some osteomalacic patients suffering from kidney failure, have responded to therapy with 25 $(OH)_2D_3$.[26,57,70] This treatment might result in the production of 24,25 $(OH)_2D_3$[69] which may have an ameliorating effect on bone. A direct action of pharmacological amounts of 25 $(OH)D_3$ on bone could also mediate the beneficial effect.

Three controlled studies evaluating 1,25 $(OH)_2D_3$ therapy in hemodialysis patients have been reported. In a multicenter study, 98 patients without overt bone disease were treated with 1,25 $(OH)_2D_3$ or placebo for 30 months after establishing baseline parameters over a period of 5 months.[22] In addition to 1,25 $(OH)_2D_3$, patients also received $CaCO_3$ providing 1 g of elemental calcium daily. Additional therapy included vitamin $D_3$ 400 U/day and aluminum hydroxide in amounts sufficient to maintain serum phosphorus concentration between 3.5 and 5.5 mg/dl. The 1,25 $(OH)_2D_3$ dose was decreased most often to 0.25 μg/day after initial therapy with 0.5 μg/day. Serum calcium and phosphorus levels increased during 1,25 $(OH)_2D_3$ therapy but did not change in placebo-treated controls. Serum levels of the vitamin D metabolite increased from 7.7 ± 7 to 16 ± 5 pg/ml and remained unchanged in controls. PTH levels fell in vitamin D treated patients but slowly increased in controls. Follow up bone x-rays indicated that the changes of hyperparathyroidism were more frequent in the control group. Favorable results were reported in patients with high pretreatment PTH and alkaline phosphatase levels. Rapidly reversible hypercalcemic episodes occurred in 21 patients during 1,25 $(OH)_2D_3$ treatment and in eight control patients. Soft tissue calcification was not a recognized problem.

A second study describes the effects of placebo and 1,25 $(OH)_2D_3$ (0.25 to 0.50 μg daily) in 75 long-term hemodialysis patients treated for 1 to 2 years.[51] Prevention, arrest, or healing of the x-ray findings of hyperparathyroidism were evaluated. The PTH concentration slightly decreased in treated subjects while that in controls slightly increased.

No information was provided on dialysate calcium concentrations. Since suppression of PTH secretion and the bone disease it engenders is effected by increasing the serum calcium concentration, it is critical to know the bath level of calcium used in this study. Since appropriately high levels of calcium in the dialysis bath can produce serum calcium concentrations comparable to that induced by 1,25 $(OH)_2D_3$, one could theoretically achieve the same therapeutic results, that is, suppressed PTH secretion and improved bone histology by adjusting bath calcium levels in the absence of the more expensive vitamin D therapy. Our experience, and that of others, would suggest that this is indeed, quite possible. Passive intestinal absorption of calcium can be increased by the oral intake of large doses of $CaCO_3$ and luminal phosphate binding enhances this absorption.[45] In this manner, serum iPTH levels can be reduced[52] and skeletal mineralization improved,[25] while histologic changes of hyperparathyroidism are ameliorated. Absorbed $CaCO_3$ also provides alkali which helps to stabilize the patient's acid-base status.[45]

Prolonged $CaCO_3$ ingestion becomes distasteful to many patients and lack of compliance tends to limit its effectiveness.

Based on the experimental findings of Slatopolsky et al.[65] showing that secondary hyperparathyroidism did not complicate renal failure when phosphate-restricted diets prevented hyperphosphatemia, Goldsmith and colleagues gave humans with advanced renal failure low phosphorus diets.[32] This diet reduced but did not normalize serum PTH levels. In related studies, it has been shown that the low incidence of renal osteodystrophy in Israel is well correlated with the low phosphorus diet ingested by these subjects.[5]

In contrast to the two aforementioned and rather positive studies of vitamin D therapy stands our own experience with 17 asymptomatic hemodialysis patients treated for 3 to 8 months with 1 μg of 1,25 $(OH)_2D_3$. We found that PTH levels decreased when measured with an N-terminal assay but did not significantly fall when the C-terminal assay was used (Fig. 15-6). When bath dialysate calcium levels of 1.80 to 1.85 mmol/L were used, PTH concentration remained stable in control

patients and bone mineral content of the radius also remained stable in both vitamin D treated and untreated groups (Fig. 15-8). Eleven patients exhibited one or more hypercalcemic episodes despite weekly measurements of serum calcium concentration (Fig. 15-9).

In addition to these controlled studies, a number of studies, reporting on small numbers of patients, revealed that hyperparathyroidism and mixed-bone lesions can be improved with 1,25 $(OH)_2D_3$ therapy whereas pure osteomalacia is barely influenced.[1,23,48]

Prevention of renal osteodystrophy in advanced renal failure with vitamin D metabolites other than 1,25 $(OH)_2D_3$ may be helpful in treating some forms of osteomalacia. In this regard a number of studies have suggested that 25$(OH)D_3$ may cause clinical and histologic improvement in osteomalacic subjects.[26,57,70]

## CONCLUSIONS

Hyperphosphatemia is related to PTH secretion in advanced renal failure. Our own studies and those of others, suggest that PTH-induced bone lesions can be effectively stabilized by reversing the biochemical changes (hypocalcemia and hyperphosphatemia) that stimulate PTH secretion.

Pure osteomalacia is far more resistant to known therapies. While certain underlying causes have been identified, our understanding of this form of renal osteodystrophy still remains rather primitive.

Accordingly, our present approach to the prophylactic treatment of renal osteodystrophy is outlined below.

### Control of Hyperparathyroidism

Maintain serum calcium and phosphorus concentrations close to the normal range. Aluminum hydroxide and calcium

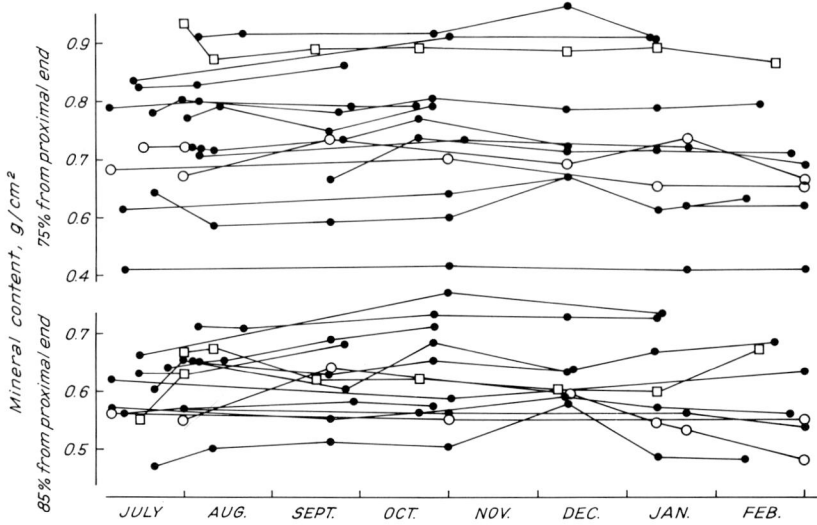

**Fig. 15-8.** Bone mineral content during treatment with 1,25 (OH)$_2$D$_3$. (●, mixed renal osteodystrophy; ○, pure renal osteomalacia; □, pure renal osteitis fibrosa.) (From Binswanger U, Fischer JA, Iselin H, et al: 1,25-dihydroxycholecalciferol treatment of clinically asymptomatic renal osteodystrophy. Min Electrol Metab 2: 103, 1979.)

(carbonate or gluconate) supplements can usually achieve these goals in nondialyzed renal failure patients. Dietary phosphorus restriction may become necessary in patients with resistant hyperphosphatemia. Dialyzed patients require similar therapy but in addition, dialysate calcium concentrations of 1.80 to 1.85 mmol/L ought to be utilized to maintain serum ionized calcium levels normal.

## Prevention of Osteomalacia

Our lack of understanding of the pathogenesis of this disorder limits devel-

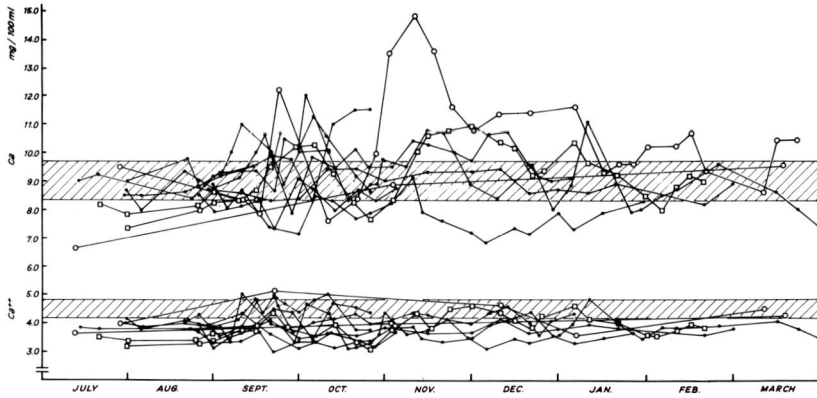

**Fig. 15-9.** Total (top) and ionized (bottom) serum calcium concentrations during 1,25 (OH)$_2$D$_3$ treatment. See legend for Fig. 15-6 for symbols. (From Binswanger U, Fischer JA, Iselin H, et al: 1,25-dihydroxycholecalciferol treatment of clinically asymptomatic renal osteodystrophy. Min Electrol Metab 2: 103, 1979.)

opment of effective therapy. We prescribe 25(OH)D$_3$ therapy to those subjects at great risk of becoming vitamin D deficient, that is, to those with inadequate diets, those receiving anticonvulsant therapy and those suffering the nephrotic syndrome.

When possible, surgically induced hypoparathyroidism is to be avoided, since it reduces bone turnover.

In selected cases of osteomalacia, therapy with aluminum-containing gels may have to be discontinued.

# ACKNOWLEDGMENTS

The expert secretarial help of Mrs. E. Singer and the assistance in preparing graphs by Mrs. F. Josuran and Mrs. I. Nänni are gratefully appreciated.

# REFERENCES

1. Ahmed KY, Wills MR, Varghese Z, et al: Long-term effects of small doses of 1,25-dihydroxycholecalciferol in renal osteodystrophy. Lancet: 2:629, 1978.
2. Alfrey AC, Hegg A, Craswell P: Metabolism and toxicity of aluminum in renal failure. Am J Clin Nutrit 33: 1509, 1980.
3. Arnaud CD: Hyperparathyroidism and renal failure. Kidney Int 4: 89, 1973.
4. Baylink D, Howard G, Ivey J, et al: Vitamin D and bone formation and mineralization. In Norman A, Schaefer K, von Herrath, et al, Eds: Vitamin D, Chemical, Biochemical and Clinical Endocrinology of Calcium Metabolism. de Gruyter, Berlin, 1982, p 363.
5. Berlyne GM, Ben-Arie J, Epstein M, et al: Rarity of renal osteodystrophy in Israel due to low phosphorus intake. Nephron 10: 141, 1973.
6. Binswanger U, Fischer J, Schenk R, et al: Osteopathie bei chronischer Niereninsuffizienz. Dtsch Med Wschr 49: 1914, 1971.
7. Binswanger U: Calcium metabolism and kidney disease (New Series) 34: 106, 1974.
8. Binswanger U, Fischer JA, Iselin H, et al: 1,25-dihydroxycholecalciferol treatment of clinically asymptomatic renal osteodystrophy. Min Electrol Metab 2: 103, 1979.
9. Binswanger U, Dambacher M, Fischer JA: Serum calcium, phosphorus and immunoreactive parathyroid hormone at various stages of renal failure. (In preparation.)
10. Bordier P, Rasmussen H, Marie P, et al: Vitamin D metabolites and bone mineralization in man. J Cli Endocrinol 2: 284, 1978.
11. Boyce BF, Elder HY, Elliot HS: Hypercalcaemic osteomalacia due to aluminum toxicity. Lancet 1:1009, 1982.
12. Bricker NS: On the pathogenesis of the uremic state. An exposition of the "trade off hypothesis." N Engl J Med 286: 1093, 1972.
13. Brickman AS, Jowsey J, Sherrard DJ, et al: Therapy with 1,25-dihydroxyvitamin D$_3$ in the management of renal osteodystrophy. In Norman AW, Schaefer K, Grigoleit HG, et al, Eds: Vitamin D and Problems Related to Uremic Bone Disease. de Gruyter, Berlin, 1975, p 241.
14. Brickman AS, Hartenbower DL, Norman AW, et al: Actions of 1α-hydroxyvitamin D$_3$ and 1,25-dihydroxyvitamin D$_3$ on mineral metabolism in man. I. Effects on net absorption of phosphorus. Am J Clin Nutr 30: 1064, 1977.
15. Brown DJ, Ham KN, Dawborn JK, et al: Treatment of dialysis osteomalacia with desferrioxamine. Lancet 2: 343, 1982.
16. Burnell JM, Teubner E, Wergedal JE, et al: Bone crystal maturation in renal osteodystrophy in humans. J Clin Invest 33: 52, 1974.
17. Chertow BS, Baylink DJ, Wergedahl JE, et al: Decrease in serum immunoreactive parathyroid hormone in rats and in parathyroid hormone secretion in vitro by 1,25 (OH)$_2$D$_3$. J Clin Invest 56: 668, 1975.
18. Christiansen C, Rødbro P, Christiansen MS, et al: Deterioration of renal function during treatment of chronic renal failure with 1,25-dihydroxycholecalciferol. Lancet 2: 700, 1978.
19. Coburn JW, Popovtzer MM, Massry SG, et al: The physiochemical state and renal handling of divalent ions in chronic renal failure. Arch Intern Med 124: 302, 1969.

20. Coburn JW, Koppel H, Brickman AS, et al: Study of intestinal absorption of calcium in patients with renal failure. Kidney Int 3: 264, 1973.

21. Coburn JW, Brickman AS, Sherrard DJ, et al: Clinical efficacy of 1,25 (OH)$_2$ Vitamin D$_3$ in renal osteodystrophy. In Norman AW, Schaefer K, Coburn JW, et al, Eds: Vitamin D: Biochemical, Chemical and Clinical Aspects Related to Calcium Metabolism. de Gruyter, Berlin, 1977, p 657.

22. Coburn JW, Di Domenico NC, Boyce GF, et al: Prospective double blind trial with calcifediol in the prophylaxis of bone disease in asymptomatic dialysis patients. In Norman AW, Schaefer K, von Herrath D, et al, Eds: Vitamin D: Biochemical, Chemical and Clinical Endocrinology of Calcium Metabolism. de Gruyter, Berlin, 1982, p 833.

23. Cordy PE, Mills DM: The early detection and treatment of renal osteodystrophy. Min Electrol Metab 5:311, 1981.

24. Dambacher A, Fischer JA, Hunziker WH, et al: Distribution of circulating immunoreactive components of parathyroid hormone in normal subjects and in patients with primary and secondary hyperparathyroidism: The role of the kidney and of the serum calcium concentration. Clin Sci Mol Med 57: 435, 1979.

25. Eastwood JB, Bordier PJ, Clarkson S, et al: The contrasting effects on bone hisology of vitamin D and of calcium carbonate in the osteomalacia of chronic renal failure. Clin Sci Mol Med 47: 23, 1974.

26. Eastwood JB, Stamp CB, de Wardener HE, et al: The effect of 25-hydroxy vitamin D$_3$ in the osteomalacia of chronic renal failure. Clin Sci Mol Med 52: 499, 1977.

27. Felsenfeld AJ, Harrelson JM, Gutman RA, et al: Osteomalacia after parathyroidectomy in patients with uremia. Ann Intern Med 96: 34, 1982.

28. Fournier AE, Arnaud CD, Johnson WJ, et al: Etiology of hyperparathyroidism and bone disease during chronic hemodialysis. II. Factors affecting serum immunoreactive parathyroid hormone. J Clin Invest 50: 599, 1971.

29. Friis T, Hahnemann S, Weeke E: Serum calcium and serum phosphorus in uremia during administration of sodium phytate and aluminum hydroxyde. Acta Med Scand 183: 497, 1968.

30. Fröhling PT, Kokot F, Vetter K, et al: Combined treatment with ketoacids and pharmacological doses of vitamin D—a new way for the prophylaxis of renal osteodystrophy. In Norman AW, Schaefer K, von Herrath D, et al, Eds: Vitamin D, Chemical, Biochemical and Clinical Endocrinology of Calcium Metabolism. de Gruyter, Berlin, 1982, p 841.

31. Galante L, Colstone KW, Grams IM, et al: The regulation of vitamin D metabolism. Nature (London) 244: 438, 1973.

32. Goldsmith RS, Furszyfer J, Johnson WJ, et al: Control of secondary hyperparathyroidism during long-term hemodialysis. Am J Med 50: 692, 1971.

33. Hahn TJ, Birge SJ, Scharp CR, Avioli LV: Phenobarbital-induced alterations in vitamin D metabolism. J Clin Invest 51: 741, 1972.

34. Haussler MR, Hughes MR, Pike JW, et al: Radioligand receptor assay for 1,25-dihydroxyvitamin D: Biochemical, physiologic and clinical applications. In Norman AW, Schaefer K, Coburn CW, Eds: Vitamin D: Chemical, Biochemical and Clinical Aspects Related to Calcium Metabolism. de Gruyter, Berlin, 1977, p 473.

35. Healy MD, Malluche HH, Goldstein DA, et al: Effects of long-term therapy with calcitriol in patients with moderate renal failure. Arch Intern Med 140: 1030, 1980.

36. Hodsman AB, Sherrard DJ, Wong EG, et al: Vitamin-D-resistant osteomalacia in hemodialysis patients lacking secondary hyperparathyroidism. Ann Intern Med 94: 623, 1981.

37. Howard GA, Turner RT, Sherrard DJ, et al: Human bone cells in culture metabolize 25-hydroxyvitamin D$_3$ to 1,25-dihydroxyvitamin D$_3$ and 24,25-dihydroxyvitamin D$_3$. J Biol Chem 256: 7738, 1981.

38. Hufnagel HD, Hausen M, Traut G, Meiser RJ: Morphometrische Untersuchungen im Frühstadium der renalen Osteopathie. Klin Wschr 52: 1070, 1974.

39. Ihle B, Buchanan M, Stevens B et al: Aluminum associated bone disease: Clinico-

pathologic correlation. Am J Kid Dis 2: 255, 1982.

40. Kerr DN, Walls J, Ellis DH, et al: Bone disease in patients undergoing regular hemodialysis. J Bone Joint Surg 51 B: 578, 1969.

41. Kleerekoper M, Cruz C, Bernstein RS, et al: The phosphaturic action of PTH in the steady state in patients with normal and impaired renal function. In Massry SG, Ritz E, Jahn H, Eds: Phosphate and Other Minerals in Health and Disease. Plenum, New York, 1980, p 145.

42. Lambert PW, Stern PH, Avioli RC, et al: Evidence for extrarenal production of 1α,25-dihydroxyvitamin D in man. J Clin Invest 69: 722, 1982.

43. Llach F, Massry SG, Singer FR, et al: Skeletal resistance to endogenous parathyroid hormone in patients with early renal failure. A possible cause for secondary hyperparathyroidism. J Clin Endocrinol Metab 41: 339, 1975.

44. Llach F, Massry SG, Koffler A, et al: Secondary hyperparathyroidism in early renal failure: Role of phosphate retention (abstr). Proc Am Soc Nephrol 10: 7, 1977.

45. Makoff DL, Gordon A, Franklin SS, et al: Chronic calcium carbonate therapy in uremia. Arch Intern Med 123: 15, 1969.

46. Malluche HH, Ritz E, Kutschera J, et al: Calcium metabolism and impaired mineralization in various stages of renal insufficiency. In Norman AW, Schaefer K, Grigoleit HG, Eds: Vitamin D and Problems Related to Uremic Bone Disease. de Gruyter, Berlin, 1975, p 513.

47. Malluche HH, Ritz E, Lange HP et al: Bone histology in incipient and advanced renal failure. Kidney Int 9: 335, 1976.

48. Malluche HH, Goldstein DA, Massry SG: Management of renal osteodystrophy with 1,25 (OH)$_2$D$_3$. II. Effects on histopathology of bone: Evidence for healing of osteomalacia. Min Electrol Metab 2: 48, 1979.

49. Maschio G, Tessitore N, D'Angelo A, et al: Early dietary phosphorus restriction and calcium supplementation in the prevention of renal osteodystrophy. Am J Clin Nutr 33: 1546, 1980.

50. Massry SG, Ritz E, Verberckmoes R: Role of phosphate in the genesis of secondary hyperparathyroidism of renal failure. Nephron 18: 77, 1977.

51. Memmos DE, Eastwood JB, Talner LB et al: Double-blind trial of oral 1,25-dihydroxy-vitamin D$_3$ versus placebo in asymptomatic hyperparathyroidism in patients receiving maintenance haemodialysis. Br Med J 282: 1919, 1981.

52. Meyrier A, Marsac J, Richet G: The influence of a high calcium carbonate intake on bone disease in patients undergoing hemodialysis. Kidney Int 4: 146, 1973.

53. Offermann G, von Herrath D, Schaefer K: Serum 25-hydroxycholecalciferol in uremia. Nephron 13: 169, 1974.

54. Pierides AM, Simpson W, Ward MK, et al: Variable response to long-term 1α-hydroxy cholecalciferol in haemodialysis osteodystrophy. Lancet 1:1092, 1976.

55. Popovtzer MM, Schainuck LI, Massry SG, et al: Bivalent ion excretion in chronic kidney disease: relation to degree of renal insufficiency. Clin Sci 38: 297, 1970.

56. Raisz LG, Niemann I: Effect of phosphate, calcium and magenesium on bone resorption and hormonal responses in tissue culture. Endocrinology 85: 446, 1969.

57. Recker R, Schoenfeld P, Letteri J, et al: The efficacy of calcifediol in renal osteodystrophy. Arch Intern Med 138: 857, 1978.

58. Reiss E, Canterbury JM, Kanter A: Circulating parathyroid hormone concentration in chronic renal insufficiency. Arch Intern Med 124: 417, 1969.

59. Ritz E, Krempien B, Mehls O, et al: Skeletal abnormalities in chronic renal insufficiency before and during maintenance hemodialysis. Kidney Int 4: 116, 1973.

60. Ritz E, Malluche HH, Krempien B, et al: Pathogenesis of renal osteodystrophy: roles of phosphate and skeletal resistance to PTH. In Massry SG, Rapado A, Ritz E, Eds: Phosphate and Other Minerals. Plenum, New York, 1978, p 443.

61. Ritz E, Malluche HH, Krempien B, et al: Calcium metabolism in renal failure. Disorders of mineral metabolism. Vol.III. Bronner FF, Coburn JW (Eds). Academic Press, 1982, p 209.

62. Schmidt-Gayk H, Schmitt W, Grawunder C, et al: 25-Hydroxyvitamin D in nephrotic syndrome. Lancet 2: 105, 1977.

63. Sherrard DJ, Coburn JW, Brickman AS, et al: An histologic comparison of 1,25 (OH)$_2$ Vitamin D$_3$ treatment with calcium supplementation in renal osteodystrophy. In Norman AW, Schaefer K, Coburn JW, et al, Eds: Vitamin D: Biochemical, Chemical and Clinical Aspects Related to Calcium Metabolism. de Gruyter, Berlin, 1977, p 719.

64. Sherrard DJ, Ott SM, Maloney NA, et al: The use of 24,25 (OH)$_2$ Vitamin D$_3$ in the refractory osteomalacia form of renal osteodystrophy. In Norman AW, Schaefer K, von Herrath D, et al, Eds: Vitamin D: Biochemical, Chemical and Clinical Aspects Related to Calcium Metabolism. de Gruyter, Berlin, 1982, p 169.

65. Slatopolsky E, Calgar S, Penell JP, et al: On the pathogenesis of hyperparathyroidism in chronic experimental renal insufficiency in the dog. J Clin Invest 50: 492, 1971.

66. Slatopolsky E, Rutherford WE, Hurska K, et al: How important is phosphate in the pathogenesis of renal osteodystrophy? Arch Intern Med 138:, 848, 1978.

67. Slatopolsky E, Gray R, Adams ND, et al: Low serum levels of 1,25 (OH)$_2$D$_3$ are not responsible for the development of secondary hyperparathyroidism in early renal failure. Kidney Int 14: 177, 1978.

68. Stanbury SW, Lumb GA, Mawer EB: Osteodystrophy developing spontaneously in the course of chronic renal failure. Arch Intern Med 124: 274, 1969.

69. Taylor CM: The measurement of 24,25 dihydroxycholecalciferol in human serum. In Norman AW, Schaefer K, Coburn JW, et al, Eds: Vitamin D: Biochemical, Chemical and Clinical Aspects Related to Calcium Metabolism. de Gruyter, Berlin, 1977, p 541.

70. Teitelbaum SL, Bone JM, Stein PM, et al: Calcifediol in chronic renal insufficiency. JAMA 235: 162, 1976.

71. Tröhler U, Bonjour JP, Fleisch H: Inorganic phosphate homeostasis. Renal adaption to the dietary intake in intact and thyroparathyroidectomized rats. J Clin Invest 57: 264, 1976.

72. Walser M: Does dietary therapy have a role in the predialysis patient? Am J Clin Nutr 33: 1629, 1980.

# The Case for Its Prophylactic Use

Jack W. Coburn, M.D.
Robert S. Wright, M.D.

In patients with far advanced renal failure, there is ample evidence that the generation of the renal hormone, 1,25-dihydroxyvitamin $D_3$,(1,25 $(OH)_2D_3$), is reduced.[27,35,41] There are several physiologic derangements, noted briefly below, which exist in advanced renal failure and which probably arise as a consequence of this deficiency. Given these established observations, it logically follows that the ideal management of patients with end-stage renal failure should include replacement of this "missing hormone."

In this review, we will consider the theoretical reasons for such therapy and review the pathophysiologic events in renal failure which arise as a consequence of the reduced generation of 1,25 $(OH)_2D_3$. Also, we will review available data on the clinical use of 1,25 $(OH)_2D_3$ in patients with end-stage renal disease, giving particular emphasis to its prophylactic use.

## PATHOPHYSIOLOGIC EFFECTS OF 1,25-DIHYDROXY-VITAMIN D$_3$ DEFICIENCY

The pathophysiologic features which contribute to altered calcium metabolism and bone disease in uremia include: (1) impaired intestinal absorption of calcium, (2) impaired mineralization of bone, (3) reduced responsiveness of the skeleton to the calcemic action of parathyroid hormone (PTH), (4) abnormal feedback suppression of PTH secretion by calcium, (5) altered degradation of PTH, (6) retention of phosphate, and (7) long-standing metabolic acidosis. There is evidence that the first four of these processes may be related, entirely or in part, to the deficiency of 1,25 $(OH)_2D_3$.[25]

Patients with end-stage renal disease and those undergoing regular dialysis treatment exhibit reduced intestinal calcium absorption, with low-normal or overtly low values.[24,45] Moreover, there are extensive data to indicate that the reduced intestinal absorption of calcium can be normalized by the administration of small quantities of 1,25 $(OH)_2D_3$, that is, 0.25 to 1.0 µg/day.[7] In the early phases of renal insufficiency, the alterations in intestinal calcium absorption are less apparent. Patients with creatinine clearances greater than 30 ml/min or serum creatinine levels below 2.5 mg/dl generally have normal intestinal calcium absorption, and it is less certain that reduced intestinal calcium absorption contributes to the abnormalities present in the early stages of renal failure.

Abnormal mineralization of bone exists in many patients with renal failure. In some instances, wide seams of unmineralized osteoid exist because of increased bone turnover, primarily with the lesions of osteitis fibrosa.[61] There are reports indicating that bone mineralization in patients with mixed features of osteitis fibrosa and osteomalacia may be improved by treatment with 1,25 $(OH)_2D_3$.[44,62] On the other hand, a number of reports have shown that treatment with 1,25 $(OH)_2D_3$ did not improve bone mineralization in end-stage uremia.[29,38,40] More recent studies in uremic patients with isolated osteomalacia and lacking the features of secondary hyperparathyroidism[38] clearly demonstrated that aluminum has accumulated in bone.[37] Furthermore, it has been possible to correlate the failure of response of such patients to 1,25 $(OH)_2D_3$ with the magnitude of aluminum accumulation.[53] Further evidence that aluminum accumulation plays an important pathogenic role is provided by experimental evidence in animals indicating that aluminum can produce osteomalacia.[28,34,60] Moreover, data in humans indicate that aluminum accumulation produces a similar lesion in the bone of patients treated with long-term total parenteral nutrition;[54] other observations indicate that the removal of aluminum from dialysis patients by chelation with desferrioxamine can lead to improvement of this skeletal lesion.[1,12] Based on this evidence as well as our own experience, we suggest that most, if not all, of the vitamin D-refractory osteomalacia encountered in end-stage uremia has occurred secondary to the accumulation of aluminum. The non aluminum-induced abnormal mineralization in renal failure can be ameliorated by treatment with an active vitamin D sterol.

The specific actions of the vitamin D sterols on bone are not well defined. Most in vitro studies of 1,25 $(OH)_2D_3$ action indicate that this sterol enhances bone resorption.[57,58] On the other hand, extensive studies in vivo in man indicate that the primary effect of 1,25 $(OH)_2D_3$ is to augment the mineralization of bone in patients with nutritional osteomalacia.[50,55] There are also conflicting data regarding the specific vitamin D sterols required to promote normal mineralization. Thus, the report of Bordier et al.[5] suggested that 1,25$(OH)_2D$ failed to induce normal mineralization in patients with renal failure, and these authors suggested that other sterols were needed for bone mineralization. The observations of Peacock et al.[55] and Nagant de Deuxchaisnes et al.[50], however, indicate that 1,25 $(OH)_2D$ alone produced healing of vitamin D-deficiency osteomalacia in man, providing evidence that the activated vitamin alone can suffice. Other observations involving the pharmacologic application of 24,25$(OH)_2D$ to patients with dialysis osteomalacia suggest that this hormone can improve bone mineralization in certain cases.[39]

Resistance of the skeleton to the calcemic action of PTH is known to exist in renal failure, and this abnormality may be a factor contributing to the secondary hyperparathyroidism of renal insufficiency. Observations in dogs with acute renal failure indicate that administration of 1,25-$(OH)_2D_3$ alone or with 24,25$(OH)_2D_3$ can either improve or restore to normal the calcemic response to exogenous PTH.[46,47] In patients with early renal failure, there is delayed recovery from acute hypocalcemia induced by EDTA; this has occurred despite increments in serum PTH levels that are greater than those found in control subjects receiving EDTA.[42] A preliminary report indicates that the administration of 1,25 $(OH)_2D_3$ to patients with mild renal insufficiency can reduce to normal the recovery time from EDTA-induced hypocalcemia.[65] These data provide strong supporting evidence for the role of abnormal vitamin D metabolism in causing skeletal resistance to the calcemic action of PTH.

One major effect of 1,25 $(OH)_2D_3$ is the suppression of PTH secretion, presumably due, in large part, to the increase in serum calcium concentration. It is well known that treatment of patients with advanced renal failure with 1,25 $(OH)_2D_3$ causes serum calcium to increase.[7,10] This increase in serum calcium could be secondary to its increased intestinal absorption or could result from mobilization of bone calcium produced when vitamin D restored bone sensitivity to PTH. As indicated below, there may be other mechanisms whereby 1,25 $(OH)_2D_3$ might affect the secretion of PTH.

Abnormal feedback suppression of PTH secretion by serum calcium has also been demonstrated in patients with end-stage kidney disease. Data are accumulating which suggest that this abnormal suppression may be related to the deficiency of 1,25 $(OH)_2D_3$, including the following observations. First, specific cytosolic receptors for 1,25 $(OH)_2D_3$ have been demonstrated in parathyroid cells, and such receptors are characteristic of target tissues.[14] Second, there are studies in animals which suggest that 1,25-$(OH)_2D_3$ may directly cause supression of PTH secretion. Thus, Chertow et al.[16] observed that 1,25 $(OH)_2D_3$ decreases serum PTH within four hours of its administration to rats, and blocks the rise in serum PTH otherwise provoked by hypocalcemia. In addition, Oldham et al.[52] found that for a given serum calcium concentration, the addition of 1,25 $(OH)_2D_3$ to calcium infusions more effectively reduced serum PTH in vitamin D-deficient puppies. Thus, the vitamin acted synergistically with calcium to reduce PTH secretion. It should be noted, however, that there have been studies, largely carried out in vitro, indicating that 1,25 $(OH)_2D_3$, when added directly to suspensions of parathyroid cells, failed to alter the secretion of PTH.[30] Finally, several studies carried out in uremic patients suggest that 1,25 $(OH)_2D_3$ may have a direct effect on the parathyroid glands. Thus, Madsen et al.[43] carried out continuous peritoneal dialysis in ten patients with acute renal failure utilizing a dialysate calcium con-

centration reduced to only 3.2 mg/dl thereby maintaining patients hypocalcemic. After 24 hours, one subgroup of hypocalcemic patients was given 1,25-$(OH)_2D_3$, 0.25 μg intravenously every six hours, while the hypocalcemic "control" group received no vitamin D. Both subgroups continued to receive peritoneal dialysis as noted. The group treated with 1,25 $(OH)_2D_3$ showed a significant fall in serum PTH levels despite persistent hypocalcemia while the serum PTH levels in the control patients, who were equally hypocalcemic but untreated with vitamin D, remained elevated (Fig. 15-10). Also, preliminary data[64] have shown that the thrice weekly intravenous administration of 1,25 $(OH)_2D_3$ to patients on regular hemodialysis produced a fall in serum PTH that occurred before there was any increase in serum calcium levels. Such data provide strong evidence that 1,25-$(OH)_2D_3$ may directly affect the parathyroid glands. The lack of such an action in uremia could be an important factor leading to persistent and often progressive secondary hyperparathyroidism in patients with longstanding renal failure.

Of interest, the alteration in PTH suppressibility of parathyroid cells from uremic patients has recently been quantitated. Thus, PTH secretion by suspensions of parathyroid cells isolated from patients with end-stage renal failure is not inhibited appropriately by an increase in a calcium concentration in the media that decreases the PTH secretion by parathyroid cells from controls.[13] Thus, there is a shift in the "setpoint," or the level of calcium causing 50 percent suppression of PTH secretion, in the parathyroid cells from most of the uremic patients studied (Fig. 15-11). Preliminary data suggest that alterations in the intracellular calcium concentration may account for this change in "setpoint."[63] Thus, it seems possible that 1,25 $(OH)_2D_3$, perhaps by stimulating the transcellular flux of calcium in a man-

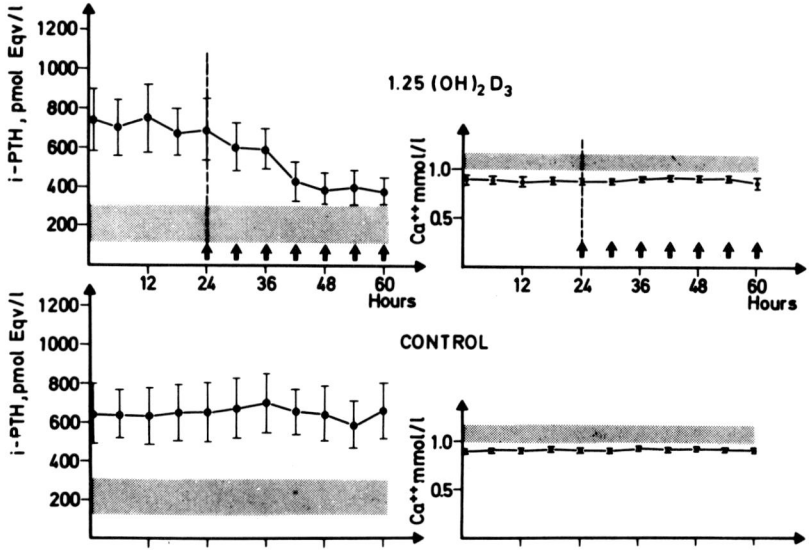

**Fig. 15-10.** Serial PTH and ionized calcium levels measured during continuous peritoneal dialysis utilizing a low-calcium dialysate. The arrows indicate the intravenous injections of 1,25 $(OH)_2D_3$, 0.25 µg/day. The upper panel represents the group of patients receiving 1,25 $(OH)_2D_3$, while the lower panel represents the control group. The normal ranges for $Ca^{++}$ and iPTH are indicated by the shaded areas. (From Madsen S, Olgaard K, Ladefoged J: Direct feed-back regulation of PTH-secretion by 1,25-dihydroxyvitamin $D_3$ in renal failure: A controlled trial Proc EDTA 17:557, 1980.)

ner analogous to its action in the intestine,[51,59] could enhance intracellular calcium activity. Such an effect might produce greater inhibition of PTH secretion at any given level of calcium in the blood or extracellular fluid. The deficiency of 1,25 $(OH)_2D_3$ in uremic patients could thus contribute to such a shift in "setpoint."

## CLINICAL EFFECTS OF 1,25 $(OH)_2D_3$ IN UREMIA

In reviewing the effects of the vitamin D sterols in patients with advanced renal failure, it seems appropriate to consider the effects that have been attributed to their use. These include observations in uncontrolled open studies as well as those from highly controlled and even double blind studies. Thus, there are a number of features of uremia that have improved following the administration of an active vitamin D sterol. For example, either 1,25-$(OH)_2D_3$ or 1-α-hydroxyvitamin D has produced dramatic and rapid improvement of the proximal myopathy that occasionally develops in patients with advanced uremia.[10,36]

Alterations in vitamin D metabolism could account for other symptoms that occur in advanced uremia. It has been shown that the vitamin D-dependent calcium binding proteins exist in several tissues of the body that are not usually considered target tissues for this hormone. These include the parotid glands, the islets of the pancreas and the central nervous system receptors.[19] The effects of 1,25 $(OH)_2D_3$ on the metabolism or func-

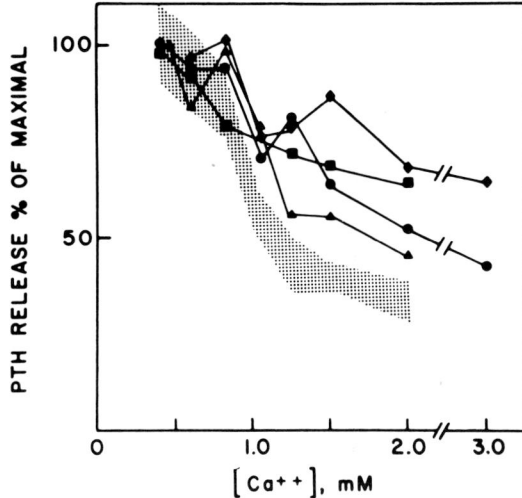

**Fig. 15-11.** The calcium-regulated release of PTH by suspensions of parathyroid cells from a uremic patient with secondary hyperparathyroidism; there is a rightward shift in the "set point." The shaded area indicates suppression of PTH release by increasing concentrations of calcium in suspensions of normal cells. Each symbol represents results from parathyroid cells from a different parathyroid gland in the same patient. (From Brown EM, Set-point for calcium: Its role in normal and abnormal parathyroid secretion. In Cohn DV, Talmage RV, Matthews JL, Eds: Hormond Control of Calcium Metabolism. Excerpta Medica, Amsterdam, 1981.)

tion of these tissues remain unclear, but it is possible that subtle alterations in their function might occur due to the deficiency of the vitamin that occurs in end-stage uremia.

Other effects of 1,25 $(OH)_2D_3$ or another active vitamin D sterol, largely noted during open and uncontrolled studies, have included the following: (1) improvement of various musculoskeletal symptoms, (2) normalization of certain abnormal biochemical finding, and (3) improvement of the skeletal abnormalities related to secondary hyperparathyroidism.[11,31,33,36] Thus, patients with substantial disability caused by bone pain and muscle weakness often show dramatic improvement. Moreover, in a number of instances, there has been the recurrence of symptoms within 2 to 3 months after withdrawal of the vitamin D sterol. In certain patients these effects were associated with improvement in the general feeling of well-being, increased appetite, and weight gain. In patients with preexisting hypocalcemia, increments in serum calcium level have been noted, and there have been significant decreases in serum PTH levels.[20] Radiographic lesions of secondary hyperparathyoidism have improved substantially in many patients, and bone biopsies have shown either a reversal of the features of osteitis fibrosa or there was marked improvement.[62] Bone biopsies showing features of "mixed" lesions (osteitis fibrosa and osteomalacia) often exhibited improvement.[62] Thus, the major effect observed has been substantial reversal of the features of secondary hyperparathyroidism. However, other effects have also been seen; for example, the mucosa of the small intestine of uremic patients has shown thickening and normalization after the administration of 1,25 $(OH)_2D_3$, evidence of increased growth of this epithelial surface.[31]

In children with advanced renal failure, symptomatic and severe renal osteodystrophy is much more common than in adults, with as many as 60 percent to 80 percent of children exhibiting overt disease.[17] Prior to the fusion of the epiphyses, the turnover and remodelling of bone is much higher in children than in adults. Thus, stunted growth, slipped epiphyses and metaphyseal fractures result in severe deformities of bone and abnormalities in gait.[67] There have been reports that the use of various active vitamin sterols, including 1-α(OH)$D_3$, 1,25 $(OH)_2D_3$, and 25(OH)$D_3$ (calcifediol), has led to substantial improvement in serum PTH, alkaline phosphatase activity, and skeletal X-rays; moreover, there have been reports of substantial improvement in the growth retar-

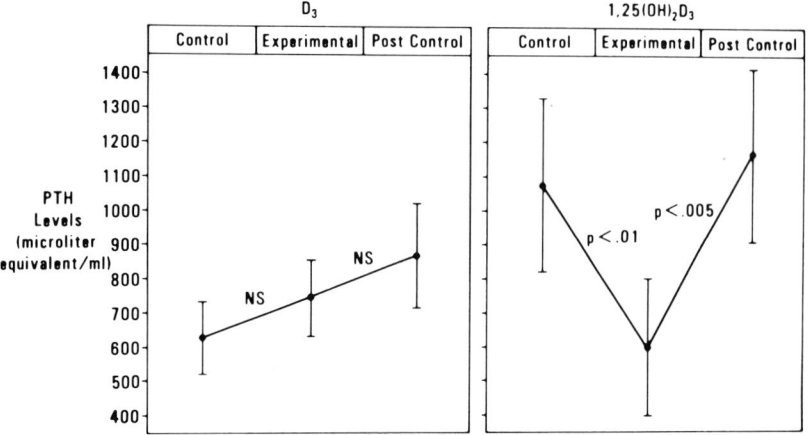

**Fig. 15-12** Mean levels of serum immunoreactive parathyroid hormone (PTH) in dialysis patients assigned to vitamin $D_3$ (400 IU/day) or 1,25-dihydroxy vitamin $D_3$ (1,25 $(OH)_2D_3$). Values are indicated for the control period, experimental period and for the post-treatment period. Only the patients receiving 1,25 $(OH)_2D_3$ demonstrated a significant decrease in serum PTH levels. (From Berl T, Berns AS, Huffer WE, et al: 1,25-dihydroxycholecalciferol effects in chronic dialysis. A double-blind controlled study. Ann Intern Med 88,774,1978.)

dation in uremic children treated with 1,25 $(OH)_2D_3$.[15,17] Although controlled studies comparing 1,25 $(OH)_2D_3$ to placebo are not available in children, the high frequency of overt bone disease and its biochemical and clinical improvement following treatment with the vitamin or another active vitamin D sterol, would indicate that the prophylactic use of such agents should be routine in all children with advanced renal failure, unless there is a specific contraindication.

## Controlled Studies Utilizing Vitamin D Sterols

In a study of 31 adult dialysis patients, selected without regard to clinical or biochemical features of renal osteodystrophy, Berl et al.[3] gave either 1,25 $(OH)_2D_3$ or vitamin $D_3$ in a "placebo" dose of 400 IU/day, for 12 weeks in a double-blind study. The dose of 1,25-$(OH)_2D_3$ averaged 0.82 μg/day. They noted an increase in serum calcium from 9.05 ± 0.15 to 10.25 ± 0.20 mg/dl ($p<0.01$), in those receiving 1,25-$(OH)_2D_3$, while there was no change in serum calcium in those receiving the capsules containing vitamin $D_3$. There were significant reductions in serum PTH in 11 of the 13 patients receiving 1,25 $(OH)_2D_3$ and these effects reverted toward control after the vitamin $D_3$ capsules were substituted for 1,25 $(OH)_2D_3$ (Fig. 15-12). Serum alkaline phosphatase, elevated in most patients, did not change in either group of patients. There were significant differences in the histologic response of bone in those receiving 1,25 $(OH)_2D_3$ compared to those receiving the vitamin $D_3$. The major change in bone was improvement of osteitis fibrosa, while the osteomalacia failed to improve. Of the patients entering the study, four had bone pain and weakness associated with features of renal osteodystrophy. Three of these patients were randomly assigned to 1,25 $(OH)_2D_3$ and they all exhibited remarkable amelioration of their symptoms.

Maxwell et al.[48] followed a protocol similar to that of Berl et al.[3] in 22 dialysis patients, except that serum PTH levels were not measured and bone biopsies were not performed. They noted a significant increase in serum calcium in those taking 1,25 $(OH)_2D_3$ compared to the effect in those taking vitamin $D_3$. Unlike the findings of Berl et al., they noted a significant decrease in plasma alkaline phosphatase activity in those receiving activated vitamin compared to the group receiving vitamin $D_3$. They also showed that when hypercalcemia occurred in those taking 1,25 $(OH)_2D_3$, this rapidly reversed after withdrawal of the drug.

In a study carried out in asymptomatic patients who had undergone hemodialysis for at least one year, Memmos et al.[49] gave either 1,25 $(OH)_2D_3$ or placebo in a double blind manner for one to two years. The patients assigned to the 1,25-$(OH)_2D_3$ group received 0.50 μg/day initially; if serum calcium exceeded 12.0 mg/dl, the drug was discontinued until the serum calcium normalized, and then the drug was reinstituted at a dose of 0.25 μg/day. Fifty-seven patients completed 1 year of study, and 32 were in the trial for 2 years. At the end of one year, 16 of the 30 patients receiving placebo but only one of 27 patients receiving 1,25 $(OH)_2D_3$ showed bony deterioration in the roentgenograms taken of their hands. Among the patients who entered the trial with abnormal skeletal roentgenograms, none of the 16 patients receiving placebo showed improvement after 2 years, while five of 11 given 1,25 $(OH)_2D_3$ exhibited improvement during this period. Serum PTH levels, which were closely related to the severity of radiographic evidence of hyperparathyroidism, showed a slight increase in the placebo group but fell in the 1,25 $(OH)_2D_3$-treated patients; the mean values were significantly different in the two groups at the end of the trial. Also, a larger proportion of those receiving placebo showed an increment in serum PTH

levels than did those receiving 1,25-$(OH)_2D_3$. Plasma alkaline phosphatase activity fell significantly in patients who entered the study with abnormal roentgenographs and received 1,25 $(OH)_2D_3$. Serum calcium exceeded 12.0 mg/dl in 16 of the original 27 patients receiving 1,25 $(OH)_2D_3$ and the values rapidly returned to normal levels after withholding therapy.

In a preliminary report of a double blind trial with either 1,25 $(OH)_2D_3$ or placebo in dialysis patients, Baker et al.[2] progressively increased the daily dosage from 0.25 μg/day to 1.0 μg/day over a 4-week period if the serum calcium did not exceed 11.0 mg/dl. Serum calcium was assessed monthly. When hypercalcemia developed, the dose was gradually reduced. This protocol resulted in prolonged hypercalcemia, which persisted for more than 15 weeks in three patients who received 1,25 $(OH)_2D_3$. The high incidence of hypercalcemia was probably related to the rapid progression to 1.0 μg/day, and it may have persisted because the dosage was gradually reduced, rather than being totally discontinued. We believe that the sustained hypercalcemia may reflect either marked hyperparathyroidism or the existence of aluminum-associated osteomalacia.[21]

In a double-blind, controlled study of asymptomatic dialysis patients with normal skeletal x-rays, Coburn et al.[22] assigned 98 patients to either 1,25 $(OH)_2D_3$ or placebo; the dosage was increased in a stepwise manner from 0.25 to 1.0 μg/day at two monthly intervals, and the patients were followed for up to 30 months. All patients received oral calcium carbonate, providing 1.0 g calcium/day, in addition to their usual dietary intake. Serum biochemical parameters, serum PTH, serial radiographs and photon absorptiometry were evaluated. The mean serum calcium increased from 9.4 ± 0.6 (mean ± SD) to 10.2 ± 0.5 mg/dl in those receiving 1,25 $(OH)_2D_3$, while the serum calcium levels changed insignificantly in the placebo group from 9.5 ± 0.6 mg/dl prior to the study, to 9.7 ± 0.6 mg/dl after treatment. Serum phosphorus levels were 4.7 ± 0.9 mg/dl and 5.1 ± 0.7 mg/dl at the beginning and end of the study, respectively, in those receiving 1,25 $(OH)_2D_3$. Initial and final values in the placebo-treated group were 4.7 ± 0.9 and 4.9 ± 0.7 mg/dl, respectively. The differences in serum phosphorus were not statistically significant, either within or between groups.[23] The distribution of patients showing changes in serum PTH varied with the treatment assigned. Thus, there was a significant reduction in serum PTH in 60 percent of those receiving 1,25 $(OH)_2D_3$, while serum PTH levels were unchanged in 31 percent and 11 percent exhibited a rise in serum PTH. In those receiving placebo, 27 percent had a reduction in serum PTH values, 34 percent showed no change, and there was a rise in 39 percent. The distribution of patients into groups according to observed changes in serum PTH was significantly influenced by 1,25-$(OH)_2D_3$ (p<0.01).[23] The development of skeletal erosions on radiographs was also related to the serum PTH levels when the patient entered the study, independent of the treatment given. Thus, 20 percent of those with serum PTH levels above 130 μlEq/ml developed erosions, while none developed in those with serum PTH levels below 130 μlEq/ml. Of interest, another "predictive" parameter for the development of skeletal erosions were the serum alkaline phosphatase levels on entry. Patients subsequently developing bony erosions entered the study with alkaline phosphatase values greater than 70 IU/L.[22] More rapid loss of bone mineral content also was related to the changes in serum PTH. Indeed, 65 percent of those whose serum PTH levels increased showed a significant decrease in bone mineral content, while only seven percent

of those whose serum PTH levels decreased manifested significant loss of bone mineral content.

These data indicate that the prophylactic administration of 1,25 $(OH)_2D_3$ to asymptomatic dialysis patients can prevent the development of radiographic features of secondary hyperparathyroidism, particularly in "high risk" patients, that is, those with higher serum PTH and alkaline phosphatase activity.

Hypercalcemia (serum calcium levels above 11.8 mg/dl), the major risk factor with the use of 1,25 $(OH)_2D_3$, occurred in eight placebo-treated patients and in 21 patients receiving the activated vitamin. The hypercalcemia did not elicit symptoms in 82 percent and resolved within 4 days after withdrawal of the drug and calcium carbonate supplements in most patients. Hypercalcemia persisted for longer than 14 days in three patients, one taking placebo and two receiving 1,25 $(OH)_2D_3$.

In another controlled study, Binswanger et al.[4] assigned 13 dialysis patients with no skeletal symptoms to either placebo or 1,25 $(OH)_2D_3$ and treated four other patients with symptomatic bone disease with 1,25 $(OH)_2D_3$, following them separately in an open trial. The 1,25-$(OH)_2D_3$ was initially given in a dose of 1.0 μg/day; when either total or ionized serum calcium increased into the upper half of the normal range, the dose was reduced by 50 percent; if both ionized and total calcium values increased, the drug was discontinued. Over the 3 to 8 months of study, the average dose of 1,25-$(OH)_2D_3$ was 0.61 μg/day. Total serum calcium increased to above the normal range in 28 percent of the measurements during the study, whereas ionized serum calcium exceeded the normal range in only 4 percent of determinations. Serum PTH, measured by an amino-terminal PTH assay, decreased significantly in the patients receiving 1,25 $(OH)_2D_3$ (p<0.05) while there was no change in those assigned to placebo. Bone mineral content of the forearm, measured by photon absorptiometry at intervals of 1 to 2 months, did not change significantly in patients in either treatment group.

The major side effect, hypercalcemia, was without clinical side effects in most patients; however serum calcium increased as high as 15 mg/dl in one patient, and the hypercalcemia persisted for 2 months after withdrawal of the 1,25-$(OH)_2D_3$. Serum PTH levels were normal in this patient and a bone biopsy disclosed severe osteomalacia with very little cellular activity. These features are similar to those present in dialysis osteomalacia due to aluminum accumulation,[37,38] and the occurrence of hypercalcemia in such cases is not at all surprising.[6,21]

## Side Effects of Vitamin D Sterols

A known and often desirable effect of treatment with an active vitamin D sterol is the observed increase in serum calcium levels. Indeed, the increase in serum calcium plays a major role in mediating the suppression of secondary hyperparathyroidism in renal failure. In most of the clinical trials, open or controlled, with 1,25 $(OH)_2D_3$ or other active sterols, hypercalcemia has been common, as described above. However, in most instances, the patients were either totally asymptomatic or the symptoms were mild and rapidly reversed. Moreover, the design of the majority of the long-term studies described above[2,4,22] either utilized initial doses as high as 1.0 µg/day or there was a progressive increase in dosage until *hypercalcemia* appeared. With the use of such a protocol, it is not surprising that hypercalcemia was common. These patients were either asymptomatic during the hypercalcemia or the symptoms were only mild and did not necessitate hospitalization.

Situations predisposing to the development of hypercalcemia in patients with end-stage renal failure include the following. (1) the presence of marked and overt secondary hyperparathyroidism[66] and, (2) the syndrome of aluminum-associated dialysis osteomalacia.[37,38] In cases with overt hyperparathyroidism, mild hypercalcemia often existed prior to the initiation of treatment with 1,25 $(OH)_2D_3$. In one group of patients, overt hypercalcemia developed within $3.3 \pm 1.3$ weeks after initiation of treatment and with the use of an average dose of 1,25 $(OH)_2D_3$ of only $0.21 \pm 0.04$ µg/day.[66] When many of the trials with the active vitamin D sterols were being carried out the role of aluminum in producing osteomalacia and predisposing to hypercalcemia was unknown. However, it was recognized early in trials of 1,25 $(OH)_2D_3$ that cases of refractory osteomalacia were prone to hypercalcemia.[21,56] In one series of those with refractory osteomalacia,[38] hypercalcemia developed with an average dose of 1,25 $(OH)_2D_3$ of $0.32 \pm 0.02$ µg/day. It seems very likely that the instances of prolonged and marked hypercalcemia that developed during treatment of osteomalacic dialysis patients with 1,25 $(OH)_2D_3$ most likely represented patients with this syndrome.

There is concern about the effects of the vitamin D sterols on phosphate metabolism in uremic patients. Active vitamin D sterols clearly augment phosphate absorption in renal failure patients,[9] and sudden increments in serum phosphorus levels caan develop during prolonged treatment.[8] In many of the controlled studies,[22,49] the doses of aluminum hydroxide or aluminum carbonate were adjusted to maintain serum phosphorus within a specific range, which may account for the lack of significant change in serum phosphorus levels. On the other hand, Binswanger et al.[4] reported problems with the control of hyperphosphatemia in the patients receiving 1,25-

$(OH)_2D_3$; this may have arisen, in part, because of rather poor control of serum phosphorus levels prior to treatment, with a mean serum phosphorus level of $6.9 \pm 1.9$ mg/dl. It has been our policy not to initiate therapy with an active vitamin D sterol unless the serum phosphorus level can be maintained below 5.5 mg/dl.

With a tendency toward increments in the levels of both serum calcium and phosphorus, an increased risk of extraskeletal calcification would be a concern in patients with advanced renal failure. To date, it is not clear that this has definitely occurred, although Binswanger et al.[4] noted that a "red-eye" syndrome developed in a dialysis patient who was not taking his phosphate-binding gels and thus developed marked hyperphosphatemia. Memmos et al. did not find radiographic evidence of soft-tissue calcifications in patients treated with $1,25$-$(OH)_2D_3$ compared to placebo,[49] and we also found no differences between the incidence of new or worsened soft-tissue or vascular calcifications in the dialysis patients treated with $1,25$ $(OH)_2D_3$ compared to placebo.[26]

## SUMMARY

On the basis of presently available data, it is our view that the prophylactic treatment of dialysis patients with $1,25$-$(OH)_2D_3$ or another equivalent active vitamin D sterol is justified. Such therapy is effective in preventing the progression of subclinical, asymptomatic disease, or preventing the appearance of overt manifestations of secondary hyperparathyroidism. When rapid hypercalcemia does develop, this may indicate the presence of marked parathyroid hyperplasia, which may be approached therapeutically only by parathyroidectomy. On the other hand, the early development of hypercalcemia may be a clue to the presence of aluminum accumulation.

The available vitamin D sterols are safe to use, the only major risk being hypercalcemia which, in general, is rapidly reversible. Moreover, we believe that the judicious monitoring of serum calcium and phosphorus levels and the dosage of the vitamin sterol can minimize this risk. It might be argued that the use of oral calcium supplements would be equally effective in raising serum calcium and suppressing secondary hyperparathyroidism; moreover, the use of a calcium salt such as calcium carbonate would be less expensive. There are several problems with this approach: first, oral calcium salts are not always effective; in our double-blind study, 39 percent of patients receiving 1 gram of calcium as calcium carbonate plus placebo rather than calcitriol exhibited a progressive rise in serum iPTH, with a greater risk of bone erosions and loss of bone mineral mass.[22] Larger doses of calcium carbonate might be effective but compliance would become a problem, and side effects, such as constipation, and even hypercalcemia, might then ensue. Finally, there are the data, which have been previously cited,[43,52,64] suggesting that $1,25$ $(OH)_2D_3$ may directly suppress the parathyroid glands. For these reasons, we believe that therapy with $1,25$-$(OH)_2D_3$ is superior to oral calcium supplementation, despite its greater cost. Moreover, the long-term greater efficacy of $1,25$ $(OH)_2D_3$ may prove more cost effective in preventing complications of secondary hyperparathyroidism.

In adults, there are certain circumstances when use of the active vitamin D sterols may either be contraindicated or of uncertain value. Patients who are noncompliant and who show persistant hyperphosphatemia clearly have an increased risk for developing extraskeletal calcifications. These patients should not receive therapy with $1,25$ $(OH)_2D_3$ until serum phosphorus is controlled. There also may be a small population of dialysis patients who have normal or only minimal elevation of serum PTH levels. Over the relatively short period of two to three years, these patients did not develop radiographic evidence of secondary hyperparathyroidism, whether they were treated with 1,25-dihydroxy-vitamin $D_3$ or not.[22] The means of identifying such patients is tentative, at best, and since they developed few side effects there appeared to be little risk in using 1,25 $(OH)_2D_3$.

Since children with chronic renal failure are at very high risk of developing overt bone disease, we recommend that the "prophylactic" administrative of an active vitamin D sterol be used in all instances, unless, of course, a definite contraindication exists.

# REFERENCES

1. Ackrill P, Ralston AJ, Day JP, et al: Successful removal of aluminum from patients with dialysis encephalopathy. Lancet 2:692, 1980.
2. Baker LRI, Muir JW, Cattell WR, et al: Use of 1,25$(OH)_2$-Vitamin $D_3$ in prevention of renal osteodystrophy: Preliminary observations. Contr Nephrol 18:147, 1980.
3. Berl T, Berns AS, Huffer WE, et al: 1,25 dihydroxycholecalciferol effects in chronic dialysis. A double-blind controlled study. Ann Intern Med 88:774, 1978.
4. Binswanger U, Fischer JA, Iselin H, et al: 1,25-dihydroxycholecalciferol treatment of clinically asymptomatic renal osteodystrophy. Min Electrolyte Metab 2:103, 1979.
5. Bordier P, Zingraff J, Gueris J, et al: The effect of 1$\alpha$ $(OH)D_3$ and 1$\alpha$,25$(OH)_2D_3$ on the bone in patients with renal osteodystrophy. Am J Med 64:101,1978.
6. Boyce BF, Fell GS, Elder HY, et al: Hypercalcaemic osteomalacia due to aluminum toxicity. Lancet 2:1009, 1982.
7. Brickman AS, Coburn JW, Massry SB, Norman AW: 1,25-dihydroxyvitamin $D_3$ in normal man and patients with renal failure. Ann Intern Med 80:161, 1974.
8. Brickman AS, Coburn JW Sherrard, DJ et al: Clinical effects of 1,25-dihydroxyvitamin $D_3$ in uremic patients with overt osteodystrophy. Contr Nephrol 18:29, 1980.
9. Brickman AS, Hartenbower DL, Norman AW, et al: Actions of 1$\alpha$-hydroxy- and 1,25-dihydroxy-vitamin $D_3$ on mineral metabolism in man. I. Effects on net absorption of phosphorus. Am J Clin Nutr 30:1064, 1977.
10. Brickman AS, Jowsey J, Sherrard DJ, et al: Therapy with 1,25-dihydroxy-vitamin $D_3$ in the management of renal osteodystrophy. In Norman AW, Schaefer K, Grigoleit HG, et al: Vitamin D and Problems Related to Uremic Bone Disease. de Gruyter, Berlin, 1975.
11. Brickman AS, Sherrard DJ, Jowsey J, et al: 1,25-dihydroxycholecalciferol: Effect on skeletal lesions and plasma parathyroid hormone levels in uremic osteodystrophy. Arch Intern Med 134:883, 1974.
12. Brown DJ, Dawborn JK, Ham KN, et al: Treatment of dialysis osteomalacia with desferrioxamine. Lancet 2:343, 1982.
13. Brown EM: Set-point for calcium: Its role in normal and abnormal parathyroid secretion. In Cohn DV, Talmage RV, Matthews JL, Eds: Hormonal Control of Calcium Metabolism. Excerpta Medica, Amsterdam, 1981, p 35.
14. Brumbaugh PF, Hughes MR, Haussler MR: Cytoplasmic and nuclear binding components for 1$\alpha$,25-dihydroxyvitamin $D_3$ in chick parathyroid glands. Proc Natl Acad Sci 72:4871, 1975.
15. Chan JCM, DeLuca HF: Growth velocity in a child on prolonged hemodialysis: Beneficial effect of 1$\alpha$-hydroxyvitamin $D_3$. JAMA 238:2053, 1977.
16. Chertow BS, Baylink DJ, Wergedal JF, et al: Decrease in serum immunoreactive parathyroid hormone in rats and in parathyroid hormone secretion in vitro by 1,25-dihydroxycholecalciferol. J Clin Invest 56:668, 1975.
17. Chesney RW: Modified vitamin D compounds in the treatment of certain bone diseases. In Spiller GA, Ed: Nutritional Pharmacology (Current Topics in Nutrition and Disease. Vol 4). Alan R Liss, New York, 1981, p 147.

18. Chesney RW, Moorthy AV, Jax DK: Increased linear growth after long-term oral 1,25(OH)$_2$-vitamin D therapy in childhood renal osteodystrophy. N Engl J Med 298:238, 1978.

19. Christakos S, Friedlander EJ, Frandsen BR, et al: Studies on the mode of action of calciferol. XIII. Development of a radioimmunoassay for vitamin D-dependent chick intestinal calcium-binding protein and tissue distribution. Endocrinology 104:1495, 1979.

20. Coburn JW: Renal osteodystrophy. Kidney Int 17:677, 1980.

21. Coburn JW, Brickman AS, Sherrard DJ, et al: Renal osteodystrophy and its relation to vitamin D: Identification of a mineralizing defect in uremia unrelated to vitamin D. In Endocrinology of Calcium Metabolism. Excerpta Medica, Amsterdam, 1977, p 27.

22. Coburn JW, DiDomenico NC, Bryce GF, et al: Prospective, double blind trial with calcitriol in the prophylaxis of bone disease in asymptomatic dialysis patients. In Norman AW, Schaefer K, von Herrath D, et al, Eds: Vitamin D: Chemical, Biochemical and Clinical Endocrinology of Calcium Metabolism. de Gruyter, Berlin 1982, p 833.

23. Coburn JW, DiDomenico NC, Bryce GG, et al: Use of calcitriol in prophylaxis of bone disease in dialysis patients. Kidney Int 23:145, 1983.

24. Coburn JW, Koppel MH, Brickman AS, et al: Study of intestinal absorption of calcium in patients with renal failure. Kidney Int 3:264, 1973.

25. Coburn JW, Slatopolsky E: Vitamin D, parathyroid hormone, and renal osteodystrophy. In Brenner BM, Rector FC Jr, Eds: The Kidney. 2nd Ed. Vol 2. Saunders, Philadelphia, 1981, p 2213.

26. DiDomenico NC, Bassett LW, Gold RH, et al: Course of x-rays and mineral content of bone during dialysis: Biochemical determinants. In Norman AW, Schaefer K, von Herrath D, et al: Eds: Vitamin D: Chemical, Biochemical and Clinical Endocrinology of Calcium Metabolism. de Gruyter, Berlin, 1982, p 877.

27. Eisman JA, Hamstra AJ, Kream BE, et al: 1,25-dihydroxyvitamin D in biological fluids: A simplified and sensitive assay. Science 193:1021, 1976.

28. Ellis HA, McCarthy JH, Herrington J: Bone aluminum in hemodialyzed patients and in rats injected with aluminum chloride: Relationship to impaired bone mineralization. J Clin Pathol 32:832, 1979.

29. Ellis HA, Pierides AM, Feest TG, et al: Histopathology of renal osteodystrophy with particular reference to the effects of 1-alpha-hydroxyvitamin D in patients treated by long-term hemodialysis. Clin Endocrinol 7[suppl]: 315, 1977.

30. Golden P, Mazey R, Greenwalt A, et al: Vitamin D: A direct effect on the parathyroid gland? Mineral Electrolyte Metab 2:1, 1979.

31. Goldstein DA, Horowitz RE, Petit S, et al: The duodenal mucosa in patients with renal failure: Response to 1,25 (OH)$_2$D$_3$. Kidney Int 19:324, 1981.

32. Goldstein DA, Malluche HH, Massry SG: Management of renal osteodystrophy with 1,25 (OH)$_2$D$_3$: I. Effects on chemical, radiographic and biochemical parameters. Mineral Electrolyte Metab 2:35, 1979.

33. Goldstein DA, Malluche HH, Massry SG: Long-term effects of 1,25 (OH)$_2$D$_3$ on clinical and biochemical derangements of divalent ions in dialysis patients. Contribution Nephrol 18:42, 1980.

34. Goodman WG, Henry DA, Nudelman RA, et al: Induction of osteomalacia in dogs following short-term injections of aluminum. Kidney Int 23:100, 1983.

35. Haussler MR, McCain TA: Basic and clinical concepts related to vitamin D metabolism and action. N Engl J Med 297:974, 1041, 1977.

36. Henderson RG, Russell RGG, Ledingham JGG, et al: Effects of 1,25-dihydroxycholecalciferol on calcium absorption, muscle weakness, and bone disease in chronic renal failure. Lancet 1:379, 1974.

37. Hodsman AB, Sherrard DJ, Alfrey AC, et al: Bone aluminum and histomorphometric features of renal osteodystrophy. J Clin Endocrinol 54:539, 1982.

38. Hodsman AB, Sherrard DJ, Wong EGC, et al: Vitamin D resistant osteomalacia in hemodialysis patients lacking secondary hyperparathyroidism. Ann Intern Med 94:629, 1981.

39. Hodsman AB, Wong EGC, Sherrard DJ, et

al: Preliminary trials with 24,25-dihydroxy-vitamin D$_3$ in dialysis osteomalacia. Am J Med 74:407, 1983.

40. Krempien B, Ritz E, Tschope W: The effect of 1,25(OH)$_2$D$_3$ on bone mineralization: Ultrastructural studies in patients with renal osteodystrophy. Contrib Nephrol 18:122, 1980.

41. Lambert PW, Stern PH, Avioli RC, et al: Evidence for extrarenal production of 1α,25-dihydroxyvitamin D in man. J Clin Invest 69:722, 1982.

42. Llach F, Massry SG, Singer FR, et al: Skeletal resistance to endogenous parathyroid hormone in patients with early renal failure: A possible cause for secondary hyperparathyroidism. J Clin Endocrinol Metab 41:339, 1975.

43. Madsen S, Olgaard K, Ladefoged J: Direct feed-back regulation of PTH-secretion by 1,25-dihydroxyvitamin D$_3$ in renal failure: A controlled trial. Proc EDTA 17:557, 1980.

44. Malluche HH, Goldstein DA, Massry SG: Management of renal osteodystrophy with 1,25 (OH)$_2$D$_3$ II. Effects on histopathology of bone: evidence for healing of osteomalacia. Mineral Electrolyte Metab 2:48, 1979.

45. Malluche HH, Werner E, Ritz E: Intestinal absorption of calcium and whole body calcium retention in incipient and advanced renal failure. Mineral Electrolyte Metab 1:263, 1978.

46. Massry SG, Stein R, Garty J, et al: Skeletal resistance to the calcemic action of parathyroid hormone in uremia: Role of 1,25 (OH)$_2$D$_3$. Kidney Int 9:467, 1976.

47. Massry SG, Tuma S, Dua S, et al: Reversal of skeletal resistance to parathyroid hormone in uremia by vitamin D metabolites. Evidence for the requirement of 1,25 (OH)$_2$D$_3$ and 24,25(OH)$_2$D$_3$. J Lab Clin Med 94:152, 1979.

48. Maxwell DR, Benjamin DM, Donahay SL, et al: Calcitriol in dialysis patients. Clin Pharmacol Ther 23:515, 1978.

49. Memmos DE, Eastwood JB, Talner LB, et al: Double-blind trial of oral 1,25-dihydroxy vitamin D$_3$ versus placebo in asymptomatic hyperparathyroidism in patients receiving maintenance haemodialysis. Br Med J 282:1919, 1981

50. Nagant de Deuxchaisnes C, Rombouts-

Lindemans C, Huaux JP, et al: Healing of vitamin D-deficient osteomalacia by the administration of 1,25 (OH)$_2$D$_3$. In McIntyre I, Syelke M, Eds: Molecular Endocrinology. Elsevier–North Holland, Amsterdam, 1979, p 375.

51. Nellans HN, Kimber DV: Cellular and paracellular calcium transport in rat ileum: effects of dietary calcium. Am J Physiol 236:E726, 1978.

52. Oldham SB, Smith R, Hartenbower DL, et al: The acute effects of 1,25-dihydroxycholecalciferol on serum immunoreactive parathyroid hormone in the dog. Endocrinology 104:248, 1979.

53. Ott SM, Maloney NA, Coburn JW, et al: The prevalence of bone aluminum deposition in renal osteodystrophy and its relations to the response to calcitriol therapy. N Engl J Med 307:709, 1982.

54. Ott SM, Maloney NA, Klein GL, et al: Aluminum is associated with low bone formation in patients receiving chronic parenteral nutrition. Ann Intern Med 98:910, 1983.

55. Peacock M, Heyburn PJ, Aaron JE, et al: Osteomalacia treated with 1-hydroxy or 1,25-dihydroxy vitamin D. In Norman AW, Schaefer K, Herrath DV, et al, Eds: Vitamin D Basic Research and its Clinical Application. de Gruyter, Berlin, 1979, p 1177.

56. Pierides AM, Ellis HA, Simpson W, et al: Variable response to long term 1-α-hydroxycholecalciferol in haemodialysis osteodystrophy. Lancet 1:1092, 1976.

57. Raisz LG, Maina DM, Gworek SC, et al: Hormonal control of bone collagen synthesis *in vitro*: Inhibitory effect of 1-hydroxylated vitamin D metabolites. Endocrinology 102:731, 1978.

58. Raisz LG, Trummel CL, Holick MF, et al: 1,25-dihydroxycholecalciferol: A potent stimulator of bone resorption in tissue culture. Science 175:768, 1972.

59. Rasmussen H, Fontaine O, Max EE, et al: The effect of 1α-hydroxyvitamin D$_3$ administration on calcium transport in chick intestine brush border membrane vesicles. J Biol Chem 254:2993, 1979.

60. Robertson JA, Felsenfeld AJ, Haygood CC, et al: Animal model of aluminum-induced

osteomalacia: Role of chronic renal failure. Kidney Int 23, 327, 1983.

61. Sherrard DJ, Baylink DJ, Wergedal JE, et al: Quantitative histological studies on the pathogenesis of uremic bone disease. J Clin Endocrinol 39: 119, 1974.

62. Sherrard DJ, Coburn JW, Brickman AS, et al: Skeletal response to treatment with 1,25-dihydroxyvitamin D in renal failure. Contrib Nephrol 18:92, 1980.

63. Shoback DM, Brown EM: Direct determination of cytosolic calcium concentration in dispersed cells from neonatal and adult bovine and abnormal human parathyroid tissue. Cal Tissue Int 35:687, 1983.

64. Slatopolsky E, Weerts C, Thielan J, et al: Marked suppression of secondary hyperparathyroidism by intravenous 1,25-(OH)$_2$D$_3$ in uremic patients. Kidney Int 23: 162, 1983.

65. Wilson L, Lam M, Felsenfeld A, et al: Role of 1,25-Dihydroxy-vitamin D$_3$ in patients with early renal failure. Kidney Int 23:219, 1983.

66. Winkler SN, Brickman AS, Wong EGC, et al: Hypercalcemia during treatment of uremic patients with 1,25 (OH)$_2$D$_3$: analysis of 43 cases. In Norman AW, Schaefer K, von Herrath D, et al, Eds: Vitamin D Basic Research and Its Clinical Application. de Gruyter, Berlin, 1979, p 851.

67. Wright RS, Mehls O, Ritz E, Coburn JW: Musculoskeletal manifestations of chronic renal failure, dialysis and transplantation. In Bacon PA, Hadler NM, Eds: The Kidney and Rheumatic Disease. Butterworth Scientific, London, 1982, p 342.

# Section V

## Controversies in Physiology and Pathophysiology

# 16

## The Pathogenesis of Progressive Renal Failure

# The Case for Tubulointerstitial Factors

Allen C. Alfrey, M.D.
Robert C. Tomford, M.D.

It has been reasonably well established that when a critical level of renal functional deterioration has occurred there is almost invariable progression to end-stage renal disease, even if the disease or condition initially responsible for the injury is eradicated or corrected.[1,37] Ahlmen found that the median time for progression to end-stage renal disease after the plasma creatinine had increased to 5 mg/dl was 6 months in patients with diabetic nephropathy, 10 months in patients with glomerulonephritis and 14 months in patients with nonobstructive pyelonephritis.[1] Therefore, it seems possible that these various forms of renal disease share a late common pathogenic mechanism which accelerates functional deterioration after a critical degree of renal damage has occurred from the initiating cause.

As a parallel to observations in the human experience, there are a number of animal models which show progression to terminal renal failure when a critical number of nephrons are destroyed by disease or injury.[14,20] In the remnant kidney (RK) model when 80 to 85 percent of the kidney is surgically removed the remaining nephrons hypertrophy and maintain a glomerular filtration rate (GFR) adequate for survival for a period of time.[14] Thereafter, proteinuria develops, progressive glomerulosclerosis occurs, and the animal dies of uremia.[14] In the nephrotoxic serum nephritis (NSN) model there is a similar course. Following the heterologous and autologous immunologic injury, GFR, although reduced, remains stable for a period of weeks and then shows progressive decline to end-stage renal diseases (ESRD).[20] In streptozotocin-induced diabetes in rats maintained on low-dose insulin there is an initial period of increased GFR lasting months followed by proteinuria, mesangial and glomerular basement membrane (GBM) morphologic and compositional changes, alterations in size and charge selective properties of the ultrafiltration barrier, decreased glomerular filtration and uremia.[13]

## THE ROLE OF ALTERED GLOMERULAR HEMODYNAMICS IN THE PROGRESSION OF RENAL DISEASE

One mechanism explaining the subsequent destruction of surviving nephron function currently receiving wide attention is the compensatory alterations in glomerular hemodynamics which occur secondary to losses of or injury to functioning nephrons. Hostetter et al. have demonstrated that the adaptive changes in the RK model consist of a reduction in afferent and efferent arteriolar resistances accompanied by increased glomerular plasma flow (GPF), glomerular transcapillary hydraulic pressure ($P_{GC}$) and single nephron GRF (SNGFR).[12] Associated with these alterations in glomerular hemodynamics was evidence of early glomerular structural damage which included focal areas of detached epithelial cells along the GBM, and expansion of the mesangial area with the deposition of circulating macromolecules.[12] It was suggested that the adaptive decrease in arteriolar resistances to maintain GFR exposed the glomerular tuft to elevated intracapillary pressures and flows which resulted in glomerular damage and glomerulosclerosis.[12] Further support for this hypothesis was produced by the same group who demonstrated that restricting RK rats' dietary protein consumption, which had previously been demonstrated to prevent uremia in RK animals,[26,38] also prevented the aforementioned hemodynamic and morphologic changes.[12] Similarly, if the adaptive hemodynamic changes are prevented in the remnant kidney by leaving the contralateral kidney in place the animal develops neither persistent histological changes nor proteinuria.[36]

Hypertensive animal models would tend to support these observations. The superimposition of hypertension upon various experimental immune glomerulonephritides worsens the morphologic glomerular disease and increases the degree of proteinuria and sclerosis.[19,27,33,40,42]

The studies of Maddox et al.[30] further support the suggestion that intrarenal hemodynamic alterations may cause renal injuries. In NSN it was found that although GPF and SNGFR were normal $P_{GC}$ was elevated, indicating a decreased afferent arteriolar resistance in this disease which allows the increased pressure to be transmitted to the glomerulus. Similarly, in streptozotocin-induced diabetic rats with moderate hyperglycemia $P_{GC}$ is also increased, as well as GPF.[13] It has also been shown that maneuvers which tend

to accentuate these vascular changes, unilateral nephrectomies,[41] and contralateral renal artery clip hypertension[31] accelerate the progression of renal failure and morphologic changes in this disease.

While the data cited provide strong evidence supporting the pathogenetic role of altered glomerular hemodynamics in progressive renal failure, regardless of inciting event, several questions remain regarding its actual role in the development of chronic renal failure (CRF). Many of the studies concerning the role of glomerular dynamics have been carried out relatively early in the course of disease.[12] More specifically, in contrast to the RK model, when the contralateral kidney is left intact in a unilateral model of NSN, the diseased kidney is not protected and progresses to ESRD.[46,47] This suggests either that renal hemodynamic changes are not important in this model or that any vascular alterations are a direct effect of the NSN and not necessarily an adaptive response to the loss of renal mass or function. In addition, severe streptozotocin-diabetes with marked elevation of blood sugar does not alter glomerular hemodynamics[13] but presumably is as likely as less severe drug-induced diabetes to cause CRF.

# THE ROLES OF PHOSPHATE RESTRICTION, PROTEIN RESTRICTION, AND THYROID ABLATION IN THE PROGRESSION OF RENAL DISEASE

Factors other than altered intrarenal hemodynamics may accelerate the rate of renal damage. These data are derived from nutritional studies and other apparently nonspecific maneuvers. Two independent groups have shown that patients with advanced renal insufficiency from various etiologies maintained on low protein nutritional therapy have a significant reduction in the rate of further renal functional loss.[9,3,49] Giordano showed that patients fed a 24 g protein diet had a slower rate of renal functional deterioration than a group of patients with comparable renal disease fed a normal 70 g protein diet.[9] Although both groups of patients had an average plasma creatinine of 5.0 mg/dl at the initiation of the above diet, the low protein group averaged 7.6 years to the development of ESRD as compared to 16 months for those on the normal protein diet. Walser's group has also demonstrated that reduced dietary protein plus essential amino acid or ketoacid analog supplementation decrease the rate of development of renal insufficiency.[49] In both studies, however, the phosphorus as well as protein intake was decreased, and, in fact, the plasma phosphorus levels were reduced from the high normal to low normal range in Walser's study. This led Walser, in reviewing the literature, to interpret the data to imply that phosphorus restriction alone might exert a similar beneficial effect.[49] At variance with this opinion, Barrientos et al.[2] failed to elicit a protective effect from phosphate restriction on renal insufficiency when initial serum creatinines were $\geq$ 2.0 mg/dl. Numerous factors could explain the lack of effect of phosphate restriction in this study since it is unknown when in the course of human renal failure phosphate restriction could be effective, how much phosphate restriction must be imposed to be effective or whether a combination of phosphate restriction and protein deprivation is required for the mediation of this effect.

Nutritional studies have been extended to experimental models of CRF to attempt to elucidate the mechanisms through which these dietary manipulations prevent and retard functional deterioration. Low protein diets prevent the development of renal failure in experimental anti-GBM nephritis,[6] the RK model of CRF,[26,38] and in a lupuslike nephritis, in NZB mice.[7,8] In addition, low caloric diets decrease the degree of glomerulosclerosis associated with aging in mice.[45] Thus, although inorganic dietary constituents were not well controlled and a role for phosphate restriction has not been entirely eliminated, it seems well documented that low protein dietary regimens alter processes involved in both immunologically and nonimmunologically mediated renal disease.

The mechanism through which protein restriction is protective was investigated in recent studies by Hostetter et al. as previously described.[12] Their data in the RK model suggested that protein restriction is protective through its prevention of altered renal hemodynamics. However, protein deprivation may be expected to have multiple systemic effects on such parameters as metabolism and the immune response, to be discussed later.

Dietary phosphate restriction (PR) has been found to be equally as protective as protein restriction in rats.[14,20] This manipulation has been shown not only to prevent histological damage and functional deterioration in NSN and RK but also to reverse proteinuria and histologic damage when instituted 30 days after the establishment of the remnant kidney.[14] These latter studies suggest that the protective effect afforded by PR may be mediated by mechanisms different from that of protein restriction, since it would have been expected at 30 days following the establishment of the RK, when PR was instituted, that the adaptive hemodynamic alterations of the RK model would have been in effect. If PR had reversed these adaptive increases in GPF and SNGFR it

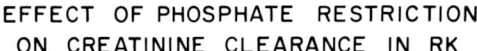

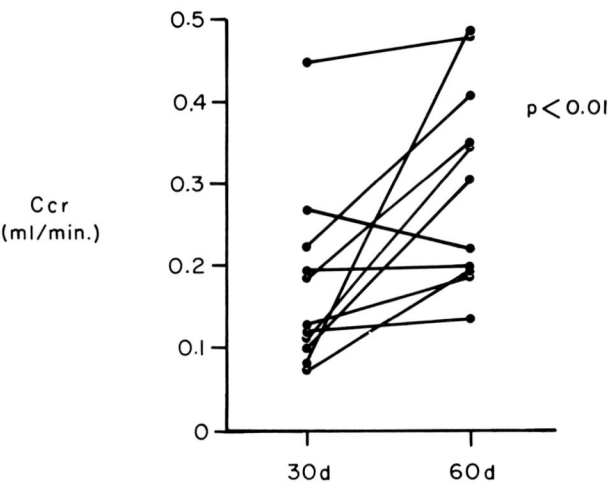

EFFECT OF PHOSPHATE RESTRICTION
ON CREATININE CLEARANCE IN RK

$p < 0.01$

**Fig. 16-1.** Animals with a remnant kidney were maintained on a normal diet for 30 days after which they were placed on a low phosphate diet for another 30 days. After being placed on a low phosphorus diet creatinine clearance increased in almost all animals.

would be expected, as found with protein restriction, that renal function should decrease.[12] However, renal function was actually found to improve following PR which suggests a pathway other than altered intrarenal dynamics[14,20] (Fig. 16-1).

Recently two other maneuvers which have been shown to have a major effect on NSN are thyroparathyroidectomy (TPTX) and selective thyroidectomy (TX). These two procedures are equally as protective against functional deterioration and histological damage as PR in NSN.[43,44] Furthermore, the protective effect of these procedures is mediated through the removal of thyroid hormone, since, if T4 is replaced, neither TX nor TPTX prevents CRF.[43]

### Underlying Mechanisms

It is somewhat difficult to envision a unifying concept to explain the protective effect that protein restriction, PR and thyroid ablation have on a diseased kidney. However, the fact that PR and protein restriction are effective in two widely dissimilar renal diseases with respect to etiology (RK and NSN) would suggest that they are exerting their protective effect by inhibiting some adaptive or secondary process that is common to injured kidneys. Although the effect of PR and thyroid ablation on glomerular dynamics and filtration in the diseased or damaged kidney is unknown it is apparent that all of these protective maneuvers could have multiple systemic effects.

It has largely been assumed that renal functional deterioration and tubule injury occur secondarily to glomerular damage. However, there is evidence to suggest that the converse can occur as well. In chronic interstitial nephritis and reflux nephropathy there is ample evidence showing that glomerulosclerosis develops and renal function deteriorates. The mechanism translating interstitial and tubular damage into glomerular injury and functional deterioration, is unknown.[25,51] One such mechanism which could promote progressive destruction of a diseased or damaged kidney is renal parenchymal calcification. Calcium phosphate deposits which could incite an inflammatory and fibrotic reaction and accelerate the rate of functional loss are commonly found in end-stage kidneys of animals and humans.[22,29,32,35] The pattern of calcification, primarily involving cortical tubular cells

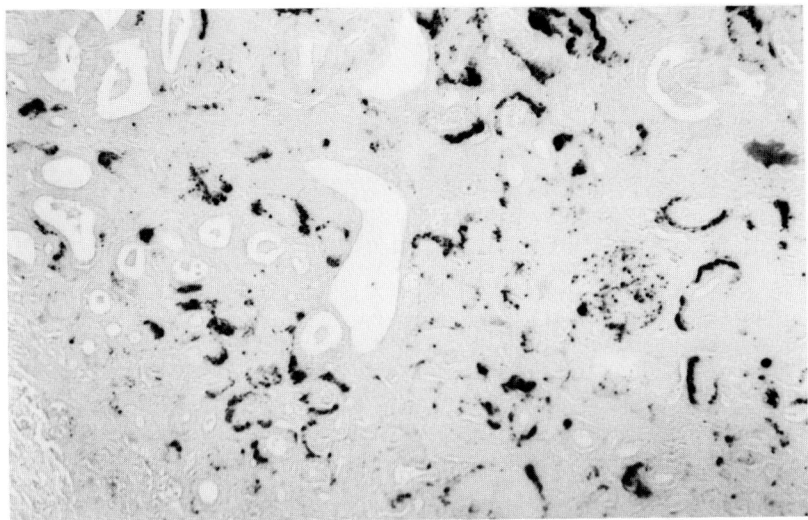

**Fig. 16-2.** Distinctive type of calcification which occurs in end-stage kidneys mainly involving cortical tubular cells and their basement membranes. (Reprinted by permission of the New England Journal of Medicine from Ibels LS, Alfrey AC, Huffer WE, et al: Preservation of function in experimental renal disease by dietary restriction of phosphate. N Engl J Med 298:122, 1978.)

and basement membrane[22,23,29,35] is similar to that noted in animals given toxic doses of parathyroid hormone,[39] suggesting that the secondary hyperparathyroidism present in renal insufficiency could cause these deposits (Fig. 16-2).

The protective effect of PR would be consistent with this mechanism since PR prevented renal parenchymal calcification[14,20] and suppressed parathyroid hormone secretion by causing hypercalcemia in rats.[20] However, parathyroidectomy has been found to have no effect on the rate of functional deterioration or the degree and pattern of renal calcification in ESRD animals with NSN.[43] Furthermore, significant functional deterioration and histological damage occur prior to the development of renal parenchymal calcification in NSN[43] (Fig. 16-3). These studies clearly demonstrate that PR does not exert its early protective effect by suppression of parathyroid hormone secretion and suggest that parathyroid hormone may not be involved in the pathogenesis of renal

parenchymal calcification in end-stage kidneys. Although the PR protective effect is not mediated through the prevention of renal parenchymal calcification, the possibility remains that renal calcification may accelerate renal parenchymal damage late in the course of renal failure.

It is of interest that all maneuvers known to accelerate or be permissive in the destruction of nephrons when renal mass is reduced (increased protein intake, thyroid hormone, phosphate and loss of nephron population) increase the energy requirements of remaining nephrons.[21,24,28] In contrast, the protective maneuvers (protein restriction, phosphate depletion and thyroid ablation) would all decrease energy requirements and oxygen consumption by the tubules.[21,24,28] Protein restriction exerts this effect by reducing glomerular filtration, sodium reabsorption and Na-K-ATPase activity.[21] Thyroid ablation would have a similar effect on sodium reabsorption and Na-K-ATPase[24] and has also been shown to de-

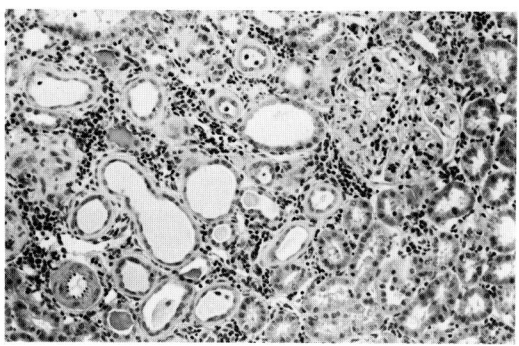

**Fig. 16-3.** Marked tubulo-interstitial disease in NSN at 30 days which preceded overt calcification. (From Tomford RC, Karlinsky ML, Buddington B, et al: Effect of thyroparathyroidectomy and parathyroidectomy on renal function and the nephrotic syndrome in rat nephrotoxic serum nephritis. J Clin Invest 68:655, 1981. By permission of the American Society for Clinical Investigation.)

crease mitochondrial respiration.[11] By removing substrate, phosphate depletion would also reduce mitochondrial respiration.[28]

Studies in hypoxic and chronic alcohol-induced liver disease seem to show that altered energy metabolism is also a possible mechanism for renal damage. Rats fed normal protein diets develop hepatocellular necrosis when exposed to 5 percent oxygen tension for 6 or more hours, whereas prior placement on a low protein diet markedly reduces the severity of liver lesions.[16] Pretreatment of these rats with 6-M-propylthiouracil (PTU), an antithyroid drug, completely suppressed the liver lesions produced by hypoxia even when the rats were fed a normal protein diet.[17] Furthermore, chronic alcohol-induced liver damage in rats, which results from increased oxygen requirements (increased Na-K-ATPase activity[17]), was also prevented by thyroidectomy and PTU.[18]

It is suggested that as a consequence of loss of renal functional units there are enhanced energy requirements on the re-

maining nephrons with resulting injury. It is well recognized that with reduction in renal mass Na-K-ATPase activity can be markedly increased.[21] Since 40 to 60 percent of the cell's ATP is consumed by Na-K-ATPase, an increased amount of Na-K-ATPase in association with enhanced single nephron sodium reabsorption could markedly increase the cell's requirement for ATP and mitochondrial respiration.

Tubule mitochondrial injury has been found to occur early in the course of NSN (Alfrey AC: unpublished observations). Since the majority of mitochondria are obtained from the tubule cells, these studies suggest an alteration in mitochondrial metabolism in this nephron segment in NSN. Since tubulointerstitial disease is a major part of NSN and precedes major glomerular disease,[44] we might conclude that this dysfunction plays a role in the pathogenesis of tubular damage. It is suggested that there is progressive deterioration in mitochondrial function which ultimately results in calcification of the mitochondria, leading to cellular death and inciting additional tissue injury. This would explain the distinctive pattern of calcification found in virtually all end-stage kidneys[15] (Fig. 16-4). The mechanism of mitochondrial injury in NSN is unknown. However, there are several possibilities. It seems possible that early in the course of renal disease the mitochondria were overactive, with this overactivity ultimately resulting in mitochondrial injury. This could especially be present in the remnant kidney model where, probably as a consequence of hyperfiltration, renal Na-K-ATPase activity would be markedly increased. A second possibility is that glomerular injury resulting from nephrotoxic serum somehow mediates injury to the mitochondria, possibly through decreased blood flow and ischemia. Irrespective of the cause, a reduction in energy requirements may exert a beneficial effect on mitochondrial

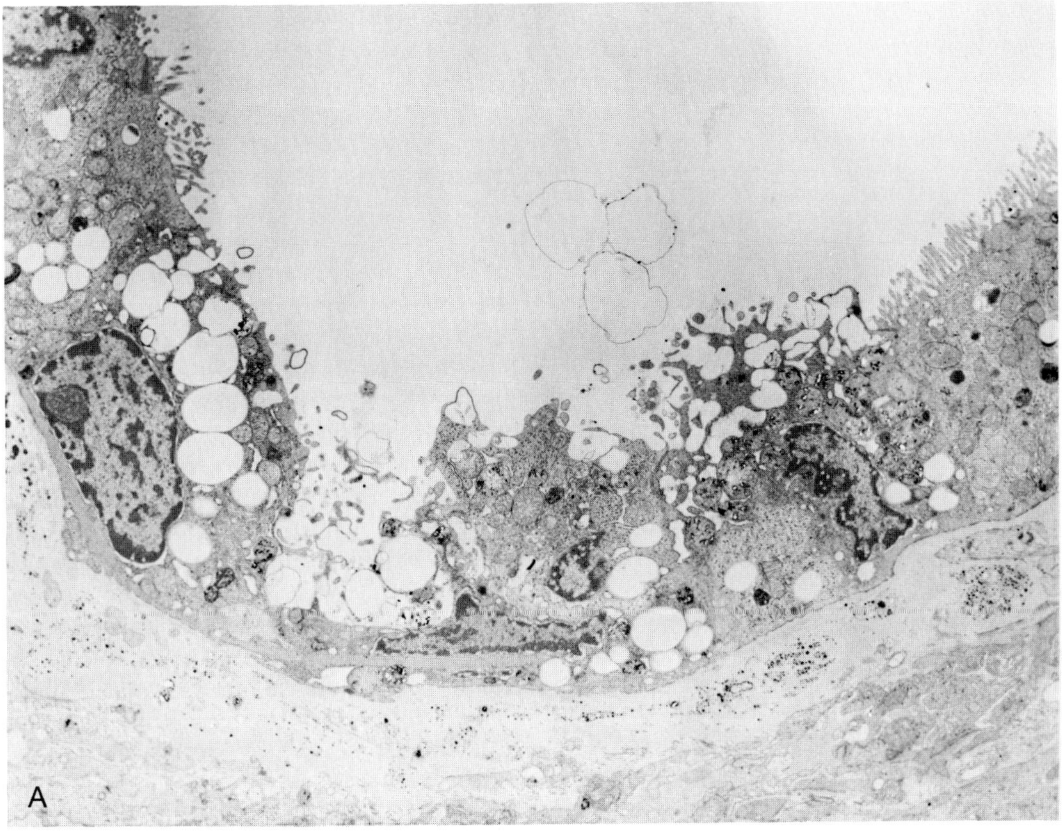

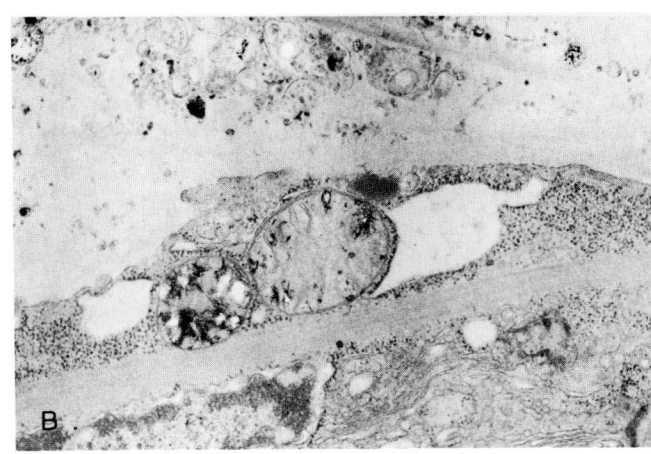

**Fig. 16-4.** (A) Electromicroscopic changes in the proximal tubule prior to marked functional deterioration in NSN. (B) Higher power view demonstrating mitochondrial calcification.

and renal damage. Another mechanism by which these three procedures could alter the course of renal functional deterioration is by blunting the intensity of the immune response. This would indicate that their effect on the RK model must be different from that in the NSN model since there is no solid evidence of a role for cell mediated and/or humoral immunity in RK renal disease. Hypophosphatemia has been demonstrated to depress chemotactic, phagocytic, and bactericidal activity of granulocytes.[5] The effect of hypothyroidism on the immune response has only recently been investigated. It has been demonstrated to have little or no effect on polymorphonuclear leukocytes (PMN) phagocytic and migratory capabilities[34] and B- and T-cell responses to salmonella[4] in humans, although the PMN bactericidal activity was suppressed.[34] Recently Wall et al. examined the effect of hypothyroidism on the various parameters of humoral and cellular immunity in rats and guinea pigs.[48] Their studies demonstrated that the antibody response was unaffected in guinea pigs but was decreased approximately 50 percent in rats. Delayed hypersensitivity to candida and PPD and in vitro macrophage function was unaffected. At this point it appears that hypothyroidism may decrease antibody production in rats but has no detectable effect on cell-mediated immunity or on the phagocytic and migratory properties of PMNs.

Studies have shown that protein depletion can also modify the immune response. In investigating the effect of dietary protein on murine lupus erythematosus, Friend et al. demonstrated that low protein diets decreased the histological severity of the glomerulonephritis and tended to decrease the DNA binding titers.[8] The degree of protein restriction appears to be important since severe malnutrition produces immunologic abnormalities involving both humoral and cellular mechanisms,[50,10] while moderate degrees of restriction depress antibody production without alterations in cell mediated responses.[32] Thus, it appears that one possible common mechanism for the effect of all the manipulations on renal function in immune mediated renal disease may be modulation of the immune response, and this aspect deserves further investigation.

Finally, it is possible that protein restriction, PR and thyroid ablation have separate and distinct protective effects on experimental renal disease. This is suggested by the fact that whereas thyroid ablation prevents proteinuria and functional deterioration in NSN,[43] it prevents neither in the RK model. This might indicate that several of the secondary or compensatory events suggested are important in promoting progressive renal damage in an already diseased kidney or that different mechanisms promoting destruction are involved in the various types of experimental renal diseases.

To conclude, it is becoming evident that there are secondary factors shared by renal diseases which are initiated by a variety of different etiologies and mechanisms which cause progressive destruction of the diseased kidney. These would appear to involve adaptive, secondary, or compensatory mechanisms resulting from renal damage or loss of nephron population. More encouraging is the fact that this late or secondary destruction of the diseased kidney is not necessarily inevitable in that several different manipulations have been found to prevent it from occurring. As this knowledge expands, it seems increasingly possible that it will be feasible to prevent or retard the progression of chronic renal failure to end-stage disease in humans.

# REFERENCES

1. Ahlmen J: Incidence of chronic renal insufficiency. Acta Med Scan [Suppl] 582:1, 1975.
2. Barrientos A, Arteaga J, Rodicio T, et al: Role of control of phosphate in the progression of chronic renal failure. Mineral Elec Metab 7:127, 1982.
3. Barsotti G, Guiducci A, Ciardella F, et al: Effects on renal function of a low-nitrogen diet supplemented with essential amino acids and ketoanalogues and of hemodialysis and free protein supply in patients with chronic renal failure. Nephron 27:113, 1981.

4. Chatterjee S, Chandel AS: Immunoregulatory role of thyroid and its hormones. Proc 4th Int Congr Immunology, Paris, 18-3-10, 1980.

5. Craddock PR, Yawata Y, VanSauten L, et al: Acquired phagocyte dysfunction: A complication of the hypophosphatemia of parenteral hyperalimentation. N Engl J Med 290:1403, 1974.

6. Farr LE, Smadel JE: The effect of dietary protein on the course of nephrotoxic nephritis in rats. J Exp Med 70:615, 1939.

7. Fernandes G, Yunis EJ, Good RA: Influence of diet on survival of mice. Proc Natl Acad Sci USA 73:1279, 1976.

8. Friend P, Fernandes G, & Good RA: Dietary restrictions early and late: effects on the nephropathy of the NZB × NZW mouse. Lab Invest 38:629, 1978.

9. Giordano C: Early diet to slow the course of chronic renal failure. Proc 8th Int Congr Nephrol. Athens:71, 1981.

10. Good RA, Fernandes G, Yunis EJ, et al: Nutritional deficiencies, immunologic function, and disease. Am J Pathol 84:599, 1976.

11. Gufstaffson R, Tata JR, Linsberg O, et al: The relationship between structure and activity of rat skeletal mitochondria after thyroidectomy and thyroid hormone treatment. J Cell Biol 26:555, 1965.

12. Hostetter TH, Olson JL, Rennke HG, et al: Hyperfiltration in remnant nephrons: a potentially adverse reaction to renal ablation. Am J Physiol 241:F85, 1981.

13. Hostetter TH, Troy JL, Brenner BM: Glomerular hemodynamics in experimental diabetes. Kidney Int 19:410, 1981.

14. Ibels LS, Alfrey AC, Haut L, et al: Preservation of function in experimental renal disease by dietary restriction of phosphate. N Engl J Med 298:122, 1978.

15. Ibels LS, Alfrey AC, Huffer WE, et al: Calcification in end-stage kidneys. Am J Med 71:33, 1981.

16. Israel Y, Kalant H, Orrego H, et al: Experimental alcohol-induced hepatic necrosis: suppression by propylthiouracil. Proc Natl Acad Sci USA 72:1137, 1975.

17. Israel Y, Videla L, Bernstein J: Liver hypermetabolic state after chronic ethanol consumption, hormonal interrelationships and pathogenic implications. Fed Proc 34:2052, 1975.

18. Israel Y, Videla L, Fernandez VV: Effects of chronic ethanol treatment and thyroxine administration on ethanol metabolism and liver oxidative capacity. J Pharmacol Exp Ther 192:565, 1975.

19. Iversen BM, Ofstad J: Influence of hypertension on the course of experimental renal failure in rats (abstr). Kidney Int 18:142, 1980.

20. Karlinsky ML, Haut L, Buddington B, et al: Preservation of renal function in experimental glomerulonephritis. Kidney Int 17:293, 1980.

21. Katz AI, Epstein FH: Physiologic role of sodium-potassium-activated adenosine triphosphatase in the transport of cations across biologic membranes. N Engl J Med 278:253, 1968.

22. Katz AI, Hampers CL, Merrill JP: Secondary hyperparathyroidism and renal osteodystrophy in chronic renal failure: analysis of 195 patients, with observations on the effects of chronic dialysis, kidney transplantation and subtotal parathyroidectomy. Medicine (Baltimore) 43:333, 1969.

23. Katz AI, Hampers CL, Wilson RE, et al: The place of subtotal parathyroidectomy in the management of patients with chronic renal failure. Trans Am Soc Artif Intern Organs 14:376, 1968.

24. Katz AI & Lindheimer MD: Renal sodium and potassium-activated adenosine triphosphatase and sodium reabsorption in the hypothyroid rat. J Clin Invest 52:796, 1973.

25. Kincaid-Smith P, & Becker GJ: Reflux nephropathy in adults. In Hodson CJ, Kincaid-Smith P, Eds: Reflux Nephropathy. Masson Publishing, New York, 1979.

26. Kleinknecht C, Salusky I, Broyer M, et al: Effect of various protein diets on growth, renal function and survival of uremic rats. Kidney Int 15:534, 1979.

27. Knowlton AL, Stoerk H, Seegal BC, et al: Influence of adrenal cortical steroids upon the blood pressure and the rate of progression of experimental nephritis in rats. Endocrinology 38:315, 1946.

28. Kreusser WJ, Kurokawa K, Aznar E, et al:

Phosphate depletion. Effect on renal inorganic phosphorus and adenine nucleotides, urinary phosphate and calcium, and calcium balance. Mineral and Elect Metab 5:30, 1978.

29. Kuzela DC, Huffer WE, Conger JD, et al: Soft tissue calcification in chronic dialysis patients. Am J Pathol 86:403, 1977.

30. Maddox DA, Bennett CM, Deen WM, et al: Determinants of glomerular filtration in experimental glomerulonephritis in the rat. J Clin Invest 55:305, 1975.

31. Mauer SM, Steffes MW, Azar S, et al: The effect of Goldblatt hypertension on the development of glomerular lesions of diabetes mellitus. Diabetes 27:738, 1978.

32. McMurray DN, Yetley EA: Immune responses in malnourished guinea pigs. J Nutr 112:167, 1982.

33. Neugarten J, Feiner HD, Schact RG, et al: Aggravation of experimental glomerulonephritis by superimposed clip hypertension. Proc Am Soc Nephrol 14:81a, 1981.

34. Palmblad J, Adamson U, Rosenqvist U, et al: Neutrophil function in hypothyroid patients. Acta Med Scand 210:287, 1981.

35. Pollak VE, Schneider AF, Freund G, et al: Chronic renal disease with secondary hyperparathyroidism, Arch Intern Med 103: 200, 1959.

36. Purkerson ML, Hoffsten PE, Klahr S: Pathogenesis of the glomerulopathy associated with renal infarction in rats. Kidney Int 9:407, 1976.

37. Rutherford WE, Blondin J, Miller JP, et al: Chronic progressive renal disease: rate of change of serum creatinine concentration. Kidney Int 11:62, 1977.

38. Salusky I, Kleinknecht C, Broyer M, et al: Prolonged renal survival and stunting with protein deficient diets in experimental amino acids. J Lab Clin Med 97:21, 1981.

39. Schneider AF, Reaven EP, Reaven G: A comparison of renal calcification produced by parathyroid extract or calcium gluconate. Endocrinology 67,733, 1960.

40. Steffs MW, Brown DM, Basgen JM, et al: The volume and surface of the mesangium prior to and following islet transplantation

in uninephrectomized and diabetic rats. Diabetes 29:509, 1980.

41. Steffes MW, Brown DM, Mauer SM: Diabetic glomerulopathy following unilateral nephrectomy in the rat. Diabetes 27:53, 1978.

42. Tikkanen I, Fryquist F, Miettinen A, et al: Autologous immune complex nephritis and DOCA-NaCl load: a new model of hypertension. Acta Pathol Microbiol Scand 88:241, 1980.

43. Tomford RC, Buddington B, Alfrey AC: Thyroidectomy prevents chronic renal insufficiency in nephrotoxic serum nephritis in rats. Kidney Int 21:231a, 1982.

44. Tomford RC, Karlinsky ML, Buddington B, et al: Effect of thyroparathyroidectomy and parathyroidectomy on renal function and the nephrotic syndrome in rat nephrotoxic serum nephritis. J Clin Invest 68:655, 1981.

45. Tucker SM, Mason RL, Beauchene R: Influence of diet and feed restrictions on kidney function in aging male rats. J Gerontol 31:264, 1976.

46. Wagnild JP, Gutmann FD, Burkholder PM: Unilateral glomerulonephritis in the split bladder dog. Lab Invest 29:642, 1973.

47. Wagnild JP, Gutmann FD, Rieselbach RE: Functional characterization of chronic unilateral glomerulonephritis in the dog. Kidney Int 5:422, 1975.

48. Wall JR, Twohig P, Chartier B: Effects of experimental hyper and hypothyroidism on the numbers of blood mononuclear cells and immune function in rats and guinea pigs. J Endocrinol 91:61, 1981.

49. Walser M: Does dietary therapy have a role in the predialysis patient? Am J Clin Nutr 33:1629, 1980.

50. Watson RR, McMurray DN: The effects of malnutrition on secretory and cellular immune processes. CRC Crit Rev Food Sci Nutr 13:113, 1979.

51. Zimmerman SW, Uehling DT, Burkholder PM: Vesicoureteral reflux nephropathy: evidence for immunologically-mediated glomerular injury. Urology 2:534, 1973.

# The Role of Intrarenal Hypertension and Hyperperfusion in Progressive Glomerular Injury

Timothy W. Meyer, M.D.
Sharon Anderson, M.D.
Barry M. Brenner, M.D.

Serious chronic renal insufficiency generally progresses to end-stage renal failure. Patients in whom glomerular filtration rate is reduced to about 25 ml/min may expect eventually to require dialysis or transplantation, regardless of the original cause of reduced function. Time plots of the reciprocal of serum creatinine generally reveal steady erosion of glomerular function at rates peculiar to individual patients but not characteristic of the underlying disease (Fig. 16-5).[51,64] Furthermore, renal function may ultimately cease even when disease processes such as hypertension or vesicoureteric reflux have been therapeutically controlled. These observations suggest that, after a certain point, reduction in functioning nephron number leads to failure of the remaining units. Hope of interrupting this process has stimulated investigation into the mechanism(s) responsible for progressive injury to functioning nephrons in kidneys damaged by disease. Recent experimental evidence suggests that continuing loss of these residual nephron units may be a predictable consequence of the glomerular hemodynamic response to widespread renal injury.

## GLOMERULAR HYPERPERFUSION AND THE PROGRESSION OF EXPERIMENTAL RENAL DISEASE

The simplest model of reduced nephron number is provided by surgical nephrectomy. As is well known, reduction of renal mass induces an increase in the single nephron glomerular filtration rate of remnant nephrons.[30] Vascular resistance is reduced in both afferent and efferent arterioles, allowing an increase in single nephron glomerular plasma flow rate.[13] Furthermore, the reduction in afferent arteriolar resistance is proportionately greater than the reduction in efferent arteriolar resistance, so that the average glomerular transcapillary hydraulic pressure gradient is increased. Together, the in-

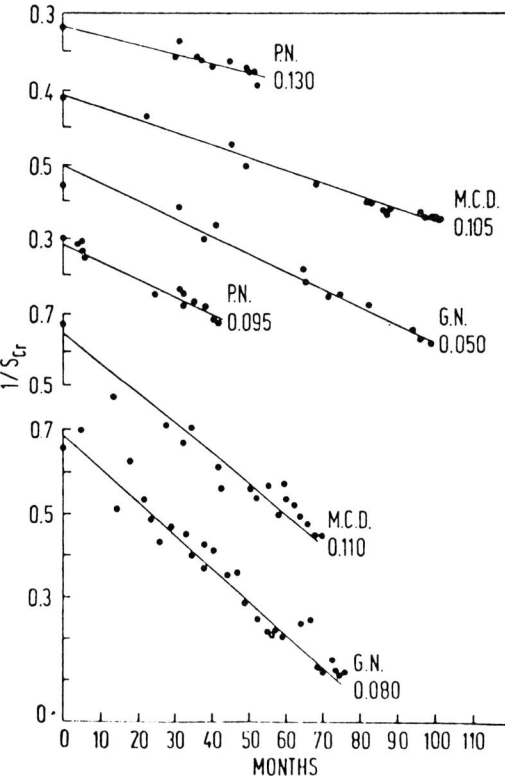

**Fig. 16-5.** Plots of reciprocol serum-creatinine concentrations (in mg/dl) versus months of observation in 6 patients with chronic renal insufficiency. Diagnoses: PN, pyelonephritis; MCD, medullary cystic disease; GN, glomerulonephritis. Reprinted with permission from Mitch WE, Walser M, Buffington GA, et al.: A simple method for estimating progression of chronic renal failure. Lancet 2:1326, 1976.)

creases in capillary plasma flow and hydraulic pressure account for the elevation in glomerular filtration rate of remnant nephrons. The magnitude of the increase in remnant nephron glomerular filtration rate, and of the underlying reductions in arteriolar resistance, correlates closely with the amount of renal mass which has been ablated. Thus, in the rat, removal of 80 percent of the renal mass results in an increase in remnant nephron glomerular filtration rate to more than twice normal, while with uninephrectomy the increment averages 40 to 50 percent.[13]

Increased filtration by remnant nephrons has been generally regarded as "adaptive" since it partially offsets the loss of function which would otherwise follow nephrectomy. A growing body of evidence, however, suggests that the hemodynamic changes which cause remnant nephron hyperfiltration eventually prove injurious to residual glomeruli. Fifty years ago Chanutin and Ferris[11] showed that removal of three-fourths of the renal mass in rats led to a syndrome of proteinuria and progressive glomerular sclerosis, ultimately resulting in uremic death. Shimamura and Morrison[65] profiled the development of pathologic changes in initially normal remnant glomeruli following approximately 85 percent renal ablation. Early glomerular hypertrophy was accompanied at 3 months by ultrastructural changes including vacuolization of epithelial cells and "fusion" of epithelial cell foot processes. By 6 months there was notable expansion of the mesangium along with focal areas of denudation of endothelial and epithelial cells from the glomerular basement membrane. Progressive mesangial expansion and collapse of capillary lumina eventually resulted in the appearance of focal sclerosis (Fig. 16-6).

In rats, the pace of injury to remnant glomeruli, like the magnitude of remnant glomerular hemodynamic changes, increases in proportion to the loss of renal mass.[33,59,65] Uninephrectomy, which results in a modest increase in glomerular capillary hydraulic pressure and a 40 to 50 percent increase in glomerular capillary plasma flow rate, is associated with moderate acceleration of the glomerular sclerosis normally seen in aging rats with two kidneys.[67] Following 90 to 95 percent nephrectomy, however, increases in glomerular capillary pressures and flows are more dramatic, and glomerular morphologic changes can be detected within two weeks of the ablation procedure.[33] Evidence that increased capillary pressures

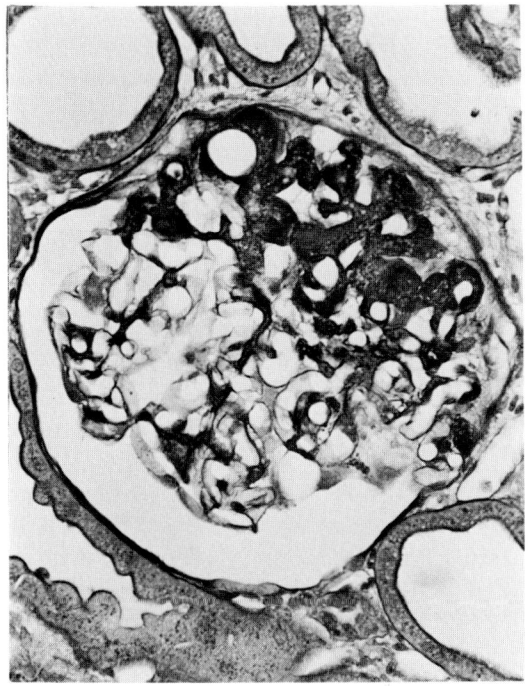
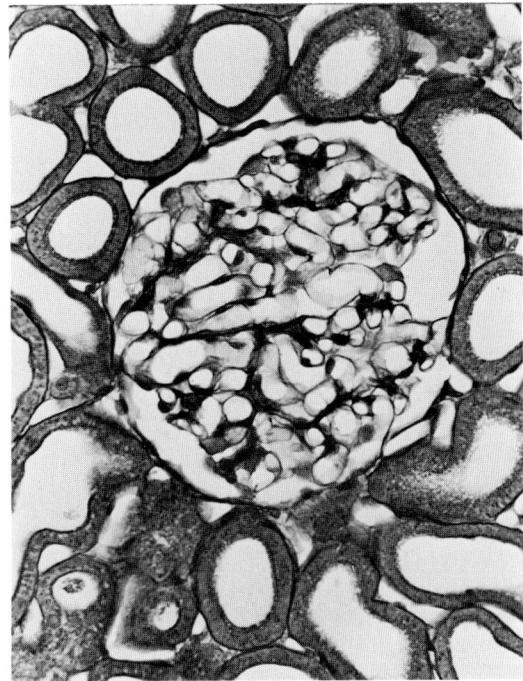

**Fig. 16-6.** Left: Segmental glomerular sclerosis observed 8 months after unilateral nephrectomy and infarction of approximately one-third of the remaining kidney of a Munich-Wistar rat. Right: Normal glomerular architecture seen in an age-matched control animal with intact kidneys. (Magnification × 330, photomicrographs courtesy of Dr. H.G. Rennke.)

and flows initiate glomerular injury has been obtained from studies of such extensive renal ablation. Severe restriction of dietary protein intake, which lowers glomerular filtration rate in intact animals,[36] was used to blunt adaptive hyperfiltration following reduction of renal mass.[33] In animals fed a 6 percent protein diet, capillary flows and pressures were maintained at near normal values following renal ablation, so that the average value of the single nephron glomerular filtration rate in the remnant kidney was restricted to 38 ± 6 nl/min. This was markedly lower than the average single nephron glomerular filtration rate of 62 ± 6 nl/min found in rats which had undergone a similar degree of ablation but had been fed standard laboratory chow containing 24 percent protein. Limitation of glomerular hyperfiltration and prevention of glomer-

ular capillary hypertension and hyperperfusion by protein restriction was associated with preservation of glomerular structure. Within 2 weeks following ablation, remnant kidneys of animals fed standard chow showed protein reabsorption droplets in glomerular epithelial cells with attenuation of epithelial cell bodies and focal fusion of foot processes. These epithelial cell changes were associated with lifting of endothelial cells from the inner aspect of the glomerular basement membrane and with increases in mesangial area. Glomerular morphologic abnormalities were much less extensive in remnant kidneys of protein restricted rats. In addition, remnant kidney proteinuria was limited in protein restricted rats, suggesting preservation of the glomerular permselectivity barrier. More recent studies have shown that dietary protein restriction also lowers remnant kidney glomerular filtration rate and retards development of proteinuria and glomerular sclerosis in rats subjected to less extensive renal ablation.[47,49] The beneficial effects of protein restriction have been demonstrated not only in these functional and morphologic studies but in other studies showing that reduction of protein intake increases the life span of rats subjected to renal ablation.[44]

Increased glomerular pressures and flows have been observed not only following surgical nephrectomy but in various experimental models of diffuse renal disease.[32] The ability of remnant glomeruli in the midst of injury to respond to reductions in renal mass was initially demonstrated in animals with unilateral renal disease. Removal of the normal kidney promptly induced hyperfiltration in residual functioning nephrons of the diseased kidney.[46] Hyperfiltration has since been shown to occur when the number of functioning nephrons is reduced by advancing disease rather than by nephrectomy. Like hyperfunctioning glomeruli of remnant kidneys, hyperperfused residual glomeruli of diseased kidneys may presumably be damaged by increased capillary pressures and flows. Support for this concept has been provided by Azar and coworkers,[3,4] who have demonstrated that premature glomerular sclerosis is associated with elevated glomerular capillary pressures and flows in "post-salt" hypertensive rats. An association between glomerular capillary hypertension and hyperperfusion and glomerular pathology has also been established in "DOCA-salt" hypertensive rats by Dworkin et al.[16]

Studies of protein restriction in "DOCA-salt" hypertension appear to confirm the importance of glomerular hemodynamic changes in the initiation of glomerular pathology. In DOCA-salt treated rats, as in rats subjected to extensive renal ablation, protein restriction lowers glomerular capillary pressures and flows,

limits proteinuria, and lessens the extent of glomerular morphologic changes.[16] Variation of dietary protein content has not been studied extensively in other disease models, but protein restriction has been shown to retard the progression of nephrotoxic serum nephritis in rats,[18,20,54] and the lupus-like nephropathy of the NZB/NZW mouse.[23] While the effects of protein restriction could be due to suppression of immune responsiveness, other manipulations that affect the progression of experimental disease suggest the importance of altered glomerular hemodynamic parameters. Thus, uninephrectomy worsens histopathology and increases mortality in the NZB/NZW mouse[8] and in rabbits given nephrotoxic serum.[68] Presumably, an increase in capillary pressures and flows induced by nephrectomy accelerates glomerular destruction. Other maneuvers that increase glomerular capillary pressures and flows likewise magnify pathologic changes in experimental glomerular disease. Heyman nephritis can be aggravated by DOCA salt treatment[69] while in Dahl rats experimental immune complex disease is made more severe when glomerular capillary pressure is raised above control levels by salt feeding.[61] Likewise, when a clip is placed around one renal artery ("two kidney" Goldblatt hypertension) glomerular capillary pressures and flows are higher in the unclipped than in the clipped kidney. As might be expected, when unilateral clip hypertension is superimposed on nephrotoxic serum nephritis lesions are more severe in the unclipped than in the clipped kidney.[55]

## THE PROGRESSION OF HUMAN RENAL DISEASE

Taken together, the experimental studies described above suggest that increased glomerular capillary pressures and flows initiate glomerular injury when nephron number is reduced and accelerate glomerular injury following other insults to the kidney. Studies in humans, though necessarily less direct, support the view that hyperperfused nephrons ultimately fail. Morphologic studies in human renal disease have demonstrated hypertrophy (presumably reflecting hyperperfusion and hyperfiltration) of those nephrons least damaged by disease.[29] Clinical studies have demonstrated progressive loss of renal function associated with increasing glomerular sclerosis in patients whose initiating disease process has remitted spontaneously or been controlled therapeutically. Patients with bilateral cortical necrosis may temporarily recover stable, albeit reduced, renal function, before proceeding to end-stage renal failure.[43] Recovery of renal function is frequently incomplete in acute renal failure of other etiologies, and in some of these cases progressive loss of renal function also follows initial recovery.[22] Patients with vesicoureteric reflux who have developed significant impairment of renal function and glomerular disease manifested by proteinuria may progress to renal failure despite control of systemic hypertension, prevention of urinary tract infection, and surgical correction of the reflux.[71] Likewise, patients with analgesic nephropathy, sometimes said to exhibit stable renal insufficiency, in fact often progress to renal failure despite discontinuation of analgesic medications.[41] Progressive glomerular sclerosis in the absence of continuing immunologic injury has been demonstrated in certain patients after initial recovery from acute poststreptococcal glomerulonephritis.[5] Moreover, in analogy with animal experiments illustrating the effects of renal artery constriction on experimental nephritis, patients with coincident glomerulonephritis and renal artery stenosis have been shown to have less severe glomerulonephritic lesions in the hypofunctioning kidney "protected"

by the arterial stenosis.[15,27,57] Hemodynamic factors might also explain the observation that pregnancy, which raises glomerular filtration and renal blood flow rates in normal women, frequently accelerates loss of renal function in women with preexisting renal disease.[40]

These clinical studies add support to the hypothesis that progressive glomerular injury is hemodynamically mediated. Fueled by this hypothesis, a number of relevant questions emerge. First, how much renal mass must be lost in humans to induce progressive glomerular disease in the absence of ongoing renal injury? An increased incidence of focal glomerular sclerosis has been reported in patients with unilateral renal agensis;[42] but it is possible that the solitary kidneys of these patients, like the kidneys of patients with bilateral reduction in nephron number ("oligomegonephronia"[17]), are congenitally abnormal. Preliminary reports of patients followed from 10 to 20 years after nephrectomy for transplant donation suggest an increased incidence of hypertension and mild proteinuria but no major reduction in the glomerular filtration rate over this time period.[14,28] Longer-term follow-up studies of patients who have had one kidney removed for trauma or localized tumor and of patients who have had uninephrectomy and partial resection of the other kidney for bilateral tumor are required to establish the consequences of reducing nephron number in humans.

A second question is whether increased glomerular capillary pressures and flows can initiate progressive glomerular disease when the number of functioning nephrons is normal. Normal subjects show a progressive decline in glomerular filtration and renal blood flow rates after the third decade; values in the eighth decade are only one-half to two-thirds those measured in young adults.[12,63] Progressive loss of renal function with aging is associated with sclerosis of an increasing portion of the total glomerular population.[38] We have recently suggested that age-related glomerular sclerosis is caused by sustained elevations in glomerular capillary pressures and flows associated with current dietary practices, in particular with ad libitum intake of protein rich foods.[9] Certain disease processes may further increase the hemodynamic burden of an initially normal glomerular population. Patients with sickle cell anemia have markedly increased glomerular filtration and renal plasma flow rates during the first decade of life, but by the third decade renal function is reduced.[19] Sickle cell nephropathy is usually attributed to medullary and papillary ischemia but glomerular sclerotic lesions, accompanied by notable proteinuria, occur often.[1] Presumably, sustained glomerular hyperperfusion early in life contributes to later development of glomerular pathology. The glomerular filtration rate is also increased in juvenile onset diabetics at the time of diagnosis and throughout the first decade of the disease.[52] Equivalent hyperfiltration in rats with experimental diabetes has been shown to result from elevations in glomerular capillary pressures and flows similar to those seen in the remnant kidney.[34] These observations have prompted the suggestion that glomerular hyperperfusion in diabetes initiates a cycle of glomerular injury causing exaggerated glomerular hemodynamic changes and leading, in turn, to accelerated glomerular destruction.[35] Why renal failure ultimately develops in about one out of three juvenile diabetic patients is unknown; studies correlating the magnitude of early hyperfiltration in juvenile diabetics with later development of diabetic nephropathy remain to be performed. Early glomerular sclerosis in familial dysautonomia, occasionally severe enough to cause renal insufficiency, could likewise be related to glomerular hemodynamic abnormalities in this disorder.[58]

A third question concerns the role of hyperperfusion of individual glomerular capillary loops in progressive glomerular disease. Hyperperfusion of capillary segments may occur not only when perfusion of structurally normal glomeruli is increased but also when glomerular blood flow is channeled through a reduced number of capillary loops. Reduction in the number of glomerular capillary loops—so-called glomerular simplification—has been observed in DOCA-salt hypertension and may contribute to accelerated glomerular sclerosis in this condition.[31] Likewise, reduction in the number of capillary channels could contribute to progressive glomerular sclerosis following recovery from acute glomerulonephritis. Ongoing glomerular damage reflected by proteinuria appears to occur in such patients when total nephron number is reduced by less than 50 percent, that is, with a lesser reduction in nephron number than would result from uninephrectomy.[24] The role of glomerular simplification in this process, however, remains to be established.

## ALTERNATIVE EXPLANATIONS OF THE PROGRESSIVE NATURE OF RENAL DISEASE

Factors other than glomerular capillary hypertension and hyperperfusion have been considered to account for progressive glomerular sclerosis following surgical nephrectomy and in diffuse renal disease. Early workers believed that systemic hypertension induced by renal ablation was responsible for pathologic changes in the remnant kidney.[74] Later studies, however, showed that glomerular sclerotic changes were poorly correlated with elevations in systemic blood pressure.[45] Moreover, while early glomerular sclerosis occurs in "post-salt" and "DOCA-salt" hypertensive rats, it is not prominent in spontaneously hypertensive rats (SHRs) which have equally elevated systemic pressures but more normal glomerular capillary pressures and flows.[2] Early proteinuria and glomerular sclerosis in this strain are confined to juxtamedullary nephrons which have higher filtration rates and presumably higher pressures and/or flows than those of the outer cortex.[6,21] Finally, following renal ablation preservation of glomerular architecture in the remnant kidney by protein restriction is achieved without reduction in systemic blood pressure[33,47] while normalization of blood pressure with antihypertensive drug therapy only moderately reduces the extent of glomerular lesions.[59]

Alfrey and coworkers have suggested that deposition of calcium salts in the renal interstitium causes progressive loss of renal function in rats with remnant kidneys[37] or nephrotoxic serum nephritis.[39] This suggestion was supported by the demonstration that restriction of phosphorus intake preserved renal function, prolonged life span, and reduced ultimate renal tissue calcium content in both groups. Excess calcification in animals maintained on normal chow, confined largely to the tubules and interstitium, was considered to result from an increase in the calcium-phosphorus product, an increase in the single nephron inorganic phosphate load, and/or an increase in the level of parathormone. Later studies by this group, however, proved that parathyroid ablation does not protect against progressive loss of renal function in nephrotoxic serum nephritis.[70] Moreover, in these studies, marked interstitial pathology, proteinuria, and functional deterioration were shown to precede any increase in renal calcium content. The efficacy of phosphate restriction in preventing these manifestations of progressive disease, therefore, must not depend entirely on in-

hibition of intrarenal calcification. Moreover, rats with nephrotoxic serum nephritis developing terminal uremia while maintained on routine phosphate intake in one study had elevations of kidney calcium content to only three times normal, suggesting that the earlier finding of a 20-fold elevation in kidney calcium content in remnant kidney animals maintained on routine phosphorous intake was due largely to calcification of scar tissue.[2,21] Finally, the degree of phosphate restriction shown to preserve renal function in rats with remnant kidneys or nephrotoxic serum nephritis was stringent enough to reduce plasma phosphate levels below normal and to reduce kidney weight in the nephritic animals. When these studies are considered together it appears that the well-documented protective effect of phosphate restriction may not have been related to prevention of intrarenal calcium salt deposition but to some other effect of phosphate deprivation, including possibly reduction of the glomerular filtration rate[10] or suppression of immune responsiveness.

The presence of immunoglobulins (particularly IgM) in diseased glomeruli of remnant kidneys has raised the possibility that an immune response directed against renal antigens could cause progressive loss of kidney function following renal ablation. Immune complexes, however, have not been noted in damaged glomeruli of remnant kidneys. Furthermore, when part of one kidney is infarcted and the contralateral kidney is left intact rather than excised, accelerated glomerular damage does not occur.[73,59]

It has also been suggested recently that progression of chronic renal disease may be mediated by abnormalities of lipid metabolism.[53] According to this hypothesis levels of circulating lipids are increased in response to initial renal injury. Various lipid fractions, primarily low density lipoproteins, are hypothesized to then cause further progressive damage to the glomerular basement membrane and to mesangial structures. To the best of our knowledge, current evidence favoring of the nephrotoxicity of circulating lipids is slim. Hyperlipidemia in early renal insufficiency is most clearly related to nephrotic proteinuria and hypoalbuminemia. Rates of decline in renal function, however, are poorly related to rates of protein excretion. In patients without primary renal disease, hyperlipidemia is not usually associated with early loss of renal function, though a rare familial syndrome of lecithin:cholesterol acyltransferase deficiency, characterized by an abnormal low density lipoprotein fraction and chronic anemia, does lead to renal failure in middle life.[26]

## THERAPIES AIMED AT INTERRUPTING THE PROGRESSION OF RENAL DISEASE

If elevated glomerular capillary pressures and flows cause progressive glomerular sclerosis in patients with renal insufficiency, therapies aimed at an initial reduction in glomerular perfusion may be required to preserve renal function over the long term. An obvious possible therapy is restriction of dietary protein intake, implemented early in the course of intrinsic renal disease. Promising results suggesting that protein restriction indeed slows the progression of a variety of renal disorders have recently been published.[28,45] Other therapies directed toward limiting glomerular capillary pressures and flows may ultimately prove more effective or more palatable than protein restriction. The mechanisms responsible for the reduction in afferent arteriolar resistance which causes hyperfiltration when nephron number is reduced are as

yet unknown. Elucidation of these mechanisms is of obvious importance to the design of therapeutic intervention aimed at preventing glomerular hyperperfusion and hyperfiltration.

It is conceivable that injury to hyperfiltering remnant glomeruli can be prevented by means other than reducing capillary pressures and flows. In this regard, it is worth considering how elevated pressures and flows damage the glomerulus (Fig. 16-7). One possible mechanism is mechanical injury to the glomerular endothelium. Denudation of endothelial cells from the glomerular basement membrane has been noted following extensive renal ablation.[33] Endothelial damage may, in turn, result in exposure of circulating proteins to basement membrane constituents, thereby precipitating intracapillary coagulation. Capillary thrombosis has been demonstrated in glomeruli of remnant kidneys following renal ablation in rats and heparin therapy has been shown to retard the progression of glomerular disease in this model.[59,60]

Increased capillary pressures and flows may also damage the glomerulus by promoting increased movement of macromolecules through the glomerular capillary wall and into the glomerular mesangium. Rats subjected to high-grade nephrectomy eventually excrete several hundred milligrams of protein per day as compared to approximately 10 mg/day in control animals.[11] Studies employing tracer macromolecules have shown that remnant kidney proteinuria results from defects in both the charge and size-selective properties of the glomerular capillary wall.[56,62] It is not clear that passage of macromolecules through the capillary wall and into the urinary space by itself aggravates glomerular injury. Damage to the filtration barrier has, however, been associated with increased deposition of tracer macromolecules into the mesangium both

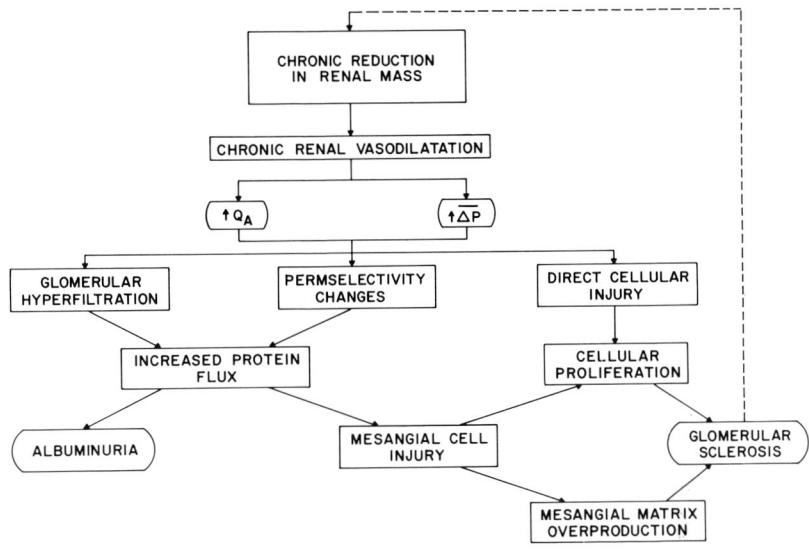

**Fig. 16-7.** Role of sustained increases in glomerular pressures and flows in the progression of glomerular sclerosis when nephron number is reduced. (Modified, by permission of the New England Journal of Medicine, from Brenner BM, Meyer TW, Hotstetter TH: Dietary protein intake and the progressive nature of kidney disease, N Engl J Med 307:652, 1982.)

in the remnant kidney[56] and in other disease models.[66] An increase in mesangial "trafficking" of macromolecules may in turn promote increases in mesangial matrix area and cellularity leading eventually to glomerular sclerosis.[50,66]

Clearly, much remains to be learned about the mechanisms responsible for progressive glomerular injury when nephron number is reduced. Exciting but as yet unexplained recent findings include the observations that increasing dietary intake of the prostaglandin precursor linoleic acid preserves renal function in remnant kidney rats,[7] while inhibition of prostaglandin synthesis retards development of proteinuria and glomerular sclerosis in aging rats with intact kidneys.[72] Further experimental studies relating both nutritional and pharmacologic maneuvers to glomerular function should ultimately enable us to prevent progressive loss of renal function in patients whose kidneys have been damaged by disease.

# REFERENCES

1. Alfrey AC: The renal response to vascular injury. In Brenner BM, Rector FC Jr, Eds: The Kidney. Saunders, Philadelphia, 1981, pp 1668–1718.
2. Arendshorst WJ, Beierewaltes WH: Renal and nephron hemodynamics in spontaneously hypertensive rats. Am J Physiol 236:F246, 1979.
3. Azar S, Johnson MA, Hertel B, et al: Single-nephron pressures, flows and resistances in hypertensive kidneys with nephrosclerosis. Kidney Int 12:28, 1977.
4. Azar S, Johnson MA, Junichi I, et al: Single-nephron dynamics in "post-salt" rats with chronic hypertension. J Lab Clin Med 91:156, 1978.
5. Baldwin DA: Poststreptococcal glomerulo-

nephritis: A progressive disease? Am J Med 62:1, 1977.

6. Bank N, Allerman L, Aynedjian HS: Selective JM nephron hyperfiltration in SHR rats with reduced renal mass (abstr). Proc Am Soc Nephrol 15:118A, 1982.

7. Barcelli UO, Weiss M, Pollak VE: Effects of a dietary prostaglandin precursor on the progression of experimentally induced chronic renal failure. J Lab Clin Med 100:786, 1982.

8. Beyer MM, Steinberg AD, Nicastri AD, Friedman EA: Unilateral nephrectomy: Effect on survival in NZB/NZW mice. Science 198:511, 1977.

9. Brenner BM, Meyer TW, Hostetter TH: Dietary protein intake and the progressive nature of kidney disease. N Engl J Med 307:652, 1982.

10. Carter HR, Merado A, Rutherford WE, et al: Effects of phosphate depletion and parathyroid hormone on glucose reabsorption. Am J Physiol 227:1422, 1974.

11. Chanutin A, Ferris EB: Experimental renal insufficiency produced by partial nephrectomy. I. Control diet. Arch Intern Med 49:767, 1932.

12. Davies DF, Shock NW: Age changes in glomerular filtration rate, effective renal plasma flow, and tubular excretory capacity in adult males. J Clin Invest 29:496, 1950.

13. Deen WM, Maddox DA, Robertson CR, et al: Dynamics of glomerular ultrafiltration in the rat. VII. Response to reduced renal mass. Am J Physiol 227:556, 1974.

14. Delano BG, Lazar IL, Friedman EA: Hypertension, a late consequence of kidney donation (abstr). Proc Am Soc Nephrol 15:75A, 1982.

15. Dikman SH, Strauss L, Berman LJ, et al: Unilateral glomerulonephritis. Arch Pathol Lab Med 100:480, 1976.

16. Dworkin LD, Hostetter TH, Rennke HG, Brenner BM: Evidence for a hemodynamic basis for glomerular injury in hypertension (abstr). Kidney Int 21:229, 1982.

17. Elema JD: Is one kidney sufficient (abstr)? Kidney Int 9:308, 1976.

18. El-Nahas AM, Zoob S, Evans DJ, et al: Modification of the course of nephrotoxic nephritis by diet (abstr). Kidney Int 22:219, 1982.

19. Etteldorf JN, Smith JS, Tuttle AH, et al: Renal hemodynamic studies in adults with sickle cell anemia. Am J Med 18:243, 1955.

20. Farr LE, Smadel JE: The effect of dietary protein on the course of nephrotoxic nephritis in rats. J Exp Med 70:615, 1939.

21. Feld LG, van Liew JB, Galaske RG, et al: Selectivity of renal injury and proteinuria in the spontaneously hypertensive rat. Kidney Int 12:332, 1977.

22. Finn WF: Recovery from acute renal failure. In Brenner BM, Ed: Acute Renal Failure. Saunders, Philadelphia, 1983.

23. Friend PS, Fernandes G, Good RA, et al: Dietary restrictions early and late: Effects on the nephropathy of the NZB × NZW mouse. Lab Invest 38:629, 1978.

24. Gallo GR, Feiner HD, Steele JM, et al: Role of intrarenal vascular sclerosis in progression of poststreptococcal glomerulonephritis. Clin Nephrol 13:49, 1980.

25. Giordano C: Protein restriction in chronic renal failure. Kidney Int 22:401, 1982.

26. Gjone E, Blomhoff JP, Skarbonk AJ: Possible association between an abnormal low density lipoprotein and nephropathy in lecithin: Cholesterol acyltransferase deficiency. Clinica Chimica Acta 54:11, 1974.

27. Godin M, Fillastre JP, Ducastelle T, et al: Sarcoidosis: Retroperitoneal fibrosis, renal artery involvement, and unilateral focal glomerulosclerosis. Arch Intern Med 140:1240, 1980.

28. Goldszer RC, Hakim RM, Brenner BM: Long-term follow up of renal function in kidney transplant donors (abstr). Proc Am Soc Nephrol 15:31a, 1982.

29. Gottschalk CW: Function of the chronically diseased kidney: The adaptive nephron. Circ Res 28:Suppl 1:1, 1971.

30. Hayslett JP: Functional adaptation to reduction in renal mass. Physiol Rev 59:137, 1979.

31. Hill GS, Heptinstall RH: Steroid-induced hypertension in the rat. Am J Pathol 52:1, 1968.

32. Hostetter TH, Brenner BM: Glomerular adaptations to renal injury. P. 1–27. In Brenner BM, Stein JH, Eds: Contemporary Is-

sues in Nephrology. Vol 7. Chronic Renal Failure. Churchill Livingstone, New York, 1981.

33. Hostetter TH, Olson JL, Rennke HG, et al: Hyperfiltration in remnant nephrons: A potentially adverse response to renal ablation. Am J Physiol 241:F85, 1981.

34. Hostetter TH, Troy JL, Brenner BM: Glomerular hemodynamics in experimental diabetes. Kidney Int 19:410, 1981.

35. Hostetter TH, Rennke GH, Brenner BM: The case for intrarenal hypertension in the initiation and progression of diabetic and other glomerulopathies. Am J Med 72:375, 1982.

36. Ichikawa I, Purkerson ML, Klahr S, et al: Mechanism of reduced glomerular filtration rate in chronic malnutrition. J Clin Invest 65:982, 1980.

37. Ibels LS, Alfrey AC, Haut L, Huffer WE: Preservation of function in experimental renal disease by dietary restriction of phosphate. N Engl J Med 298:122, 1978.

38. Kappel B, Olsen S: Cortical interstitial tissue and sclerosed glomeruli in the normal human kidney, related to age and sex. Virchows Arch (Pathol Anat) 387:271, 1980.

39. Karlinsky ML, Haut L, Buddington B, et al: Preservation of renal function in experimental glomerulonephritis. Kidney Int 17:293, 1982.

40. Kincaid-Smith P: The Kidney, a Clinico-Pathological Study. Blackwell, Oxford, pp 222–239.

41. Kincaid-Smith P: Analgesic abuse and the kidney. Kidney Int 17:250, 1980.

42. Kiprov DD, Colvin RB, McCluskey RT: Focal and segmental glomerulosclerosis and proteinuria associated with unilateral renal agenesis. Lab Invest 46:275, 1982.

43. Kleinknecht D, Grünfeld JP, Gomez PC, et al: Diagnostic procedures and long-term prognosis in bilateral renal cortical necrosis. Kidney Int 4:390, 1973.

44. Kleinknecht C, Salusky I, Broyer M, et al: Effect of various protein diets on growth, renal function, and survival of uremic rats. Kidney Int 15:534, 1979.

45. Koletsky S: Role of salt and renal mass in experimental hypertension. AMA Arch Pathol 68:11, 1959.

46. Lubowitz H, Purkerson ML, Sugita M, et al: GFR per nephron and per kidney in chronically diseased (pyelonephritic) kidney of the rat. Am J Physiol 217:853, 1969.

47. Madden MA, Zimmerman SW: Protein restriction and renal function in the uremic rat (abstr). Proc Am Soc Nephrol 15:124A, 1982.

48. Maschio G, Oldrizzi L, Tessiture N, et al: Effects of dietary protein and phosphorus restriction on the progression of early renal failure. Kidney Int 22:371, 1982.

49. Meyer TW, Hostetter TH, Rennke HG, et al: Preservation of renal structure and function by long term protein restriction in rats with reduced nephron mass (abstr). Proc Am Soc Nephrol 15:125A, 1982.

50. Michael AF, Keane WF, Raij L, et al: The glomerular mesangium. Kidney Int 17:141, 1980.

51. Mitch WE, Walser M, Buffington GA, et al: A simple method for estimating progression of chronic renal failure. Lancet 2:1326, 1976.

52. Mogensen CE: Renal function changes in diabetes. Diabetes 25:872, 1976.

53. Moorehead JF, El-Nahas M, Chan MK, et al: Lipid nephrotoxicity in chronic progressive glomerular and tubulo-interstitial disease. Lancet 2:1309, 1982.

54. Neugarten J, Feiner H, Schacht RG, et al: Ameliorative effect of dietary protein restriction on the course of nephrotoxic serum nephritis (abstr). Clin Res 30:541A, 1982.

55. Neugarten J, Feiner HD, Schacht RG, et al: Aggravation of experimental glomerulonephritis by superimposed clip hypertension. Kidney Int 22:257, 1982.

56. Olson JL, Hostetter TH, Rennke HG, et al: Altered glomerular permselectivity and progressive sclerosis following extreme ablation of renal mass. Kidney Int 22:112, 1982.

57. Palmer JH, Eversole SL, Stamey TA: Unilateral glomerulonephritis. Am J Med 40:816, 1966.

58. Pearson J, Gallo G, Gluck M, Axelrod F: Renal disease in familial dysautonomia. Kidney Int 17:102, 1980.

59. Purkerson ML, Hoffsten PE, Klahr S: Path-

ogenesis of the glomerulopathy associated with renal infarction in rats. Kidney Int 9:407, 1976.

60. Purkerson ML, Joist JH, Greenberg JM, et al: Inhibition of anticoagulant drugs of the progressive hypertension and uremia associated with renal infarction in rats. Thrombosis Res 26:227, 1982.

61. Jaij L, Azar S, Keane WF: Role of hypertension and mesangial injury in progressive glomerular damage. Proc Am Soc Nephrol 15:126A, 1982.

62. Robson AM, Mor J, Root ER, et al: Mechanism of proteinuria in nonglomerular disease. Kidney Int 16:416, 1979.

63. Rowe JW, Andres R, Tobin JD, et al: The effect of age on creatinine clearance in man: A cross sectional and longitudinal study. J Gerontol 31:155, 1976.

64. Rutherford WE, Blondin J, Miller JP, et al: Chronic progressive renal disease: Rate of change of serum creatinine. Kidney Int 11:62, 1977.

65. Shimamura T, Morrison SB: A progressive glomerulosclerosis occurring in partial five-sixths nephrectomized rats. Am J Pathol 79:95, 1975.

66. Sterzel RB, Lovett DH, Stein HD, et al: The mesangium and glomerulonephritis. Klin Wochenschr 60:1077, 1982.

67. Striker GE, Nagle RB, Kohnen PW, et al: Response to unilateral nephrectomy in old rats. Arch Pathol 87:439, 1969.

68. Teoduru CV, Saifer A, Frankel H: Conditioning factors influencing evolution of experimental glomerulonephritis in rabbits. Am J Physiol 196:457, 1959.

69. Tikkanen I, Fyhrquist F, Miettinen A, et al: Autologous immune complex nephritis and DOCA-NaCl load: A new model of hypertension. Acta Path Microbiol Scand 88:241, 1980.

70. Tomford RC, Karlinsky ML, Buddington B, et al: Effect of thyroparathyroidectomy and parathyroidectomy on renal function and the nephrotic syndrome in rat nephrotoxic serum nephritis. J Clin Invest 68:655, 1981.

71. Torres VE, Velosa JA, Holley KE, et al: The progression of vesicoureteral reflux. Ann Intern Med 92:776, 1980.

72. Vanrenterghem Y, Roels L, VanDamme B, et al: Influence of indomethacin treatment on the spontaneous glomerulosclerosis of the rat. Kidney Int 61:659, 1979.

73. White FN, Grollman A: Autoimmune factors associated with infarction of the kidney. Nephron 1:93, 1964.

74. Wood JE Jr, Ethridge C: Hypertension with arteriolar changes in the albino rat following subtotal nephrectomy. Proc Soc Exp Biol Med 30:1039, 1933.

# 17

# The Mechanism of Action of Aldosterone and Glucocorticoids and Their Effects on Fluid– Electrolyte Metabolism: Review of Ongoing and Emerging Controversies

Christine P. Bastl, M.D.
Diana Marver, Ph.D.

## INTRODUCTION

In recent years the interplay between adrenal steroids and electrolyte transport has undergone a revolution. With identification of steroid structure in the 1950s came their functional classification into glucocorticoids which modulate metabolic functions and mineralocorticoids which control external electrolyte balance. As knowledge of steroid receptor physiology matured, it became clear that corticosteroids showed crossover binding of mineralocorticoids to glucocorticoid receptors and vice versa.[32,34,71,124] More recent experiments have controlled for this phenomenon, thereby allowing for more precise designation of given biochemical and physiologic process as mineralocorticoid or glucocorticoid functions.

Despite marked differences in their spectrum of physiologic effects and in their target sites, gluco- and mineralocorticoids may act synergistically on kidney and gastrointestinal (GI) tract to influence sodium reabsorption and potassium excretion. Where it has been examined closely, however, mineralocorticoids appear to regulate acute transport changes while glucocorticoids modulate steady-state electrolyte handling.

The overall intent of this chapter is to

compare and contrast the interplay of these two classes of steroids on fluid-electrolyte metabolism in the two steroid-responsive organs, kidney and colon, and to discuss controversies regarding their actions.

# ADRENAL STEROIDS AND ELECTROLYTE TRANSPORT: GENERAL ASPECTS

The consequences of adrenal insufficiency include hyponatremia, hyperkalemia, renal sodium wasting, hypotension, impairment of maximal renal concentration and dilution, metabolic acidosis and hemoconcentration.[52] Selective replacement of glucocorticoids corrects the impaired ability to both maximally concentrate and dilute urine and consequent osmolality disturbances. Correction of the electrolyte disturbances and acidosis, although classically considered to require aldosterone, may actually require *both* mineralocorticoids and glucocorticoids.

It should be noted that both classes of steroid modify renal and intestinal electrolyte transport. The kidney's contribution to fluid-electrolyte homeostasis is an order of magnitude greater that that of the GI tract and may increase further in times of stress. Nevertheless, examination of the effects of these hormones on intestinal and renal transport is important since it allows us to compare and contrast the actions of corticosteroids in these two mammalian target epithelia.

## Cellular Mechanism of Action

The mechanism by which aldosterone stimulates sodium and potassium transport is still under investigation. Figure 17-1 depicts several important features of the most widely held model for aldosterone-stimulated sodium/potassium trans-port. In the upper panel, aldosterone is shown to freely enter the cell and bind to a cytoplasmic receptor. The binding of the hormone activates the receptor and the hormone-receptor complex enters the nucleus, where it, in turn, binds to specific acceptor sites on chromatin. Existing evidence suggests that various spirolactones compete with aldosterone for cytoplasmic receptor sites and once bound, prevent receptor activation and thereby, preclude binding to key chromatin sites.[84] The attachment of the aldosterone-activated receptor complex to chromatin acceptor sites leads to the biochemical construction of messenger RNAs (mRNAs) coding for specific proteins.[32,36,37,52,81]

Existing evidence suggests that the effects of glucocorticoids on their target epithelia are mediated by receptor mechanisms very similar to that of aldosterone[36,52] (Fig. 17-2). Glucocorticoids bind to a unique cytoplasmic receptor; the latter is activated and the complex is translocated into the nucleus where it attaches to a chromatin acceptor and codes for specific proteins. Doses of spirolactones which strongly inhibit mineralocorticoid action, exert little effect on the interaction of glucocorticoids with its receptor.[124] Although these models are attractive, to date no mineralocorticoid and relatively few glucocorticoid-induced proteins have been isolated or identified. Aldosterone has been shown, however, to increase the apparent activity of several mitochondrial enzymes. Furthermore, several changes in cellular transport capacity occur which suggest that mineralocorticoid induced membrane:membrane protein alterations have taken place.[32]

Most studies of mineralocorticoid action have focused on four potential rate-limiting steps in cation transport.[32,52,81] First, aldosterone may influence either the synthesis or recruitment of amiloride-inhibitable sodium channels in the apical membrane.[93] Second, mineralocorticoids

**Fig. 17-1.** Schematic representation of target cells for aldosterone. The upper panel depicts a target cell which mediates aldosterone-stimulated sodium reabsorption while the bottom panel depicts a target cell which mediates aldosterone-stimulated hydrogen secretion. The luminal PD profile is negative with respect to blood in the sodium-reabsorbing cell while it is positive in the hydrogen-secreting cell. In the models, aldosterone (A) freely enters the cell and binds to a receptor (R). This aldosterone: receptor complex (AR) undergoes an activation step (AR') which enhances its affinity for specific acceptor sites on chromatin. This process initiates a cascade of events which includes the synthesis of mRNAs and eventually new proteins. The possible identity of the induced proteins and how the processes might differ in the two types of cells are discussed in the text.

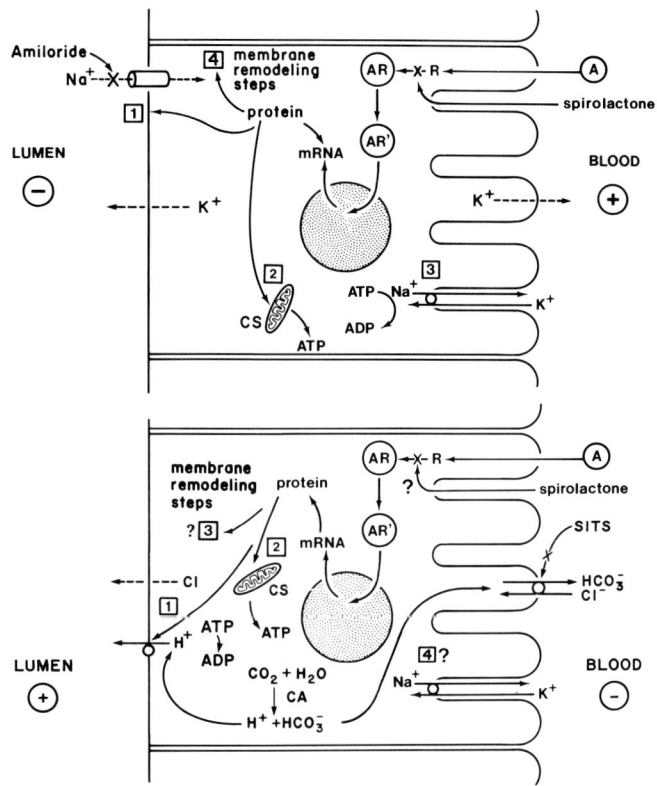

may induce or activate a series of rate-limiting enzymes involved in the delivery of reducing equivalents to the mitochondrial respiratory chain leading to the generation of ATP. Third, aldosterone may activate or induce NaK-ATPase. This enzyme is a translocator of sodium and potassium which utilizes ATP to achieve transport against an electrochemical gradient. Fourth, the hormone may influence the phospholipid composition of specific membranes within target cells. The cellular locale of membranes altered by aldosterone is unknown since reported studies using toad bladder did not discriminate between the various classes of membranes within the cell nor did they identify the specific cell types so affected.[44] Thus, it is conceivable that modifications of membrane phospholipid content induced by aldosterone might influence sodium and potassium permeability of the luminal membrane, facilitate the action of NaK-ATPase in the basolateral membrane, or influence another aldosterone-mediated process, proton secretion, detailed below. Stimulation of all of these mechanisms simultaneously however, would facilitate transcellular sodium reabsorption and potassium entry into cells.

The fate of potassium once in the cell depends on the intrinsic permeabilities of luminal and antiluminal membranes to the cation and the electrochemical driving force for potassium secretion. Whether or not steroids asymmetrically influence the intrinsic potassium permeability of the luminal and antiluminal membranes is a debate which will be considered in succeeding sections.

Aldosterone also influences renal acid excretion. Recent work in both toad bladder and in mammalian kidney has indi-

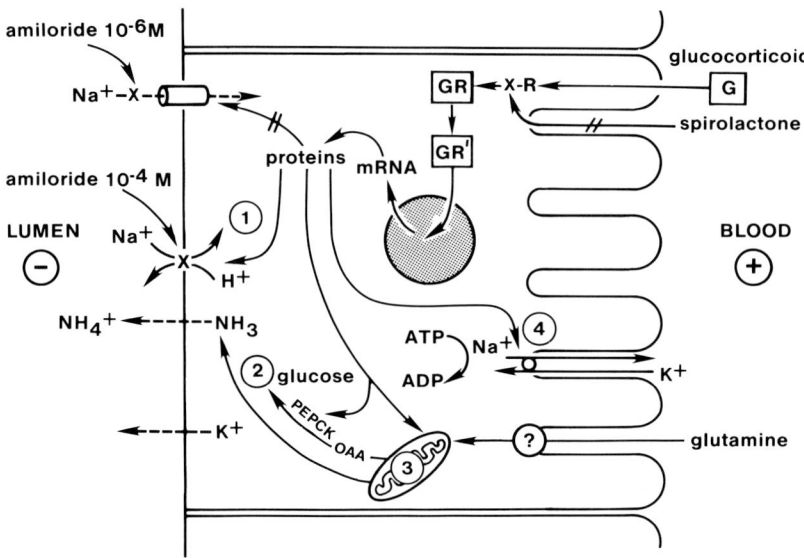

**Fig. 17-2.** Schematic representation of target cells for glucocorticoids. All processes need not occur in all cell types affected by the steroid. Again the lumen potential is negative with respect to blood in the sodium-reabsorbing cell. In this model, glucocorticoids (G) freely enter their target cells and bind to receptors (R) for which spirolactones have comparatively little affinity. The steroid-receptor complex is activated and translocated to specific nuclear acceptor chromatin resulting in synthesis of mRNA and new proteins. As discussed in the text, cell processes (1–4) have been suggested as glucocorticoid inducible sites of action.

cated that aldosterone-responsive proton secretion is isolated to distinct cell types.[115] Unlike the mediation of steroid-induced changes in sodium and potassium transport, there is uncertainty as to whether the response of proton secretion is receptor related. Both spironolactone and aldosterone stimulate acid secretion by toad bladder.[88] Since receptor agonist and antagonist both stimulate secretion, it follows that aldosterone mediated acid secretion is likely to be receptor-independent. On the other hand, that segmental site along the mammalian nephron which is responsive to mineralocorticoid-stimulated acid secretion is rich in aldosterone-specific receptors. Furthermore, the classical inhibitors of mineralocorticoid receptor mediated sodium transport, actinomycin D and cycloheximide, have been found to have little effect on aldosterone-stimulated acid secretion, and in fact tend to stimulate rather than block acid secretion when given in the absence of steroids.[73,75] Thus, the role of the receptor in acid secretion is still unresolved.[29,115]

Present data would suggest that ATP driven proton pumps are responsible for active acid secretion in both toad bladder and in the distal nephron.[12] Such a process may not be as simple as that delineated in Fig. 17-1 since these pumps may be coupled to redox reactions in the membrane. Although proton secretion in some portions of the nephron may occur via a sodium-hydrogen antiport system, the sodium independence of the event in the distal nephron suggests that acid secretion by the medullary collecting duct is not mediated via such exchangers.[115]

Using the model depicted in Fig.

17-1, aldosterone could either influence shuttling of membrane containing proton pumps, analagous to the system presented by Al-Awqati and colleagues to explain $CO_2$ stimulation of proton secretion[1,2,43]; it could influence energy or substrate production; or as Fanestil has suggested, aldosterone could reverse the action of a preexisting inhibitor protein.[75] Again, membrane remodeling steps could ultimately prove to be very important. In fact, a recent finding by Al-Awqati et al. further emphasizes this possibility. They demonstrated that $PCO_2$ influenced the fusion of intracellular vesicles with the luminal membrane and coincident with this fusion hydrogen ion secretory activity was enhanced.[43] Thus, it is conceivable that alterations in the nature of the phospholipids at either the luminal membrane or in intracellular membrane-limited bodies following aldosterone could ultimately influence acid secretion.

The cellular model for the mechanism of action of glucocorticoids is even more speculative than that for aldosterone (Fig. 17-2). Studies with the aldosterone receptor antagonist spironolactone indicate that glucocorticoids increase sodium absorption in the colon through binding to its specific receptor, not to the aldosterone receptor.[9,18,19] (1) There is evidence suggesting that glucocorticoids increase uptake of sodium into colonic epithelial cells by a pathway separate from that stimulated by aldosterone.[8,39] Unlike aldosterone, low-dose glucocorticoid-induced sodium transport is insensitive to blockade of the luminal sodium conductive channel by amiloride.[8,41,61] In keeping with this concept is a recent study using luminal membrane vesicles from the proximal tubule which suggest that glucocorticoids, but not mineralocorticoids, increase the activity of the sodium-hydrogen antiport system,[39] a system affected by amiloride only at high doses.

There are few data defining the effect of the glucocorticoids on mitochondrial enzyme induction. Increased citrate synthase activity has been used as a marker of epithelial cell response to aldosterone. When the effect of physiologic doses of glucocorticoids on this enzyme's activity has been examined in glucocorticoid-responsive tissue or in tissue that is primarily aldosterone responsive, no acute increase in activity is detectable with or without measurable stimulation of sodium absorption.[49,85,135] This observation, of course, does not rule out a pivotal influence of glucocorticoids on cellular and/or organ energy production. (2) Glucocorticoids, indeed, are well known to increase gluconeogenesis and this effect is mediated via enhancement of such enzymes as phosphoenolpyruvate carboxykinase.[35,101] (3) There is also evidence that they increase ammonia production via the glutaminase I mitochondrial pathway.[127] (4) In specific target cells, glucocorticoids may increase the activity of NaK-ATPase at the basolateral membrane. There is little question that they are potent modulators of this enzyme in kidney and colon and experiments with spironolactone again support the tenet that this modulation is independent of aldosterone mediated pathways.[18,19] Whether the glucocorticoid effect on NaK-ATPase activity is primary or secondary to increased luminal sodium uptake remains currently unresolved.

## Corticosteroid Target Sites

Renal target sites for aldosterone and glucocorticoids have been characterized by studies utilizing both biochemical and physiological techniques (Tables 17-1 and 17-2). The biochemical analyses include both receptor and enzyme assays, the latter involving either the putative mineralocorticoid marker enzyme, citrate synthase, or NaK-ATPase.[80] Both the absolute dose of steroid and duration of steroid

**Table 17-1.** Evaluation of Renal Target Sites

| Segment | Index | Adx? | Mineralo-Corticoid Dose | Exposure | Result | Gluco-Corticoid Dose | Exposure | Result | Ref # |
|---|---|---|---|---|---|---|---|---|---|
| PCT & PST | Receptors | Yes | aldo-L | A in vitro | – | dex-L | A in vitro | + | 29,87,105 |
| | | No | aldo-L | A in vivo | – | dex-L | A in vivo | + | 33,34,121 |
| | Citrate synthase | Yes | aldo-L | A in vivo | – | | | | 85 |
| | Na-K-ATPase | Yes | aldo-L | A in vivo | – | | | | 28 |
| | | | | A in vitro | – | | | | 28 |
| | Na-K-ATPase | No | DOCA-H | C in vivo | – | dex-L | C in vivo | + | 5,42 |
| | Na reabsorption | | | | | | | | |
| | Micropuncture | Yes | aldo-L | A in vivo | –? | | | | 52,53 |
| | Luminal membrane | Yes | aldo-L | C in vivo | – | dex-L | C in vivo | + | 39 |
| | Luminal membrane | No | | | | dex-H | C in vivo | + | 39 |
| MTALH | Cytosol receptors | Yes | aldo-L | A in vitro | – | dex-L | A in vitro | + | 29 |
| | | No | aldo-L | A in vitro | ± | dex-L | A in vivo | + | 33,34,121 |
| | Citrate synthase | Yes | aldo-L | A in vivo | + | dex-L | A in vivo | | 82,85 |
| | Na-K-ATPase | Yes | aldo-L | A in vitro | – | dex-L | A in vitro | + | 28,100 |
| | Na-K-ATPase | No | DOCA-H | C in vivo | – | | | | 42 |
| CTALH | Receptors | Yes | aldo-L | A in vitro | – | dex-L | A in vitro | + | 29,121 |
| | | No | aldo-L | A in vitro | ± | dex-L | A in vitro | + | 33,34 |
| | Citrate synthase | Yes | aldo-L | A in vivo | | | | | 85 |
| | Na-K-ATPase | Yes | aldo-L | A in vitro | + | | | | 56 |
| | Na-K-ATPase | No | DOCA-H | C in vivo | – | | | | 42 |
| DCT | Receptors | Yes | aldo-L | A in vitro | – | | | | 29 |
| | | No | aldo-L | A in vitro | + | dex-L | A in vitro | + | 33,34,121 |
| | Citrate synthase | Yes | aldo-L | A in vivo | – | | | | 83,85 |
| | Na-K-ATPase | Yes | aldo-L | A in vivo | – | | | | 28 |
| | Na-K-ATPase | No | DOCA-H | C in vivo | – | | | | 42 |
| | Na-K-ATPase | No | DOCA-L | C in vivo | – | | | | 47 |
| | PD microperfusion | | aldo-L | A in vitro | – | | | | 46 |
| CCT | Receptors | Yes | aldo-L | A in vitro | + | dex-L | A in vitro | + | 29 |
| | | No | aldo-L | A in vitro | + | dex-L | A in vitro | + | 33,34,121 |
| | Citrate synthase | Yes | aldo-L | A in vivo | + | dex-L | A in vivo | – | 85 |
| | Na-K-ATPase | Yes | aldo-L | A in vivo | + | dex-L | A in vivo | – | 28,96 |
| | | Yes | aldo-L | A in vitro | + | dex-L | A in vitro | – | 28,56 |
| | Na-K-ATPase | Yes | aldo-L | C in vivo | + | cort-L | C in vivo | + | 89 |
| | | No | DOCA-H | C in vivo | + | | | | 42,72,93 |
| | Basolateral Infoldings | No | DOCA-H | C in vivo | + | dex-H | C in vivo | + | 123 |

| | | | | | | | | |
|---|---|---|---|---|---|---|---|---|
| **Na reabsorption** | | | | | | | | |
| Micropuncture | Yes | aldo-L | C in vivo | + | dex-H | C in vivo | − | 52,53 |
| Microperfusion | No | DOCA-H | A in vitro | − | | | | 93,106,111 |
| | Yes | aldo-L | C in vivo | + | | | | 106,136 |
| **K secretion** | | | | | | | | |
| Micropuncture | Yes | aldo-L | A in vivo | + | dex-H | C in vivo | + | 129,131,132 |
| Microperfusion | No | DOCA-H | C in vivo | + | dex-H | C in vivo | − | 93,106,111 |
| | | | | | | | | |
| PD micropuncture | Yes | aldo-L | C in vivo | + | dex-H | C in vivo | − | 47,93,106 |
| Microperfusion | No | DOCA-H | C in vivo | + | | | | |
| **MCT** Receptors | Yes | aldo-L | A in vitro | + | dex-L | A in vitro | + | 29 |
| | No | aldo-L | A in vitro | + | | | | 33,34,121 |
| Citrate synthase | Yes | aldo-L | A in vivo | + | | | | 82,85 |
| Na-K-ATPase | Yes | aldo-L | A in vivo | + | | | | 28 |
| Na-K-ATPase | No | DOCA-H | C in vivo | − | | | | 42 |
| Microperfusion | | | | | | | | |
| Na reabsorption | No | DOCA-H | C in vivo | − | | | | 111 |
| K secretion | No | DOCA-H | C in vivo | − | | | | 111 |
| Transmural PD | No | DOCA-H | C in vivo | − | | | | 111 |

A:acute, up to 24 hrs; Aldo:aldosterone; C:chronic, >24 hrs; CCT:cortical collecting tubule; Cort:corticosterone; CTALH:cortical thick ascending limb of Henle; DCT:distal convoluted tubule; Dex:dexamethasone; H:high; L:low; MCT:medullary collecting duct; MTALH:medullary thick ascending limb of Henle; PCT:proximal convoluted tubule; PST:proximal straight tubule.

**Table 17-2.** Evaluation of Gastrointestinal Target Sites

| Segment | Index | Adx? | Mineralo-Corticoid Dose | Exposure | Result | Gluco-Corticoid Dose | Exposure | Result | Ref # |
|---|---|---|---|---|---|---|---|---|---|
| Jejunum | Receptors | Yes | aldo-L | A in vitro | ?[a] | dex-L | A in vitro | + | 33,50,97 |
| | Citrate synthase | Yes | aldo-H | A in vivo | − | dex-H | A in vivo | − | 135 |
| | Na-K-ATPase | Yes | aldo-H | A in vivo | − | dex-H | A in vivo | + | 135 |
| | Na-K-ATPase | No | DOCA-H | C in vivo | − | MP-H | C in vivo | + | 17 |
| | Na reabsorption | No | DOCA-H | C in vivo | − | MP-H | C in vivo | + | 17 |
| | K secretion | No | DOCA-H | C in vivo | − | MP-H | C in vivo | + | 17 |
| | Transmural PD | No | DOCA-H | C in vivo | − | MP-H | C in vivo | + | 17 |
| Ileum | Receptors | Yes | aldo-L | A in vitro | ?[a] | dex-L | A in vitro | + | 97 |
| | Citrate synthase | Yes | aldo-H | A in vivo | − | dex-H | A in vivo | − | 135 |
| | Na-K-ATPase | Yes | aldo-H | A in vivo | − | dex-H | A in vivo | + | 135 |
| | Na-K-ATPase | Yes | DOCA-H | C in vivo | − | MP-H | C in vivo | + | 17 |
| | Na reabsorption | Yes | aldo-H | A in vivo | ± | dex-H | A in vivo | + | 135 |
| | Na reabsorption | No | DOCA-H | C in vivo | − | MP-H | C in vivo | + | 17 |
| | K secretion | No | DOCA-H | C in vivo | − | MP-H | C in vivo | + | 17 |
| | Transmural PD | No | DOCA-H | C in vivo | − | MP-H | C in vivo | + | 17 |
| | Transmural PD | Yes | aldo-H | A in vivo | − | dex-H | A in vivo | + | 135 |
| Colon | Receptors | Yes | aldo-L | A in vitro | ?[a] | dex-L | A in vitro | + | 3,33,79,97 |
| | Citrate synthase | Yes | aldo-H | A in vivo | − | dex-H | A in vivo | − | 135 |
| | Na-K-ATPase | Yes | aldo-H | A in vivo | + | dex-H | A in vivo | + | 14,135 |
| | Na-K-ATPase | No | DOCA-H | C in vivo | + | MP-H | C in vivo | + | 17 |
| | Na reabsorption | Yes | aldo-H | A in vivo | + | dex-L | A in vivo | + | 7,31 |
| | Na reabsorption | Yes | aldo-H | A in vivo | + | dex-H | A in vivo | + | 14,22,135 |
| | Na reabsorption | No | DOCA-H | C in vivo | + | MP-H | C in vivo | + | 17,19,20 |
| | K secretion | Yes | aldo-L | A in vitro | + | dex-L | A in vitro | + | 40,61 |
| | K secretion | Yes | aldo-L | A in vivo | + | dex-L | A in vivo | + | 7,31 |
| | K secretion | No | DOCA-H | C in vivo | + | MP-H | C in vivo | + | 17,19,20 |
| | Transmural PD | Yes | aldo-L | A in vitro | + | dex-L | A in vitro | + | 40,61 |
| | Transmural PD | Yes | aldo-L | A in vivo | + | dex-L | A in vivo | + | 7,31 |
| | Transmural PD | Yes | aldo-H | A in vivo | + | dex-H | A in vivo | + | 14,135 |
| | Transmural PD | No | DOCA-H | C in vivo | + | MP-H | C in vivo | + | 17,19,20 |
| | Basolat. infolding | No | aldo-L | C in vivo | + | dex-H | C in vivo | + | 64 |

[a]Either competitive binding assay does not demonstrate specificity or binding characteristics could not be established.
*Abbreviations*: MP:methylprednisolone. See Table 17-1.

therapy influence the results. Three types of corticosteroid receptors, Types I-III have been identified.[36] These sites are characterized in part, by their interaction with the following steroids: deoxycorticosterone (DOCA), corticosterone, aldosterone, cortisol and the synthetic glucocorticoid, dexamethasone. The relative effectiveness with which these steroids interact with receptors I-III clarifies some of the confusing and conflicting reports regarding target analyses. Importantly, the Type I site may be considered the "classical" mineralocorticoid receptor, that is, it mediates acute actions of steroid on sodium reabsorption.[36] Thus, the affinity of aldosterone for this site exceeds that of all other steroids indicated above. Type II is the classical glucocorticoid receptor and has a high affinity for dexamethasone and corticosterone. Type III sites are most interesting in that they have a high affinity for corticosterone and DOCA and a very low affinity for aldosterone and dexamethasone.[36] Inherent in most reported studies is the tacit assumption that these steroids bind only to a single class of receptors. It turns out, however, that all the above steroids have *some* affinity for each site making it critical to identify the exact dose of steroid utilized in a given study since large doses promote crossover binding. Thus, experiments are easiest to interpret when modest doses of aldosterone or dexamethasone are used to examine Type I and Type II sites and the data contrasted with those after corticosterone or DOCA, here used to determine additional functions which might be attributable to site III activity.

It is assumed that in order for steroids to produce a direct tissue effect they must first bind to their cytosolic receptor. In most biologic systems studied, the physiologic effect has correlated well with receptor affinity and density.[36,81] Thus, in kidney and colon, receptor density and specificity should parallel the physiologic response both in intensity of response and anatomic localization of response. Recently developed techniques have allowed localization of the renal aldosterone (Type I receptor) to a part of the nephron which does indeed correspond to its area of biochemical and physiologic effect.[29,34,105,121] Scholer et al. studied isolated cortical tubules from rat kidney, enriched either in proximal or distal segments.[105] They showed that there was a 9- to 14-fold greater quantity of mineralocorticoid receptors in distal segments compared to proximal segments, implying that mineralocorticoid receptors are confined almost entirely to the distal nephron. Doucet and Katz were able to more specifically localize the site of high specific binding in microdissected rabbit nephron segments to only the branched collecting tubule, cortical collecting tubule, and outer medullary collecting tubule with neglible binding in all other segments.[29] These data strongly suggest that the collecting tubule is indeed the prime site of mineralocorticoid action.

Farman, Bonvalet, and Vandewalle monitored nuclear localization of $^3$H-aldosterone receptors using three different concentrations of $^3$H-aldosterone.[34,121] Nephron binding studies with $10^{-10}$ M-labeled hormone indicated little activity in the thick ascending limb, essentially none in the distal convoluted tubule, and very little in the medullary collecting tubule. However, the connecting tubule as well as the cortical collecting tubule contained moderate amounts of labeling. As these investigators raised the aldosterone concentration to $10^{-9}$ M, they noted a significant increase in labeled sites in the distal convoluted and medullary collecting tubules. At even higher concentrations, the cortical collecting tubule and connecting tubule became saturated, while the cortical thick ascending limb and medullary collecting duct now first became labeled. While such findings could be interpreted in a number of ways, it is quite conceivable that as the dosage of aldosterone was increased, occupancy of different classes of receptors in turn increased. However, the Type I sites (at low doses of steroid) were localized to the connecting segment and collecting duct.

Few studies have examined the localization of the glucocorticoid (Type II) receptor along the nephron. Mishina reported a three- to sixfold increase in glucocorticoid receptor sites in proximal tubules compared to distal tubules.[87] In contrast to aldosterone's effects being localized to the distal tubule, sufficient glucocorticoid receptors were identified in distal tubules as well as in proximal tubules, providing evidence for a direct physiologic effect in both segments of the nephron.[33,87] The widespread distribution of glucocorticoid receptors throughout the nephron is echoed by studies of this receptor in the intestine where it appears that receptors have been identified in every segment studied.[50,79,97]

The above differential localization of effect is supported by enzyme assays. Administration of aldosterone to adrenalectomized rabbits acutely returns citrate synthase activity in cortical and medullary collecting tubules to normal levels.[80,82,83,85] Citrate synthase activity is influenced by both adrenalectomy and aldosterone administration in another segment, namely, medullary thick ascending limb of Henle.[82] However, the exact relationship between aldosterone and the biochemistry of this segment is unclear since receptor assays do not report a concentration of Type I sites in this area.[29,34] In all other segments citrate synthase activity does not decrease with adrenalectomy or increase with aldosterone therapy.[80,85] Several studies have shown that aldosterone but not glucocorticoids increases NaK-ATPase in the cortical collecting tubule.[42,80,89,96] Morphometric studies of this segment have demonstrated that following high dose chronic DOCA administration or low sodium diets there is a specific enhancement of the basolateral surface area, site of NaK-ATPase, caused by increased basolateral infoldings of the principal cells but not of the intercalated cells.[109,123] The increase may be localized to only this segment.[42,72] A similar anatomic localization of the effect of mineralocorticoids on NaK-ATPase in the GI tract has been noted.[17,135] Aldosterone repletion enhances enzyme activity only in colon and not in more proximal intestinal segments.

Localization of glucocorticoid effect by change in enzyme levels has been less rigorous. There is no evidence to suggest that glucocorticoids acutely alter citrate synthase activity. However, the bulk of evidence does suggest that glucocorticoids are potent inducers of NaK-ATPase.[17,18,100,102] Assay of glucocorticoid stimulation of NaK-ATPase using isolated nephron segments has indicated that at least the proximal convoluted tubules (developing animals) and medullary thick ascending limb of Henle's loop, are the steroids' major sites of action with respect to this enzyme.[5,100] Thus mapping studies comparable to those reported for aldosterone have not yet been reported. In the GI tract, glucocorticoids enhance NaK-ATPase activity in all anatomic segments.[17,135]

## Physiologic Effects of Corticosteroids on Sodium Transport

The main renal impairment in adrenal insufficiency is the inability to conserve sodium.[52] Mineralocorticoids in physiologic doses reverse this defect, and the induced sodium retention is a direct tubular effect of the steroid.[46,47,52,81,96,136] It also seems clear that aldosterone's effect on the reabsorption of sodium, is localized to the distal nephron, and probably is carried out in the main by the cortical collecting tubule.[46,49,96] Any changes in proximal sodium handling are most likely secondary to changes previously noted by investigators in intravascular volume and glomerular filtration rate or due to occupancy and activation of glucocorticoid receptors.[52,81,105]

Micropuncture and microperfusion experiments support this contention.[47,53] The acute and chronic actions of aldosterne on transepithelial PD and sodium transport appear localized to the cortical collecting tubule.[46,47,93,105,111,136] Furthermore the hormonal effect is blocked by spironolactone.[45]

It seems clear that in the cortical collecting tubule, aldosterone stimulates transepithelial sodium transport and that this transport is active and electrogenic in nature.[93,106,111] The elements that impede our understanding of how aldosterone affects these demonstrated changes in cation transport include the following. Numerous aldosterone-induced proteins have been indentified at various locations within epithelial cells and various physiologic and anatomic changes are induced by the hormone.[32,52] It is currently not clear which biosynthetic changes are primary and which occur secondary to initial alterations in transport. The time course of each of these changes has yet to be clarified. Which biochemical and which physiologic changes are caused by acute exposure to the hormone and which require prolonged exposure, have yet to be convincingly defined. The uncertainty surrounding the mechanism of aldosterone action is best focused by the interplay between the hormone and its potential target, NaK-ATPase.

Aldosterone enhances sodium reabsorption, a process mediated by an increase in the turnover of this ion by NaK-ATPase. The two main theories that have been proposed to explain this finding are: (1) An increase in the turnover of sodium by existing pumps as a result of an aldosterone-dependent increase in the cellular entry of sodium, a limiting substrate for NaK-ATPase. (2) Aldosterone increases NaK-ATPase synthesis or the number of functioning units by activation of latent enzyme. In the case of the latter proposal, the question would still remain whether the rise in activity was a direct action of aldosterone, or secondary to either sodium per se, or to increases in sodium transport. For instance, much evidence strongly supports a role for this enzyme pump in the chronic adaptation to altered sodium loads. NaK-ATPase decreases after adrenalectomy[18,28,96] but this decline takes days and can be ameliorated by salt loading.[60] Chronic administration of large doses of DOCA appears to increase the sodium reabsorptive capacity in specific nephron segments.[65,72] However, these increases are not seen if animals on low sodium diets are given DOCA.[18,128] Petty et al. provided strong evidence of the sodium dependence of acute NaK-ATPase elevations in cortical collecting tubules of adrenalectomized rabbits exposed in vivo to physiologic doses of aldosterone.[96] NaK-ATPase was acutely increased in exposed tubules and this increase could be prevented by spirolactones. However, if amiloride was administered in vivo prior to aldosterone injection this sodium channel blocking agent prevented the rise in NaK-ATPase, suggesting that acutely increases in intracellular sodium play a role in the induction/activation of this enzyme by aldosterone. In contrast to the instances noted above, Garg et al. were able to show a 200 percent rise in cortical collecting tubule NaK-ATPase with chronic sodium deprivation.[42] Thus, the composite role of sodium and steroid remains speculative.

It is widely recognized that the colon is an aldosterone responsive tissue.[7,17,21,31,40,41,134,135] Numerous experiments have demonstrated that adrenalectomy decreases and aldosterone administration increases colonic sodium absorption in vivo and in vitro and increases colonic short circuit current in vitro.[7,22,31,61,134,135] The bulk of evidence suggests that this response by the GI tract is strictly limited to the colon and perhaps only the distal colon and rectum.[17,41,134,135] In distal colon, aldosterone specifically induces amiloride sensitive sodium absorption and short circuit current and increases luminal membrane sodium conductance.[22,40,134,135] It is striking that only the distal portions of the nephron and distal intestine respond to mineralocorticoids.

Will et al. studied the effect of amiloride on in vitro short circuit current of rat colon.[134] They found that normal rats had an amiloride-resistant short circuit current but rats with high endogenous aldosterone levels or rats that received exogenous aldosterone rapidly induced an almost completely amiloride sensitive short circuit current in the distal part of the colon. Thus, as in other aldosterone sensitive tissues, the hormone specifically affects the luminal sodium conductance pathways.[22,40,134] Although proximal colon short circuit current increased, only 20 percent of the increment was amiloride sensitive. The lack of amiloride sensitivity suggests that this is not a physiologic pathway of aldosterone transport and indeed, may be due to crossover binding to glucocorticoid receptors since in vivo and in vitro studies using low-dose glucocorticoids have suggested that these hormones induce transport that is amiloride resistant.[8,61] An alternative explanation would be that aldosterone increases proximal colon sodium absorption via pathways that are distinct from those enhanced by the mineralocorticoid in other tissues. The latter explanation seems less likely. Induction of distal amiloride sensitive short circuit current was inhibitable by spironolactone.[134] NaK-ATPase was increased in both the amiloride sensitive

distal colon and the amiloride resistant proximal colon only by chronic exposure to high aldosterone levels.[134] This study suggests that initially aldosterone acts on colonic epithelia by increasing sodium transport without altering the peritubular pump.

The distribution of aldosterone receptors in the colon is less certain than that of glucocorticoids, because previous studies failed to exclude binding to Type II receptors or had difficulty in stabilizing the fragile receptor.[3,79,97] If indeed the receptor density does parallel its physiologic effect as in the kidney, one would postulate the Type I receptor should be limited to colon and perhaps only to the distal colon.[41]

The effect of glucocorticoids on renal sodium handling has received comparatively little study. On balance it appears that acute glucocorticoid administration results in no change or in an increase in sodium excretion in either adrenal steroid depleted or intact animals.[10,24,48] Chronic glucocorticoid administration also appears to be associated with mild renal sodium wasting which becomes most apparent with sodium restriction.[24,26,48] Since chronic glucocorticoid treatment significantly increases glomerular filtration rate (GFR) and thus the filtered load of sodium, net sodium reabsorption actually increases either by a direct tubular effect or indirectly as a consequence of hyperfiltration.[24,48,98]

In this regard the earlier studies on the effect of adrenal steroids on proximal tubule sodium absorption are of interest. The time required to establish proximal transtubular sodium gradients is markedly prolonged in adrenalectomized rats and the rate of fluid reabsorption is reduced.[114] These defects are reportedly normalized with either large doses of aldosterone or glucocorticoid.[53,114,132] In addition, Freiberg et al. have recently reported that the rate of sodium-hydrogen exchange across rat proximal tubule apical membranes is increased when adrenalectomized rats are given replacement doses of glucocorticoids or when intact rats are treated with dexamethasone.[39] Aldosterone in the same molar dose as dexamethasone did not increase proximal tubule sodium-hydrogen exchange in adrenalectomized rats.

A defect in sodium reabsorption in Henle's loop has been inferred from the finding of abnormally high TF/P sodium ratios at the first accessible part of the distal tubule of adrenalectomized rats.[53] Cortisol administration is necessary to restore sodium absorption along Henle's loop.[90] Further evidence supporting glucocorticoid action at this site includes the receptor data and the NaK-ATPase data cited above and the reduced concentrating capacity complicating adrenal insufficiency[52,100] However, a direct effect of glucocorticoids on sodium absorption has yet to be established. As with the sodium-dependent argument for augmentation of cortical collecting tubule NaK-ATPase, glucocorticoid-induced NaK-ATPase activity in the medulla, occurring over hours to days, may result from enhanced delivery of sodium to the enzyme site consequent to steroid-induced increments in GFR.[24,52] Jorgensen asserted that sodium availability is partly responsible for the steady-state levels of this enzyme.[40] He noted that the fall in medullary NaK-ATPase activity was hastened by a low salt diet postadrenalectomy. His conclusion is suspect, however, since adrenalectomized rats usually succumb within 72 hours unless sodium balance is maintained by administering saline in their drinking water. Lethal restriction of salt may have so compromised renal function as to render Jorgenson's conclusions uninterpretable. Nonetheless, several investigators have questioned if glucocorticoids modify medullary NaK-ATPase activity in the absence of elevations in GFR.[38,100,108] It

should be noted, however, that although glucocorticoids increased NaK-ATPase activity without altering the *delivery* of sodium to the segment in some studies,[38] and also increased NaK-ATPase when added to isolated tubules in vitro,[100] no one has examined whether glucocorticoids directly enhance sodium uptake in the thick ascending limb of Henle, or if increases in GFR would augment the response.

Although glucocorticoids are potent stimulators of renal NaK-ATPase, to date the bulk of evidence suggests that they have no acute effect on sodium transport or on NaK-ATPase in the cortical collecting tubule, the aldosterone responsive site.[89,96,106]

In contrast to the paucity of information regarding glucocorticoid-stimulated renal sodium absorption, these hormones have been shown to markedly influence intestinal sodium transport when administered in vivo or in vitro, and to stimulate absorption in other asymmetric transporting epithelia such as toad bladder and cultured A6 toad kidney cells.[21,49,61,125]

In 1975, Charney et al. reported that large doses of methylprednisolone increased in vivo sodium and water absorption and transmural potential difference (PD) in the jejunum, ileum and colon of intact rats.[17] NaK-ATPase activity was also shown to increase in all three intestinal segments. In contrast to glucocorticoids, large doses of DOCA increased cation transport and NaK-ATPase only in the colon, suggesting that mineralocorticoid and glucocorticoid effects could be differentiated by their specific sites of action. Binder et al. demonstrated that doses of dexamethasone as small as 10 to 25 µg/100 gbw increased distal colon transmural PD and colonic NaK-ATPase activity.[14] The increase in sodium absorption and transmural PD significantly preceded a detectable increase in NaK-ATPase activity. Spironolactone only partially inhibited the increase in transmural PD provoked by dexamethasone.

Bastl et al. extended these observations by demonstrating in adrenalectomized rats that glucocorticoids were critically important to maintenance of normal basal transport.[7] Small replacement doses of either aldosterone, 10 μg/100 gbw/d, or dexamethasone, 10 μg/100 gbw/d, were used in the latter study. Adrenalectomy alone markedly decreased cation transport and transmural PD. Aldosterone replacement at these or larger doses increased but did not normalize net potassium secretion, sodium absorption and transmural PD. Administration of small doses of dexamethasone in the absence of any mineralocorticoids maintained normal colonic electrolyte movement and electrical properties in adrenalectomized rats. In addition, spironolactone administration to intact rats decreased sodium absorption by only 22 percent without significantly decreasing potassium secretion or transmural PD.[7] This marked sensitivity of the adrenal steroid deficient colon to glucocorticoids in comparison to aldosterone has recently been confirmed in vitro.[61]

Will et al. compared the effect of in vivo glucocorticoids and mineralocorticoids on short circuit current in the distal colon of adrenalectomized rats.[135] In both ileum and colon the effects of dexamethasone were two to three times greater than that of aldosterone. In the terminal portion of the distal colon amiloride inhibited 80 percent of the increased short circuit current provoked by both steroids. In the ileum both steroids increased short circuit current, but amiloride inhibited only four percent of the dexamethasone-induced increase and only 12 percent of the aldosterone-induced increase. Both hormones increased NaK-ATPase activity in distal colon but only dexamethasone increased the enzyme's activity in the ileum. The in-

creased enzyme activity in dexamethasone-treated rats showed a closer temporal correlation with the increase in short circuit current than that seen in aldosterone-treated rats. As determined by these investigators, citrate synthase activity was unchanged throughout the intestine. The doses of steroids used in this study were large in comparison to normal production rates, leaving open the question of whether crossover binding effects occurred.[120]

Using very low doses of dexamethasone either in vivo or in vitro, two studies have demonstrated that glucocorticoid induced sodium absorption in the colon is amiloride-resistant at doses which markedly decrease aldosterone-induced sodium absorption.[8,61] If adrenalectomized rats are maintained on low doses of dexamethasone, only the very distal portion of the intestine responds to administered aldosterone with an increase in sodium absorption and only this segment develops amiloride sensitive transport.[41]

The aldosterone inhibitor, spironolactone, prevents the increase in transport seen when low or high doses of mineralocorticoids are administered to adrenalectomized or intact rats but has no effect on glucocorticoid-induced sodium absorption nor does it modify the increase in NaK-ATPase activity elicited by the latter hormones.[9,19] These findings suggest that glucocorticoid-induced sodium absorption is not mediated by binding to aldosterone receptors.

## Adrenal Steroids: Miscellaneous Effects

**Effects Of Corticosteroids On Potassium Transport.** The role of the adrenal steroids in potassium excretion has recently come under close scrutiny.[13,51,137] It is well recognized that hyperkalemia and decreased potassium excretion complicate adrenal insufficiency.[52,98] It is also well recognized that hypokalemia is an almost invariable complication of hyperaldosteronism.[58] However, aldosterone's role in modulating basal renal potassium secretory rates and in modulating the renal response to acute hyperkalemia, has recently been questioned.[13,51] It should be mentioned, however, that the lack of an effect of aldosterone on urinary potassium does not preclude an effect at the level of the cortical collecting tubule which is countered at more distal collecting duct site.

Many of the previous data suggesting that aldosterone exerted an acute kaliuretic effect were derived from induced changes in the urinary Na/K ratio, a value which is difficult to interpret in light of the hormone's antinatriuretic effect and lack of correlation with effect at the cortical collecting tubule.[106] Dietary potassium markedly modifies the acute effect of aldosterone on potassium excretion. Aldosterone did not increase potassium excretion when administered to adrenalectomized rats maintained on a normal potassium diet, but did result in a kaliuresis when the rats were kept on a low potassium diet.[37,114] Lowering plasma potassium below a critical value eliminated aldosterone's kaliuretic effect.[130] In addition, rats on a sodium restricted diet do not have a kaliuretic response to aldosterone.[130]

Hiatt et al. found that acutely adrenalectomized dogs maintained on aldosterone infusions were not able to excrete potassium at the rate of nonadrenalectomized controls in response to an acute potassium load.[51] Bia et al. demonstrated in chronically adrenalectomized rats maintained on saline, that acute administration of aldosterone in doses sufficient to produce antinatriuresis had no effect on potassium excretion.[13] In this study the animals had been on a normal potassium diet and had serum potassium concentrations of 5 mEq/liter.

Data from these two studies also supported a kaliuretic effect for glucocorticoids. When these hormones were administered with potassium loads to the adrenalectomized dogs in the former study, potassium was excreted at twice the rate of intact controls and at three times the rate of the group receiving only aldosterone.[51] In adrenalectomized rats, doses of dexamethasone as low as 2 $\mu$g/100 gbw, produced a 70 percent increase in urinary potassium excretion.[13] The increase in potassium excretion was not associated with elevations in GFR, sodium excretion or urine flow rates. In a follow-up study the same group demonstrated that adrenalectomized rats chronically exposed to dexamethasone had similar renal excretory responses to an acute potassium load as did intact controls although extrarenal potassium tolerance appeared to be impaired.[15]

The kaliuretic effect of glucocorticoids had been previously recognized.[52] While this may result from a renal effect of the hormone, it is also possible that the catabolic effects of steroids cause increased tissue release of potassium, which may account for the kaliuresis. However, balance studies in adrenalectomized rats maintained on low doses of dexamethasone demonstrate no increased turnover.[12,25]

While effect of glucocorticoids on renal epithelial potassium transport has not been extensively explored, micropuncture experiments have demonstrated decreased distal tubular secretion of potassium in adrenalectomized rats.[52,53,129,130] Maintenance of the animals on 50 $\mu$g/100 gbw/day of dexamethasone restores delivery of potassium out of the distal tubule and enhances potassium excretion in the final urine.[132] Although this normalization of potassium secretion could be attributed to an increased distal flow rate, the above study by Bia[13] and studies in the colon cited below, suggest that enhanced flow is not necessary for glucocorticoids to increase potassium excretion. Chronic high dose dexamethasone administration to intact rabbits does not alter potassium secretion by their isolated cortical collecting tubules.[106] It should be noted that aldosterone levels were markedly suppressed by dexamethasone compared to control levels, so this study does not rule out a permissive effect of the glucocorticoid at this site.

Glucocorticoids appear to exert a stimulatory effect on potassium secretion in the colon.[7,14,17] Administration of glucocorticoids either acutely or chronically to intact or adrenalectomized animals is associated with increased potassium secretion in distal colon. Use of this model allows the steroid effect to be dissociated from the effect of flow rate since this variable is controlled in the catheterized colon. Whether this steroid effect is primary or secondary to the increase in sodium absorption and transmural PD has not been established.[7,14,17]

In colon and cortical collecting tubule high-dose glucocorticoids produce increases in basolateral infolding and peritubular membrane surface area.[64,123] Similar changes are seen in potassium adaptation in both colonic epithelia and in the principal cells of the cortical collecting tubule.[64,109]

In distinct contrast to the apparent resistance of the whole kidney of adrenalectomized animals to the effects of aldosterone on potassium secretion, micropuncture studies and isolated perfused tubule studies convincingly demonstrate a striking effect of aldosterone on potassium secretion by the cortical collecting tubule.[93,106,111] Earlier micropuncture studies identified the distal tubule as the main site of action of aldosterone on potassium secretion. Experiments with isolated perfused tubules have convincingly demonstrated that the cortical collecting tubule is the site of net potassium addition, ac-

companied by changes in transmural PD and increases in the surface area of the basolateral membrane of principal cells.[111,123] Several micropuncture studies have demonstrated that net secretion along this segment is reduced with adrenalectomy and TF/P potassium ratios are markedly reduced.[53,130,131] Administration of aldosterone corrects these abnormalities. Luminal permeability to potassium, intracellular potassium activity and peritubular membrane PD are all decreased by adrenalectomy.[129-131] Acute administration of aldosterone (2 to 4 hours) normalizes only luminal permeability, an effect which is independent of dietary intake of potassium and is not blocked by cycloheximide administration. Administration of aldosterone for five days normalizes intracellular potassium concentration, peritubular PD, and blood to lumen potassium flux.[129,131] These acute and chronic effects have been confirmed in isolated cortical collecting tubules.[92,121] The obvious conclusion from these experiments is that aldosterone increases luminal membrane passive permeability and chronically aldosterone stimulates peritubular uptake of potassium into epithelial cells.[129] One might conclude that an adaptive secondary response may alter membrane permeabilities in such a way that an apparently nonelectrogenic sodium reabsorptive process is, in time, converted to an electrogenic one. However, this conclusion regarding the isolated cortical collecting tubule does not fit with the known in vivo influence of aldosterone on potassium secretion. If small doses of aldosterone are given to adrenalectomized animals and care is taken to reduce dietary potassium just prior to the experiment, potassium excretion increases as sodium reabsorption increases. To resolve this finding, it is important to resurrect the observation that actinomycin D given in vivo, 30 minutes prior to administering the hormone, inhibits aldosterone mediated sodium reabsorption but does not interfere with hormone-stimulated potassium or hydrogen secretion.[37,73] However, actinomycin D alone was also found to enhance potassium secretion. Therefore, potassium excretion was increased equally by aldosterone alone or actinomycin D alone or by the combination of both drugs. Two important and interesting properties of actinomycin D help to explain these findings. In addition to blocking RNA synthesis the drug prolongs the half-life of certain mRNAs. It is therefore difficult to know if actinomycin D inhibited the synthesis of an endogenous inhibitor of potassium secretion or prolonged the half-life of an endogenous stimulator. Nevertheless, aldosterone could not stimulate potassium secretion beyond that effected by actinomycin D alone. Perhaps actinomycin D inhibited aldosterone dependent potassium secretion while stimulating another process of similar magnitude and similar time course. These observations also reflect upon the dependence of changes in potassium secretion on altered sodium transport. Since actinomycin D blocked aldosterone-induced increments in sodium transport, but did not alter the enhancement of potassium secretion, one might conclude that *acutely*, the reabsorptive and secretory processes are independently affected by the hormone. Indeed, aldosterone may have posttranscriptional effects and the site of its acute affect on potassium secretion may or may not be localized to the cortical collecting tubule.

*Chronically*, however, it is clear that potassium secretion by the cortical collecting tubule is stimulated by the lumen negative PD established by mineralocorticoids.[93] The ability of amiloride, the sodium conductance channel blocker, to decrease cortical collecting tubule potassium secretion in DOCA-stimulated rats also suggests that aldosterone-induced potassium secretion must be linked, at least partially, to sodium absorption and/or to the resultant increase in transmural PD.[93] However, this segment also undergoes chronic potassium adaptation which is independent of the presence of mineralocorticoids.[187] Indeed, the increased NaK-ATPase activity in the cortical collecting tubule found with chronic potassium adaptation, cannot be blocked by spironolactone.[27] To further support the independence of sodium and potassium transport in cortical collecting tubule epithelia, certain steroids have been isolated which acutely affected sodium reabsorption but do not alter potassium excretion.[120]

Numerous experiments in the colon have demonstrated that adrenalectomy decreases and aldosterone administration increases net potassium secretion.[7,17,19,37] The effect of aldosterone on the GI tract again appears to be limited to the colon.

**Effects Of Corticosteroids On Acid-Base Metabolism.** Metabolic acidosis stimulates the release of glucocorticoids and mineralocorticoids.[95,126] Adrenalectomized animals and patients with Addison's disease often have mild to moderate metabolic acidosis.[26] Conversely, both hyperaldosteronism and hypercortisolism are characterized by the development of hypokalemic, metabolic alkalosis.[52,58] Adrenal insufficiency diminishes urinary acidification and the excretion of titratable acid and ammonia. These effects are especially evident in the presence of systemic acidemia when maximal lowering of urinary pH and enhanced excretion of titratable acid and ammonia are to be expected.

Existing evidence strongly suggests that ammonia production and excretion are influenced by glucocorticoids.[58,118,127,133] Adrenalectomized animals have decreased circulating levels of the ammoniagenic precursor, glutamine, and manifest impaired ability to normally increase plasma levels of this amino acid during acute acidosis.[57] Renal extraction of glutamine is also decreased by adrenal insufficiency.[57] Adrenalectomized animals given glucocorticoids but not mineralocorticoids continue to excrete diminished quantities of ammonia only if volume depleted or hyperkalemic.[26,133] Normovolemic, normokalemic, adrenalectomized animals normalize their ammonia excretion when physiologic doses of glucocorticoids are administered but physiologic doses of aldosterone are without effect.[117] Aldosterone's influence on ammonia production thus appears to be secondary to changes in ECF volume, sodium excretion, reabsorption and to potassium metabolism.[26,133]

The defect in excretion of titratable acids in adrenalectomized animals also appears to be related to glucocorticoid rather than mineralocorticoid deficiency.[133] Titratable acid excretion increases with physiologic replacement.[133] Large doses of glucocorticoids, however, increase renal acid excretion and this is associated with increased systemic acid production due to increased tissue catabolism.[38] The resultant systemic pH and bicarbonate concentration is usually normal.[58]

The proximal tubule is surely a major target for glucocorticoids. This segment is the primary locus of gluconeogenic and ammoniagenic enzymes, the activities of which are stimulated by glucocorticoids.[23,35,122,127] Augmentation of phosphoenolpyruvate carboxykinase biosynthesis by glucocorticoids may enhance both pathways since converting the carbon products of glutamine catabolism to glucose relieves feedback inhibition on glutamine catabolism.[35,118] Ammoniagenesis is also stimulated by the following renal and extrarenal actions of glucocorticoids. Liver glutamine synthetase activity is stimulated by these hormones, resulting in the provision of more substrate for renal ammoniagenesis.[57,70,118] Steroids also stimulate renal glutamine uptake.[70,127] As previously mentioned, dexamethasone increases the level or "activity" of an Na:H exchanger located in proximal tu-

bule brush border membranes of adrenalectomized and intact animals.[39] Since this exchanger also countertransports $Na^+$ and $NH_4^+$,[66] it has been suggested that glucocorticoids may exert their effect on ammonia excretion by influencing this exchanger.[39] Freiberg also demonstrated that glucocorticoids simultaneously decreased Na-gradient dependent phosphate uptake by luminal membranes from both adrenalectomized and intact rats.[39] This increased phosphate clearance could explain glucocorticoid enhancement of the excretion of titratable acid.

The physiologic importance of these findings are as yet undetermined, but these observations fit well with the cited effects of glucocorticoids on whole kidney acid excretion. However, as Tannen has pointed out, the renal biochemistry can adapt to situations of metabolic acidosis in the absence of glucocorticoids, suggesting that these hormones are supportive but not crucial for renal acid excretion.[118]

It does appear that aldosterone is necessary for the maximal rate of acid secretion in medullary collecting duct.[118,133] Most studies suggest that mineralocorticoids do not increase the maximal tubular fluid to blood pH gradients but rather increase the maximum capacity to secrete acid.[1,2,133] This appears to be a direct effect of aldosterone and not a secondary effect of altered systemic fluid-electrolyte balance since it can be demonstrated in vitro in a controlled environment with isolated medullary collecting tubules.[115] The effect of aldosterone on net hydrogen ion flux and TF/P gradients have been confirmed in turtle and toad bladder where aldosterone stimulates net hydrogen ion secretion.[1,2] As previously discussed, net hydrogen secretion may be controlled by a separate cell type and at a different tubular location than net sodium absorption.[115]

**Effects of Corticosteroids On Water Metabolism.** The role of adrenal steroids in controlling renal water handling remains controversial. It is well established that adrenal insufficiency is associated with a defect in free water clearance as well as an inability to generate a maximally concentrated urine.[98] Thus, the latitude of urinary concentration and dilution is narrowed by adrenal insufficiency.

It is generally, but not universally, accepted that the defect in free water excretion and reabsorption is largely related to the interplay of glucocorticoids with ADH release and the permeability of the distal nephron to water.[16,98,138] Deficiency of mineralocorticoids appears to exert its effects on water balance via the hypovolemia and resulting hemodynamic consequences of negative sodium balance.[59,98] However, a permissive effect of mineralocorticoids on ADH-stimulated water absorption in the cortical collecting tubule has been suggested.[107] Three different mechanisms have been proposed to explain how glucocorticoids alter free water generation[52]: (1) Glucocorticoids may modulate the release of ADH from the hypothalamus. (2) Glucocorticoids may antagonize the effects of ADH on the nephron. (3) Glucocorticoids may have a direct effect on water permeability of collecting duct, independent of the presence of ADH.

Recent studies have demonstrated that plasma vasopressin levels are persistently increased in glucocorticoid deficient animals, despite hypoosmolality and normal or expanded ECF volume.[16,74,76] Studies, however, have documented compromised systemic and renal hemodynamics despite normovolemia.[16,74,98] Glucocorticoid deficiency, therefore, represents a persistent, nonosmotic stimulus to vasopressin release which may be baroreceptor mediated.[16]

Evidence has been cited to indicate that glucocorticoids have a direct effect on the water permeability of the distal tubular epithelia. Green et al. adrenalectomized rats with diabetes insipidus and demonstrated a defect in water excretion despite total absence of vasopressin.[45]

Hemodynamic factors, however, were not entirely excluded in this study. Linas et al. repeated these experiments and showed that the vasopressin-independent defect in water excretion was associated with marked changes in systemic and renal hemodynamics, thus, leaving unsettled the question of whether glucocorticoids exert a direct tissue effect.[74] Ishikawa and Schrier using an AVP antagonist have demonstrated a vasopressin, GFR independent defect in free water excretion with glucocorticoid deficiency.[59]

Results both supporting and refuting a direct effect of glucocorticoids on toad bladder water permeability have been reported.[52] While in vivo micropuncture studies have shown an increased water permeability in cortical collecting ducts of rats with adrenal insufficiency,[98] no such increase was documented in collecting ducts from isolated papillae of adrenalectomized rats.[99]

Basal cyclic AMP (cAMP) levels have been reported to be elevated in the medullary collecting duct of adrenalectomized animals, a finding that possibly reflected the increased ADH levels complicating adrenal insufficiency.[99] However, the increment in cAMP generation caused by the addition of ADH to the isolated collecting duct is decreased. In vivo but not in vitro administration of glucocorticoids increases the synthesis of cAMP in response to a given amount of ADH.[99] These results are in direct opposition to what would be expected if glucocorticoids opposed the action of ADH. However, these findings may partially explain the concentrating defect of adrenal insufficiency. Adrenal steroids, cyclic AMP or phosphodiesterase inhibitors can restore water reabsorption in response to ADH in the cortical collecting tubule[85,107] suggesting that the defect is either due to decreased production or increased breakdown of cAMP.

Since medullary thick ascending limb NaK-ATPase activity appears to be dependent on the presence of glucocorticoids, glucocorticoids could participate in water metabolism by enhancing the capacity of the medullary thick ascending limb to maintain medullary hypertonicity and to generate free water.[100] Correction of sodium reabsorption in this segment by glucocorticoids would explain why steroids correct both the inability to maximally dilute urine and maximally concentrate urine in adrenal insufficiency.

**Interaction Of Corticosteroids With Renal Prostaglandins.** Recent experiments have increased our understanding of glucocorticoid inhibition of prostaglandin (PG) synthesis. Isolated renal interstitial cells have been found to synthesize PG and this synthetic process is inhibitable by glucocorticoids.[138,139] This effect of glucocorticoids is, in turn blocked by actinomycin D.[104] A key factor involved in this interaction is lipomodulin, a nondialyzable protein ($\approx$40,000 MW), which inhibits phospholipase $A_2$ activity, an important enzyme in PG formation.[55,103] Interestingly, lipomodulin undergoes phosphorylation-dephosphorylation reactions that are catalyzed by a $Ca^{2+}$-dependent protein kinase.[54] Phosphorylation inactivates lipomodulin and thus activates of phospholipase $A_2$ thereby increasing PG synthesis.

Purified lipomodulin inhibits bradykinin-stimulated arachidonate release.[54] Bradykinins, in turn, are natriuretic, enhance renal blood flow, and increase PG synthesis. It is likely that PG and not bradykinin is directly responsible for the natriuresis.[30,117] Small doses of aldosterone, like dexamethasone, appear to inhibit PG synthesis.[94,138] However, chronic administration of high doses of DOCA enhances distal nephron release of kallikrein, formation of bradykinin, activation of phospholipase $A_2$, and PG synthesis.[15,30,77,78,91,92] Thus, it is conceivable that chronic administration of mineralocorticoids could result in "escape" by a brady-

kinin-induced inactivation of lipomodulin and the resulting increase in natriuretic PGs could return sodium excretion to baseline.

**Effects Of Corticosteroids On Internal Electrolyte Balance.** Evidence that adrenal corticosteroids may influence the internal distribution of cation as well as modulating renal cation excretion, has existed for decades but the issue remains controversial. Thatcher and Radike noted in 1947 that adrenal hormones protected rats from acute potassium intoxication.[119] Alexander and Levinsky demonstrated that rats chronically fed large amounts of potassium had markedly improved survivals and manifested lesser increments in serum potassium concentration when challenged with a large parenteral load of KCl.[4] The acute dose of KCl proved lethal to control rats not chronically exposed to potassium enriched diets. The bulk of protection afforded by chronic potassium loading was from facilitation of extrarenal potassium uptake that was dependent upon the presence of aldosterone.[4,111] Several experimental observations have further strengthened the suggestion that chronic exposure to aldosterone enhances potassium uptake by cells. Hyperkalemia is a well recognized complication of adrenal insufficiency and potassium loads are acutely lethal to the adrenalectomized animal.[51,119] It is known that the immediate defense against suddenly increased extracellular potassium cannot be renal but must represent rapid redistribution of potassium from the small extracellular potassium space to the large intracellular potassium space.[4,11,12] This redistribution is markedly impaired by adrenal insufficiency.[4,12,25] This defect is apparently present in adrenalectomized animals maintained on glucocorticoids although basal urinary potassium excretion is higher than controls not receiving steroids, suggesting that part of the basal hyperkalemia is due to increased tissue release or redistribution.[11,12,25] During acute potassium administration no defect in potassium excretion is manifest in glucocorticoid replete rats or dogs yet serum potassium concentration tends to be higher.[12,13,25,51] Acute administration of aldosterone has a small hypokalemic effect while chronic aldosterone replacement restores basal serum potassium levels and normalizes the increment attending acute KCl infusion.[12] These changes cannot be explained by renal potassium excretion.[4,12] The human counterpart of this experiment is the observation that patients with hyporeninemic hypoaldosteronism become normokalemic when given mineralocorticoids without increasing their renal or fecal potasssium excretion.[11]

The mechanism by which aldosterone affects potassium distribution remains largely unexplored, but does not appear to be related to the state of ECF volume, blood pressure, or blood pH.[11,12,25] The effects of aldosterone on muscle potassium content have been variable depending on experimental conditions.[11]

The effect of glucocorticoids on internal potassium distribution has been even more difficult to unravel. It is a well recognized clinical observation that addisonian patients maintained on glucocorticoids without mineralocorticoids but given adequate salt and water, do not become hyperkalemic except under severely stressful conditions.[98] Large doses of glucocorticoids indeed may cause hyperkalemia both acutely in normals and chronically in adrenalectomized individuals, possibly because of the catabolic effects of the steroid.[11] However, Roberts and Pitts demonstrated that cortisone corrects hyperkalemia in adrenalectomized dogs with only minimal increase in potassium excretion.[10] A study of human erythrocytes taken from individuals treated chronically with glucocorticoids demonstrated increased intracellular potassium

with a reciprocal decrease in intracellular sodium.[63] This exchange was associated with increased numbers of membrane Na-K pump sites as measured by ouabain binding.

Thus, although the exact role of the adrenal steroids in the control of internal potassium balance remains unmapped, the evidence suggesting that they modulate potassium movement across cell membranes continues to grow.

**The Interplay Between Glucocorticoids And Mineralocorticoids With Renin, Angiotensin And Aldosterone.** An area which has not been extensively explored is the relationship between glucocorticoids and the renin-angiotensin, aldosterone axis. Hypertension is a frequent complication of hypercortisolism[68] and hypotension is frequently seen in Addison's disease even with adequate mineralocorticoid replacement.[10]

Studies of the renin-angiotensin system in pure mineralocorticoid deficiency, show that renin levels are markedly increased.[10,110] With pure glucocorticoid deficiency, renin levels tend to be normal or slight increased.[10,110] However, renin substrate levels are consistently decreased in glucocorticoid deficiency and consistently increased in hypercortisolism.[68,110] Levels of renin substrate may be rate limiting since substrate levels appear to influence the rate of angiotensin formation in man and the ratio of angiotensin generation to renin concentration.[68] There is also a reduced vascular responsiveness to pressor agents in glucocorticoid deficiency and increased vascular responsiveness to angiotensin in hypercortisolism.[10,68]

Recent studies have investigated the importance of glucocorticoids in regulating angiotensin converting enzyme (ACE) activity.[86] Studies strongly suggest that glucocorticoids specifically stimulate this enzyme in endothelial cells and lung at physiologic concentrations.[86] Although it is assumed that ACE activity is not an important regulatory step in the control of angiotensin II production this assumption has not been rigorously tested. The hypertension produced by hypercortisolism is inhibitable by angiotensin II blockade.[68] In adrenalectomized animals peripheral vascular resistance falls with angiotensin II blockade only when animals are given glucocorticoids and not in those given mineralocorticoids and the decrease in blood pressure is greater in the former group.[10]

# ACKNOWLEDGMENT

Both C.P. Bastl and D. Marver are Established Investigators of the American Heart Association.

# REFERENCES

1. Al-Awqati Q, Norby LH, Mueller A, et al: Characteristics of stimulation of H$^+$ transport by aldosterone in turtle urinary bladder. J Clin Invest 58:351, 1976.
2. Al-Awqati Q: Effect of aldosterone on the coupling between H$^+$ transport and glucose oxidation. J Clin Invest 60:1240, 1977.
3. Alberti KGMM, Sharp GWG: The isolation of bound aldosterone from the nuclei of human toad and rat colon. Ann Endocrinol (Paris) 31, 4 supp 777, 1970.
4. Alexander EA, Levinsky NG: An extrarenal mechanism of potassium adaptation. J Clin Invest 47:740, 1968.
5. Aperia A, Larssen L, Letterstrom R: Hormonal induction of Na-K-ATPase in developing proximal tubular cells. Am J Physiol 241:F356, 1981.
6. Baggio B, Bordin D, de Giorgi G, et al: DOCA administration increases renal phospholipase activity in the rat. Experientia 30:366, 1980.
7. Bastl CP, Binder HJ, Hayslett JP: Role of glucocorticoids and aldosterone in maintenance of colonic cation transport. Am J Physiol 238 7:F181, 1980.
8. Bastl CP, Kapoor V: Amiloride distinguishes glucocorticoid from aldosterone stimulated sodium transport. Clin Res 30:2, 441A, 1982.
9. Bastl C, Kapoor V: Glucocorticoid-mediated sodium transport is independent of aldosterone receptor binding. Kidney Int 21:258, 1982.
10. Berns AS, Pluss RG, Erickson AL, et al: Renin-angiotensin system and cardiovascular homeostasis in adrenal insufficiency. Am J Physiol 233:F509, 1977.
11. Bia MJ, DeFronzo RA: Extrarenal potassium homeostasis. Am J Physiol 240:F257, 1981.
12. Bia MJ, Tyler KA, DeFronzo RA: Regulation of extrarenal potassium homeostasis by adrenal hormones in rats. Am J Physiol 242:F641, 1982.
13. Bia MJ, Tyler K, DeFronzo RA: The effect of dexamethasone on renal electrolyte excretion in the adrenalectomized rat. Endocrinology 111:3, 882, 1982.
14. Binder HJ: Effect of dexamethasone on electrolyte transport in the large intestine of the rat. Gastroenterology 75:212, 1978.
15. Bonner G, Autenrieth R, Marin-Grez W, et al: Effects of Na loading, DOCA and corticosterone on urinary kallikrein activity. Hormone Res 14:87, 1981.
16. Boykin J, DeTorrenté A, Erickson A, et al: Role of plasma vasopressin in impaired water excretion of glucocorticoid deficiency. J Clin Invest 62:738, 1978.
17. Charney AN, Kinsey MD, Myers L, et al: Na$^+$-K$^+$ activated, adenosine triphosphatase and intestinal electrolyte transport: Effect of adrenal steroids. J Clin Invest 56:653, 1975.
18. Charney AN, Silva P, Besarab A, et al: Separate effects of aldosterone, DOCA and methylprednisolone on renal Na-K-ATPase. Am J Physiol 227:345, 1974.
19. Charney AN, Wallach J, Ceccarelli S, et al: Effects of spironolactone and amiloride on corticosteroid-induced changes in colonic function. Am J Physiol 241:G300, 1981.
20. Charney AN, Wallach J, Donowitz M: Effect of cycloheximide on corticosteroid-induced changes in colonic function. Am J Physiol 243:6112, 1982.

21. Crabbé J: Decreased effectiveness of aldosterone on active sodium transport by the isolated toad bladder in the presence of other steroids. Acta Endocrinol 47:419, 1964.

22. Cofré G, Crabbé J: Active sodium transport by the colon of Bufo Marinus: stimulation by aldosterone and antidiuretic hormone. J Physiol 188:177, 1967.

23. Curthoys NP, Lowry OH: The distribution of glutaminase isoenzymes in the various structures of the nephron in normal, acidotic and alkalotic rat kidney. J Biol Chem 248:162, 1973.

24. deBermudez L, Hayslett JP: Effect of methylprednisolone on renal function and the zonal distribution of blood flow in the rat. Circ Res 31:44, 1972.

25. DeFronzo RA, Lee R, Jones A, et al: Effect of insulinopenia and adrenal hormone deficiency on acute potassium tolerance. Kidney Int 17:586, 1980.

26. DiTella PJ, Sodhi B, McCreary J, et al: Mechanism of the metabolic acidosis of selective mineralocorticoid deficiency. Kidney Int 14:466, 1978.

27. Doucet A, Katz AI: Renal potassium adaptation: Na-K-ATPase activity along the nephron after chronic potassium loading. Am J Physiol 238:F380, 1980.

28. Doucet A, Katz AI: Short-term effect of aldosterone on Na-K-ATPase in single nephron segments. Am J Physiol 241:F273, 1981.

29. Doucet A, Katz AI: Mineralocorticoid receptors along the nephron: $^3$H aldosterone binding in rabbit tubules. Am J Physiol 237:F105, 1979.

30. Durr J, Favre L, Gailliard R, et al: Mineralocorticoid escape in man: role of renal prostaglandins. Acta Endocrinol 99:474, 1982.

31. Edmonds CJ, Marriot JC: The effect of aldosterone and adrenalectomy on the electrical potential difference of rat colon and in the transport of sodium potassium chloride and bicarbonate. J Endocrinol 39:517, 1967.

32. Fanestil DD, Kipnowski CL: Molecular action of aldosterone. Klin Wochenschr 60:1180, 1982.

33. Farman N, Vandewalle A, Bonvalet LP: Autoradiographic determination of dexamethasone binding sites along the rabbit nephron. Am J Physiol 244:F325, 1983.

34. Farman N, Vandewalle A, Bonvalet JP: Aldosterone binding in isolated tubules. II. An autoradiographic study of concentration dependence in the rabbit nephron. Am J Physiol 242:F69, 1982.

35. Feldman D: Glucocorticoid receptors and regulation of PEPCK activity in rat kidney and adipose tissue. Am J Physiol 233:E147, 1977.

36. Feldman D, Funder JW, Edelman IS: Subcellular mechanisms in the action of adrenal steroids. Am J Med 53:545, 1972.

37. Fimognari GM, Fanestil DD, Edelman IS: Induction of RNA and protein synthesis in the action of aldosterone in the rat. Am J Physiol 213:954, 1967.

38. Fisher KW, Welt LG, Hayslett JP: Dissociation of Na-K-ATPase specific activity and net reabsorption of Na. Am J Physiol 228:1745, 1975.

39. Freiberg JM, Kinsella J, Sacktor B: Glucocorticoids increase the Na:H exchange and decrease the Na gradient-dependent phosphate-uptake systems in renal brush border membrane vesicles. Proc Natl Acad Sci USA 79:4932, 1982.

40. Frizzell RA, Schultz SG: Effect of aldosterone on ion transport by rabbit colon in vitro. J Membrane Biol 39:1, 1978.

41. Fromm M, Hegel U: Segmental heterogeneity of epithelial transport in rat large intestine. Pflügers Arch 378:71, 1978.

42. Garg LC, Knepper MA, Burg MB: Mineralocorticoid effects in Na-K-ATPase in individual nephron segments. Am J Physiol 240:F536, 1981.

43. Gluck S, Cannon C, Al-Awqati Q: Exocytosis regulates urinary acidification in turtle bladder by rapid insertion of H pumps into the luminal membrane. Proc Natl Acad Sci 79:4327, 1982.

44. Goodman DBP: The role of lipid metabolism in the response of the toad urinary bladder to aldosterone. Ann NY Acad Sci 372:30, 1981.

45. Green HH, Harrington AR, Valtin H: On the role of antidiuretic hormone in the inhibition of acute water diuresis in adrenal insufficiency and the effects of gluco- and

mineralocorticoids in reversing the inhibition. J Clin Invest 41:1078, 1970.

46. Gross JB, Kokko JP: Effects of aldosterone and potassium-sparing diuretics on electrical potential differences across distal nephron. J Clin Invest 59:82, 1977.

47. Gross JB, Imai M, Kokko JP: A functional comparison of the cortical collecting tubule and the distal convoluted tubule. J Clin Invest 55:1284, 1975.

48. Hall JE, Morse CL, Smith MJ, et al: Control of arterial blood pressure and renal function during glucocorticoid excess in dogs. Hypertension 2, 2:139, 1980.

49. Handler JS, Preston AS, Perkins FM, et al: The effect of adrenal steroid hormones on epithelia formed in culture by A6 cells. Ann NY Acad Sci 372:442, 1981.

50. Henning SJ, Ballard PL, Kretchmer N: A study of the cytoplasmic receptors for glucocorticoids in intestine of pre and post weanling rats. J Biol Chem 220: 6:2073, 1975.

51. Hiatt N, Chapman L, Davidson MB, et al: Adrenal hormones and the regulation of serum potassium in potassium-loaded adrenalectomized dogs. Endocrinology 105:215, 1979.

52. Hierholzer K, Lange S: The effects of adrenal steroids on renal function. In MTP International Review of Science: Kidney and Urinary Tract Physiology. Vol 6. Baltimore. University Park Press, Baltimore, 1974, p 273.

53. Hierholzer K, Wiederholt M, Holzgreve, H, et al. Micropuncture study of renal transtubular concentration gradients of sodium and potassium in adrenalectomized rats. Pflügers Arch 285:193, 1965.

54. Hirata F: The regulation of lipomodulin, a phospholipase inhibitory protein in rabbit neutrophils by phosphorylation. J Biol Chem 256:7730, 1981.

55. Hirata F, Schiffman E, Venkatasubramanian K, et al: A phospholipase $A_2$ inhibitory protein in rabbit neutrophils induced by glucocorticoids. Proc Natl Acad Sci 77:2533, 1980.

56. Horster M, Schmid H, Schmidt U: Aldosterone in vitro restores nephron Na-K-ATPase of distal segments from adrenalectomized rabbits. Pflügers Arch 384:203, 1980.

57. Hughey RA, Rankin BB, Curthoys NP: Acute acidosis and renal arteriovenous differences of glutamine in normal and adrenalectomized rats. Am J Physiol 238:F199, 1980.

58. Hulter HN, Licht JH, Bonner EL, et al: Effects of glucocorticoid steroids on renal and systemic acid-base metabolism. Am J Physiol 239:F30, 1980.

59. Ishikawa S, Schrier RW: Effect of arginine vasopressin antagonist on renal water excretion in glucocorticoid and mineralocorticoid deficient rats. Kidney Int 22:587, 1982.

60. Jorgensen PL: The role of aldosterone in the regulation of Na-K-ATPase in rat kidney. J Steroid Biochem 3:181, 1972.

61. Jorkasky D, Cox M, Feldman G: Differential effects of aldosterone and dexamethasone on rat colon in vitro. Clin Res 31:283A, 1983.

62. Kaissling B, LeHir M: Distal tubular segments of the rabbit kidney after adaptation to altered Na and K intake. Cell Tissue Res 224:469, 1982.

63. Kaji DM, Thakkar U, Kahn T: Glucocorticoid-induced alterations in the sodium potassium pump of the human erythrocyte. J Clin Invest 68:422, 1981.

64. Kashgarian M: Changes in cell membrane surfaces associated with alterations of transepithelial ion movement. In Current Topics in Membrane and Transport. Vol 13. Boulpaep EL, Ed: Cellular Mechanisms of Renal Tubular Ion Transport. Academic Press, New York, 1980, p 149.

65. Katz AI, Lee SK, Chekal MA: Corticosteroid binding along the rat nephron. In Morel F, Ed: Biochemistry of Kidney Functions. Elsevier Biomedical Press, Amsterdam, 1982, pp 277–283.

66. Kinsella JL, Aronson PS: Interaction of $NH_4^+$ and $Li^+$ with the renal microvillus membrane $Na^+$-$H^+$ exchanger. Am J Physiol 241:C220, 1981.

67. Kirschenbaum MA, Lowe AG, Trizna W, et al: Regulation of ADH action by prostaglandins. Evidence for prostaglandin synthesis in the rabbit cortical collecting tubule. J Clin Invest 70:1193, 1982.

68. Krakoff L, Nicolis G, Amsel B: Pathogenesis of hypertension in Cushing's syndrome. Am J Med 58:216, 1975.

69. Krozowski ZS, Hamilton CA, Funder JW: Heterogeneity of corticosterone binding sites in rat hippocampus: implications for mineralocorticoid and glucocorticoid specificity. Endocrine Soc, San Francisco, June, 1982, Abstract No. 754.

70. Kulka RC, Cohen H: Regulation of glutamine synthetase activity of hepatoma tissue culture cells by glutamine and dexamethasone. J Biol Chem 248:6738, 1973.

71. Lan NC, Graham B, Bartter FC, et al: Binding of steroids to the mineralocorticoid receptors: implications for in vivo occupancy by glucocorticoids. J Clin Endocrinol Metab 54:332, 1982.

72. LeHir M, Kaissling B, Dubach UC: Distal tubular segments of the rabbit kidney after adaptation to altered Na and K intake. II. Changes in Na-K-ATPase activity. Cell Tissue Res 224:493, 1982.

73. Lifschitz MD, Schrier RW, Edelman IS: Effect of actinomycin D on aldosterone-mediated changes in electrolyte excretion. Am J Physiol 224:376, 1973.

74. Linas SL, Berl T, Robertson GL, et al: Role of vasopressin in the impaired water excretion of glucocorticoid deficiency. Kidney Int 18:58, 1980.

75. Ludens JH, Vaughn DA, Fanestil DD: Stimulation of urine acidification by aldosterone and inhibitors of mRNA and protein synthesis. J Membr Biol 40: Spec 191, 1978.

76. Mandell IN, DeFronzo RA, Robertson GL, et al: Role of arginine vasopressin in the impaired water diuresis of isolated glucocorticoid deficiency in the rat. Kidney Int 17:186, 1980.

77. Margolius HS, Horwitz D, Geiter RG, et al: Urinary kallikrein excretion in normal man. Circ Res 35:812, 1974.

78. Marin-Grez M: Multihormonal regulation of renal kallikrein. Biochem Pharmacol 31:3941, 1982.

79. Marusic ET, Hayslett JP, Binder HJ: Corticosteroid binding studies in cytosol of colonic mucosa of the rat. Am J Physiol 240:G417, 1981.

80. Marver D: Aldosterone action in target epithelia. In Munson P, Ed: Vitamins and Hormones. Vol 18. Academic Press, New York, 1980, pp 55–117.

81. Marver D, Kokko JP: Renal target sites and the mechanism of action of aldosterone. Mineral Electr Metab 9:1, 1983.

82. Marver D, Lombard WE: Localization of aldosterone target sites in rabbit renal medulla. Kidney Int 19:248A, 1981.

83. Marver D, Schwartz MJ: Identification of mineralocorticoid target sites in the isolated rabbit cortical nephron. Proc Natl Acad Sci USA 77:3672, 1980.

84. Marver D, Stewart JW, Funder JW, et al: Renal aldosterone receptors: Studies with [3]H aldosterone and the antimineralocorticoid [3]H spirolactone (SC 26304). Proc Natl Acad Sci USA 71:1431, 1974.

85. Marver D, Schwartz MJ, Kokko JP: Multiple effects of corticoid hormones on the mammalian nephron. Ann NY Acad Sci 372:39, 1981.

86. Mendelsohn FAO, Lloyd CJ, Kachel C, et al: Induction by glucocorticoids of angiotensin converting enyzme production from bovine endothelial cells in culture and rat lung in vivo. J Clin Invest 70:684, 1982.

87. Mishina T, Scholar DW, Edelman IS: Glucocorticoid receptors in rat kidney cortical tubules enriched in proximal and distal segments. Am J Physiol 240:F38, 1981.

88. Mueller A, Steinmetz PR: Spironolactone: An aldosterone agonist in stimulation of $H^+$ secretion by turtle urinary bladder. J Clin Invest 61:1666, 1978.

89. Mujais SK, Chekal MA, Jones WJ, et al: Is renal Na-K-ATPase under mineralocorticoid or glucocorticoid control? Clin Res 31:2, 437A, 1983.

90. Murayama J, Suzuki A, Tadokozo M, et al: Microperfusion of Henle's Loop in the kidney of the adrenalectomized rat. Jap J Pharmacol 18:518, 1968.

91. Nishimura K, Alhinc-Gilas F, White A, et al: Activation of membrane-bound kallikrein and renin in the kidney. Proc Natl Acad Sci USA 77:4975, 1980.

92. Omata K, Carretero OA, Scicli AG, et al: Localization of active and inactive kallikrein in the microdissected rabbit nephron. Kidney Int 22:602, 1982.

93. O'Neil RG, Helman SI: Transport characteristics of renal collecting tubules: Influences of DOCA and diet. Am J Physiol 233:F544, 1977.

94. Papanicolaou N, Lefkos N, Masourides E,

et al: Interaction between aldosterone and renomedullary prostaglandins. Competitive action between aspirin and spirolactone. Experientia 33: 1632, 1977.

95. Perez GO, Oster JR, Vaamonde CA, et al: Effect of NH₄Cl on plasma aldosterone cortisol and renin activity in supine man. J Clin Endocrinol Metab 45:762, 1977.

96. Petty KJ, Kokko JP, Marver D: Secondary effect of aldosterone on Na-K-ATPase activity in the rabbit cortical collecting tubule. J Clin Invest 68:1514, 1981.

97. Pressley L, Funder JW: Glucocorticoid and mineralocorticoid receptors in gut mucosa. Endocrinology 97:588, 1975.

98. Quintanilla AP, Delgado-Butron C, Zeballos J: Renal hemodynamics and water excretion in Addison's disease. Metabolism 25:419, 1976.

99. Rayson BMR, Ray C, Morgan T: The effect of adrenocortical hormones on water permeability of the collecting duct of rat. Pflügers Arch 373:105, 1978.

100. Rayson BM, Edelman IS: Glucocorticoid stimulation of Na-K-ATPase in superfused distal segments of kidney tubules in vitro. Am J Physiol 243:F463, 1982.

101. Roberts KE, Pitts RF: The effects of cortisone and deoxycorticosterone on the renal tubular reabsorption of phosphate and the excretion of titratable acid and potassium in dogs. Endocrinology 50:324, 1953.

102. Rodriguez HJ, Sinha SK, Starling J, et al: Regulation of Na-K-ATPase in the rat by adrenal steroids. Am J Physiol 241:F186, 1981.

103. Russo-Marie F, Duval D: Dexamethasone-induced inhibition of prostaglandin production does not result from a direct action on phospholipase activities but is mediated through a steroid-inducible factor. Biochim Biophys Acta 712:177, 1982.

104. Russo-Marie R, Paing M, Duval D. Involvement of glucocorticoid receptors in steroid-induced inhibition of prostaglandin secretion. J Biol Chem 254: 8498, 1979.

105. Scholer DW, Mishina T, Eldeman IS: Distribution of aldosterone receptors in rat kidney cortical tubules enriched in proximal and distal segments. Am J Physiol 237:F360, 1979.

106. Schwartz GJ, Burg MB: Mineralocorticoid effects on cation transport by cortical collecting tubules in vitro. Am J Physiol 235: F576, 1978.

107. Schwartz MJ, Kokko JP: Urinary concentrating defect on adrenal insufficiency. Permissive role of adrenal steroids on the hydroosmotic response across the rabbit cortical collecting tubule. J Clin Invest 66: 234, 1980.

108. Sinha SK, Rodriguez HJ, Hogan WC, et al: Mechanisms of activation of renal Na-K-ATPase in the rat. Effect of acute and chronic administration of dexamethasone. Biochim Biophys Acta 641:20, 1981.

109. Stanton BA, Boomesderfu D, Wade JB, et al: Structural and functional study of the rat distal nephrons: Effect of potassium adaptation and potassium depletion. Kidney Int 19:36, 1981.

110. Stockigt JR, Hewett MJ, Topliss SJ, et al: Renin and renin substrate in primary adrenal insufficiency. Contrasting effects of glucocorticoid and mineralocorticoid deficiency. Am J Med 66:915, 1979.

111. Stokes JB, Ingram MJ, Williams AD, et al: Heterogeneity of the rabbit collecting tubule: Localization of mineralocorticoid hormone action to the cortical portion. Kidney Int 20:340, 1981.

112. Stokes JV, Kokko JP: Inhibition of Na transport by PGE₂ across the isolated, perfused rabbit collecting tubule. J Clin Invest 59:1099, 1977.

113. Stolte H, Bracht JP, Wiederholt M, et al: Einfluss von adrenalektomie und glucocorticoiden auf die wasserpermeabilitat corticaler nephronabschnitte der rattenniere. Pflügers Arch 299:99, 1968.

114. Stolte H, Wiederholt M, Fuchs G, et al: Time course of development of transtubular sodium concentrations differences in proximal surface tubules of the rat kidney. Pflügers Arch 313, 252, 1969.

115. Stone DK, Kokko JP, Jacobson HR: In vitro stimulation of proton secretion by aldosterone. Kidney Int 21:240, 1982.

116. Stone DK, Seldin D, Kokko JP, et al: Anion-dependence of rabbit medullary collecting duct acidification. J Clin Invest 71:1505, 1983.

117. Strand JC, Gilmore JP: Prostaglandins do

not mediate the renal effects of brady-kinin. Renal Physiol 5:286, 1982.

118. Tannen RL: Ammonia metabolism. Am J Physiol 235:F265, 1978.

119. Thatcher JS, Radike AW: Tolerance to potassium intoxication in the albino rat. Am J Physiol 151:138, 1947.

120. Thomas CJ, Gomez-Sanchez CE, Marver D, et al: 19-Oxo-deoxycorticosterone binds to renal mineralocorticoid receptor and stimulates Na retention but not K excretion. Endocrinology, 113:517, 1983.

121. Vandewalle A, Farman N, Bencsath P, et al: Aldosterone binding along the rabbit nephron: An autoradiographic study on isolated tubules. Am J Physiol 240:F172, 1981.

122. Vandewalle A, Wirthensohn G, Heidrick H, et al: Distribution of hexokinase and PEPCK along the rabbit nephron. Am J Physiol 240:F492, 1981.

123. Wade JB: Hormonal modulator of epithelial structure. In Current Topics in Membrane and Transport. Vol 13. Boulpaep E, Ed: Cellular Mechanisms of Renal Tubular Ion Transport. Academic Press, New York, 1980, pp 123–160.

124. Warnock DG, Edelman IS: Occupancy of aldosterone binding sites in rat kidney cytosol. Mol Cell Endocrin 12:221, 1978.

125. Watlington CO, Perkins FM, Munson PJ, et al: Aldosterone and corticosteroid binding and effects on $Na^+$ transport in cultured kidney cells. Am J Physiol 242: F610, 1982.

126. Welbourne TC: Acidosis activation of the pituitary adrenal-renal glutaminase I axis. Endocrinology 99:1071, 1976.

127. Welbourne TC, Phenix P, Thornley-Brown C, et al: Triamcinolone activation of renal ammonia production. Proc Soc Exp Biol Med 153:539, 1976.

128. Westenfelder C, Arevalo GJ, Baranowski RL, et al: Relationship between mineralocorticoids and renal Na-K-ATPase: Na reabsorption. Am J Physiol 233:F593, 1977.

129. Wiederholt M, Auglian SK, Khuri RN: Intracellular potassium in the distal tubule of the adrenalectomized and aldosterone treated rat. Pflügers Arch 347:117, 1974.

130. Wiederholt M, Behn NC, Schoormans W, et al: Effect of aldosterone on sodium and potassium transport in the kidney. J Steroid Biochem 3:151, 1972.

131. Wiederholt M, Schoormans W, Fischer F, et al: Mechanism of action of aldosterone on potassium transfer in the rat kidney. Pflügers Arch 345:159, 1973.

132. Wiederholt M, Wiederholt B: The influence of dexamethasone on water and electrolyte excretion in adrenalectomized rats. Pflügers Arch 302:57, 1968.

133. Wilcox CS, Cemerikic DA, Giebisch G: Differential effects of acute mineralo- and glucocorticoid administration on renal acid elimination. Kidney Int 21:546, 1982.

134. Will PC, Lebowitz JL, Hopfer U: Induction of amiloride sensitive sodium transport in rat colon by mineralocorticoids. Am J Physiol 238:F261, 1980.

135. Will PC, DeLisle RC, Cortright RN, et al: Induction of amiloride-sensitive sodium transport in the intestines by adrenal steroids. Proc NY Acad Sci 372:64, 1981.

136. Wingo CS, Kokko JP, Jacobson HR: Evidence for different acute and chronic actions of mineralocorticoids on the rabbit cortical collecting tubule. Clin Res 29: 481A, 1981.

137. Wingo CS, Seldin DW, Kokko JP, et al: Dietary modulation of active $K^+$ secretion in the cortical collecting tubule of adrenalectomized rabbits. J Clin Invest 70:579, 1982.

138. Zusman RM, Keiser HR, Handler JS: Effect of adrenal steroids on ADH-stimulated PGE synthesis and water flow. Am J Physiol 234:F532, 1978.

139. Zusman RM, Keiser HR: Prostaglandin $E_2$ biosynthesis by rabbit renomedullary interstitial cells in tissue culture. J Biol Chem 252:2069, 1977.

# Index

Page numbers followed by *f* refer to figures; page numbers followed by *t* refer to tables.